Edition **13**

Criminalistics
An Introduction
to Forensic Science

Richard Saferstein, Ph.D.

Forensic Science Consultant, Mt. Laurel, New Jersey

Tiffany Roy

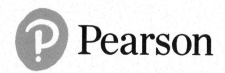

Pearson

Library of Congress Cataloging-in-Publication Data
Names: Saferstein, Richard, author.
Title: Criminalistics : an introduction to forensic science / Richard
    Saferstein, Ph.D., Forensic Science Consultant, Mt. Laurel, New Jersey.
Other titles: An introduction to forensic science | Pearson education book.
Description: Thirteenth Edition. | New York : Pearson, 2020. | Includes bibliographical
    references and index.
Identifiers: LCCN 2019033731 | ISBN 9780135218310 (Paperback) |
    ISBN 0135218314 (Paperback) | ISBN 9780135268797 (ePUB)
Subjects: LCSH: Criminal investigation. | Forensic ballistics. | Chemistry,
    Forensic. | Medical jurisprudence.
Classification: LCC HV8073 .S2 2020 | DDC 363.25—dc23
LC record available at https://lccn.loc.gov/2019033731

11 2022

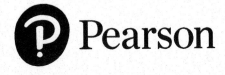

Revel Access Code
ISBN 10:   0-13-526825-7
ISBN 13: 978-0-13-526825-4

Rental Edition
ISBN 10:   0-13-521831-4
ISBN 13: 978-0-13-521831-0

Instructor's Review Copy
ISBN 10:   0-13-670658-4
ISBN 13: 978-0-13-670658-8

To the memory of Fran, Michael and Richard

Brief Contents

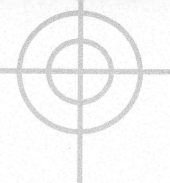

Contents

Chapter 5

Chapter 6

Chapter 7

Chapter 8

Chapter 14

Metals, Paint, and Soil   349

Chapter 15

Forensic Serology   375

Chapter 16

DNA: The Indispensable Forensic Science Tool   399

Chapter 17

Forensic Aspects of Fire and Explosion Investigation   431

Chapter 18

Chapter 19

Chapter 20

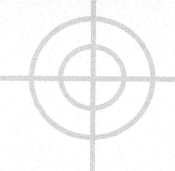

Preface

Public Fascination with Forensic Science

Many readers of this book have been drawn to the subject of forensic science by the assortment of television shows about scientific crime investigation. Story lines depicting the crime-solving abilities of forensic scientists have greatly excited the imagination of the general public. Furthermore, a constant of forensic science is how frequently its applications become front-page news. Whether the story is the sudden death of pop music superstar Michael Jackson, sniper shootings, or the tragic consequences of the terrorist attacks of 9/11, forensic science is at the forefront of the public response.

During the highly publicized O. J. Simpson criminal and civil trials, forensic scientists systematically placed Simpson at the crime scene through DNA analyses, hair and fiber comparisons, and footwear impressions. As millions of Americans watched the case unfold, they, in a sense, became students of forensic science. Intense media coverage of the crime-scene search and investigation, as well as the ramifications of findings of physical evidence at the crime scene, became the subject of study, commentary, and conjecture.

For instructors who have taught forensic science in the classroom, it comes as no surprise that forensic science can grab and hold the attention of those who otherwise would have no interest in any area of science. The O. J. Simpson case, for example, amply demonstrates the extent to which forensic science has intertwined with criminal investigation.

Perhaps we can attribute our obsession with forensic science to the yearnings of a society bent on apprehending people who commit crimes but desirous of a system of justice that ensures the correctness of its verdicts. The level of sophistication that forensic science has brought to criminal investigations is formidable. But once one puts aside all the drama of a forensic science case, what remains is *an academic subject emphasizing logic and technology.*

Purpose of This Book

It is to this end—revealing that essence of forensic science—that the thirteenth edition of *Criminalistics* is dedicated. The basic aim of the book is still to make the subject of forensic science clear and comprehensible to a wide variety of readers who are or plan to be aligned with the forensic science profession, as well as to those who have a curiosity about the subject's underpinnings.

DNA profiling has altered the complexion of criminal investigation. DNA collected from saliva on a cup or from dandruff or sweat on a hat exemplifies the emergence of nontraditional forms of evidence collection at crime scenes. Currently, the criminal justice system is creating vast DNA data banks designed to snare people who commit crimes who are unaware of the consequences of leaving the minutest quantity of biological material behind at a crime scene.

New to This Edition

- Numerous case files have been added to select chapters to illustrate how forensic technology has been applied to solving crimes of notoriety.
- Chapter 4 "Crime scene Reconstruction: Bloodstain Pattern Analysis" has been updated to reflect changes in terminology and interpretation of blood stain pattern evidence.
- Chapter 16, "DNA: The Indispensable Forensic Science Tool," has been updated to including information on the use of Rapid DNA systems, Probabilistic Genotyping and Forensic Genetic Genealogy.
- Chapter 1, "Introduction," has been expanded to cover the discussion of the reliability and controversy surrounding forensic bite mark comparison.

- Chapter 20, "Mobile Device Forensics," has been updated to discuss the impact of Carpenter v. United States and an overview of the use of a StingRay device.
- Information throughout the text has been updated and many new figures have been added to illustrate concepts discussed in the chapters.

Focus on Cutting-Edge Tools and Techniques

Through thirteen editions, *Criminalistics* has strived to depict the role of the forensic scientist in the criminal justice system. The current edition builds on the content of its predecessors and updates the reader on the latest technologies available to crime laboratory personnel.

A new chapter has been added to this edition dealing with the subject of forensic biometrics. The reader is introduced to the FBI's recently implemented Next Generation Identification System which houses its fingerprint and facial recognition databases.

The computer, the Internet, and mobile electronic devices have influenced all aspects of modern life, and forensic science is no exception. Chapter 19, "Computer Forensics," and Chapter 20, "Mobile Devices Forensics," explore the retrieval of computerized information thought to be lost or erased during the course of a criminal investigation and delve into the investigation of hacking incidents.

A major portion of the text centers on discussions of the common items of physical evidence encountered at crime scenes. Various chapters include descriptions of forensic analysis, as well as updated techniques for the proper collection and preservation of evidence at crime scenes. The reader is offered the option of delving into the more difficult technical aspects of the subject by reading the "Inside the Science" features. This option can be bypassed without detracting from a basic comprehension of the subject of forensic science.

The implications of DNA profiling are important enough to warrant their inclusion in a separate chapter in *Criminalistics*. Chapter 16 describes the topic of DNA in a manner that is comprehensible and relevant to readers who lack a scientific background. The discussion defines DNA and explains its central role in controlling the body's chemistry. Finally, Chapter 16 explains the process of DNA typing and illustrates its application to criminal investigations through the presentation of actual case histories.

A Grounded Approach

The content of *Criminalistics* reflects the author's experience as both an active forensic scientist and an instructor of forensic science at the college level. The author assumes that readers have no prior knowledge of scientific principles or techniques. The areas of chemistry and biology relating to the analysis of physical evidence are presented with a minimum of scientific terminology and equations. The discussion involving chemistry and biology is limited to a minimum core of facts and principles that make the subject matter understandable and meaningful to the nonscientist. Although it is not the intent of this book to turn readers into scientists or forensic experts, the author would certainly be gratified if the book motivates some students to seek further scientific knowledge and perhaps direct their education toward careers in forensic science.

Although *Criminalistics* is an outgrowth of a one-semester course offered as part of a criminal justice program at many New Jersey colleges, the value of the book is not limited to college students. Optimum utilization of crime laboratory services requires that criminal investigators have knowledge of the techniques and capabilities of the laboratory. That awareness extends beyond any summary that may be gleaned from departmental brochures dealing with the collection and packaging of physical evidence. Investigators must mesh knowledge of the principles and techniques of forensic science with logic and common sense to gain comprehensive insight into the meaning and significance of physical evidence and its role in criminal investigations. Forensic science begins at the crime scene. If the investigator cannot recognize, collect, and package evidence properly, no amount of equipment or expertise will salvage the situation.

Likewise, there is a dire need to bridge the "communication gap" that currently exists among lawyers, judges, and forensic scientists. An intelligent evaluation of the scientist's data and any subsequent testimony will again depend on familiarity with the underlying principles of forensic science. Too many practitioners of the law profess ignorance of the subject or attempt to gain a superficial understanding of its meaning and significance only minutes before meeting the expert witness. It is hoped that the book will provide a painless route to comprehending the nature of the science.

In order to merge theory with practice, actual forensic case histories are included in the text. The intent is for these illustrations to move forensic science from the domain of the abstract into the real world of criminal investigation.

Key Features of the Thirteenth Edition

The Thirteenth edition, which is now available in a variety of print and electronic formats, presents modern forensic science approaches and techniques with the aid of real-life examples, up-to-date information, and interactive media. Key features include the following:

Headline News stories at the beginning of each chapter introduce readers to the chapter topics by describing high-profile crimes and the related forensic science techniques used in the investigations.

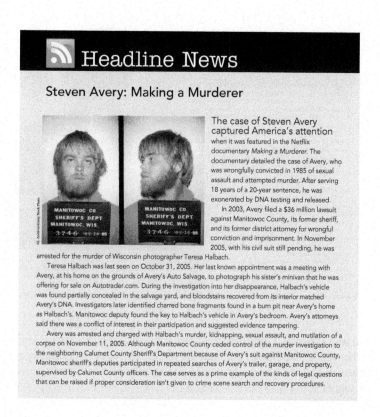

Headline News

Steven Avery: Making a Murderer

The case of Steven Avery captured America's attention when it was featured in the Netflix documentary *Making a Murderer*. The documentary detailed the case of Avery, who was wrongfully convicted in 1985 of sexual assault and attempted murder. After serving 18 years of a 20-year sentence, he was exonerated by DNA testing and released.

In 2003, Avery filed a $36 million lawsuit against Manitowoc County, its former sheriff, and its former district attorney for wrongful conviction and imprisonment. In November 2005, with his civil suit still pending, he was arrested for the murder of Wisconsin photographer Teresa Halbach.

Teresa Halbach was last seen on October 31, 2005. Her last known appointment was a meeting with Avery, at his home on the grounds of Avery's Auto Salvage, to photograph his sister's minivan that he was offering for sale on Autotrader.com. During the investigation into her disappearance, Halbach's vehicle was found partially concealed in the salvage yard, and bloodstains recovered from its interior matched Avery's DNA. Investigators later identified charred bone fragments found in a burn pit near Avery's home as Halbach's. Manitowoc deputy found the key to Halbach's vehicle in Avery's bedroom. Avery's attorneys said there was a conflict of interest in their participation and suggested evidence tampering.

Avery was arrested and charged with Halbach's murder, kidnapping, sexual assault, and mutilation of a corpse on November 11, 2005. Although Manitowoc County ceded control of the murder investigation to the neighboring Calumet County Sheriff's Department because of Avery's suit against Manitowoc County, Manitowoc sheriff's deputies participated in repeated searches of Avery's trailer, garage, and property, supervised by Calumet County officers. The case serves as a prime example of the kinds of legal questions that can be raised if proper consideration isn't given to crime scene search and recovery procedures.

Inside the Science boxes throughout the text explore scientific phenomena and technology in relation to select chapter topics, and are accompanied by Review Questions for Inside the Science at the end of the chapter.

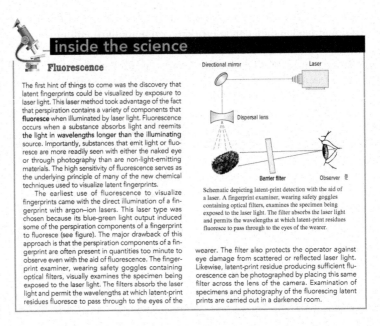

inside the science

Fluorescence

The first hint of things to come was the discovery that latent fingerprints could be visualized by exposure to laser light. This laser method took advantage of the fact that perspiration contains a variety of components that **fluoresce** when illuminated by laser light. Fluorescence occurs when a substance absorbs light and reemits the light in **wavelengths longer than the illuminating** source. Importantly, substances that emit light or fluoresce are more readily seen with either the naked eye or through photography than are non-light-emitting materials. The high sensitivity of fluorescence serves as the underlying principle of many of the new chemical techniques used to visualize latent fingerprints.

The earliest use of fluorescence to visualize fingerprints came with the direct illumination of a fingerprint with argon–ion lasers. This laser type was chosen because its blue-green light output induced some of the perspiration components of a fingerprint to fluoresce (see figure). The major drawback of this approach is that the perspiration components of a fingerprint are often present in quantities too minute to observe even with the aid of fluorescence. The fingerprint examiner, wearing safety goggles containing optical filters, visually examines the specimen being exposed to the laser light. The filters absorb the laser light and permit the wavelengths at which latent-print residues fluoresce to pass through to the eyes of the

Schematic depicting latent-print detection with the aid of a laser. A fingerprint examiner, wearing safety goggles containing optical filters, examines the specimen being exposed to the laser light. The filter absorbs the laser light and permits the wavelengths at which latent-print residues fluoresce to pass through to the eyes of the wearer.

wearer. The filter also protects the operator against eye damage from scattered or reflected laser light. Likewise, latent-print residue producing sufficient fluorescence can be photographed by placing this same filter across the lens of the camera. Examination of specimens and photography of the fluorescing latent prints are carried out in a darkened room.

Case File boxes throughout the text present brief, real-life case examples that are illustrative of the forensic science topics and techniques described in the chapters.

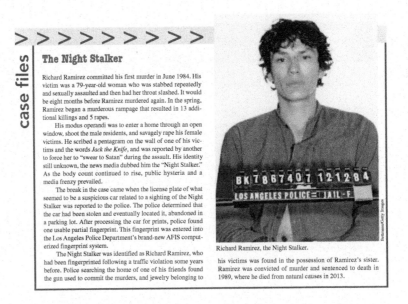

case files

The Night Stalker

Richard Ramirez committed his first murder in June 1984. His victim was a 79-year-old woman who was stabbed repeatedly and sexually assaulted and then had her throat slashed. It would be eight months before Ramirez murdered again. In the spring, Ramirez began a murderous rampage that resulted in 13 additional killings and 5 rapes.

His modus operandi was to enter a home through an open window, shoot the male residents, and savagely rape his female victims. He scribed a pentagram on the wall of one of his victims and the words *Jack the Knife*, and was reported by another to force her to "swear to Satan" during the assault. His identity still unknown, the news media dubbed him the "Night Stalker." As the body count continued to rise, public hysteria and a media frenzy prevailed.

The break in the case came when the license plate of what seemed to be a suspicious car related to a sighting of the Night Stalker was reported to the police. The police determined that the car had been stolen and eventually located it, abandoned in a parking lot. After processing the car for prints, police found one usable partial fingerprint. This fingerprint was entered into the Los Angeles Police Department's brand-new AFIS computerized fingerprint system.

The Night Stalker was identified as Richard Ramirez, who had been fingerprinted following a traffic violation some years before. Police searching the home of one of his friends found the gun used to commit the murders, and jewelry belonging to

Richard Ramirez, the Night Stalker.

his victims was found in the possession of Ramirez's sister. Ramirez was convicted of murder and sentenced to death in 1989, where he died from natural causes in 2013.

Application and Critical Thinking questions at the end of each chapter challenge students to demonstrate their understanding of the material through a variety of question types, including hypothetical scenarios and sets of images for visual identification and analysis. Answers to these questions are provided in the Instructor's Manual.

Webextras serve to expand the coverage of the book through video presentations, Internet-related information, animations, and graphic displays keyed to enhancing reader's understanding of the subject's more difficult concepts. Webextras are accessible on the book website at www.pearsonhighered.com/careersresources.

application and critical thinking

1. Indicate the phase of growth of each of the following hairs:
   a. The root is club-shaped
   b. The hair has a follicular tag
   c. The root bulb is flame-shaped
   d. The root is elongated

2. A criminalist studying a dyed sample hair notices that the dyed color ends about 1.5 centimeters from the tip of the hair. Approximately how many weeks before the examination was the hair dyed? Explain your answer.

3. Following are descriptions of several hairs; based on these descriptions, indicate the likely race of the person from whom the hair originated:
   a. Evenly distributed, fine pigmentation
   b. Continuous medullation
   c. Dense, uneven pigmentation
   d. Wavy with a round cross-section

4. Criminalist Pete Evett is collecting fiber evidence from a murder scene. He notices fibers on the victim's shirt and trousers, so he places both of these items of clothing in a plastic bag. He also sees fibers on a sheet near the victim, so he balls up the sheet and places it in a separate plastic bag. Noticing fibers adhering to the windowsill from which the attacker gained entrance, Pete carefully removes them with his fingers and places them in a regular envelope. What mistakes, if any, did Pete make while collecting this evidence?

5. For each of the following human hair samples, indicate the medulla pattern present.

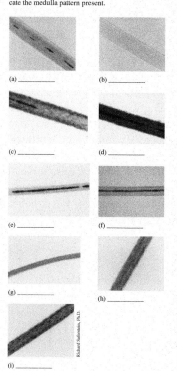

(a) _____   (b) _____

(c) _____   (d) _____

(e) _____   (f) _____

(g) _____   (h) _____

(i) _____

Richard Saferstein, Ph.D.

Instructor Supplements

Instructor's Manual with Test Bank. Includes content outlines for classroom discussion, teaching suggestions, and answers to selected end-of-chapter questions from the text. This also contains a Word document version of the test bank.

TestGen. This computerized test generation system gives you maximum flexibility in creating and administering tests on paper, electronically, or online. It provides state-of-the-art features for viewing and editing test bank questions, dragging a selected question into a test you are creating, and printing sleek, formatted tests in a variety of layouts. Select test items from test banks included with TestGen for quick test creation, or write your own questions from scratch. TestGen's random generator provides the option to display different text or calculated number values each time questions are used.

PowerPoint Presentations. Our presentations are clear and straightforward. Photos, illustrations, charts, and tables from the book are included in the presentations when applicable.

To access supplementary materials online, instructors need to request an instructor access code. Go to www.pearsonhighered.com/irc, where you can register for an instructor access code. Within 48 hours after registering, you will receive a confirming email, including an instructor access code. Once you have received your code, go to the site and log on for full instructions on downloading the materials you wish to use.

Alternate Versions

eBooks. This text is also available in multiple eBook formats. These are an exciting new choice for students looking to save money. As an alternative to purchasing the printed textbook, students can purchase an electronic version of the same content. With an eTextbook, students can search the text, make notes online, print out reading assignments that incorporate lecture notes, and bookmark important passages for later review. For more information, visit your favorite online eBook reseller or visit www.mypearsonstore.com.

Revel *Criminalistics*, Thirteenth Edition by Richard Saferstein and Tiffany Roy

Designed for how you want to teach — and how your students want to learn

Revel is an interactive learning environment that engages students and helps them prepare for your class. Reimagining their content, our authors integrate media and assessment throughout the narrative so students can read, explore, and practice, all at the same time. Thanks to this dynamic reading experience, students come to class prepared to discuss, apply, and learn about criminal justice — from you and from each other.

Revel seamlessly combines the full content of Pearson's bestselling criminal justice titles with multimedia learning tools. You assign the topics your students cover. Author Explanatory Videos, application exercises, survey questions, and short quizzes engage students and enhance their understanding of core topics as they progress through the content. Through its engaging learning experience, Revel helps students better understand course material while preparing them to meaningfully participate in class.

Author Explanatory Videos

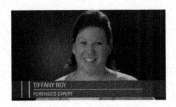

Short 2-3 minute Author Explanatory Videos, embedded in the narrative, provide students with a verbal explanation of an important topic or concept and illuminating the concept with additional examples.

Criminalistics Virtual Laboratory Exercises

The *Criminalistics* virtual laboratory exercises are intended to give the student a first-hand look at the types of tests and examinations performed in the crime lab. Using 360-degree photography, microscope imagery and explanatory videos, these laboratory exercises will bring the content to life and give students an opportunity to experience a day in the life of a forensic scientist.

Point/CounterPoint Videos

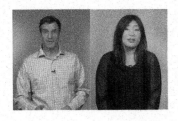

Instead of simply reading about criminal justice, students are empowered to think critically about key topics through Point/Counterpoint videos that explore different views on controversial issues such as the effectiveness of the fourth amendment, privacy, search and seizure, Miranda, prisoner rights, death penalty and many other topics.

Student Survey Questions

Student Survey Questions appear within the narrative asking students to respond to questions about controversial topics and important concepts. Students then see their response versus the responses of all other students who have answered the question in the form of a bar chart.

Track time-on-task throughout the course

The Performance Dashboard allows you to see how much time the class or individual students have spent reading a section or doing an assignment, as well as points earned per assignment. This data helps correlate study time with performance and provides a window into where students may be having difficulty with the material.

Learning Management System Integration

Pearson provides Blackboard Learn™, Canvas™, Brightspace by D2L, and Moodle integration, giving institutions, instructors, and students easy access to Revel. Our Revel integration delivers streamlined access to everything your students need for the course in these learning management system (LMS) environments.

The Revel App

The Revel mobile app lets students read, practice, and study—anywhere, anytime, on any device. Content is available both online and offline, and the app syncs work across all registered devices automatically, giving students great flexibility to toggle between phone, tablet, and laptop as they move through their day. The app also lets students set assignment notifications to stay on top of all due dates. Available for download from the App Store or Google Play. Visit www.pearson-highered.com/revel/ to learn more.

Acknowledgments

I would like to express my most sincere thanks to Dr. Richard Saferstein and his family for the opportunity to work on this text. It is an honor and privilege. I will work hard to ensure it is up to the high standard set by Richard in his lifetime.

I am most appreciative of my former students, now forensic science colleagues, who worked closely with me on this project. Thank you to Tatum Price of the Palm Beach Sheriff's Office Crime Lab DNA Unit for her work in the development of the interactive content. Thanks to Taj Laing of the West Palm Beach Police Department CSI Unit and Karlee Jonas for their assistance with case selection and text revision.

I would like to thank the subject matter experts who reviewed this text content and recommended updates, including Dr. Michael McCutcheon of the Londonderry, NH Police Department; James Palma of the Palm Beach County Sheriff's Office Firearms Unit; Melissa O'Meara of Vuyronx Technology/Federal Resources, and Jeremiah Morris of the Johnson County Crime Lab in Mission, Kansas. Additionally, I would like to thank Andrew Donofrio and Dr. Peter Stephenson for their previous contributions to this book on the subject of mobile and digital forensics.

I would like to thank Michael Dosmann and the staff at Arnold Arboretum at Harvard University for their assistance.

Many people provided assistance and advice in the preparation of this book. I would like to acknowledge the contributions of Michael Marciano of Syracuse University; Kristi Barba of the Onondaga County Health Department for comments on the DNA and Toxicology chapters, respectively. A big thanks to Amy Brodeur, Dr. Robin Cotton, Dr. Sean Tallman, Dr. Adam Hall, Dr. Sabra Botch-Jones and Robert Bouchie from Boston University School of Medicine for the use of their laboratory facilities in the development of the Revel product for this text. Thank you to everyone who assisted Richard in making this book a success by providing photos and materials including Robert Thompson, Roger Ely, Jose R. Almirall, Darlene Brezinski, Michael Malone, Robert J. Phillips, David Pauly, Dr. Barbara Needell, Marla Carroll, Robin D. Williams, Peter Diaczuk, Jacqueline A. Joseph, John Lentini and Robert Welsh. I'm appreciative for the contributions, reviews, and comments that Dr. Claus Speth, Dr. Mark Taff, Dr. Elizabeth Laposata, Thomas P. Mauriello, and Michelle D. Miranda.

I'm appreciative of the assistance provided by Dr. Adam Freeman, DDS in the area of forensic odontology for guidance on peer reviewed, published literature in the area of forensic bitemark comparison.

Pearson Education and I would like to thank the reviewers of this edition for their input and guidance:

Gail Anderson, Simon Fraser University; Lisa Dadio, University of New Haven; Barry Michael, University of Memphis; and Charla Perdue, Florida State University - Panama City.

I am grateful to the law enforcement agencies, governmental agencies, private individuals, and equipment manufacturers cited in the text for contributing their photographs and illustrations.

Finally, I would like to thank my family, friends and colleagues for all they have done to support me in my academic and professional pursuits. Any successes I achieve in my lifetime, I owe to the family and friends who love and support me through hard times and celebrate with me in the good.

Tiffany Roy, JD, MSFS

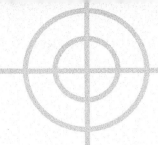

About the Author

Richard Saferstein, Ph.D., retired after serving 21 years as the chief forensic scientist of the New Jersey State Police Laboratory, one of the largest crime laboratories in the United States. He currently acts as a consultant for attorneys and the media in the area of forensic science. During the O. J. Simpson criminal trial, Dr. Saferstein provided extensive commentary on forensic aspects of the case for the *Rivera Live* show, the E! television network, ABC radio, and various radio talk shows. Dr. Saferstein holds degrees from the City College of New York and earned his doctorate degree in chemistry in 1970 from the City University of New York. From 1972 to 1991, he taught an introductory forensic science course in the criminal justice programs at the College of New Jersey and Ocean County College. These teaching experiences played an influential role in Dr. Saferstein's authorship in 1977 of the widely used introductory textbook *Criminalistics: An Introduction to Forensic Science*, currently in this thirteenth edition. Saferstein's basic philosophy in writing *Criminalistics* is to make forensic science understandable and meaningful to the nonscience reader, while giving the reader an appreciation for the scientific principles that underlie the subject.

Dr. Saferstein has authored or co-authored more than 45 technical papers and chapters covering a variety of forensic topics. Dr. Saferstein has co-authored *Lab Manual for Criminalistics* (Pearson, 2015) to be used in conjunction with this text. He is also the author of *Forensic Science: An Introduction* (Pearson, 2008 and 2011) and *Forensic Science: From the Crime Scene to the Crime Lab* (2009 and 2015). He has also edited the widely used professional reference books *Forensic Science Handbook*, Volumes I, II, and III, 2nd edition (published in 2002, 2005, and 2010, respectively, by Pearson).

Dr. Saferstein is a member of the American Chemical Society, the American Academy of Forensic Sciences, the Canadian Society of Forensic Scientists, the International Association for Identification, the Northeastern Association of Forensic Scientists, and the Society of Forensic Toxicologists. He is the recipient of the American Academy of Forensic Sciences 2006 Paul L. Kirk Award for distinguished service and contributions to the field of criminalistics.

Tiffany Roy, MSFS, JD is a Forensic DNA expert with over thirteen years of forensic biology experience in both public and private laboratories in the United States. She has processed thousands of DNA samples and thousands of cases over the course of her career. She has provided expert witness testimony in more than one hundred cases in state, federal and international courts. She instructs undergraduates at Palm Beach Atlantic University; University of Maryland Global Campus; and Southern New Hampshire University. She currently acts as a consultant for attorneys and the media in the area of forensic biology through her firm, *ForensicAid, LLC*.

Roy holds degrees from Syracuse University, Massachusetts School of Law and University of Florida in the areas of Biology, Law and Forensic Science. Her teaching, legal writing and testimonial experience help her to take complex scientific concepts and make them easily understandable for the nonscientist. Roy assisted Dr. Saferstein in completing *Forensic Science: From the Crime Scene to the Crime Lab 4e* (Pearson 2019) and has authored the text *The Complete Guide to the American Board of Criminalistics Molecular Biology Examination (CRC Press 2020) to assist working forensic scientists achieve the goal of certification.*

Roy is a member of the American Academy of Forensic Sciences, the Northeastern Association of Forensic Scientists and the Massachusetts Board of Bar Examiners. She is a certified Diplomate in the area of Forensic Biology by the American Board of Criminalistics. Aside from her teaching, writing and consulting, Roy also assists with international capacity building initiatives, providing subject matter expertise for trainings for criminal justice stakeholders in the Middle East and Africa.

Introduction

Learning Objectives

After studying this chapter, you should be able to:

1.1 Distinguish between forensic science and criminalistics

1.2 Describe the organization and services of a typical comprehensive crime laboratory in the criminal justice system

1.3 Explain how physical evidence is analyzed and presented in the courtroom by the forensic scientist, and how admissibility of evidence is determined in the courtroom

1.4 Explain the role and responsibilities of the expert witness and what specialized forensic services, aside from the crime laboratory, are generally available to law enforcement personnel

KEY TERMS

expert witness
Locard's exchange
  principle
scientific method

Go to www.pearsonhighered.com/careersresources to access Webextras for this chapter.

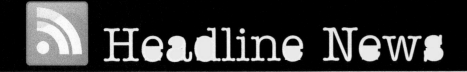

Steven Avery: Making a Murderer

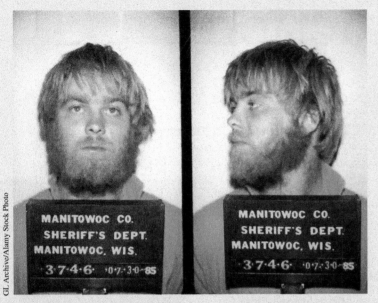

GL Archive/Alamy Stock Photo

The case of Steven Avery captured America's attention when it was featured in the Netflix documentary *Making a Murderer*. The documentary detailed the case of Avery, who was wrongfully convicted in 1985 of sexual assault and attempted murder. After serving 18 years of a 20-year sentence, he was exonerated by DNA testing and released.

In 2003, Avery filed a $36 million lawsuit against Manitowoc County, its former sheriff, and its former district attorney for wrongful conviction and imprisonment. In November 2005, with his civil suit still pending, he was arrested for the murder of Wisconsin photographer Teresa Halbach.

Teresa Halbach was last seen on October 31, 2005. Her last known appointment was a meeting with Avery, at his home on the grounds of Avery's Auto Salvage, to photograph his sister's minivan that he was offering for sale on Autotrader.com. During the investigation into her disappearance, Halbach's vehicle was found partially concealed in the salvage yard, and bloodstains recovered from its interior matched Avery's DNA. Investigators later identified charred bone fragments found in a burn pit near Avery's home as belonging to Halbach's. A Manitowoc deputy found the key to Halbach's vehicle in Avery's bedroom. Avery's attorneys assert said there was a conflict of interest in the participation of the Manitowoc Sheriff's Department and suggested evidence tampering.

Avery was arrested and charged with Halbach's murder, kidnapping, sexual assault, and mutilation of her corpse on November 11, 2005. Although Manitowoc County ceded control of the murder investigation to the neighboring Calumet County Sheriff's Department because of Avery's law suit, Manitowoc sheriff's deputies participated in repeated searches of Avery's trailer, garage, and property, supervised by Calumet County officers. The case serves as a prime example of the kinds of legal questions that can be raised if proper consideration isn't given to crime scene search and recovery procedures.

Definition and Scope of Forensic Science

Forensic science in its broadest definition is the application of science to law. As our society has grown more complex, it has become more dependent on rules of law to regulate the activities of its members. Forensic science applies the knowledge and technology of science to the definition and enforcement of such laws.

Each year, as government finds it increasingly necessary to regulate the activities that most intimately influence our daily lives, science merges more closely with civil and criminal law. Consider, for example, the laws and agencies that regulate the quality of our food, the nature and potency of drugs, the extent of automobile emissions, the kind of fuel oil we burn, the purity of our drinking water, and the pesticides we use on our crops and plants. It would be difficult to conceive of a food or drug regulation or environmental protection act that could be effectively monitored and enforced without the assistance of scientific technology and the skill of the scientific community.

Laws are continually being broadened and revised to counter the alarming increase in crime rates. In response to public concern, law enforcement agencies have expanded their patrol and investigative functions, hoping to stem the rising tide of crime. At the same time, they are looking more to the scientific community for advice and technical support for their efforts. Can the technology that put astronauts on the moon, split the atom, and eradicated most dreaded diseases be enlisted in this critical battle?

Unfortunately, science cannot offer final and authoritative solutions to problems that stem from a maze of social and psychological factors. However, as the content of this book attests, science occupies an important and unique role in the criminal justice system—a role that relates to the scientist's ability to supply accurate and objective information about the events that have occurred at a crime scene. A good deal of work remains to be done if the full potential of science as applied to criminal investigations is to be realized.

Because of the vast array of civil and criminal laws that regulate society, forensic science, in its broadest sense, has become so comprehensive a subject that a meaningful introductory textbook treating its role and techniques would be difficult to create and probably overwhelming to read. For this reason, we have narrowed the scope of the subject according to the most common definition: **Forensic science is the application of science to the criminal and civil laws that are enforced by police agencies in a criminal justice system.** *Forensic science* is an umbrella term encompassing a myriad of professions that use their skills to aid law enforcement officials in conducting their investigations.

The diversity of professions practicing forensic science is illustrated by the 11 sections of the American Academy of Forensic Science, the largest forensic science organization in the world:

1. Criminalistics
2. Digital and Multimedia Sciences
3. Engineering Science
4. General
5. Jurisprudence
6. Odontology
7. Pathology/Biology
8. Physical Anthropology
9. Psychiatry/Behavioral Science
10. Questioned Documents
11. Toxicology

Even this list of professions is not exclusive. It does not encompass skills such as fingerprint examination, firearm and tool mark examination, and photography.

Obviously, to author a book covering all of the major activities of forensic science as they apply to the enforcement of criminal and civil laws by police agencies would be a major undertaking. Thus, this book will further restrict itself to discussions of the subjects of chemistry, biology, physics, geology, and computer technology, which are useful for determining the evidential value of crime-scene and related evidence. Forensic psychology, anthropology, and odontology also encompass important and relevant areas of knowledge and practice in law enforcement, each being an integral part of the total forensic science service that is provided to any up-to-date criminal justice system. However, these subjects go beyond the intended scope of this book, and except for brief discussions, along with pointing the reader to relevant websites, the reader is referred elsewhere for discussions of their applications and techniques. Instead, this book focuses on the services of what has popularly become known as the crime laboratory, where the principles and techniques of the physical and natural sciences are practiced and applied to the analysis of crime-scene evidence.

For many, the term *criminalistics* seems more descriptive than *forensic science* for describing the services of a crime laboratory. Regardless of his or her title—criminalist or forensic scientist—the trend of events has made the scientist in the crime laboratory an active participant in the criminal justice system.

Prime-time television shows like *CSI: Crime Scene Investigation* have greatly increased the public's awareness of the use of science in criminal and civil investigations (Figure 1–1). However, by simplifying scientific procedures to fit the allotted airtime, these shows have created within both the public and the legal community unrealistic expectations of forensic science. In these shows, members of the CSI team collect evidence at the crime scene, process all evidence, question witnesses, interrogate suspects, carry out search warrants, and testify in court. In the real world, these tasks are almost always delegated to different people in different parts of the criminal justice system. Procedures that in reality could take days, weeks, months, or years appear on these shows to take mere minutes. This false image is significantly responsible for the public's high interest in and expectations for DNA evidence.

The dramatization of forensic science on television has led the public to believe that every crime scene will yield forensic evidence, and it produces unrealistic expectations that a prosecutor's case should always be bolstered and supported by forensic evidence. This phenomenon is known as the "CSI effect." Some jurists have come to believe that this phenomenon ultimately detracts from the search for truth and justice in the courtroom.

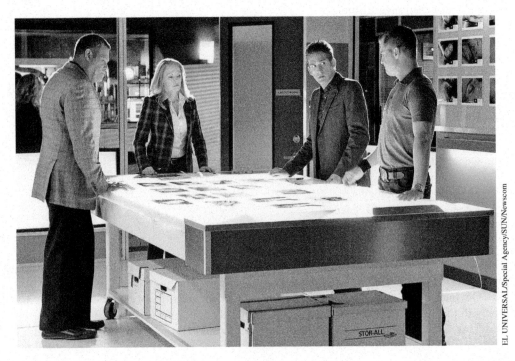

EL UNIVERSAL/Special Agency/SUN/Newscom

FIGURE 1–1

A scene from *CSI*, a forensic science television show.

History and Development of Forensic Science

Forensic science owes its origins first to the individuals who developed the principles and techniques needed to identify or compare physical evidence and second to those who recognized the need to merge these principles into a coherent discipline that could be practically applied to a criminal justice system.

Literary Roots

Today many believe that Sir Arthur Conan Doyle had a considerable influence on popularizing scientific crime-detection methods through his fictional character Sherlock Holmes (see Figure 1–2), who first applied the newly developing principles of serology (see Chapter 14), fingerprinting, firearms identification, and questioned document examination long before their value was first recognized and accepted by real-life criminal investigators. Holmes's feats excited the imagination of an emerging generation of forensic scientists and criminal investigators. Even in the first Sherlock Holmes novel, *A Study in Scarlet,* published in 1887, we find examples of Doyle's uncanny ability to describe scientific methods of detection years before they were actually discovered and implemented. For instance, here Holmes probes and recognizes the potential usefulness of forensic serology to criminal investigation:

"I've found it. I've found it," he shouted to my companion, running towards us with a test tube in his hand. "I have found a reagent which is precipitated by hemoglobin and by nothing else. . . . Why, man, it is the most practical medico-legal discovery for years. Don't you see that it gives us an infallible test for blood stains?. . . The old guaiacum test was very clumsy and uncertain. So is the microscopic examination for blood corpuscles. The latter is valueless if the stains are a few hours old. Now, this appears to act as well whether the blood is old or new. Had this test been invented, there are hundreds of men now walking the earth who would long ago have paid the penalty of their crimes. . . . Criminal cases are continually hinging upon that one point. A man is suspected of a crime months perhaps after it has been committed. His linen or clothes are examined and brownish stains discovered upon them. Are they blood stains, or rust stains, or fruit stains, or what are they? That is a question which has puzzled many an expert, and why? Because there was no reliable test. Now we have the Sherlock Holmes test, and there will no longer be any difficulty."

Important Contributors to Forensic Science

Many people can be cited for their specific contributions to the field of forensic science. The following is just a brief list of those who made the earliest contributions to formulating the disciplines that now constitute forensic science.

MATHIEU ORFILA (1787–1853) Orfila is considered the founder of forensic toxicology. A native of Spain, he ultimately became a renowned teacher of medicine in France. In 1814, Orfila published the first scientific treatise on the detection of poisons and their effects on animals. This treatise established forensic toxicology as a legitimate scientific endeavor.

ALPHONSE BERTILLON (1853–1914) Bertillon devised the first scientific system of personal identification. In 1879, Bertillon began to develop the science of *anthropometry* (see Chapter 6), a systematic procedure of taking a series of body measurements as a means of distinguishing one individual from another (see Figure 1–3).

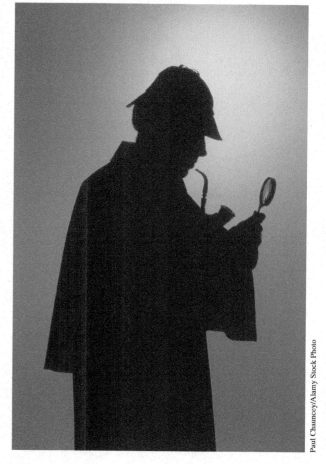

Paul Chauncey/Alamy Stock Photo

FIGURE 1–2

Sir Arthur Conan Doyle's legendary detective Sherlock Holmes applied many of the principles of modern forensic science long before they were adopted widely by police.

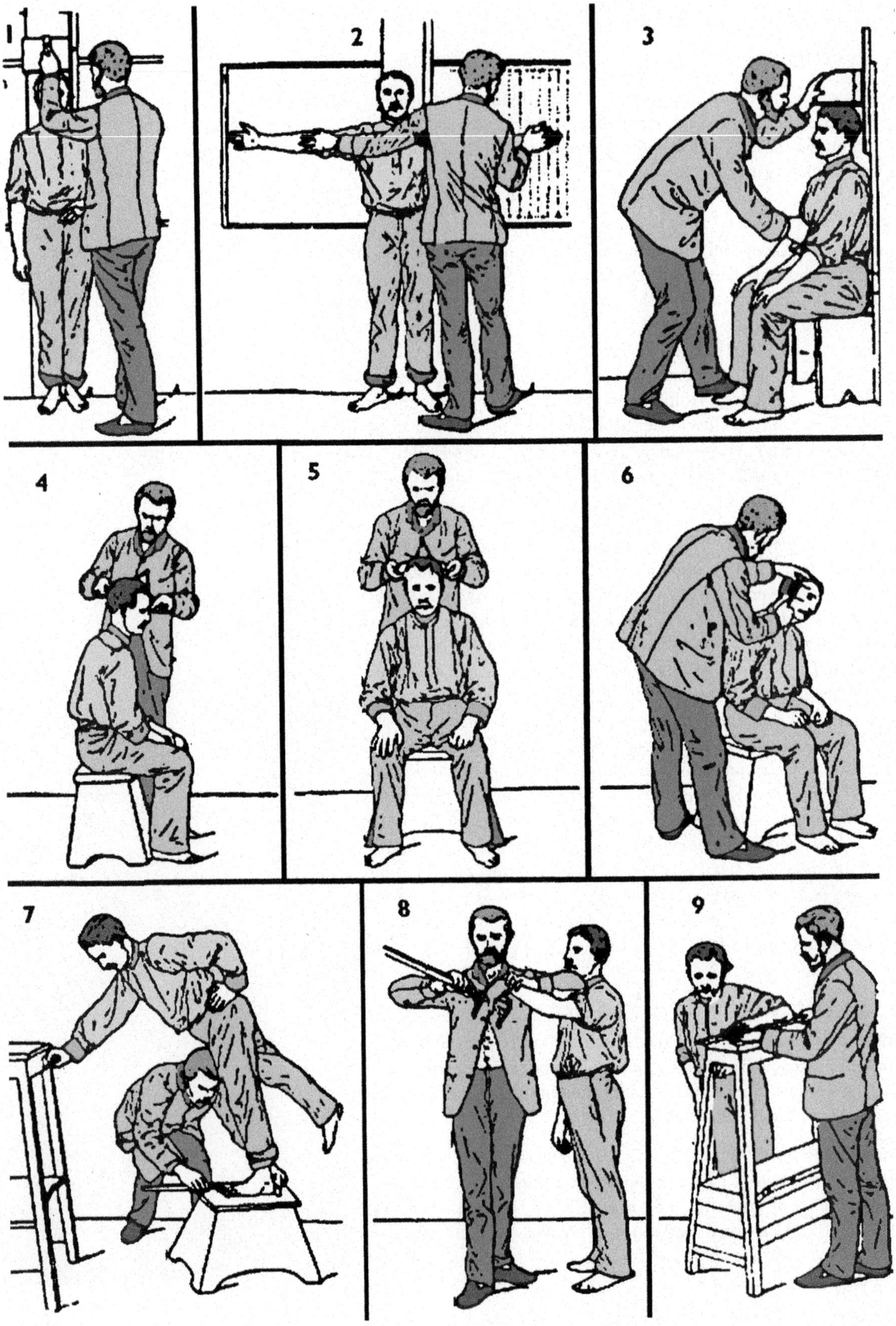

Courtesy Sirchie Fingerprint Laboratories, Youngsville, NC, *www.sirchie.com*

FIGURE 1–3
Bertillon's system of bodily measurements as used for the identification of an individual.

For nearly two decades, this system was considered the most accurate method of personal identification. Although anthropometry was eventually replaced by fingerprinting in the early 1900s, Bertillon's early efforts have earned him the distinction of being known as the founder of criminal identification.

FRANCIS GALTON (1822–1911) Galton undertook the first definitive study of fingerprints and developed a methodology of classifying them for filing. In 1892, he published a book titled *Finger Prints,* which contained the first statistical proof supporting the uniqueness of his method of personal identification. His work went on to describe the basic principles that form the present system of identification by fingerprints.

LEONE LATTES (1887–1954) In 1901, Dr. Karl Landsteiner discovered that blood can be grouped into different categories. These blood groups or types are now recognized as A, B, AB, and O. The possibility that blood grouping could be a useful characteristic for the identification of an individual intrigued Dr. Lattes, a professor at the Institute of Forensic Medicine at the University of Turin in Italy. In 1915, he devised a relatively simple procedure for determining the blood group of a dried bloodstain, a technique that he immediately applied to criminal investigations.

CALVIN GODDARD (1891–1955) To determine whether a particular gun has fired a bullet requires a comparison of the bullet with one that has been test-fired from the suspect's weapon. Goddard, a U.S. Army colonel, refined the techniques of such an examination by using the comparison microscope. From the mid-1920s on, Goddard's expertise established the comparison microscope as the indispensable tool of the modern firearms examiner.

ALBERT S. OSBORN (1858–1946) Osborn's development of the fundamental principles of document examination was responsible for the acceptance of documents as scientific evidence by the courts. In 1910, Osborn authored the first significant text in this field, *Questioned Documents.* This book is still considered a primary reference for document examiners.

WALTER C. MCCRONE (1916–2002) Dr. McCrone's career paralleled startling advances in sophisticated analytical technology. Nevertheless, during his lifetime McCrone became the world's preeminent microscopist. Through his books, journal publications, and research institute, McCrone was a tireless advocate for applying microscopy to analytical problems, particularly forensic science cases. McCrone's exceptional communication skills made him a much-sought-after instructor, and he was responsible for educating thousands of forensic scientists throughout the world in the application of microscopic techniques. Dr. McCrone used microscopy, often in conjunction with other analytical methodologies, to examine evidence in thousands of criminal and civil cases throughout a long and illustrious career.

HANS GROSS (1847–1915) Gross wrote the first treatise describing the application of scientific disciplines to the field of criminal investigation in 1893. A public prosecutor and judge in Graz, Austria, Gross spent many years studying and developing principles of criminal investigation. In his classic book *Handbuch für Untersuchungsrichter als System der Kriminalistik* (later published in English under the title *Criminal Investigation*), he detailed the assistance that investigators could expect from the fields of microscopy, chemistry, physics, mineralogy, zoology, botany, anthropometry, and fingerprinting. He later introduced the forensic journal *Archiv für Kriminal Anthropologie und Kriminalistik,* which still serves as a medium for reporting improved methods of scientific crime detection.

EDMOND LOCARD (1877–1966) Although Gross was a strong advocate of the use of the scientific method in criminal investigation, he did not make any specific technical contributions to this philosophy. Locard, a Frenchman, demonstrated how the principles enunciated by Gross could be incorporated within a workable crime laboratory. Locard's formal education was in both medicine and law. In 1910, he persuaded the Lyons police department to give him two attic rooms and two assistants to start a police laboratory.

During Locard's first years of work, the only available instruments were a microscope and a rudimentary spectrometer. However, his enthusiasm quickly overcame the technical and monetary deficiencies he encountered. From these modest beginnings, Locard's research and accomplishments became known throughout the world by forensic scientists and criminal investigators. Eventually he became the founder and director of the Institute of Criminalistics at the University of Lyons; this quickly developed into a leading international center for study and research in forensic science.

Locard's exchange principle
Whenever two objects come into contact with one another, there is exchange of materials between them.

Locard believed that when a person comes in contact with an object or person, a cross-transfer of materials occurs (**Locard's exchange principle**). Locard maintained that every person who commits a crime can be connected to a crime by dust particles carried from the crime scene. This concept was reinforced by a series of successful and well-publicized investigations. In one case, presented with counterfeit coins and the names of three suspects, Locard urged the police to bring the suspects' clothing to his laboratory. On careful examination, he located small metallic particles in all the garments. Chemical analysis revealed that the particles and coins were composed of exactly the same metallic elements. Confronted with this evidence, the suspects were arrested and soon confessed to the crime. After World War I, Locard's successes served as an impetus for the formation of police laboratories in Vienna, Berlin, Sweden, Finland, and Holland.

Crime Laboratories

The most ambitious commitment to forensic science occurred in the United States with the systematic development of national and state crime laboratories. This development greatly hastened the progress of forensic science.

Crime Labs in the United States

In 1932, the Federal Bureau of Investigation (FBI), under the directorship of J. Edgar Hoover, organized a national laboratory that offered forensic services to all law enforcement agencies in the country. During its formative stages, agents consulted extensively with business executives, manufacturers, and scientists whose knowledge and experience were useful in guiding the new facility through its infancy. The FBI Laboratory is now the world's largest forensic laboratory, performing more than one million examinations every year. Its accomplishments have earned it worldwide recognition, and its structure and organization have served as a model for forensic laboratories formed at the state and local levels in the United States as well as in other countries. Furthermore, the opening of the FBI's Forensic Science Research and Training Center in 1981 gave the United States, for the first time, a facility dedicated to conducting research to develop new and reliable scientific methods that can be applied to forensic science. This facility is also used to train crime laboratory personnel in the latest forensic science techniques and methods.

The oldest forensic laboratory in the United States is that of the Los Angeles Police Department, created in 1923 by August Vollmer, a police chief from Berkeley, California. In the 1930s, Vollmer headed the first U.S. university institute for criminology and criminalistics at the University of California at Berkeley. However, this institute lacked any official status in the university until 1948, when a school of criminology was formed. The famous criminalist Paul Kirk (see Figure 1–4) was selected to head its criminalistics department. Many graduates of this school have gone on to help develop forensic laboratories in other parts of the state and country.

California has numerous federal, state, county, and city crime laboratories, many of which operate independently. However, in 1972 the California Department of Justice embarked on an ambitious plan to create a network of state-operated crime laboratories. As a result, California has created a model system of integrated forensic laboratories consisting of regional and satellite facilities. An informal exchange of information and expertise is facilitated among California's criminalist community through a regional professional society, the California Association of Criminalists. This organization was the forerunner of a number of regional organizations that have developed throughout the United States to foster cooperation among the nation's growing community of criminalists.

The publication of *Strengthening Forensic Science in the United States* in 2009 by the National Academy of Sciences has served as a catalyst for

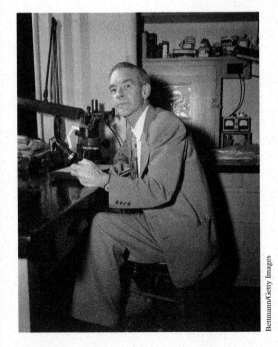

FIGURE 1–4
Paul Leland Kirk, 1902–1970.

Bettmann/Getty Images

improving the quality of research and development and standardization in the forensic sciences. The National Institute for Standards and Technology (NIST) within the Department of Commerce has emerged as a leading governmental agency in promoting the objectives advocated by *Forensic Science: A Path Forward*. Currently, NIST is active in these efforts by cochairing the National Commission of Forensic Science within the Department of Justice which is aimed at coordinating federal policies surrounding the practice of forensic science. It also leads the Organization of Scientific Area Committees (OSAC) a series of committees and subcommittees designed to standardize forensic practices across numerous forensic science disciplines. NIST also has an active forensic research program carried out within the institute.

International Crime Labs

In contrast to the American system of independent local laboratories, Great Britain had developed a national system of regional laboratories under the direction of the government's Home Office. In the early 1990s, the British Home Office reorganized the country's forensic laboratories into the Forensic Science Service and instituted a system in which police agencies are charged a fee for services rendered by the laboratory. The fee-for-service concept encouraged the creation of a number of private laboratories that provide services to both police and criminal defense attorneys. One such organization is LGC. In 2010, the British government announced the closure of the Forensic Science Service, citing financial losses. The laboratories closed in 2012, and forensic work in England and Wales is now contracted out to the private sector. Since privatization, LGC has grown to be the largest forensic science provider in the United Kingdom, employing more than 700 forensic scientists servicing both police agencies and the private sector.

In Canada, forensic services are provided by three government-funded institutes: (1) three Royal Canadian Mounted Police regional laboratories, (2) the Centre of Forensic Sciences in Toronto, and (3) the Institute of Legal Medicine and Police Science in Montreal. The Royal Canadian Mounted Police opened its first laboratory in Regina, Saskatchewan, in 1937. Altogether, more than a hundred countries throughout the world have at least one laboratory facility offering services in the field of forensic science.

Organization of a Crime Laboratory

The development of crime laboratories in the United States has been characterized by rapid growth accompanied by a lack of national and regional planning and coordination. It is estimated that more than 411 publicly funded crime laboratories currently operate at various levels of government (federal, state, county, and municipal)—more than three times the number of crime laboratories operating in 1966. They employ more than 14,000 full-time personnel.

The size and diversity of crime laboratories make it impossible to select any one model that best describes a typical crime laboratory. Although most of these facilities function as part of a police department, others operate under the direction of the prosecutor's or district attorney's office; some work with the laboratories of the medical examiner or coroner. Far fewer are affiliated with universities or exist as independent agencies in government. Laboratory staff sizes range from one person to more than a hundred, and their services may be diverse or specialized, depending on the responsibilities of the agency that houses the laboratory.

The Growth of Crime Laboratories

Crime laboratories have mostly been organized by agencies that either foresaw their potential application to criminal investigation or were pressed by the increasing demands of casework. Several reasons explain the unparalleled growth of crime laboratories during the past 35 years. Supreme Court decisions in the 1960s were responsible for greater police emphasis on securing scientifically evaluated evidence. The requirement to advise criminal suspects of their constitutional rights and their right of immediate access to counsel has all but eliminated confessions as a routine investigative tool. Successful prosecution of criminal cases requires a thorough and professional police investigation, frequently incorporating the skills of forensic science experts. Modern technology has provided forensic scientists with many new skills and techniques to meet the challenges accompanying their increased participation in the criminal justice system.

Coinciding with changing judicial requirements has been the staggering increase in crime rates in the United States over the past 40 years. This factor alone would probably have accounted for the increased use of crime laboratory services by police agencies, but only a small percentage of police investigations generate evidence requiring scientific examination. There is, however, one important exception to this observation: drug-related arrests. All illicit drug seizures must be sent to a forensic laboratory for confirmatory chemical analysis before the case can be adjudicated. Since the mid-1960s, drug use has accelerated to nearly uncontrollable levels and has resulted in crime laboratories being inundated with drug specimens. Current estimates indicate that nearly half of all requests for examination of forensic evidence deal with drugs.

Future Challenges

A more recent impetus leading to the growth and maturation of crime laboratories has been the advent of DNA profiling. Since the early 1990s, this technology has progressed to the point at which traces of blood, semen stains, hair, and saliva residues left behind on stamps, cups, bite marks, and so on have made possible the individualization or near-individualization of biological evidence. To meet the demands of DNA technology, crime labs have expanded staff and in many cases modernized their physical plants. The labor-intensive demands and sophisticated requirements of the technology have affected the structure of the forensic laboratory as has no other technology in the past 50 years. Likewise, DNA profiling has become the dominant factor in explaining how the general public perceives the workings and capabilities of the modern crime laboratory.

In coming years, an estimated 10,000 forensic scientists will be added to the rolls of both public and private forensic laboratories to process crime-scene evidence for DNA and to acquire DNA profiles, as mandated by state laws, from the hundreds of thousands of individuals convicted of crimes. This endeavor has already added many new scientists to the field and will eventually more than double the number of scientists employed by forensic laboratories in the United States.

A major problem facing the forensic DNA community is the substantial backlog of unanalyzed DNA samples from crime scenes. The number of unanalyzed casework DNA samples reported by state and national agencies is more than 57,000. The estimated number of untested convicted offender samples is more than 500,000. In an attempt to eliminate the backlog of convicted offender or arrestee samples to be analyzed and entered into the Combined DNA Index System (CODIS), the federal government has initiated funding for in-house analysis of samples at the crime laboratory or outsourcing samples to private laboratories for analysis.

Beginning in 2008, California began collecting DNA samples from all people arrested on suspicion of a felony, not waiting until a person is convicted. The state's database, with approximately one million DNA profiles, is already the third largest in the world, behind those maintained by the United Kingdom and the FBI. The federal government plans to begin doing the same.

Types of Crime Laboratories

Historically, a federal system of government, combined with a desire to retain local control, has produced a variety of independent laboratories in the United States, precluding the creation of a national system. Crime laboratories to a large extent mirror the fragmented law enforcement structure that exists on the national, state, and local levels.

FEDERAL CRIME LABORATORIES   The federal government has no single law enforcement or investigative agency with unlimited jurisdiction. Four major federal crime laboratories have been created to help investigate and enforce criminal laws that extend beyond the jurisdictional boundaries of state and local forces.

The FBI (Department of Justice) maintains the largest crime laboratory in the world. An ultramodern facility housing the FBI's forensic science services is located in Quantico, Virginia (see Figure 1–5). Its expertise and technology support its broad investigative powers. The Drug Enforcement Administration laboratories (Department of Justice) analyze drugs seized in violation of federal laws regulating the production, sale, and transportation of drugs. The laboratories of the Bureau of Alcohol, Tobacco, Firearms, and Explosives (Department of Justice) analyze

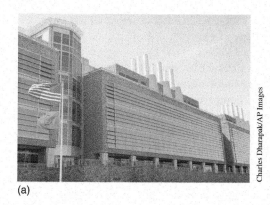
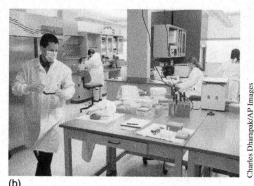

(a)   (b)

FIGURE 1–5

(a) Exterior and (b) interior views of the FBI crime laboratory in Quantico, Virginia.

alcoholic beverages and documents relating to alcohol and firearm excise tax law enforcement and examine weapons, explosive devices, and related evidence to enforce the Gun Control Act of 1968 and the Organized Crime Control Act of 1970. The U.S. Postal Inspection Service maintains laboratories concerned with criminal investigations relating to the postal service. Each of these federal facilities will offer its expertise to any local agency that requests assistance in relevant investigative matters.

The Defensive Forensic Science Center in the Department of Defense located in the state of Georgia provides traditional forensic capabilities to support worldwide criminal investigation across all military services. This organization also provides research and development to meet the military's forensic needs, as well as providing training to investigators and military attorneys.

STATE AND LOCAL CRIME LABORATORIES   Most state governments maintain a crime laboratory to service state and local law enforcement agencies that do not have ready access to a laboratory. Some states, such as Alabama, California, Illinois, Michigan, New Jersey, Texas, Washington, Oregon, Virginia, and Florida, have developed a comprehensive statewide system of regional or satellite laboratories. These operate under the direction of a central facility and provide forensic services to most areas of the state. The concept of a regional laboratory operating as part of a statewide system has increased the accessibility of many local law enforcement agencies to a crime laboratory, while minimizing duplication of services and ensuring maximum interlaboratory cooperation through the sharing of expertise and equipment.

Local laboratories provide services to county and municipal agencies. Generally, these facilities operate independently of the state crime laboratory and are financed directly by local government. However, as costs have risen, some counties have combined resources and created multicounty laboratories to service their jurisdictions. Many of the larger cities in the United States maintain their own crime laboratories, usually under the direction of the local police department. Frequently, high population and high crime rates combine to make a municipal facility, such as that of New York City, the largest crime laboratory in the state.

Services of the Crime Laboratory

Bearing in mind the independent development of crime laboratories in the United States, the wide variation in total services offered in different communities is not surprising. There are many reasons for this, including (1) variations in local laws, (2) the different capabilities and functions of the organization to which a laboratory is attached, and (3) budgetary and staffing limitations.

In recent years, many local crime laboratories have been created solely to process drug specimens. Often these facilities were staffed with few personnel and operated under limited budgets. Although many have expanded their forensic services, some still primarily perform drug analyses. However, even among crime laboratories providing services beyond drug identification, the diversity and quality of services rendered vary significantly. For the purposes of this text, I have taken the liberty of arbitrarily designating the following units as those that should constitute a "full-service" crime laboratory.

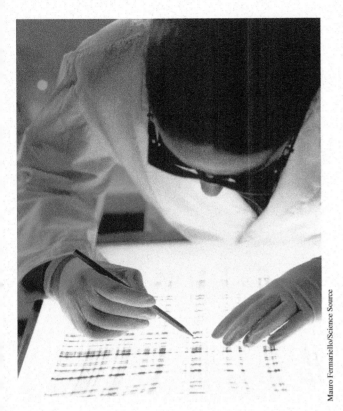

FIGURE 1–6
A forensic scientist performing DNA analysis.

Mauro Fermariello/Science Source

Basic Services Provided by Full-Service Crime Laboratories

PHYSICAL SCIENCE UNIT   The physical science unit applies principles and techniques of chemistry, physics, and geology to the identification and comparison of crime-scene evidence. It is staffed by criminalists who have the expertise to use chemical tests and modern analytical instrumentation to examine items as diverse as drugs, glass, paint, explosives, and soil. In a laboratory that has a staff large enough to permit specialization, the responsibilities of this unit may be further subdivided into drug identification, soil and mineral analysis, and examination of a variety of trace physical evidence.

BIOLOGY UNIT   The biology unit is staffed with biologists and biochemists who identify and perform DNA profiling on dried bloodstains and other body fluids, compare hairs and fibers, and identify and compare botanical materials such as wood and plants (see Figure 1–6).

FIREARMS UNIT   The firearms unit examines firearms, discharged bullets, cartridge cases, shotgun shells, and ammunition of all types. Garments and other objects are also examined to detect firearms discharge residues and to approximate the distance from a target at which a weapon was fired. The basic principles of firearms examination are also applied here to the comparison of marks made by tools (see Figure 1–7).

DOCUMENT EXAMINATION UNIT   The document examination unit studies the handwriting and typewriting on questioned documents to ascertain authenticity and/or source. Related responsibilities include analyzing paper and ink and examining indented writings (the term usually applied to the partially visible depressions appearing on a sheet of paper underneath the one on which the visible writing appears), obliterations, erasures, and burned or charred documents.

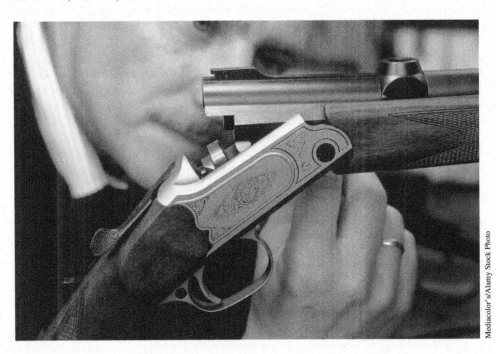

Mediacolor's/Alamy Stock Photo

FIGURE 1–7
A forensic analyst examining a firearm.

PHOTOGRAPHY UNIT   A complete photographic laboratory examines and records physical evidence. Its procedures may require the use of highly specialized photographic techniques, such as digital imaging, infrared, ultraviolet, and X-ray photography, to make invisible information visible to the naked eye. This unit also prepares photographic exhibits for courtroom presentation.

Optional Services Provided by Full-Service Crime Laboratories

TOXICOLOGY UNIT   The toxicology group examines body fluids and organs to determine the presence or absence of drugs and poisons. Frequently, such functions are shared with or may be the sole responsibility of a separate laboratory facility placed under the direction of the medical examiner's or coroner's office.

In most jurisdictions, field instruments such as the Intoxilyzer are used to determine the alcoholic consumption of individuals. Often the toxicology section also trains operators and maintains and services these instruments.

LATENT FINGERPRINT UNIT   The latent fingerprint unit processes and examines evidence for latent fingerprints when they are submitted in conjunction with other laboratory examinations.

POLYGRAPH UNIT   The polygraph, or lie detector, has come to be recognized as an essential tool of the criminal investigator rather than the forensic scientist. However, during the formative years of polygraph technology, many police agencies incorporated this unit into the laboratory's administrative structure, where it sometimes remains today. In any case, its functions are handled by people trained in the techniques of criminal investigation and interrogation.

VOICEPRINT ANALYSIS UNIT   In cases involving telephoned threats or tape-recorded messages, investigators may require the skills of the voiceprint analysis unit to tie the voice to a particular suspect. To this end, a good deal of casework has been performed with the sound spectrograph, an instrument that transforms speech into a visual display called a *voiceprint*. The validity of this technique as a means of personal identification rests on the premise that the sound patterns produced in speech are unique to the individual and that the voiceprint displays this uniqueness.

CRIME-SCENE INVESTIGATION UNIT   The concept of incorporating crime-scene evidence collection into the total forensic science service is slowly gaining recognition in the United States. This unit dispatches specially trained personnel (civilian and/or police) to the crime scene to collect and preserve physical evidence that will later be processed at the crime laboratory.

Whatever the organizational structure of a forensic science laboratory may be, specialization must not impede the overall coordination of services demanded by today's criminal investigator. Laboratory administrators need to keep open the lines of communication between analysts (civilian and uniform), crime-scene investigators, and police personnel. Inevitably, forensic investigations require the skills of many individuals. One notoriously high-profile investigation illustrates this process—the search to uncover the source of the anthrax letters mailed shortly after September 11, 2001. Figure 1–8 shows one of the letters and illustrates the multitude of skills required in the investigation—skills possessed by forensic chemists and biologists, fingerprint examiners, and forensic document examiners.

> > > > > > > > > >

Case Files

Forensic Science Helps Unravel the Mystery of the Anthrax Letters*

In September and October 2001, at least five envelopes containing significant quantities of anthrax were mailed to United States Senators Patrick Leahy and Thomas Daschle in the District of Columbia and to media organizations located in New York City and Boca Raton, Florida. The two letters addressed to Senators Leahy and Daschle had the same fictitious return address. The four envelopes each contained a Trenton, New Jersey, postmark. Swabbing of 621 mailboxes for Anthrax allowed investigators to identify a heavily contaminated blue street-side box located across the street from the main entrance to Princeton University.

By 2007, investigators conclusively determined that a single spore-batch created and maintained by Dr. Bruce E. Ivins at the United States Army Medical Research Institute of Infectious Diseases, located in Frederick, Maryland, was the parent material for the letter spores. An intensive investigation of individuals with access to that material ensued. Evidence developed from

(continued)

that investigation established that Dr. Ivins, alone, mailed the anthrax letters.

The four envelopes used in the attacks were all 6¾ inch "Federal Eagle" pre-franked 34¢ envelopes. The "Federal Eagle" name was derived from the postage frank in the upper right-hand corner of the envelope, which consisted of an image of an eagle perched on a bar bearing the letters "USA." Underneath those letters was the number 34, which denoted the 34¢ postage. The envelopes were manufactured exclusively for, and sold solely by, the United States Postal Service between January 8, 2001, and June 2002.

The printing on these envelopes was applied by a process called flexography. This was a form of relief printing, where a plate containing a raised image area was inked and then transferred the image directly onto the envelope via impact. These printing plates were composed of a flexible polymer material and could cause printing defects due to, among other things, excess ink or abrasions on the plate which arose and departed during envelope production, and which could impart a distinctive characteristic.

In January 2005, forensic examiners at the United States Secret Service Laboratory identified a number of defects in the pre-printed Eagle and wording on the envelopes used in the attacks. Based on this discovery, investigators implemented their plan to compare these defects to other envelopes recovered from post offices across the country in an effort to locate a point of purchase. Investigators collected as many pre-franked Federal Eagle envelopes as possible from post offices that had received them for comparison to the evidence. In total 290,245 known Federal Eagle envelopes were collected and examined.

Close scrutiny of the evidentiary envelopes revealed that the envelopes mailed to Tom Brokaw and Senator Leahy had the same print defects. The envelopes mailed to the NY Post and Senator Daschle shared the same print defects as each other, but different from the print defects observed on the envelopes mailed to Brokaw and Senator Leahy. As it turned out, during manufacturing/printing, two plates on a single printing machine drum were used to print the envelopes, in an alternating pattern. This is evidence that the envelopes mailed to both Brokaw and Senator Leahy were stamped by the same plate, while the envelopes mailed to the NY Post and Senator Daschle were stamped by the same plate, but different from the plate that stamped the envelopes to Brokaw and Senator Leahy. The logical inference was that these four envelopes were produced in succession and grouped this way because they were pulled from the box of envelopes in the order in which they were printed on the machine.

In the course of their examination of the known Eagle envelopes, experts determined that a particular box of envelopes from the Elkton, Maryland, office had alternating print defects strikingly similar to those observed in the evidence. Shipment records disclosed that the post offices in Elkton and Frederick, Maryland, received Eagle envelopes on the same day. Unfortunately, the envelopes from the Frederick post office had been destroyed.

Over the course of the next several months, examiners focused on how the printing defects changed over the course of the production run and how long it took for changes to start to occur. The expert examiners concluded that the same printing defects could occur on envelopes in as few as four boxes (2,000 envelopes). The occurrence of printing defects and the number of envelopes exhibiting the defect with the same morphological characteristics was quite low. It was concluded that the envelopes most similar to those used in the attacks were also distributed to the Elkton and Frederick, Maryland, post offices. The latter was located just a few blocks from the home of Dr. Ivins, and where Dr. Ivins maintained a post office box at the time of the mailings.

The anthrax letters were mailed from a collection box near Princeton University outside of an office building that housed a particular sorority with which Dr. Ivins was admittedly obsessed dating back 40 years to his college days. This mailbox was located approximately three hours from his house in Frederick, Maryland.

Aware of the FBI investigation and the prospect of being indicted, Dr. Ivins took an overdose of over-the-counter medications and died shortly thereafter.

Source: Amerithrax Investigative Summary: Released Pursuant to the Freedom of Information Act. The United States Department of Justice, 2010.

Functions of the Forensic Scientist

Although a forensic scientist relies primarily on scientific knowledge and skill, only half of the job is performed in the laboratory. The other half takes place in the courtroom, where the ultimate significance of the evidence is determined. The forensic scientist must not only analyze physical evidence but also persuade a jury to accept the conclusions derived from that analysis.

Analysis of Physical Evidence

First and foremost, the forensic scientist must be skilled in applying the principles and techniques of the physical and natural sciences to analyze the many types of physical evidence that may be recovered during a criminal investigation. Of the three major avenues available to police investigators for assistance in solving a crime—confessions, eyewitness accounts by victims or witnesses, and the evaluation of physical evidence retrieved from the crime scene—only physical evidence is free of inherent error or bias.

THE IMPORTANCE OF PHYSICAL EVIDENCE   Criminal cases are replete with examples of individuals who were incorrectly charged with and convicted of committing a crime because of

Indented writing may be deposited on paper left underneath a sheet of paper being written upon. Electrostatic imaging is used to visualize indented impressions on paper.

Handwriting examination reveals that block lettering is consistent with a single writer who wrote three other anthrax letters.

DNA may be recovered from saliva used to seal an envelope.

Cellophane tape was used to seal four envelopes containing the anthrax letters. The fitting together of the serrated ends of the tape strips confirmed that they were torn in succession from the same roll of tape.

Photocopier toner may reveal its manufacturer through chemical and physical properties.

Fingerprints may be detectable on paper using a variety of chemical developing techniques.

Paper examination may identify a manufacturer. General appearance, watermarks, fiber analysis, and chemical analysis of pigments, additives, and fillers may reveal a paper's origin.

DNA may be recovered from saliva residues on the back of a stamp. However, in this case, the stamp is printed onto the envelope.

Typescript comparison of transient defects imparted to the envelopes from printing plates impacting with the envelope.

Ink analysis may reveal a pen's manufacturer.

Trace evidence, such as hairs and fibers, may be present within the contents of the envelope.

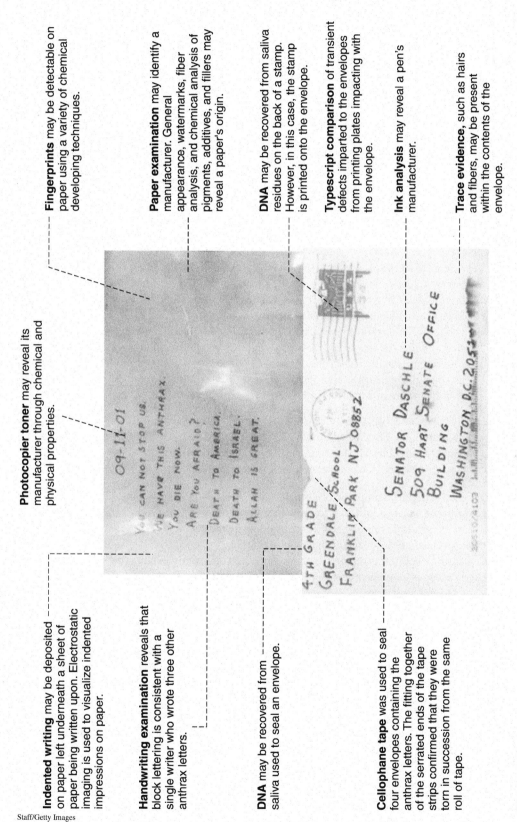

Staff/Getty Images

FIGURE 1–8

An envelope containing anthrax spores along with an anonymous letter was sent to the office of Senator Tom Daschle shortly after the terrorist attacks of September 11, 2001. A variety of forensic skills were used to examine the envelope and letter. Also, bar codes placed on the front and back of the envelope by mail-sorting machines contain address information and information about where the envelope was first processed.

faulty memories or lapses in judgment. For example, investigators may be led astray during their preliminary evaluation of the events and circumstances surrounding the commission of a crime. These errors may be compounded by misleading eyewitness statements and inappropriate confessions. These same concerns don't apply to physical evidence.

What about physical evidence that allows investigators to sort out facts as they are and not what one wishes they were? The hallmark of physical evidence is that it must undergo scientific inquiry. Science derives its integrity from adherence to strict guidelines that ensure the careful and systematic collection, organization, and analysis of information—a process known as the **scientific method**. The underlying principles of the scientific method provide a safety net to ensure that the outcome of an investigation is not tainted by human emotion or compromised by distorting, belittling, or ignoring contrary evidence.

scientific method
A process that uses strict guidelines to ensure careful and systematic collection, organization, and analysis of information.

The scientific method seeks answers by adhering to the systematic collection, organization, and analysis of information. The particular question to be examined is called the *hypothesis*. Scientific methodology is based on testing the hypothesis to see if it can be disproven or falsified. A scientific hypothesis is tentative and testable by experimentation and must be capable of being supported or not supported by experimental evidence. Hypotheses of durable explanatory power that have been tested over a wide variety of conditions are incorporated into theories. Theories represent the best explanations for various natural and physical phenomena and are capable of being tested and re-tested by multiple independent research.

The scientific method serves as a model for the criminal investigator. It begins by formulating a question worthy of investigation, such as who committed a particular crime. The investigator next formulates a hypothesis, a reasonable explanation proposed to answer the question. What follows is the basic foundation of scientific inquiry—the testing of the hypothesis through experimentation. The testing process must be thorough and recognized by other scientists and investigators as valid. Scientists and investigators must accept the findings even when they wish they were different. Finally, when the hypothesis is validated by experimentation, it becomes suitable as scientific evidence, appropriate for use in a criminal investigation and ultimately available for admission in a court of law.

DETERMINING ADMISSIBILITY OF EVIDENCE   In rejecting the scientific validity of the lie detector (polygraph), the District of Columbia Circuit Court in 1923 set forth what has since become a standard guideline for determining the judicial admissibility of scientific examinations. In *Frye* v. *United States*,[1] the court stated the following:

> Just when a scientific principle or discovery crosses the line between the experimental and demonstrable stages is difficult to define. Somewhere in this twilight zone the evidential force of the principle must be recognized, and while the courts will go a long way in admitting expert testimony deduced from a well-recognized scientific principle or discovery, the thing from which the deduction is made must be sufficiently established to have gained general acceptance in the particular field in which it belongs.

To meet the *Frye* standard, the court must decide whether the questioned procedure, technique, or principle is "generally accepted" by a meaningful segment of the relevant scientific community. In practice, this approach required the proponent of a scientific test to present to the court a collection of experts who could testify that the scientific issue before the court is generally accepted by the relevant members of the scientific community. Furthermore, in determining whether a novel technique meets criteria associated with "general acceptance," courts have frequently taken note of books and papers written on the subject, as well as prior judicial decisions relating to the reliability and general acceptance of the technique. In recent years, this approach has engendered a great deal of debate as to whether it is sufficiently flexible to deal with new and novel scientific issues that may not have gained widespread support within the scientific community.

OTHER STANDARDS OF ADMISSIBILITY   As an alternative to the *Frye* standard, some courts came to believe that the Federal Rules of Evidence espoused a more flexible standard that did not rely on general acceptance as an absolute prerequisite for admitting scientific evidence. Part of the Federal Rules of Evidence governs the admissibility of all evidence, including expert

[1] 293 Fed. 1013 (D.C. Cir. 1923).

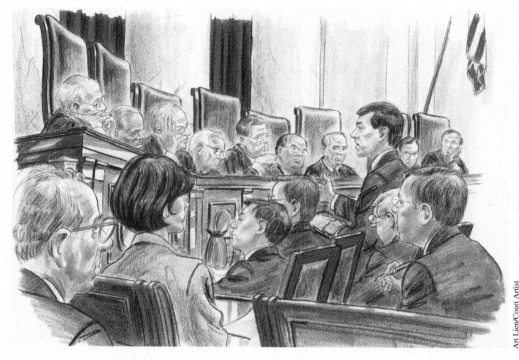

Art Lien/Court Artist

FIGURE 1–9
Sketch of a U.S. Supreme Court hearing.

testimony, in federal courts, and many states have adopted codes similar to those of the Federal Rules. Specifically, Rule 702 of the Federal Rules of Evidence deals with the admissibility of expert testimony:

> If scientific, technical, or other specialized knowledge will assist the trier of fact to understand the evidence or to determine a fact in issue, a witness qualified as an expert by knowledge, skill, experience, training, or education, may testify thereto in the form of an opinion or otherwise, if (1) the testimony is based upon sufficient facts or data, (2) the testimony is the product of reliable principles and methods, and (3) the witness has applied the principles and methods reliably to the facts of the case.

In a landmark ruling in the 1993 case of *Daubert* v. *Merrell Dow Pharmaceuticals, Inc.,*[2] the U.S. Supreme Court asserted that "general acceptance," or the *Frye* standard, is not an absolute prerequisite to the admissibility of scientific evidence under the Federal Rules of Evidence. According to the Court, the Rules of Evidence—especially Rule 702—assign to the trial judge the task of ensuring that an expert's testimony rests on a reliable foundation and is relevant to the case. Although this ruling applies only to federal courts, many state courts are expected to use this decision as a guideline in setting standards for the admissibility of scientific evidence.

JUDGING SCIENTIFIC EVIDENCE   What the Court advocates in *Daubert* is that trial judges assume the ultimate responsibility for acting as a "gatekeeper" in judging the admissibility and reliability of scientific evidence presented in their courts (see Figure 1–9). The Court offered some guidelines as to how a judge can gauge the veracity of scientific evidence, emphasizing that the inquiry should be flexible. Suggested areas of inquiry include the following:

1. Whether the scientific technique or theory can be (and has been) tested
2. Whether the technique or theory has been subject to peer review and publication
3. The technique's potential rate of error
4. Existence and maintenance of standards controlling the technique's operation
5. Whether the scientific theory or method has attracted widespread acceptance within a relevant scientific community

[2] 509 U.S. 579 (1993).

Some legal practitioners have expressed concern that abandoning *Frye*'s general-acceptance test will result in the introduction of absurd and irrational pseudoscientific claims in the courtroom. The Supreme Court rejected these concerns:

> In this regard, the respondent seems to us to be overly pessimistic about the capabilities of the jury and of the adversary system generally. Vigorous cross-examination, presentation of contrary evidence, and careful instruction on the burden of proof are the traditional and appropriate means of attacking shaky but admissible evidence.

In a 1999 decision, *Kumho Tire Co., Ltd.* v. *Carmichael*,[3] the Court unanimously ruled that the "gatekeeping" role of the trial judge applied not only to scientific testimony but also to all expert testimony:

> We conclude that *Daubert*'s general holding—setting forth the trial judge's general "gatekeeping" obligation—applies not only to testimony based on "scientific" knowledge, but also to testimony based on "technical" and "other specialized" knowledge. . . . We also conclude that a trial court may consider one or more of the more specific factors that *Daubert* mentioned when doing so will help determine that testimony's reliability. But, as the Court stated in *Daubert,* the test of reliability is "flexible," and *Daubert*'s list of specific factors neither necessarily nor exclusively applies to all experts in every case.

A leading case that exemplifies the type of flexibility and wide discretion that the *Daubert* ruling apparently gives trial judges in matters of scientific inquiry is *Coppolino* v. *State*.[4] Here, a medical examiner testified to his finding that the victim had died of an overdose of a drug known as succinylcholine chloride. This drug had never before been detected in the human body. The medical examiner's findings were dependent on a toxicological report that identified an abnormally high concentration of succinic acid, a breakdown product of the drug, in the victim's body. The defense argued that this test for the presence of succinylcholine chloride was new, and the absence of corroborative experimental data by other scientists meant that it had not yet gained general acceptance in the toxicology profession. The court, in rejecting this argument, recognized the necessity for devising new scientific tests to solve the special problems that are continually arising in the forensic laboratory. It emphasized, however, that although these tests may be new and unique, they are admissible only if they are based on scientifically valid principles and techniques: "The tests by which the medical examiner sought to determine whether death was caused by succinylcholine chloride were novel and devised specifically for this case. This does not render the evidence inadmissible. Society need not tolerate homicide until there develops a body of medical literature about some particular lethal agent."

Providing Expert Testimony

Because the results of their work may be a factor in determining a person's ultimate guilt or innocence, forensic scientists may be required to testify about their methods and conclusions at a trial or hearing.

expert witness
An individual whom the court determines to possess knowledge relevant to the trial that is not expected of the average layperson.

Trial courts have broad discretion in accepting an individual as an **expert witness** on any particular subject. Generally, if a witness can establish to the satisfaction of a trial judge that they possess a particular skill or have knowledge in a trade or profession that will aid the court in determining the truth of the matter at issue, that individual will be accepted as an expert witness. Depending on the subject area in question, the court will usually consider knowledge acquired through experience, training, education, or a combination of these as sufficient grounds for qualification as an expert witness.

In court, an expert witness may be asked questions intended to demonstrate his or her ability and competence pertaining to the matter at hand. Competency may be established by having the witness cite educational degrees, participation in special courses, membership in professional societies, and any professional articles or books published. Also important is the number of years of occupational experience the witness has had in areas related to the matter before the court.

Most chemists, biologists, geologists, and physicists prepare themselves for careers in forensic science by combining training under an experienced examiner with independent study.

---

[3] 526 U.S. 137 (1999).

[4] 223 So. 2d 68 (Fla. App. 1968), app. dismissed, 234 So. 2d (Fla. 1969), cert. denied, 399 U.S. 927 (1970).

Of course, formal education in the physical sciences provides a firm foundation for learning and understanding the principles and techniques of forensic science. Nevertheless, for the most part, courts must rely on training and years of experience as a measurement of the knowledge and ability of the expert.

Before the judge rules on the witness's qualifications, the opposing attorney may cross-examine the witness and point out weaknesses in training and knowledge. Most courts are reluctant to disqualify an individual as an expert even when presented with someone whose background is only remotely associated with the issue at hand. The question of what credentials are suitable for qualification as an expert is ambiguous and highly subjective and one that the courts wisely try to avoid.

The weight that a judge or jury assigns to "expert" testimony in subsequent deliberations is, however, quite another matter. Undoubtedly, education and experience have considerable bearing on what value should be assigned to the expert's opinions. Just as important may be his or her demeanor and ability to explain scientific data and conclusions clearly, concisely, and logically to a judge and jury composed of nonscientists. The problem of sorting out the strengths and weaknesses of expert testimony falls to prosecution and defense counsel.

The ordinary or lay witness must testify on events or observations that arise from personal knowledge. This testimony must be factual and, with few exceptions, cannot contain the personal opinions of the witness. On the other hand, the expert witness is called on to evaluate evidence when the court lacks the expertise to do so. This expert then expresses an opinion as to the significance of the findings. The views expressed are accepted only as representing the expert's opinion and may later be accepted or ignored in jury deliberations (see Figure 1–10).

The expert cannot render any view with absolute certainty. At best, the expert may only be able to offer an opinion based on a reasonable scientific certainty derived from training and experience. Obviously, the expert is expected to defend vigorously the techniques and conclusions of the analysis, but at the same time they must not be reluctant to discuss impartially any findings that could minimize the significance of the analysis. The forensic scientist should not be an advocate of one party's cause but an advocate of truth only. An adversary system of justice

> > > > > > > > > > >

Case Files

Dr. Coppolino's Deadly House Calls

A frantic late-night telephone call brought a local physician to the Florida home of Drs. Carl and Carmela Coppolino. The physician arrived to find Carmela beyond help. Carmela Coppolino's body, unexamined by anyone, was then buried in her family's plot in her home state of New Jersey.

A little more than a month later, Carl married a money-eyed socialite, Mary Gibson. News of Carl's marriage infuriated Marjorie Farber, a former New Jersey neighbor of Dr. Coppolino who had been having an affair with the doctor. Soon Marjorie had an interesting story to recount to investigators: Her husband's death two years before, although ruled to be from natural causes, had actually been murder! Carl, an anesthesiologist, had given Marjorie a syringe containing some medication and told her to inject her husband, William, while he was sleeping. Ultimately, Marjorie claimed, she was unable to inject the full dose and called Carl, who finished the job by suffocating William with a pillow.

Marjorie Farber's astonishing story was supported in part by Carl's having recently increased his wife's life insurance. Carmela's $65,000 policy, along with his new wife's fortune, would keep Dr. Coppolino in high society for the rest of his life. Based on this information, authorities in New Jersey and Florida obtained exhumation orders for both William Farber

and Carmela Coppolino. After both bodies were examined, Dr. Coppolino was charged with the murders of William and Carmela.

Officials decided to try Dr. Coppolino first in New Jersey for the murder of William Farber. The Farber autopsy did not reveal any evidence of poisoning but seemed to show strong evidence of strangulation. The absence of toxicological findings left the jury to deliberate the conflicting medical expert testimony versus Marjorie Farber's sensational story. In the end, Dr. Coppolino was acquitted.

The Florida trial presented another chance to bring Carl Coppolino to justice. Recalling Dr. Coppolino's career as an anesthesiologist, the prosecution theorized that to commit these murders Coppolino had exploited his access to the many potent drugs used during surgery, specifically an injectable paralytic agent called succinylcholine chloride.

Carmela's body was exhumed, and it was found that Carmela had been injected in her left buttock shortly before her death. Ultimately, a completely novel procedure for detecting succinylcholine chloride was devised. With this procedure elevated levels of succinic acid were found in Carmela's brain, which proved that she had received a large dose of the paralytic drug shortly before her death. This evidence, along with evidence of the same drug residues in the injection site on her buttock, was presented in the Florida murder trial of Carl Coppolino, who was convicted of second-degree murder.

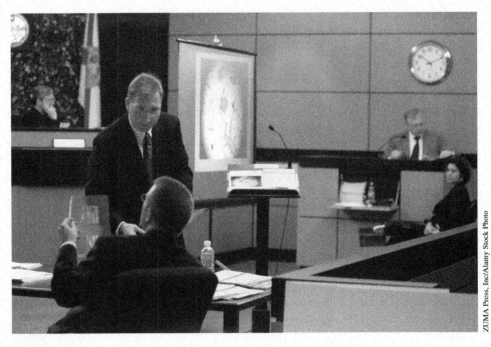

FIGURE 1–10
An expert witness testifying in court.

must give the prosecutor and defense ample opportunity to offer expert opinions and to argue the merits of such testimony. Ultimately, the duty of the judge or jury is to weigh the pros and cons of all the information presented when deciding guilt or innocence.

The U.S. Department of Justice has issued a series of guidelines defining the ethical responsibilities of forensic examiners both within the laboratory and courtroom (see Appendix II). These foundational guidelines can be expected to be adopted as universally accepted criteria by practicing forensic scientists. They will serve as a measuring rod to judge the integrity and competence of forensic science as it's practiced in the criminal justice system. The necessity for the forensic scientist to appear in court has been imposed on the criminal justice system by a 2009 U.S. Supreme Court Case, *Melendez-Diaz* v. *Massachusetts*.[5] The *Melendez-Diaz* decision addressed the practice of using evidence affidavits or laboratory certificates in lieu of in-person testimony by forensic analysts. In its reasoning, the Court relied on a previous ruling, *Crawford* v. *Washington*,[6] where it explored the meaning of the Confrontation Clause of the Sixth Amendment. In the *Crawford* case, a recorded statement by a spouse was used against her husband in his prosecution. Crawford argued that this was a violation of his right to confront witnesses against him under the Sixth Amendment, and the Court agreed. Using the same logic in *Melendez-Diaz,* the Court reasoned that introducing forensic science evidence via an affidavit or a certificate denied a defendant the opportunity to cross-examine the analyst. In 2011, the Supreme Court reaffirmed the *Melendez-Diaz* decision in the case of *Bullcoming* v. *New Mexico*[7] by rejecting a substitute expert witness in lieu of the original analyst:

WEBEXTRA 1.1
Watch a Forensic Expert Witness
Testify—I

WEBEXTRA 1.2
Watch a Forensic Expert Witness
Testify—II

> The question presented is whether the Confrontation Clause permits the prosecution to introduce a forensic laboratory report containing a testimonial certification—made for the purpose of proving a particular fact through the in-court testimony of a scientist who did not sign the certification or perform or observe the test reported in the certification. We hold that surrogate testimony of that order does not meet the constitutional requirement. The accused's right is to be confronted with the analyst who made the certification, unless that analyst is unavailable at trial, and the accused had an opportunity, pretrial, to cross-examine that particular scientist.

[5] 557 U.S. 305 (2009).
[6] 541 U.S. 36 (2004).
[7] 131 S. Ct. 2705 (2011).

Furnishing Training in the Proper Recognition, Collection, and Preservation of Physical Evidence

The competence of a laboratory staff and the sophistication of its analytical equipment have little or no value if relevant evidence cannot be properly recognized, collected, and preserved at the site of a crime. For this reason, the forensic staff must have responsibilities that will influence the conduct of the crime-scene investigation.

The most direct and effective response to this problem has been to dispatch specially trained evidence-collection technicians to the crime scene. A growing number of crime laboratories and the police agencies they service keep trained "evidence technicians" on 24-hour call to help criminal investigators retrieve evidence. These technicians are trained by the laboratory staff to recognize and gather pertinent physical evidence at the crime scene. They are assigned to the laboratory full time for continued exposure to forensic techniques and procedures. They have at their disposal all the proper tools and supplies for proper collection and packaging of evidence for future scientific examination.

Unfortunately, many police forces still have not adopted this approach. Often a patrol officer or detective collects the evidence. The individual's effectiveness in this role depends on the extent of his or her training and working relationship with the laboratory. For maximum use of the skills of the crime laboratory, training of the crime-scene investigator must go beyond superficial classroom lectures to involve extensive personal contact with the forensic scientist. Each must become aware of the other's problems, techniques, and limitations.

The training of police officers in evidence collection and their familiarization with the capabilities of a crime laboratory should not be restricted to a select group of personnel on the force. Every officer engaged in fieldwork, whether it be traffic, patrol, investigation, or juvenile control, often must process evidence for laboratory examination. Obviously, it would be difficult and time consuming to give everyone the in-depth training and attention that a qualified criminal investigator requires. However, familiarity with crime laboratory services and capabilities can be gained through periodic lectures, laboratory tours, and dissemination of manuals prepared by the laboratory staff that outline the proper methods for collecting and submitting physical evidence to the laboratory (see Figure 1–11).

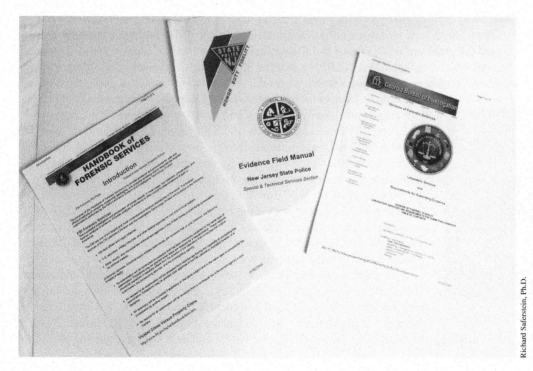

Richard Saferstein, Ph.D.

FIGURE 1–11

Representative evidence-collection guides prepared by various police agencies.

A brief outline describing the proper collection and packaging of common types of physical evidence is found in Appendix II. The procedures and information summarized in this appendix are discussed in greater detail in forthcoming chapters.

Other Forensic Science Services

Even though this textbook is devoted to describing the services normally provided by a crime laboratory, the field of forensic science is by no means limited to the areas covered in this book. A number of specialized forensic science services outside the crime laboratory are routinely available to law enforcement personnel. These services are important aids to a criminal investigation and require the involvement of individuals who have highly specialized skills.

Forensic Psychiatry

Forensic psychiatry is a specialized area in which the relationship between human behavior and legal proceedings is examined. Forensic psychiatrists are retained for both civil and criminal litigations. For civil cases, forensic psychiatrists normally determine whether people are competent to make decisions about preparing wills, settling property, or refusing medical treatment. For criminal cases, they evaluate behavioral disorders and determine whether people are competent to stand trial. Forensic psychiatrists also examine behavioral patterns of people who commit crimes as an aid in developing a suspect's behavioral profile.

Forensic Odontology

Practitioners of forensic odontology help identify victims when the body is left in an unrecognizable state. Teeth are composed of enamel, the hardest substance in the body. Because of enamel's resilience, the teeth outlast tissues and organs as decomposition begins. The characteristics of teeth, their alignment, and the overall structure of the mouth provide individual evidence for identifying a specific person. With the use of dental records such as X-rays and dental casts or even a photograph of the person's smile, a set of dental remains can be compared to a suspected victim (see Figure 1–12).

Historically, forensic odontologists have also interpreted human bitemarks as a means of identifying a potential perpetrator with a mark left on a victim. Bitemark comparison evidence was first admitted in courts in the United States in 1975 and were soon admissible in all 50 states. In light of recent scientific advancements, namely DNA testing, it has been demonstrated that there are serious flaws in the assertions made by forensic dentists during a bitemark comparison. Since the advent of DNA, a number of cases involving trial level bitemark identifications have been overturned following post-conviction DNA testing. In 2009, the National Academy of Sciences took a hard look at the scientific underpinnings of forensic bitemark identification and found glaring gaps in the scientific research.

There are two assumptions on which the practice of human bitemark comparison rests. First, that human dentition is substantially unique such that a person can be identified by marks made by their teeth. Second, that human skin is an accurate impression material for the individual marks made by the teeth, if they exist. In 2016, the U.S. American Board of Forensic Odontology published a rejection of past practices of using bitemarks for human identification. Still, some experts practicing in this area disagreed with criticisms that there was a lack of scientific evidence to support the "assumptions and assertions made by forensic dentists during bitemark comparisons."[8]

The controversy highlights an important struggle where law and science intersect. What evidence will be admitted in a criminal trial is often governed by legal precedent. Once that legal precedent is firmly established, as with human bitemark comparisons, it is hard to change what has been admissible in courts for the past 40 years. As more scientific evidence mounts rejecting the use of

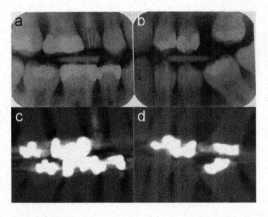

FIGURE 1–12

Images (a) and (c) and (b) and (d) are postmortem and antemortem dental X-rays taken from the same person. The images were used to positively identify the individual using dental records.

[8] Bowers, C. M., "Review of a Forensic Pseudoscience: Identification of Criminals from Bitemark Patterns," *Journal of Forensic and Legal Medicine* 61 (2019): 34–39. doi:10.1016/j.jflm.2018.11.001

bitemark comparison as a means of human identification, scientists are becoming more skeptical of its use in courtrooms, but many prosecutors and judges are proceeding undeterred.

On February12, 2016, the Texas Forensic Science Commission[9] published a report on bite mark comparison in response to a complaint filed by the National Innocence Project on behalf of Steven Mark Chaney. The Commission concluded the following: (1) at the current time, the overwhelming majority of existing research does not support the contention that bite mark comparison can be performed reliably and accurately from examiner to examiner due to the subjective nature of the analysis and (2) in addition to the foundational scientific and research issues, there are significant quality control and infrastructure differences between forensic odontology and other patterned and impression disciplines performed in accredited laboratories. The Commission recommended bite mark comparison evidence *not be admitted in criminal cases in Texas* unless and until the following are established: (1) criteria for identifying when a patterned injury constitutes a human bite mark, (2) criteria for identifying when a human bite mark was made by an adult versus a child, and (3) rigorous and appropriately validated proficiency testing.

Forensic Engineering

Forensic engineers are concerned with failure analysis, accident reconstruction, and causes and origins of fires or explosions. Forensic engineers answer questions such as these: How did an accident or structural failure occur? Were the parties involved responsible? If so, how were they responsible? Accident scenes are examined, photographs are reviewed, and any mechanical objects involved are inspected.

Forensic Computer and Digital Analysis

Forensic computer science is a new and fast-growing field that involves the identification, collection, preservation, and examination of information derived from computers and other digital devices, such as cell phones. Law enforcement aspects of this work normally involve the recovery of deleted or overwritten data from a computer's hard drive and the tracking of hacking activities within a compromised system. This field of forensic computer analysis and recovery of data from mobile devices will be addressed in detail in Chapters 18 and 19.

Exploring Forensic Science on the Internet

There are no limits to the amount or type of information that can be found on the Internet. The fields of law enforcement and forensic science have not been left behind by advancing computer technology. Extensive information about forensic science is available on the Internet. The types of information available on websites range from simple explanations of the various fields of forensics to intricate details of crime-scene reconstruction. People can also find information on which colleges offer degree programs in forensics and web pages posted by law enforcement agencies that detail their activities as well as employment opportunities.

General Forensics Sites

Reddy's Forensic Home Page (www.forensicpage.com) is a valuable starting point. This site is a collection of forensic web pages in categories such as new links in forensics; general forensic information sources; associations, colleges, and societies; literature and journals; forensic laboratories; general web pages; forensic-related mailing lists and newsgroups; universities; conferences; and various forensic fields of expertise.

Another website offering a multitude of information related to forensic science is Zeno's Forensic Site (www.forensic.to/forensic.html). Here, users can find links related to forensic education and expert consultation, as well as a wealth of information concerning specific fields of forensic science.

A comprehensive and useful website for those interested in law enforcement is Officer.com (www.officer.com). This comprehensive collection of criminal justice resources is organized into easy-to-read subdirectories that relate to topics such as law enforcement agencies, police association and organization sites, criminal justice organizations, law research pages, and police mailing-list directories.

---

[9] https://www.txcourts.gov/media/1440353/fsc-annual-report-fy2017.pdf

WEBEXTRA 1.3
An Introduction to Forensic Firearm
Identification

AN INTRODUCTION TO FORENSIC FIREARM IDENTIFICATION (http://www.firearmsid.com/) This website contains an extensive collection of information relating to the identification of firearms. An individual can explore in detail how to examine bullets, cartridge cases, and clothing for gunshot residues and suspect shooters' hands for primer residues. Information on the latest technology involving the automated firearms search system NIBIN can also be found on this site.

WEBEXTRA 1.4
Carpenter's Forensic Science
Resources

CARPENTER'S FORENSIC SCIENCE RESOURCES (http://www.tncrimlaw.com/forensic/) This site provides a bibliography involving forensic evidence. For example, the user can find references about DNA, fingerprints, hairs, fibers, and questioned documents as they relate to crime scenes and assist investigations. This website is an excellent place to start a research project in forensic science.

WEBEXTRA 1.5
Crime Scene Investigator Network

CRIME SCENE INVESTIGATOR NETWORK (http://www.crime-scene-investigator.net/index.html) For those who are interested in learning the process of crime-scene investigation, this site provides detailed guidelines and information regarding crime-scene response and the collection and preservation of evidence. For example, information concerning the packaging and analysis of bloodstains, seminal fluids, hairs, fibers, paint, glass, firearms, documents, and fingerprints can be found through this website. It explains the importance of inspecting the crime scene and the impact forensic evidence has on the investigation.

WEBEXTRA 1.6
Crimes and Clues

CRIMES AND CLUES (http://crimeandclues.com/) Users interested in learning about the forensic aspects of fingerprinting will find this to be a useful and informative website. The site covers the history of fingerprints, as well as subjects pertaining to the development of latent fingerprints. The user will also find links to other websites covering a variety of subjects pertaining to crime-scene investigation, documentation of the crime scene, and expert testimony.

WEBEXTRA 1.7
Questioned-Document Examination

QUESTIONED DOCUMENT EXAMINATION (http://www.qdewill.com/) This basic, informative web page answers frequently asked questions concerning document examination, explains the application of typical document examinations, and details the basic facts and theory of handwriting and signatures. There are also links to noted document examination cases that present the user with real-life applications of forensic document examination.

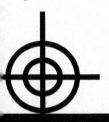

Chapter Summary > > > > > > > > > >

In its broadest definition, forensic science is the application of science to criminal and civil laws. This book emphasizes the application of science to the criminal and civil laws that are enforced by police agencies in a criminal justice system. Forensic science owes its origins to individuals such as Bertillon, Galton, Lattes, Goddard, Osborn, and Locard, who developed the principles and techniques needed to identify or compare physical evidence.

The development of crime laboratories in the United States has been characterized by rapid growth accompanied by a lack of national and regional planning and coordination. At present, approximately four hundred public crime laboratories operate at various levels of government—federal, state, county, and municipal.

The technical support provided by crime laboratories can be assigned to five basic services. The physical science unit uses the principles of chemistry, physics, and geology to identify and compare physical evidence. The biology unit uses knowledge of biological sciences to investigate blood

samples, body fluids, hair, and fiber samples. The firearms unit investigates discharged bullets, cartridge cases, shotgun shells, and ammunition. The document examination unit performs handwriting analysis and other questioned document examination. Finally, the photography unit uses specialized photographic techniques to record and examine physical evidence. Some crime laboratories offer the optional services of toxicology, fingerprint analysis, polygraph administration, voiceprint analysis, and crime-scene investigation and evidence collection.

A forensic scientist must be skilled in applying the principles and techniques of the physical and natural sciences to the analysis of the many types of evidence that may be recovered during a criminal investigation. A forensic scientist may also provide expert court testimony. An expert witness is called on to evaluate evidence based on specialized training and experience and to express an opinion as to the significance of the findings. Also, forensic scientists participate in training law enforcement personnel in proper recognition, collection, and preservation of physical evidence.

The *Frye* v. *United States* decision set guidelines for determining the admissibility of scientific evidence into the courtroom. To meet the *Frye* standard, the evidence in question must be "generally accepted" by the scientific community. However, in the 1993 case of *Daubert* v. *Merrell Dow Pharmaceuticals, Inc.,* the U.S. Supreme Court asserted that the *Frye* standard is not an absolute prerequisite to the admissibility of scientific evidence. Trial judges were said to be ultimately responsible as "gatekeepers" for the admissibility and validity of scientific evidence presented in their courts.

A number of special forensic science services are available to the law enforcement community to augment the services of the crime laboratory. These services include forensic psychiatry, forensic odontology, forensic engineering, and forensic computer and digital analysis.

Review Questions

1. The application of science to law describes _____.

2. The fictional exploits of _____ excited the imagination of an emerging generation of forensic scientists and criminal investigators.

3. A system of personal identification using a series of body measurements was first devised by _____.

4. _____ is responsible for developing the first statistical study proving the uniqueness of fingerprints.

5. The Italian scientist _____ devised the first workable procedure for typing dried bloodstains.

6. The comparison microscope became an indispensable tool of firearms examination through the efforts of _____.

7. Early efforts at applying scientific principles to document examination are associated with _____.

8. The application of science to criminal investigation was advocated by the Austrian magistrate _____.

9. One of the first functional crime laboratories was formed in Lyons, France, under the direction of _____.

10. The transfer of evidence that occurs when two objects come in contact with one another was a concept first advocated by the forensic scientist _____.

11. The first forensic laboratory in the United States was created in 1923 by the _____ Police Department.

12. The state of _____ is an excellent example of a geographical area in the United States that has created a system of integrated regional and satellite laboratories.

13. In contrast to the United States, Britain's crime laboratory system is characterized by a national system of _____ laboratories.

14. The increasing demand for _____ analyses has been the single most important factor in the recent expansion of crime laboratory services in the United States.

15. Four important federal agencies offering forensic services are _____, _____, _____, and _____.

16. A decentralized system of crime laboratories currently exists in the United States under the auspices of various governmental agencies at the _____, _____, _____, and _____ levels of government.

17. The application of chemistry, physics, and geology to the identification and comparison of crime-scene evidence is the function of the _____ unit of a crime laboratory.

18. The examination of blood, hairs, fibers, and botanical materials is conducted in the _____ unit of a crime laboratory.

19. The examination of bullets, cartridge cases, shotgun shells, and ammunition of all types is the responsibility of the _____ unit.

20. The examination of body fluids and organs for drugs and poisons is a function of the _____ unit.

21. The _____ unit dispatches trained personnel to the scene of a crime to retrieve evidence for laboratory examination.

22. The "general acceptance" principle, which serves as a criterion for the judicial admissibility of scientific evidence, was set forth in the case of _____.

23. In the case of _____, the Supreme Court ruled that in assessing the admissibility of new and unique scientific tests, the trial judge did not have to rely solely on the concept of "general acceptance."

24. True or False: The U.S. Supreme Court decision in *Kumho Tire Co., Ltd.* v. *Carmichael* restricted the "gatekeeping" role of a trial judge only to scientific testimony. _____

25. A Florida case that exemplifies the flexibility and wide discretion that the trial judge has in matters of scientific inquiry is _____.

26. A(n) _____ is a person who can demonstrate a particular skill or has knowledge in a trade or profession that will help the court determine the truth of the matter at issue.

27. True or False: The expert witness's courtroom demeanor may play an important role in deciding what weight the court will assign to his or her testimony. _____

28. True or False: The testimony of an expert witness incorporates their personal opinion relating to a matter the expert has either studied or examined. _____

29. The ability of the investigator to recognize and collect crime-scene evidence properly depends on the amount of _____ received from the crime laboratory.

30. True or False: In 2004, the U.S. Supreme Court addressed issues relating to the Confrontation Clause of the Sixth Amendment in the case of *Crawford* v. *Washington*. _____

31. The 2009 U.S. Supreme Court decision _____ addressed the practice of using affidavits in lieu of in-person testimony by forensic examiners.

Application and Critical Thinking

1. Most crime labs in the United States are funded and operated by the government and provide services free to police and prosecutors. Great Britain, however, uses private laboratories that charges fees for their services and keep any profits they make. Suggest potential strengths and weaknesses of each system.

2. Police investigating an apparent suicide collect the following items at the scene: a note purportedly written by the victim, a revolver bearing very faint fingerprints, and traces of skin and blood under the victim's fingernails. What units of the crime laboratory will examine each piece of evidence?

3. List at least three advantages of having an evidence-collection unit process a crime scene instead of a patrol officer or detective.

4. What legal issue was raised on appeal by the defense in Carl Coppolino's Florida murder trial? What court ruling is most relevant to the decision to reject the appeal? Explain your answer.

5. **A Timeline of Forensic Science** The following images depict different types of evidence or techniques for analyzing evidence. Place the images in order pertaining to the time in history (least recent to most recent) at which each type of evidence or technique was first introduced. Do this using the letters assigned to the images.

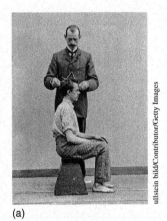
(a) *ullstein bild/Contributor/Getty Images*

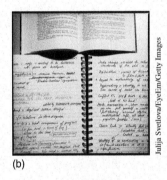
(b) *Julija Svetlova/EyeEm/Getty Images*

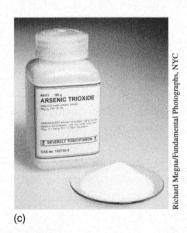
(c) *Richard Megna/Fundamental Photographs, NYC*

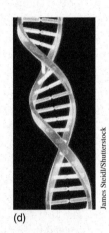
(d) *James Steidl/Shutterstock*

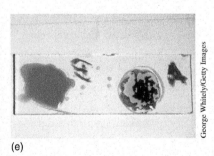
(e) *George Whitely/Getty Images*

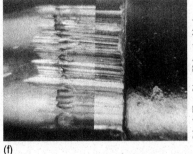
(f) *Orlando/Three Lions/Hulton Archive/Getty Images*

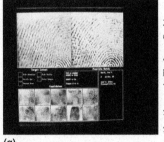
(g) *Alan Abramowitz/The Image Bank/Getty Images*

6. **Evidence Processing at the Crime Laboratory** You are the evidence technician at the front desk of the state crime lab. You receive the following items of evidence to check in on a very busy day. You must indicate which unit each piece of evidence should be sent to for analysis. Your crime lab has a criminalistics (physical science) unit, a drug unit, a biology unit, a firearms unit, a document examination unit, a toxicology unit, a latent fingerprinting unit, an anthropology unit, and a forensic computer and digital analysis unit.

(a) _____

(b) _____

(c) _____

(d) _____

(e) _____

(f) _____

(g) _____

(h) _____

(i) _____

(j) _____

(k) _____

(l) _____

(m) _____

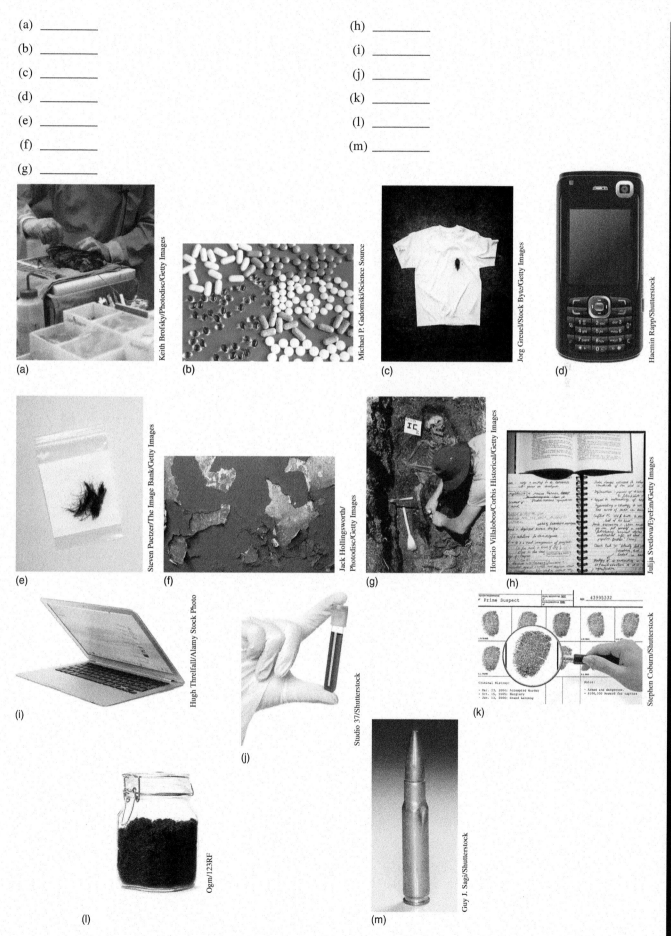

Keith Brofsky/Photodisc/Getty Images

(a)

Michael P. Gadomski/Science Source

(b)

Jorg Greuel/Stock Byte/Getty Images

(c)

Haemin Rapp/Shutterstock

(d)

Steven Puetzer/The Image Bank/Getty Images

(e)

Jack Hollingsworth/Photodisc/Getty Images

(f)

Horacio Villalobos/Corbis Historical/Getty Images

(g)

Julija Svetlova/EyeEm/Getty Images

(h)

Hugh Threlfall/Alamy Stock Photo

(i)

Studio 37/Shutterstock

(j)

Stephen Coburn/Shutterstock

(k)

Ogm/123RF

(l)

Guy J. Sagi/Shutterstock

(m)

Further References

A Simplified Guide to Forensic Science, http://www.forensicsciencesimplified.org/

Cohen, Stanley A., "The Role of the Forensic Expert in a Criminal Trial," *Canadian Society of Forensic Science Journal* 12 (1979): 75.

Doyle, Sir Arthur Conan, *The Complete Sherlock Holmes,* vol. 1. New York: Doubleday, 1956.

Kagan, J. D., "On Being a Good Expert Witness in a Criminal Case," *Journal of Forensic Sciences* 23 (1978): 190.

Lucas, D. M., "North of 49—The Development of Forensic Science in Canada," *Science & Justice* 37 (1997): 47.

National Research Council, *Strengthening Forensic Science in the United States: A Path Forward,* Washington, D.C.: National Academies Press, 2009, http://books.nap.edu/openbook.php?record_id=12589&page=R1

Sandercock, P. Mark L., "75 Years of Forensic Chemistry in the Royal Canadian Mounted Police. A Timeline for Trace Evidence, 1937–2012," *Canadian Society of Forensic Science Journal* 46 (2013): 120.

Sapir, Gil I., "Legal Aspects of Forensic Science," in R. Saferstein, ed., *Forensic Science Handbook,* vol. 1, 2nd ed. Upper Saddle River, N J: Prentice Hall, 2002.

Shelton, D. E., "The CSI Effect: Does It Really Exist?" http://www.nij.gov/journals/259/csi-effect.htm

Waggoner, Kim, "The FBI Laboratory: 75 Years of Forensic Science Service," *Forensic Science Communications* 9, no. 4 (2007). https://www2.fbi.gov/hq/lab/fsc/backissu/oct2007/index.htm

The Crime Scene

Learning Objectives

After studying this chapter, you should be able to:

2.1 Describe the various measures taken while securing, recording, and searching the crime scene

2.2 Describe proper techniques for packaging common types of physical evidence

2.3 Explain the concept of chain of custody

2.4 Relate what steps are typically required to maintain appropriate health and safety standards at the crime scene

2.5 Understand the implications of relevant U.S. Supreme Court decisions in conducting a crime scene investigation

Go to www.pearsonhighered.com/careersresources to access Webextras for this chapter.

Amanda Knox: A Flawed Case of Murder

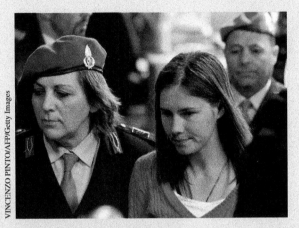

VINCENZO PINTO/AFP/Getty Images

In September 2007, Amanda Knox moved to Perugia, Italy, as a foreign exchange student. Knox shared an upstairs flat in a cottage with Meredith Kercher and two other women. Within weeks of her arrival, Knox became romantically linked to an Italian student, Raffaele Sollecito, and began spending nights at his home.

On November 1, Kercher was brutally murdered. Early that afternoon, Kercher's naked body was found inside her bedroom covered by a bedspread soaked in blood and with stab wounds to her throat. The prosecution charged Knox and Sollecito with murder and sexual assault. The case became an international media sensation, and Knox was vilified in the British and Italian news media in what some called the European "trial of the century." Knox was convicted of slander, sexual violence, and murder and sentenced to 26 years in prison. Four years later, her conviction was set aside by the Italian Supreme Court and a new trial was ordered.

The prosecution's case in the original trial focused on two key pieces of evidence; a bra clasp and a kitchen knife. The knife, found in Sollecito's kitchen purported to have Kercher's DNA on the blade and Knox's DNA on the handle. The bra, allegedly belonging to Kercher, was reported to have Knox's DNA on the clasp. Defense experts hired during the appeal process to examine the evidence questioned the protocols of the DNA lab as well as the crime scene personnel. After a review of photos and videos taken from the crime scene, it was determined that there were major failures by Italian authorities to properly control, document, and preserve evidence at the scene. For example, the bra wasn't even collected during the first search of the crime scene, but rather 40 days after the initial examination took place. In 2015, Italy's Supreme Court of Cassation, citing concerns about possible contamination of evidence, definitively exonerated Knox and Sollecito. After a review of the evidence, the court noted "stunning flaws in the investigation and increased media attention" and concluded there were no "biological traces" that connected Knox and Sollecito to the slaying.

A third suspect, Rudy Guede, whose fingerprints were found in Kercher's bedroom and whose DNA was found on and inside Kercher's body, was convicted of the murder and remains in an Italian jail until he serves out the remainder of his sentence.

Processing the Crime Scene

As automobiles run on gasoline, crime laboratories "run" on **physical evidence**. Physical evidence encompasses any and all objects that can establish that a crime has or has not been committed or can link a crime and its victim or its perpetrator. But if physical evidence is to be used effectively to aid the investigator, its presence first must be recognized at the crime scene. If all the natural and commercial objects within a reasonable distance of a crime were gathered so that the scientist could uncover significant clues from them, the deluge of material would quickly immobilize the laboratory facility. Physical evidence can achieve its optimum value in criminal investigations only when its collection is performed with a selectivity governed by the collector's thorough knowledge of the crime laboratory's techniques, capabilities, and limitations.

physical evidence
Any object that can establish that a crime has or has not been committed or can link a crime and its victim or its perpetrator.

Forthcoming chapters will be devoted to discussions of methods and techniques available to forensic scientists to evaluate physical evidence. Although current technology has given the crime laboratory capabilities far exceeding those of past decades, these advances are no excuse for complacency on the part of criminal investigators. Crime laboratories do not solve crimes; only a thorough and competent investigation conducted by professional police officers will enhance the chances for a successful criminal investigation. Forensic science is, and will continue to be, an important element of the total investigative process, but it is only one aspect of an endeavor that must be a team effort. The investigator who believes the crime laboratory to be a panacea for laxity or ineptness is in for a rude awakening.

Forensic science begins at the crime scene. If the investigator cannot recognize physical evidence or cannot properly preserve it for laboratory examination, no amount of sophisticated laboratory instrumentation or technical expertise can salvage the situation. The know-how for conducting a proper crime-scene search for physical evidence is within the grasp of any police department, regardless of its size. With proper training, police agencies can ensure competent performance at crime scenes. In many jurisdictions, police agencies have delegated this task to a specialized team of technicians. However, the techniques of crime-scene investigation are not difficult to master and certainly lie within the bounds of comprehension of the average police officer.

Not all crime scenes require retrieval of physical evidence, and limited resources and personnel have forced many police agencies to restrict their efforts in this area to crimes of a more serious nature. Once the commitment is made to completely process a crime site for physical evidence, however, certain fundamental practices must be followed.

Securing and Isolating the Crime Scene

The first officer arriving on the scene of a crime is responsible for preserving and protecting the area as much as possible. The officer should not let their guard down and must rely on their training to deal with any violent or hazardous circumstances. Special note should be taken of any vehicles or people leaving the scene.

Of course, first priority should be given to obtaining medical assistance for individuals in need of it and to arresting the perpetrator. However, as soon as possible, extensive efforts must be made to exclude all unauthorized personnel from the scene. If medical assistance is needed, the officer should direct medical workers to approach the body by an indirect route to minimize the possibility of disturbing evidence. The first responding officer must evaluate the victim's condition and record any statements made by the victim. This information should later be included in notes.

As additional officers arrive, measures are immediately initiated to isolate the area (see Figure 2–1). The boundaries should encompass the center of the scene where the crime occurred, any paths of entry or exit, and any areas where evidence may have been discarded or moved. Ropes or barricades along with strategic positioning of guards will prevent unauthorized access to the area. Efforts must be taken to identify all individuals at the scene and detain all potential suspects or witnesses still at the scene. At the same time, officers should exclude all unauthorized personnel from the scene. This includes family and friends of the victim, who should be shown as much compassion as possible. Only investigative personnel assigned to the scene should be admitted. The responding officers must keep an accurate log of who enters and exits the scene and the time at which they do so.

Sometimes the exclusion of unauthorized personnel proves more difficult than expected. Violent crimes are especially susceptible to attention from higher-level police officials and

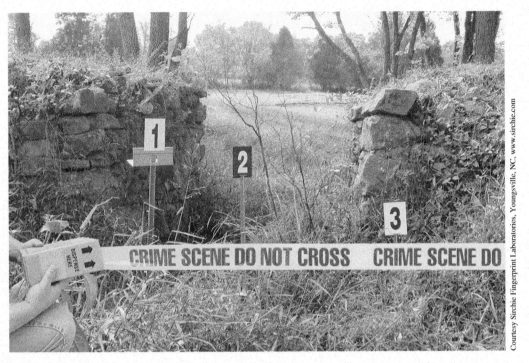

Courtesy Sirchie Fingerprint Laboratories, Youngsville, NC, www.sirchie.com

FIGURE 2–1

The first investigators to arrive must secure the crime scene and establish the crime-scene perimeter.

members of the press, as well as by emotionally charged neighbors and curiosity seekers. Every individual who enters the scene is a potential destroyer of physical evidence, even if it is by unintentional carelessness. To exercise proper control over the crime scene, the officer responsible for protecting it must have the authority to exclude everyone, including fellow police officers not directly involved in processing the site or in conducting the investigation. Seasoned criminal investigators are always prepared to relate horror stories about crime scenes where physical evidence was rendered totally valueless by hordes of people who, for one reason or another, trampled through the site. Securing and isolating the crime scene are critical steps in an investigation, the accomplishment of which is the mark of a trained and professional crime-scene investigative team.

Once the scene has been secured, a lead investigator starts evaluating the area. First, the investigator determines the boundaries of the scene and then establishes the perpetrator's path of entry and exit. Logic dictates that obvious items of crime-scene evidence will first come to the attention of the crime-scene investigator. These items must be documented and photographed. The investigator then proceeds with an initial walk-through of the scene to gain an overview of the situation and develop a strategy for systematically examining and documenting the entire crime scene.

Racial tensions in Ferguson, Baltimore, Cleveland, and Staten Island have pushed the issue of police body cameras to the national forefront. A tiny clip-on camera that can be snapped onto a uniform or glasses and monitor in real-time initial efforts at securing the crime scene seems to be a reasonable tool that can be issued to first responders. However, at this point in time, adoption of this tool is fraught with serious concerns. In general law, enforcement has not universally accepted the technology nor implemented protocols governing the deployment of body-worn cameras (BWCs). Aside from the cost of the equipment, one of the primary concerns revolves around data storage and management. BWCs produce an enormous amount of video data that must be properly and securely stored. In any case, the adoption of a BWC will not replace traditional digital and video cameras at crime scenes.

Personnel should never do anything while at the crime scene—including smoking, eating, drinking, and littering—that may alter the scene. No aspects of the scene, including a body at a death scene, should be moved or disturbed unless they pose a serious threat to investigating officers or bystanders. This means that no one should open or close faucets or flush toilets at the scene. Also, officers should avoid altering temperature conditions at the scene by adjusting windows, doors, or the heating or air conditioning.

Recording the Crime Scene

Investigators have only a limited amount of time to work a crime site in its untouched state. The opportunity to permanently record the scene in its original state must not be lost. Such records not only will prove useful during the subsequent investigation but also are required for presentation at a trial in order to document the condition of the crime site and to delineate the location of physical evidence. Notes, photography, and sketches are the three methods for crime-scene recording (see Figure 2–2). Ideally all three should be employed; however, personnel and monetary limitations often prohibit the use of photography at every crime site. Under these circumstances, departmental guidelines will establish priorities for deploying photographic resources. However, there is no reason not to make sketches and notes at the crime scene.

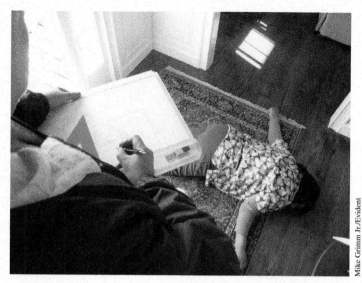

FIGURE 2–2

Sketching a victim at the crime scene to show the victim's relation to the crime scene.

NOTES   Note-taking begins with the call to a crime-scene investigator to report to a scene. The notes should start by identifying the person who contacted the investigator, the time of the contact, and any preliminary information disclosed, including the case number. When the lead investigator arrives, the notetaker should record the date and time of arrival, who is present, and the identities of any other personnel who are being contacted. If additional personnel are contacted, their names, titles, and time of arrival should be recorded. Investigators must keep a precise record of personnel movements in and out of the scene, beginning with an interview of the first responding officer in order to record their movements. It is also important to record the tasks assigned to each member of a team, as well as the beginning and ending times for the processing of the scene.

Before the scene is sketched, photographed, or searched, the lead investigator carries out the initial walk-through. During this walk-through, the investigator should take notes on many aspects of the crime scene in its original condition. These notes should be uniform in layout for all cases. The notes should be in ink (preferably black or blue) and written in a bound notebook. Most important, notes should be written at the time of the crime-scene investigation, not left to memory to record later.

Once a search for evidence has taken place, the team members mark the location of all evidence and fully describe each item in their notes. If a victim is present at a homicide scene, the investigator should observe and record the state of the body before the medical examiner or coroner moves it. Any preliminary identification of a victim or suspect should be recorded.

Audio-recording notes at a scene can be advantageous because detailed notes can be spoken much faster than they can be written. This may also leave hands free to carry out other tasks while recording the notes. Some investigators may use digital voice recorders to record their notes. These recordings are easily uploaded to a computer, but they must be copied to a disk to produce a hard copy. Another method of recording notes is by narrating a video of the crime scene. This has the advantage of combining note-taking with photography. However, at some point the video must be transcribed into a written document.

Finally, it may also be helpful to employ a crime scene checklist that can be filled out during the documentation process. Crime scene work can be chaotic, and it can be easy to miss a step. Creation of a detailed crime scene checklist can ensure that all necessary and important information is observed and collected. Checklists can be crafted which contain general information that should be collected for every type of scene, and also specific information that may be unique to certain scene types (burglaries, scenes involving motor vehicle crashes, etc.). An example of a general crime scene check list is described in Appendix III.

PHOTOGRAPHY   The most important prerequisite for photographing a crime scene is for it to be unaltered. Unless injured people are involved, objects must not be moved until they have been photographed from all necessary angles. If objects are removed, positions changed, or items

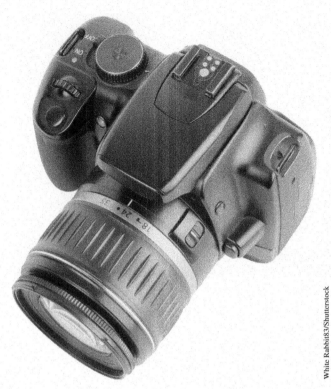

White Rabbit83/Shutterstock

FIGURE 2–3

An example of a digital single lens reflex (DSLR) camera.

added, the photographs may not be admissible as evidence at a trial, and their intended value will be lost. If evidence has been moved or removed before photography, the fact should be noted in the report, but the evidence should not be reintroduced into the scene in order to take photographs.

Crime-scene photographs have great value in their ability to show the layout of the scene, the position of evidence to be collected, and the relation of objects at the scene to one another. Photographs taken from many angles can show possible lines of sight of victims, suspects, or witnesses. An accurate description of the scene must be available to investigators for future analysis. Photography is also important for documenting biological evidence in its original condition, as this kind of evidence is often altered during testing. Photographs cannot stand alone, however, and they are complementary to notes and sketches.

Crime-scene investigators use a digital camera, such as the digital single-lens reflex camera shown in Figure 2–3, to document crime scenes, and digital photography is rapidly becoming the method of choice in the field of forensic science. A digital photograph is made when a light-sensitive microchip inside a digital camera is exposed to light coming from an object or scene. A digital camera captures light on each of millions of tiny picture elements called pixels. The light is recorded on each pixel as a specific electric charge using a charged coupled device (CCD) or complementary metal oxide semiconductor (CMOS). The camera reads this charge number as image information, then stores the image as a file on a memory card.

The number of pixels used to capture light is directly related to the resolution of the picture. Resolution is defined as the minimum distance that must separate two objects in order for them to be viewed as distinct objects. The lower the distance needed, the greater the resolution of the photograph. Photographs of increasingly higher resolution show more and more detail and sharpness. The greater the number of pixels featured on the digital camera, the better the resolution will be.

Because the number of pixels on a digital camera is in the millions, it is usually referred to in terms of *megapixels*. A camera that has four million pixels is a four-megapixel camera. A standard four-megapixel camera can create a clear image on a photographic print of up to 8 by 10 inches. As the number of megapixels increases, the clarity increases, allowing photographers to create bigger prints. Crime-scene photographers usually use cameras that feature as many as 12 megapixels or more.

The nature of digital images, however, opens digital photography to important criticisms within forensic science casework. Because the photographs are digital, they can be easily manipulated by using computer software. This manipulation goes beyond traditional photograph enhancement such as adjusting brightness and contrast or color balancing. Because the main function of crime-scene photography is to provide an accurate depiction, this is a major concern. To ensure that their digital images are admissible, many jurisdictions set guidelines for determining the circumstances under which digital photography may be used and establish and enforce strict protocols for image security and chain of custody.

Photographic Procedures Each crime scene should be photographed as completely as possible. This means that the crime scene should include the area in which the crime took place and all adjacent areas where important acts occurred immediately before or after the commission of the crime. Overview photographs of the entire scene and surrounding area, including points of exit and entry, must be taken from various angles. If the crime took place indoors, the entire room should be photographed to show each wall area. Rooms adjacent to the actual crime site must be similarly photographed. If the crime scene includes a body, photographs must be taken to show the body's position and location relative to the entire scene. Close-up photos depicting injuries and weapons lying near the body are also necessary (see Figure 2–4). After the body is removed from the scene, the surface beneath the body should be photographed.

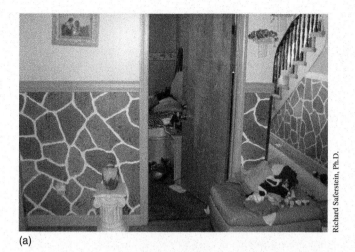

(a)

Richard Saferstein, Ph.D.

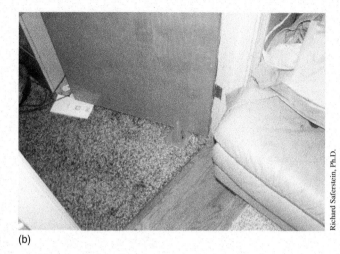

(b)

Richard Saferstein, Ph.D.

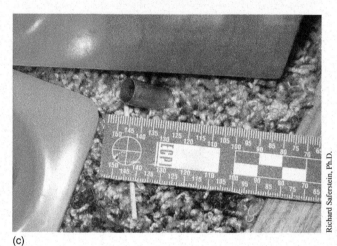

(c)

Richard Saferstein, Ph.D.

FIGURE 2–4
This sequence of crime-scene photographs shows the proper progression of photographing the scene. (a) The sequence begins with an overview photograph of the entry to the victim's bedroom showing evidence markers in place. (b) The medium-range photograph shows the evidence marker next to the door denoting a cartridge case. (c) The close-up photograph shows the cartridge in detail with a scale in the photograph.

As items of physical evidence are discovered, they are photographed to show their position and location relative to the entire scene. After these overviews are taken, close-ups should be taken to record the details of the object itself. When the size of an item is significant, a ruler or other measuring scale may be inserted near the object and included in the photograph as a point of reference. At a minimum, four photographs are required at a crime scene: an overview photograph, a medium-range photograph, a close-up photograph, and a close-up photograph with a scale. These photographs create an adequate visual record of the position and appearance of an item of evidence at a crime scene.

The digital revolution promises to bring enhanced photographic capabilities to the crime scene. For example, individual images of the crime scene captured with a digital camera can be stitched together electronically to reveal a nearly 3-D panoramic view of the crime scene (see Figure 2–5). With the advent of drone technology, aerial photography is assisting in the investigation of many crime scenes.

The digital era promises new and elegant approaches to document the crime scene. Cameras such as that shown in Figure 2–6 are capable of taking dozens of digital images while scanning the crime scene. Photographic and laser data from multiple scan locations are combined to produce 3-D models of the scene in full color that can be viewed from any vantage point, measured, and used for analysis and courtroom presentations.

Video Recording   The use of digital video at crime scenes is becoming increasingly popular because the cost of this equipment is decreasing. The same principles used in crime-scene photographs apply to digital video. As with conventional photography, digital video should include the entire scene and the immediate surrounding area. Long shots as well as close-ups should be taken in a slow and systematic manner. Furthermore, it is desirable to have one crime-scene investigator narrate the events and scenes being recorded while another does the shooting.

WEBEXTRA 2.1
Three-Dimensional Crime-Scene Imaging I

WEBEXTRA 2.2
Three-Dimensional Crime-Scene Imaging II

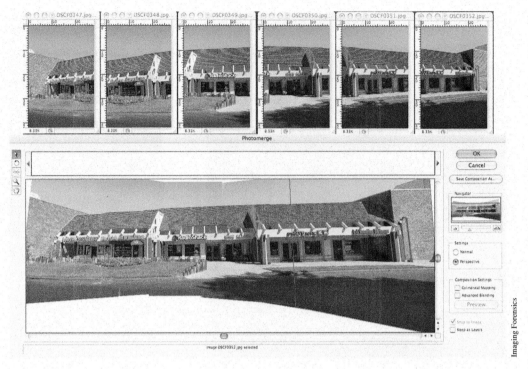

Imaging Forensics

FIGURE 2–5

Individual images (top) are shown before being electronically stitched together into a single panoramic image (bottom). Individual photographs should be taken with about a 30 percent overlap.

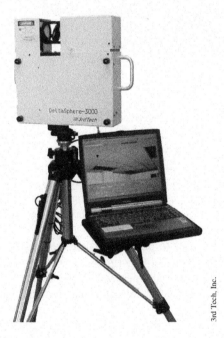

3rd Tech, Inc.

FIGURE 2–6

A computer-controlled scanner has both a high-resolution, professional digital camera and a long-range laser rangefinder. The tripod-mounted device rotates a full 360 degrees, taking dozens of photographs and measuring millions of individual points. Photographic and laser data from multiple scan locations are combined to produce 3D models of the scene.

However, there are some disadvantages to videos of crime scenes. First, although some cameras have a stabilization feature, most cameras will inevitably shake during filming. Also, zooming and panning can be sloppy; these techniques should be used only occasionally and should be done very slowly. Extra noise due to wind or other investigators talking can obscure narration or may be inappropriate and damaging. Because of the "on the spot" nature of the narration, investigators may stumble over words, which can be confusing when a video is used in court. To avoid this, some investigators record the video with the sound off and dub notes over it later.

Still images taken from videotape are usually of much poorer quality than those taken by a digital camera. Although video can capture the sounds and scenes of the crime site with relative ease, the technique cannot be used in place of still photography at this time. The still photograph remains unsurpassed in defining details for the human eye. Digital video can have advantages over still photography in certain situations. For example, modern video cameras allow the user to play back recordings of a scene and check it for completeness. In addition, many video cameras can also take still photographs, or stills can be created from the disc on a computer. Video essentially combines notes and photography.

Body-Worn Cameras Relations between police and the community have been disrupted in recent years due to a media and social movement decrying the actions of police officers during criminal investigations. Many claims have been made that police use excessive force and fail to follow proper procedure for evidence collection and processing. Cases with conflicting eyewitness accounts, like those of Michael Brown (see Figure 2-7) in Ferguson, MO, and Freddy Gray in Baltimore, MD, prompted calls for police to be outfitted with Body Worn Cameras (BWCs). After protests unfolded all over the country, President Barack Obama requested federal aid in support of new police training initiatives and BWCs to make this technology more accessible to police departments. In the last few years, there has been a dramatic increase in the use of BWCs by law enforcement personnel across the nation. There is hope this technology will increase the legitimacy and the accountability of both law enforcement and the public (Figure 2-8).

BWCs are cameras with at least one microphone and internal data storage, which allow audio/video footage to be stored and analyzed with compatible software (Figure 2-9). In recent years, technological strides have made BWCs a reality for police agencies across the United States. Every police officer within a department can be outfitted with a small camera that is lightweight and easy to operate. Training is both quick and efficient, and the portable cameras can be activated/deactivated with the press of a single button.

As police agencies begin implementing BWC programs, variation is expected in the procedures and protocols for each department. This variation is due to the different technology available and diverse companies that produce the hardware. Every department will develop its own set of policies and regulations that govern the activation and inactivation of the cameras, prohibited uses, retention and confidentiality of data recordings.

BWCs are an efficient tool for collecting evidence and recording crime scenes. When an officer reports to a chaotic scene, documentation may or may not be the priority. Scene security and assisting with medical care for victims demand immediate attention over documenting every intricate piece of evidence. During the initial phases, evidence could be moved or destroyed. A great attribute of BWCs is that they will record and document the timeline of the scene for the officer as he performs other tasks. Evidence collection can often be a very tedious and daunting task for crime-scene technicians and officers alike. Many crime-scene locations can contain hundreds of pieces of individual evidence

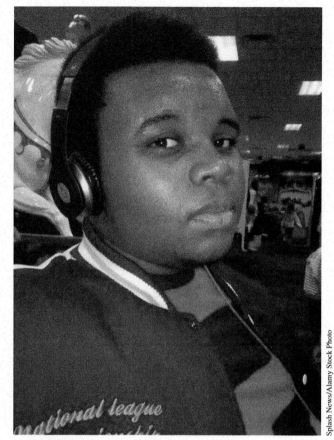

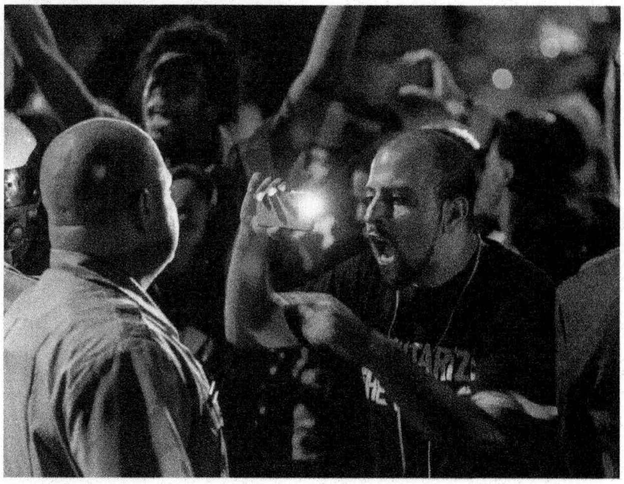

FIGURE 2-7

Michael Brown was shot and killed by Ferguson Police Officer Darren Wilson on August 9, 2014. The case brought national attention to the use of body-worn cameras by law enforcement.

Splash News/Alamy Stock Photo

FIGURE 2-8

Demonstrator Bassem Masri confronts a St. Louis police officer following an incident in which a white off-duty policeman shot and killed a black teenager in St. Louis on October 8, 2014.

Kenny Bahr/Reuters

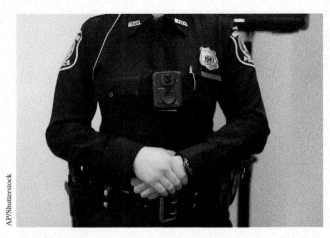

FIGURE 2-9
Example of a body-worn camera affixed to the uniform of a police officer.

rough sketch
A draft representation of all essential information and measurements at a crime scene. This sketch is drawn at the crime scene.

that needs to be documented, processed, and collected. BWCs can serve as focal point for recreating the exact dynamics of a crime scene just as it was found. When reviewing footage of an officer collecting evidence, the location of different objects can be determined by the relation of other objects in proximity to each other. BWCs can also prove in a court of law that evidence was collected properly and not tampered with by the processing officer. This can be an invaluable tool when defense attorneys attempt to discredit evidence by calling the collection or processing into question.

SKETCHES   Once photographs have been taken, the crime-scene investigator sketches the scene. The sketch serves many important functions in the legal investigation of a crime. If done correctly, a sketch can clearly show the layout of an indoor or outdoor crime scene and the relationship in space of all the items and features significant to the investigation. Sketches are especially important to illustrate the location of collected evidence. Possible paths of entry, exit, and movement through the scene may be speculated from a good sketch.

The investigator may have neither the skill nor the time to make a polished sketch of the scene. However, this is not required during the early phase of the investigation. What is necessary is a **rough sketch** containing an accurate depiction of the dimensions of the scene and showing the location of all objects having a bearing on the case. This may be achieved through the use of a sketching kit like the one shown in Figure 2–10.

A rough sketch is illustrated in Figure 2–11. It shows all recovered items of physical evidence as well as other important features of the crime scene. Objects are located in the sketch by distance measurements from two fixed points, such as the walls of a room. Distances shown on the sketch must be accurate and not the result of a guess or estimate. For this reason, all

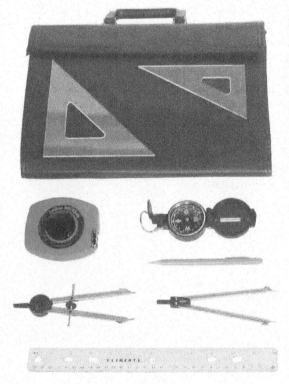
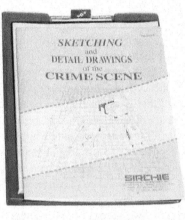
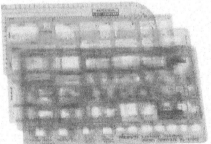

FIGURE 2-10
A basic kit for sketching the crime scene.

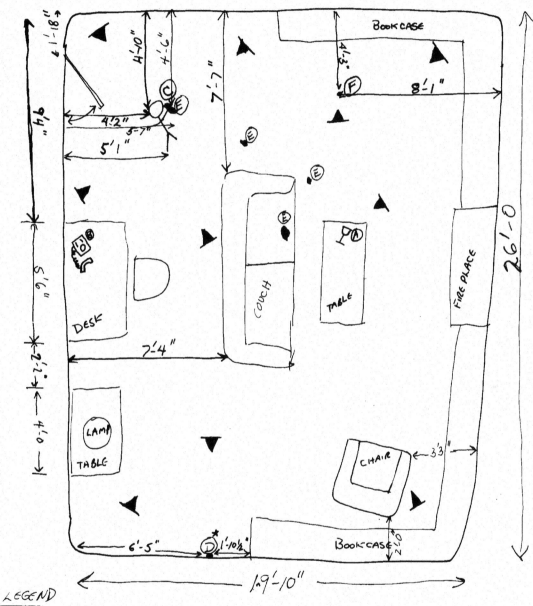

CASE 10-789-96
301 N. CENTRE ST.
OCT. 6, 1996   11:40 PM
HOMICIDE

VICTIM: LESTER W. BROWN
INVESTIGATOR: SGT. LA. DUFFY
ASS'T BY : PTLM. R.W. HICKS

BOOKCASE
BOOKCASE
DESK
LAMP
TABLE
COUCH
TABLE
FIRE PLACE
CHAIR

LEGEND
A = COCKTAIL GLASS
B = TELEPHONE
C = VICTIM
D = BULLET HOLE
E = BLOOD STAINS
F = SHELL CASING
▲ = CAMERA LOCATIONS

1/4" = 1 FOOT

* D 3'-4¾" FROM FLOOR

FIGURE 2–11
Rough-sketch diagram of a crime scene.

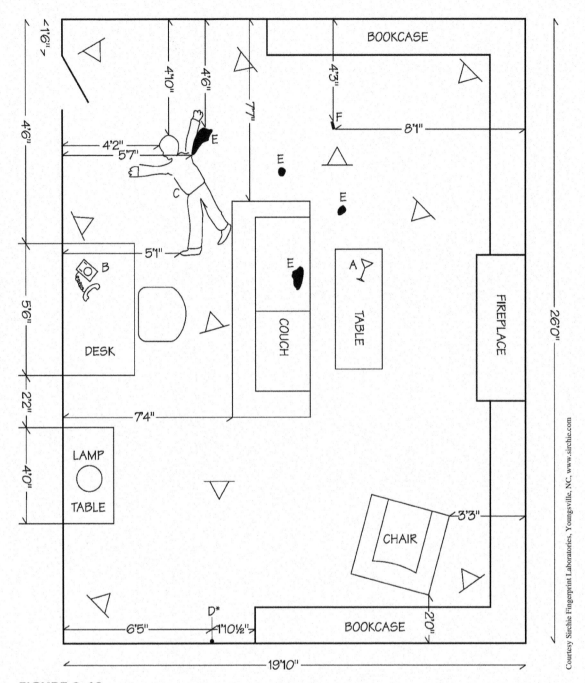

FIGURE 2–12

Finished-sketch diagram of a crime scene.

measurements are made with a tape measure. The simplest way to designate an item in a sketch is to assign it a number or letter. A legend or list placed below the sketch then correlates the letter to the item's description. The sketch should also show a compass heading designating north as well as a title block designating the location of the crime scene and any case information.

Unlike the rough sketch, the **finished sketch** in Figure 2–12 is constructed with care and concern for aesthetic appearance. When the finished sketch is completed, it must reflect information contained within the rough sketch in order to be admissible evidence in a courtroom. Computer-aided drafting (CAD) has become the norm to reconstruct crime scenes from rough sketches. The software, ranging from simple, low-cost programs to complex, expensive programs, contains predrawn intersections and roadways or buildings and rooms onto which information can be entered (see Figure 2–13). A generous symbol library provides the operator with a variety of images that can be used to add intricate details such as blood spatters to a crime-scene

finished sketch

A precise rendering of the crime scene, usually drawn to scale.

Courtesy Sirchie Fingerprint Laboratories, Youngsville, NC, www.sirchie.com

sketch. Equipped with a zoom function, computerized sketching can focus on a specific area for a more detailed picture. CAD programs allow the operator to select scale size so that the ultimate product can be produced in a size suitable for courtroom presentation.

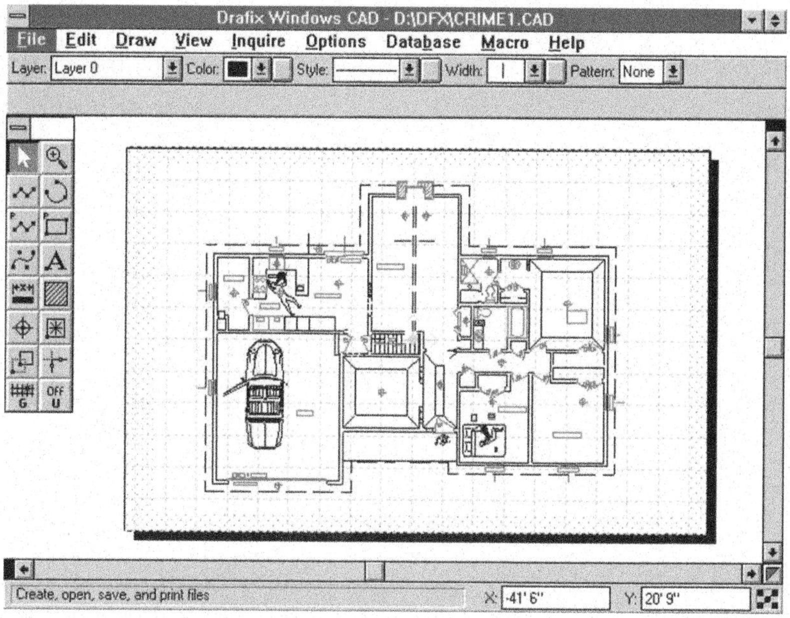

Conducting a Systematic Search for Evidence

The search for physical evidence at a crime scene must be thorough and systematic. For a factual, unbiased reconstruction of the crime, investigators, relying on their training and experience, must not overlook any pertinent evidence. Even when suspects are immediately seized and the motives and circumstances of the crime are readily apparent, a thorough search for physical evidence must be conducted at once. Failure in this, even though it may seem unnecessary, can lead to accusations of negligence or charges that the investigative agency knowingly "covered up" evidence that would be detrimental to its case.

Assigning those responsible for searching a crime scene is a function of the investigator in charge. Except in major crimes, or when the evidence is complex, the assistance forensic scientists at the crime scene is usually not necessary; their role appropriately begins when evidence is submitted to the crime laboratory. As has already been observed, some police agencies have trained field evidence technicians to search for physical evidence at the crime scene. They have the equipment and skill to photograph the scene and examine it for the presence of fingerprints, footprints, tool marks, or any other type of evidence that may be relevant to the crime.

FIGURE 2–13

Construction of a crime-scene diagram with the aid of a computer-aided drafting program.

Courtesy Sirchie Fingerprint Laboratories, Youngsville, NC, www.sirchie.com

SEARCH PATTERNS How one conducts a crime-scene search will depend on the locale and size of the area, as well as on the actions of the suspect(s) and victim(s) at the scene. When possible, one person should supervise and coordinate the collection of evidence. Without proper control, the search may be conducted in an atmosphere of confusion with needless duplication of effort. The various search patterns that may be used can be observed in Figure 2–14.

Strip or Line Search Pattern In the line or strip method, one or two investigators start at the boundary at one end of the scene and walk straight across to the other side. They then move a little farther along the border and walk straight back to the other side. This method is best used in scenes where the boundaries are well established because the boundaries dictate the beginning and end of the search lines. If the boundary is incorrectly chosen, important evidence may remain undiscovered outside the search area.

Grid Search Pattern The grid method employs two people performing line searches that originate from adjacent corners and form perpendicular lines. This method is very thorough, but the boundaries must be well established in order to use this method as well.

Spiral Search Pattern The spiral search pattern usually employs one person. The investigator moves either in an inward spiral from the boundary to the center of the scene or in an outward spiral from the center to the boundary. The inward spiral method is helpful because the searcher is moving from an area light with evidence to an area where more evidence will most likely be found. With either spiral approach the searcher can easily locate footprints leading away from the scene in any direction. However, completing a perfect spiral is often difficult, and evidence could be missed.

Wheel or Ray Search Pattern The wheel or ray method employs several people moving from the boundary straight toward the center of the scene (inward) or from the center straight to the boundary (outward). This method is not preferred because the areas between the "rays" are not searched.

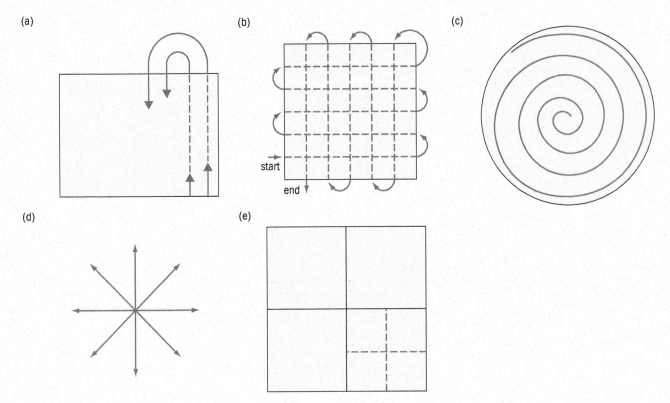

FIGURE 2–14

(a) Strip or line search pattern. (b) Grid search pattern. (c) Spiral search pattern. (d) Wheel or ray search pattern. (e) Quadrant or zone search pattern.

Quadrant or Zone Search Pattern   The quadrant or zone method divides the scene into zones or quadrants, and team members are assigned to search each section. Each of these sections can be subdivided into smaller sections for smaller teams to search thoroughly. This method is best suited for scenes that cover a large area. The areas searched must include all probable points of entry and exit used by the people who committed the crime.

LOCATING PHYSICAL EVIDENCE   What to search for will be determined by the particular circumstances of the crime. Obviously, the skill of crime-scene investigators at recognizing evidence and searching relevant locations is paramount to successful processing of the crime scene. Although training will impart general knowledge for conducting a proper crime-scene investigation, ultimately the investigator must rely on experience gained from numerous investigations to form a successful strategy for recovering relevant physical evidence.

For example, in a homicide case, the search will center on the weapon and any evidence left as a result of contact between the victim and the assailant. The cross-transfer of evidence, such as hairs, fibers, and blood, between individuals involved in the crime is particularly useful for linking suspects to the crime scene and for corroborating events that transpired during the commission of the crime. During the investigation of a burglary, efforts will be made to locate tool marks at the point of entry. In most crimes, a thorough and systematic search for latent fingerprints is required.

Vehicle searches must be carefully planned and systematically carried out. The nature of the case determines how detailed the search must be. In hit-and-run cases, the outside and undercarriage of the car must be examined with care. Particular attention is paid to looking for any evidence resulting from a cross-transfer of evidence between the car and the victim—this includes blood, tissue, hair, fibers, and fabric impressions. Traces of paint or broken glass may be located on the victim. In cases of homicide, burglary, kidnapping, and so on, all areas of the vehicle, inside and outside, are searched with equal care for physical evidence.

Collecting and Packaging Physical Evidence

Physical evidence can be anything from massive objects to microscopic traces. Often, many items of evidence are obvious in their presence, but others may be detected only through examination in the crime laboratory. For example, minute traces of blood may be discovered on garments only after a thorough search in the laboratory, or the presence of hairs and fibers may be revealed in vacuum sweepings or on garments only after close laboratory scrutiny. For this reason, it is important to collect possible carriers of trace evidence in addition to more discernible items. Hence, it may be necessary to take custody of all clothing worn by the participants in a crime.

COLLECTING PHYSICAL EVIDENCE   Each clothing item should be handled carefully and wrapped separately to avoid loss of trace materials. Critical areas of the crime scene should be vacuumed and the sweepings submitted to the laboratory for analysis. The sweepings from different areas must be collected and packaged separately. A portable vacuum cleaner equipped with a special filter attachment is suitable for this purpose (see Figure 2–15). Additionally, fingernail scrapings from individuals who were in contact with other individuals may contain minute fragments of evidence capable of linking the assailant and victim. The undersurface of each nail is best scraped with a dull object such as a toothpick to avoid cutting the skin. These scrapings will be subjected to microscopic examination in the laboratory.

The search for physical evidence must extend beyond the crime scene to the autopsy room of a deceased victim. Here, the medical examiner or coroner carefully examines the victim to establish a cause and manner of death. Tissues and organs are routinely retained for pathological and toxicological examination. At the same time, arrangements must be made between the examiner and investigator to secure a variety of items that may be obtainable from the body for laboratory examination (see p. 106).

In recent years, many police departments have gone to the expense of purchasing and equipping "mobile crime laboratories" (see Figure 2–16) for their evidence technicians. However, the term *mobile crime laboratory* is a misnomer. These vehicles carry the necessary supplies to protect the crime scene; photograph, collect, and package physical evidence; and perform latent print development. They are not designed to carry out the functions of a chemical laboratory. *Crime-scene search vehicle* would be a more appropriate but perhaps less dramatic name for such a vehicle.

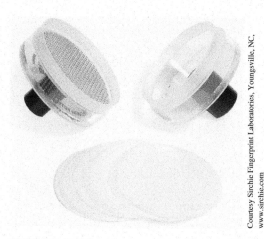
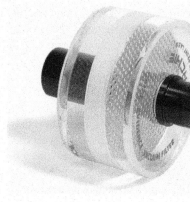

Courtesy Sirchie Fingerprint Laboratories, Youngsville, NC, www.sirchie.com

Courtesy Sirchie Fingerprint Laboratories, Youngsville, NC, www.sirchie.com

FIGURE 2–15

Vacuum sweeper attachment, constructed of clear plastic in two pieces that are joined by a threaded joint. A metal screen is mounted in one half to support a filter paper to collect debris. The unit attaches to the hose of the vacuum sweeper. After a designated area of the crime scene is vacuumed, the filter paper is removed and retained for laboratory examination.

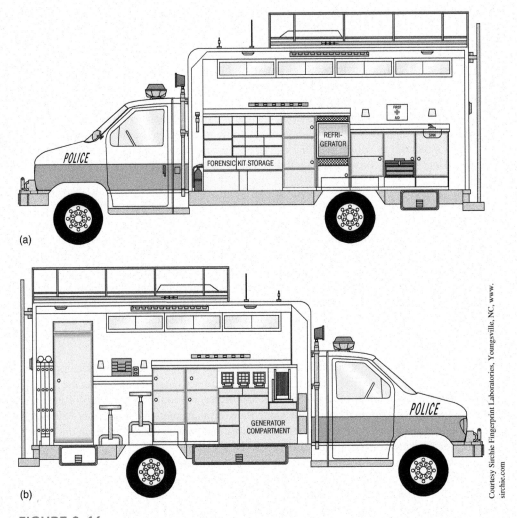

(a)

(b)

FIGURE 2–16

Inside view of a mobile crime-scene van: (a) driver's side and (b) passenger's side.

HANDLING EVIDENCE   Investigators must handle and process physical evidence in a way that prevents any change from taking place between the time the evidence is removed from the crime scene and the time it is received by the crime laboratory. Changes can arise through contamination, breakage, evaporation, accidental scratching or bending, or improper or careless packaging. The use of latex gloves or disposable forceps when touching evidence often can prevent such problems. Any equipment that is not disposable should be cleaned and/or sanitized between collecting each piece of evidence. Evidence should remain unmoved until investigators have documented its location and appearance in notes, sketches, and photographs.

Evidence best maintains its integrity when kept in its original condition as found at the crime site. Whenever possible, investigators should submit evidence to the laboratory intact. Investigators normally should not remove blood, hairs, fibers, soil particles, and other types of trace evidence from garments, weapons, or other articles that bear them. Instead, they should send the entire object to the laboratory for processing.

Of course, if evidence is adhering to an object in a precarious manner, good judgment dictates removing and packaging the item. Use common sense when handling evidence adhering to a large structure, such as a door, wall, or floor; remove the specimen with a forceps or other appropriate tool. In the case of a bloodstain, one may either scrape the stain off the surface, transfer the stain to a moistened swab, or cut out the area of the object bearing the stain.

PACKAGING EVIDENCE   The well-prepared evidence collector arrives at a crime scene with a large assortment of packaging materials and tools, ready to encounter any type of situation. Forceps and similar tools may be used to pick up small items. Unbreakable plastic pill bottles with

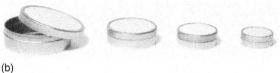

(a)

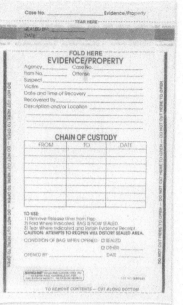

(b)

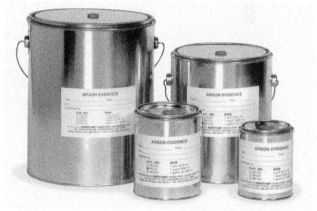

(c)

FIGURE 2–17

(a) Manila evidence envelope. (b) Metal pillboxes. (c) Sealable plastic evidence bag.

pressure lids are excellent containers for hairs, glass, fibers, and various other kinds of small or trace evidence. Alternatively, manila envelopes, screw-cap glass vials, sealable plastic bags, or metal pillboxes are adequate containers for most trace evidence encountered at crime sites (see Figure 2–17). Charred debris recovered from the scene of a suspicious fire must be sealed in an airtight container to prevent the evaporation of volatile petroleum residues. New paint cans or tightly sealed jars are recommended in such situations (see Figure 2–18).

One should not use ordinary mailing envelopes as evidence containers because powders and fine particles will leak out of their corners. Instead, small amounts of trace evidence can be conveniently packaged in a carefully folded paper, using what is known as a "druggist fold" (see Figure 2–19). This consists of folding one end of the paper over by one-third, then folding the other end (one-third) over that, and repeating the process from the other two sides. After folding the paper in this manner, tuck the outside two edges into each other to produce a closed container that keeps the specimen from falling out.

Place each different item or similar items collected at different locations in separate containers. Packaging evidence separately prevents damage through contact and prevents cross-contamination.

BIOLOGICAL MATERIALS Use only disposable tools to collect biological materials for packaging. If biological materials such as blood are stored in airtight containers, the accumulation of moisture may encourage the growth of mold, which can destroy their evidential value. In these instances, wrapping paper, manila envelopes, or paper bags are the recommended packaging materials (see Figure 2–20). As a matter of routine, all items possibly containing biological fluid evidence should be air-dried and placed individually in separate paper bags to ensure constant circulation of air around them. This will prevent the formation of mold and mildew. Paper packaging is easily

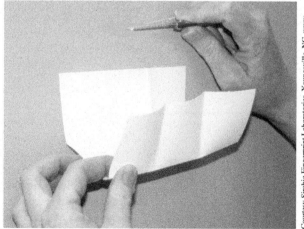

FIGURE 2–18

Airtight metal cans used to package arson evidence.

FIGURE 2–19

A druggist fold is used to package paint transfer evidence.

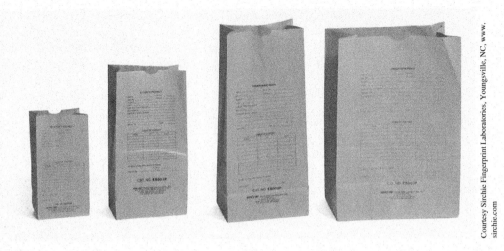

Courtesy Sirchie Fingerprint Laboratories, Youngsville, NC, www. sirchie.com

FIGURE 2–20

Paper bags are recommended evidence containers for objects suspected of containing blood and semen stains. Each object should be packaged in a separate bag.

written on, but seals may not be sturdy. Finally, place a red biohazard sticker on both the secured evidence bag and the property receipt to ensure that all handlers will be aware the item is contaminated with biological fluids, such as blood, saliva, or semen (see Table 2–1).

DNA EVIDENCE   The advent of DNA analysis brought one of the most significant recent advances in crime-scene investigation. This technique is valuable for making it possible to identify suspects through detecting and analyzing minute quantities of DNA deposited on evidence as a result of contact with saliva, sweat, or skin cells. The search for DNA evidence should include any and all objects with which the suspect or victim may have come into bodily contact. Likely sources of DNA evidence include stamps and envelopes that have been licked, a cup or can that has touched a person's lips, chewing gum, the sweatband of a hat, and a bed sheet containing dead skin cells.

TABLE 2–1

Best Practices in Biological Evidence Packaging

Containers
- Use paper bags, manila envelopes, cardboard boxes, and similar porous materials for all biological evidence.
- Use butcher paper or art paper for wrapping evidence, for padding in the evidence container, and/or as a general drop cloth to collect trace evidence.
- Package evidence and seal the container to protect it from loss, cross-transfer, contamination, and/or deleterious change.
- For security purposes, seal the package in such a manner that opening it causes obvious damage or alteration to the container or its seal.

Item Packaging
- Package each item separately; avoid commingling items to prevent cross-contamination.
- Use a biohazard label to indicate that a potential biohazard is present.
- Plastic bags are not preferred for storage because of the possibility of bacterial growth or mold.
- If drying wet evidence is not possible, place the evidence in an impermeable, nonporous container and place the container in a refrigerator that maintains a temperature of 2–8°C (approximately 35–46°F) and that is located away from direct sunlight until the evidence can be air-dried or submitted to the laboratory.
- Seal each package with evidence tape or other seals, such as heat seals and gum seals; if possible, do not use staples. Mark across the seal with the sealer's identification or initials and the date.

Reprinted in part from *The Biological Evidence Preservation Handbook: Best Practices for Evidence Handlers,* http://nvlpubs.nist.gov/nistpubs/ir/2013/NIST.IR.7928.pdf.

One key concern during the collection of a DNA-containing specimen is contamination. Contamination—in this case, introducing foreign DNA—can occur from coughing or sneezing onto evidence during the collection process. Transfer of DNA can also occur when items of evidence are incorrectly placed in contact with each other during packaging. To prevent contamination, the evidence collector must wear a face mask and lab coat, use disposable latex gloves, and work with disposable forceps. The evidence collector must also take into consideration that biological materials, such as dried blood, should be considered potentially infectious. It's recommended practice that the biological evidence collector wear disposable coveralls, shoe covers, and eye protection as an extra precaution to avoid contaminating DNA evidence and being exposed to infectious diseases.

Blood analysis has great evidential value when it allows the investigator to demonstrate a transfer between a victim and a suspect. For this reason, all clothing from both the victim and suspect should be collected and sent to the laboratory for examination, even when the presence of blood on a garment does not appear obvious to the investigator. Laboratory search procedures are far more revealing and sensitive than any that can be conducted at the crime scene.

A detailed description of the proper collection and packaging of various types of physical evidence will be discussed in forthcoming chapters.

Maintaining the Chain of Custody

Continuity of possession, or the **chain of custody**, must be established whenever evidence is presented in court as an exhibit. Adherence to standard procedures in recording the location of evidence, marking it for identification, and properly completing evidence submission forms for laboratory analysis is the best guarantee that the evidence will withstand inquiries of what happened to it from the time of its finding to its presentation in court. This means that every person who handled or examined the evidence must be accounted for. Failure to substantiate the evidence's chain of custody may lead to serious questions regarding the authenticity and integrity of the evidence and examinations of it.

chain of custody
A list of all people who came into possession of an item of evidence.

All items of physical evidence should be carefully packaged and marked upon their retrieval at crime sites. This should be done with the utmost care to avoid destroying their evidential value or restricting the number and kind of examinations to which the criminalist may subject them. If possible, the evidence itself should be marked for identification. Normally, the collector's initials and the date of collection are inscribed directly on the article. However, if the evidence collector is unsure of the necessity of marking the item itself or of where to mark it, it is best to omit this step. Once an evidence container is selected for the evidence, whether a box, bag, vial, or can, it also must be marked for identification. Evidence containers often have a preprinted identification form that the evidence collector fills out. Otherwise, the collector must attach an evidence tag to the container. The investigator who packaged the evidence must write their initials and the date on the evidence tape seal. Anyone who removes the evidence for further testing or observation at a later time should try to avoid breaking the original seal if possible so that the information on the seal will not be lost. The person who reseals the packaging should record their initials and the date on the new seal.

A minimum chain-of-custody record would show the collector's initials, location of the evidence, and date of collection. If the evidence is turned over to another individual for care or delivery to the laboratory, this transfer must be recorded in notes and other appropriate forms. In fact, every individual who possesses the evidence must maintain a written record of its acquisition and disposition. Frequently, all of the individuals involved in the collection and transportation of the evidence may be requested to testify in court. Thus, to avoid confusion and to retain complete control of the evidence at all times, the chain of custody should be kept to a minimum.

Obtaining Standard/Reference Samples

The examination of evidence, whether soil, blood, glass, hair, fibers, and so on, often requires comparison with a known **standard/reference sample**. Although most investigators have little difficulty recognizing and collecting relevant crime-scene evidence, few seem aware of the necessity and importance of providing the crime lab with a thorough sampling of standard/reference materials. Such materials may be obtained from the victim, a suspect, or other known

standard/reference sample
Physical evidence whose origin is known, such as fibers or hair from a suspect, that can be compared to crime-scene evidence.

sources. For instance, investigation of a hit-and-run incident may require the removal of standard/reference paint from a suspect vehicle. This will permit its comparison to paint recovered at the scene. Similarly, hair found at the crime scene will be of optimum value only when compared to standard/reference hairs removed from the suspect and victim. Likewise, bloodstained evidence must be accompanied by a **buccal swab** standard/reference sample obtained from all relevant crime-scene participants. The quality and quantity of standard/reference specimens often determine the evidential value of crime-scene evidence, and these standard/reference specimens must be treated with equal care.

Some types of evidence must also be accompanied by the collection of **substrate controls**. These are materials adjacent or close to areas where physical evidence has been deposited. For example, substrate controls are normally collected at arson scenes. If an investigator suspects that a particular surface has been exposed to gasoline or some other accelerant, the investigator should also collect a piece of the same surface material that is believed not to have been exposed to the accelerant. At the laboratory, the substrate control is tested to ensure that the surface on which the accelerant was deposited does not interfere with testing procedures. Another common example of a substrate control is a material on which a bloodstain has been deposited. Unstained areas close to the stain may be sampled for the purpose of determining whether this material will have an impact on the interpretation of laboratory results.

Thorough collection and proper packaging of standard/reference specimens and substrate controls are the mark of a skilled investigator.

Submitting Evidence to the Laboratory

Evidence is usually submitted to the laboratory either by personal delivery or by mail shipment. The method of transmittal is determined by the distance the submitting agency must travel to the laboratory and the urgency of the case. If the evidence is delivered personally, the deliverer should be familiar with the case, to facilitate any discussions between laboratory personnel and the deliverer concerning specific aspects of the case.

If desired, most evidence can be conveniently shipped by mail. However, postal regulations restrict the shipment of certain chemicals and live ammunition and prohibit the mailing of explosives. In such situations, the laboratory must be consulted to determine the disposition of these substances. Care must also be exercised in the packaging of evidence in order to prevent breakage or other accidental destruction while it is in transit to the laboratory.

Most laboratories require that an evidence submission form accompany all evidence submitted. One such form is shown in Figure 2–21. This form must be properly completed. Its information will enable the laboratory analyst to make an intelligent and complete examination of the evidence. Particular attention should be paid to providing the laboratory with a brief description of the case history. This information will allow the examiner to analyze the specimens in a logical sequence and make the proper comparisons, and it will also facilitate the search for trace quantities of evidence.

The particular kind of examination requested for each type of evidence is to be delineated. However, the analyst will not be bound to adhere strictly to the specific tests requested by the investigator. As the examination proceeds, new evidence may be uncovered, and as a result the complexity of the case may change. Furthermore, the analyst may find the initial requests incomplete or not totally relevant to the case. Finally, a list of items submitted for examination must be included on the evidence submission form. Each item is to be packaged separately and assigned a number or letter, which should be listed in an orderly and logical sequence on the form.

Ensuring Crime-Scene Safety

The increasing spread of AIDS and hepatitis B has sensitized the law enforcement community to the potential health hazards at crime scenes. Law enforcement officers have an extremely small chance of contracting AIDS or hepatitis at the crime scene. Both diseases are normally transmitted by the exchange of body fluids, such as blood, semen, and vaginal and cervical secretions; intravenous drug needles and syringes; and transfusion of infected blood products. However, the presence of blood and semen at crime scenes presents the investigator with biological specimens of unknown origin; the investigator has no way of gauging what health hazards they may contain. Therefore, caution and protection must be used at all times.

buccal swab
A swab of the inner portion of the cheek; cheek cells are usually collected to determine the DNA profile of an individual.

substrate control
Uncontaminated surface material close to an area where physical evidence has been deposited. This sample is to be used to ensure that the surface on which a sample has been deposited does not interfere with laboratory tests.

CRIME: Homicide; Aggravated Sexual Assault					COUNTY OF: Mercer			

VICTIM: Jane Doe (v)	Age 25	Sex F	Race C	SUSPECT: John Doe(s)	Age 30	Sex M	Race C

SUBMITTING AGENCY: (Address)
Trenton P.D. Central Evidence 225 N. Clinton Avenue, Trenton, N.J. 08609

FORWARD REPLIES TO: Capt. John Smith, Chief of Detectives	(Name) Same as above	(Address)	Telephone Number: 609 555-5555

INVESTIGATED BY: Detective John Jones	DELIVERED BY: (Signature of Person Delivering Evidence)

BRIEF HISTORY OF CASE: (Include Date and Location, if Applicable)
On March 1st, 2001 the victim was found dead in her bedroom. Victim was partially clothed and autopsy revealed that victim was stabbed numerous times and medical examiner stated that there was evidence of sexual assault. Victim was last seen drinking with suspect at a local tavern. Suspect was arrested and item # 23, a folding knife, was found in his pocket.

* Note* Suspect is HIV+

EXAMINATION REQUESTED ON SPECIMENS LISTED BELOW:

Examine items 2, 5, 8-11, 13-15, 18 and 19 for seminal material and compare to controls #'s 12 and 26. Examine #1, 2, 4, 7, 13, 14, 15, 18, 20, 21, 22 and 23 for trace evidence transfer. Examine #3 for saliva from suspect. Examine #6 for skin, blood and trace evidence. Examine #'s 20-23 for transfer blood evidence and compare to control #'s 12 and 26.

Item #	* Code	LIST OF SPECIMENS *SOURCE OF EVIDENCE CODE (V-Victim, S-Suspect, SC-Scene)
1	V	Debris collection
2	V	Clothing, white panties
3	V	Dried Secretions/bite marks
4	V	Head Hair Combings
5	V	Oral Specimens
6	V	Fingernail Specimens
7	V	Pubic Hair Combings
8	V	External Genital Specimen
9	V	Vaginal Specimens
10	V	Cervical Specimens

Right side vertical checkboxes: DRUG ☐ · TRACE ☐ · BIO/CHEM ☐ (LABORATORY USE ONLY) · TOX ☐ · ABC ☐ · EQUINE ☐ · BALLISTICS ☐

FOR ADDITIONAL INFORMATION USE FORM 631A AND ATTACH

Page 1 of 2 pages

Richard Saferstein, Criminalistics: An Introduction to Forensic Science, 12e, © 2018. Pearson Education, Inc., New York, NY.

FIGURE 2–21
An example of a properly completed evidence submission form.

Fortunately, inoculation can easily prevent hepatitis B infection in most people. Furthermore, the federal Occupational Safety and Health Administration (OSHA) requires that law enforcement agencies offer hepatitis B vaccinations to all officers who may have contact with body fluids while on the job, at no expense to the officer.

Each crime scene is unique and carries with it its own collection of hazards. Fortunately, a number of options are available to crime-scene investigators for dealing with the potential hazards that crime scenes present. More frequently than not, once the scene is secured and isolated, it should become apparent that the locale may not contain urgent safety concerns, as in burglaries and car thefts. Nevertheless, routine safety practices must be enforced. This includes donning latex or nitrite gloves. The latter provides better protection from chemicals. Gloves offer protection from inadvertent contact with blood or other biological materials. They also prevent accidental deposition of fingerprints on objects the scene investigators may touch. Gloves must be changed frequently; in fact, a new pair of gloves must be worn for each item of evidence handled by the investigator. When removed, the gloves must be disposed of in a biohazard bag.

Protective footwear is an important component of the crime-scene investigator's garb. Shoes must be covered with rubber booties when moving about indoors. The investigator should routinely wear shoes or boots that provide good traction and ample support. Inexpensive shoes are recommended, as the investigator must be prepared to dispose of them if they become contaminated with unknown liquids or chemicals.

A basic concern of the crime scene is eye protection. It's appropriate to wear eyeglasses or goggles at crime scenes. However, if concerns exist about encountering splashing liquids, a face shield should be donned to maximize eye and face protection.

Crime scenes that contain the greatest risks to health and safety typically entail exposure to potentially life-threatening biological hazards. These scenes call for maximum respiratory, eye, and skin protection. A wide variety of respiratory masks are available. They include single and double filter masks. Tyvek protective suits are a good option for keeping biohazards off the skin. These suits allow the wearer to move about with ease and flexibility.

When processing and collecting evidence at a crime scene, personnel should be alert to sharp objects, knives, hypodermic syringes, razor blades, and similar items. If such sharp objects are encountered and must be recovered as evidence, the items should be placed in a puncture-resistant container and properly labeled.

When potentially infectious materials are present at a crime scene, personnel should maintain a red biohazard plastic bag for the disposal of contaminated gloves, clothing, masks, pencils, wrapping paper, and so on. On departure from the scene, the biohazard bag must be taped shut and transported to an approved biohazardous waste pickup site.

Legal Considerations at the Crime Scene

In police work, perhaps no experience is more exasperating or demoralizing than to see valuable evidence excluded from use against the accused because of legal considerations. This situation most often arises from what is deemed an "unreasonable" search and seizure of evidence. Therefore, removal of any evidence from a person or from the scene of a crime must be done in conformity with Fourth Amendment privileges: "The right of the people to be secure in their persons, houses, papers, and effects, against unreasonable searches and seizure, shall not be violated, and no warrants shall issue, but upon probable cause, supported by oath or affirmation, and particularly describing the place to be searched, and the persons or things to be seized."

Since the 1960s, the Supreme Court has been particularly concerned with defining the circumstances under which the police can search for evidence in the absence of a court-approved search warrant. A number of allowances have been made to justify a warrantless search: (1) the existence of emergency circumstances, (2) the need to prevent the immediate loss or destruction of evidence, (3) a search of a person and property within the immediate control of the person, provided it is made incident to a lawful arrest, and (4) a search made by consent of the parties involved. In cases other than these, police must be particularly cautious about processing a crime scene without a search warrant. In 1978, the Supreme Court addressed this very issue and in so doing set forth guidelines for investigators to follow in determining the propriety of conducting a warrantless search at a crime scene. Significantly, the two cases decided on this issue related to homicide and arson crime scenes, both of which are normally subjected to the most intensive forms of physical evidence searches by police.

In the case of *Mincey* v. *Arizona*,[1] the Court dealt with the legality of a four-day search at a homicide scene. The case involved a police raid on the home of Rufus Mincey, who had been suspected of dealing drugs. Under the pretext of buying drugs, an undercover police officer forced entry into Mincey's apartment and was killed in a scuffle that ensued. Without a search warrant, the police spent four days searching the apartment, recovering, among other things, bullets, drugs, and drug paraphernalia. These items were subsequently introduced as evidence at the trial. Mincey was convicted and on appeal contended that the evidence gathered from his

[1]437 U.S. 385 (1978).

apartment, without a warrant and without his consent, was illegally seized. The Court unanimously upheld Mincey's position, stating:

> We do not question the right of the police to respond to emergency situations. Numerous state and federal cases have recognized that the Fourth Amendment does not bar police officers from making warrantless entries and searches when they reasonably believe that a person within is in need of immediate aid. Similarly, when the police come upon the scene of a homicide they may make a prompt warrantless search of the area to see if there are other victims or if a killer is still on the premises.... Except for the fact that the offense under investigation was a homicide, there were no exigent circumstances in this case.... There was no indication that evidence would be lost, destroyed or removed during the time required to obtain a search warrant. Indeed, the police guard at the apartment minimized that possibility. And there is no suggestion that a search warrant could not easily and conveniently have been obtained. We decline to hold that the seriousness of the offense under investigation itself creates exigent circumstances of the kind that under the Fourth Amendment justify a warrantless search.

In *Michigan* v. *Tyler*,[2] a business establishment leased by Loren Tyler and a business partner was destroyed by fire. The fire was finally extinguished in the early hours of the morning; however, hampered by smoke, steam, and darkness, fire officials and police were prevented from thoroughly examining the scene for evidence of arson. The building was then left unattended until 8 a.m. that day, when officials returned and began an inspection of the burned premises. During the morning search, assorted items of evidence were recovered and removed from the building. On three other occasions—4 days, 7 days, and 25 days after the fire—investigators reentered the premises and removed additional items of evidence. Each of these searches was made without a warrant or without consent, and the evidence seized was used to convict Tyler and his partner of conspiracy to burn real property and related offenses. The Supreme Court upheld the reversal of the conviction, holding the initial morning search to be proper but contending that evidence obtained from subsequent reentries to the scene was inadmissible: "We hold that an entry to fight a fire requires no warrant, and that once in the building, officials may remain there for a reasonable time to investigate the cause of a blaze. Thereafter, additional entries to investigate the cause of the fire must be made pursuant to the warrant procedures."

The message from the Supreme Court is clear: when time and circumstances permit, obtain a search warrant before investigating and retrieving physical evidence at the crime scene.

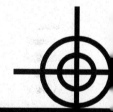

Chapter Summary >>>>>>>>>>

Physical evidence includes all objects that can establish or disprove that a crime has been committed or can link a crime and its victim or its perpetrator. Forensic science begins at the crime scene. Here, investigators must recognize and properly preserve evidence for laboratory examination. The first officer to arrive is responsible for securing the crime scene. Once the scene is secured, relevant investigators record the crime scene by using photographs, sketches, and notes. Before processing the crime scene for physical evidence, the investigator should make a preliminary examination of the scene as it was left by the perpetrator. The search for physical evidence at a crime scene must be thorough and systematic. The search pattern selected normally depends on the size and locale of the scene and the number of collectors participating in the search.

Physical evidence can be anything from massive objects to microscopic traces. Often, many items of evidence are

clearly visible, but others may be detected only through examination at the crime laboratory. For this reason, it is important to collect possible carriers of trace evidence, such as clothing, vacuum sweepings, and fingernail scrapings, in addition to more discernible items. Each different item or similar items collected at different locations must be placed in a separate container. Packaging evidence separately prevents damage through contact and prevents cross-contamination.

During the collection of evidence, the chain of custody, a record for denoting the location of the evidence, must be maintained. In addition, proper standard/reference samples, such as hairs, a buccal swab, and fibers, must be collected at the crime scene and from appropriate subjects for comparison in the laboratory. The removal of any evidence from a person or from the scene of a crime must be done in accordance with appropriate search and seizure protocols.

[2]436 U.S. 499 (1978).

Review Questions

1. The term _____ encompasses all objects that can establish or disprove whether a crime has been committed or can link a crime and its victim or its perpetrator.

2. True or False: Scientific evaluation of crime-scene evidence can usually overcome the results of a poorly conducted criminal investigation. _____

3. True or False: The techniques of physical evidence collection require a highly skilled individual who must specialize in this area of investigation. _____

4. All unauthorized personnel must be _____ from crime scenes.

5. True or False: Failure to protect a crime scene properly may result in the destruction or altering of evidence. _____

6. The _____ arriving on the scene of a crime is responsible for taking steps to preserve and protect the area to the greatest extent possible, and they must rely on their training to deal with any violent or hazardous circumstances.

7. At a crime scene, first priority should be given to obtaining _____ for individuals in need of it and attempting to minimize disturbance of evidence.

8. True or False: The boundaries of the crime scene, denoted by crime-scene tape, rope, or traffic cones, should encompass only the center of the scene where the crime occurred. _____

9. Even though no unauthorized personnel are admitted to the scene, an accurate _____ must be kept of those who do enter and exit the scene and the time they do so.

10. True or False: The lead investigator will immediately proceed to gain an overview of the situation and develop a strategy for the systematic examination of the crime scene during the final survey. _____

11. Three methods for recording the crime scene are _____, _____, and _____.

12. True or False: Note-taking begins with the call to a crime-scene investigator to report to a scene. _____

13. The crime-scene notes should include a precise record of personnel movements in and out of the scene starting with the _____.

14. True or False: Crime-scene notes should be written from memory back at the laboratory. _____

15. Before located evidence is collected, it must be fully described in the investigator's _____.

16. True or False: When an injured or deceased victim is present at the scene, the state of the body before being moved should be observed but not recorded. _____

17. The most important prerequisite for photographing a crime scene is to have it in a(n) _____ condition.

18. Photographs of physical evidence must include overviews as well as _____ to record the details of objects.

19. True or False: The value of crime-scene photographs lies in their ability to show the layout of the scene, position of witnesses, and relation of people to one another in the scene. _____

20. The most commonly used camera for crime-scene photography is the _____ camera, which can be film or digital.

21. A digital camera captures light on a light-sensitive _____.

22. True or False: Each crime scene should be photographed as completely as possible in a logical succession, and the photographs should include the area in which the crime actually took place and all adjacent areas where important acts occurred. _____

23. The succession of photographs taken at a crime scene is _____ photographs first and _____ photographs last.

24. True or False: Overview photographs should include only points of entry and points of exit. _____

25. To ensure that their digital images will be admissible, many jurisdictions have developed or are developing _____ for the use of digital photography to avoid the possibility of enhancement or doctoring of crime-scene photographs.

26. The process of _____ the crime scene essentially combines notes and photography.

27. Unlike the rough sketch, the _____ is constructed with care and concern for aesthetic appearance and must be drawn to scale.

28. _____ programs provide an extensive symbol library and may create a three-dimensional sketch.

29. An investigator need only draw a(n) _____ sketch at the crime scene to show its dimensions and pertinent objects.

30. A detailed search of the crime scene for physical evidence must be conducted in a(n) _____ manner.

31. The crime-scene search is undertaken to locate _____.

32. True or False: The search patterns that may be used to search a crime scene for evidence include the line pattern, grid pattern, polar coordinate pattern, and spiral pattern. _____

33. True or False: If the investigator does not recognize physical evidence or does not properly preserve it for laboratory examination, sophisticated laboratory

instrumentation or technical expertise can salvage the situation and attain the desired results. _____

34. Besides the more obvious items of physical evidence, possible _____ of trace evidence must be collected for detailed examination in the laboratory.

35. Whenever possible, trace evidence (is, is not) to be removed from the object that bears it.

36. Each item collected at the crime scene must be placed in a(n) _____ container.

37. True or False: An ordinary mailing envelope is considered a good general-purpose evidence container. _____

38. An airtight container (is, is not) recommended packaging material for bloodstained garments.

39. As a matter of routine, all items of clothing are to be _____ before packaging.

40. True or False: Charred debris recovered from the scene of an arson is best placed in a porous container. _____

41. The possibility of future legal proceedings requires that a(n) _____ be established with respect to the possession and location of physical evidence.

42. Most physical evidence collected at the crime scene will require the accompanying submission of _____ material for comparison purposes.

43. In the case of *Mincey* v. *Arizona*, the Supreme Court restricted the practice of conducting a(n) _____ search at a homicide scene.

44. In the case of *Michigan* v. *Tyler*, the Supreme Court dealt with search-and-seizure procedures at a(n) _____ scene.

Application and Critical Thinking

1. You are the first officer at the scene of an outdoor assault. You find the victim bleeding but conscious, with two of the victim's friends and several onlookers standing nearby. You call for backup and quickly glance around but see no one fleeing the scene. Describe the steps you would take while you wait for backup to arrive.

2. What kind of search pattern(s) would investigators be most likely to employ in each of the following situations?

   a. Two people searching a small area with well-defined boundaries

   b. Several people searching a large area

   c. A single person searching a large area

4. Officer Bill Walter arrives at the scene of an apparent murder: a body bearing several gunshot wounds lies on the floor of a small, un-air-conditioned house in late July. A pungent odor almost overwhelms him when he enters the house, so he opens a window to allow him to breathe so he can investigate the scene. While airing out the house, he secures the scene and interviews bystanders. When he inspects the scene, he discovers very little blood in the room and little evidence of a struggle. What mistake did Officer Walter make in his investigation? What conclusion did he draw about the scene from his observations?

5. Officer Martin Guajardo is the first responder at an apparent homicide scene. After securing the area, interviewing the sole witness, and calling for backup, he begins to search for evidence. He makes note of a bloody knife lying next to the body, with a small scrap of bloody cloth clinging precariously to the knife. Because it is a very windy day, Officer Guajardo removes the scrap of fabric and seals it in a plastic bag. A few moments later, a crime-scene team, including a photographer, arrives to take over the investigation. What mistakes, if any, did Officer Guajardo make before the crime-scene team arrived?

6. During his search of a homicide scene, investigator David Gurney collects evidence that includes a bloody shirt. After the crime-scene team has completely processed the scene, Investigator Gurney packages the shirt in a paper bag, seals the bag, and labels it to indicate the contents. He then delivers the shirt to the laboratory with an evidence submission form. There, a forensic scientist breaks the seal, removes the shirt, and performs a series of tests on it. He replaces the shirt, discards the old seal, and places a new seal on the package containing his initials and the date on which it was resealed. What mistakes, if any, were made in handling the shirt?

7. What important elements are missing from the following crime-scene sketch?

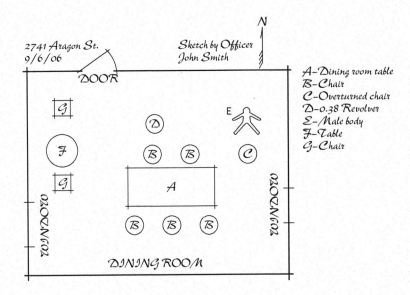

2741 Aragon St.
9/6/06

DOOR

Sketch by Officer
John Smith

A–Dining room table
B–Chair
C–Overturned chair
D–0.38 Revolver
E–Male body
F–Table
G–Chair

DINING ROOM

Further References

The Biological Evidence Preservation Handbook: Best Practices for Evidence Handlers, http://nvlpubs.nist.gov/nistpubs/ir/2013/NIST.IR.7928.pdf

Crime Scene Investigation: A Guide for Law Enforcement, 2013, http://www.nfstc.org/bja-programs/crime-scene-investigation-guide/

Gardner, R. M., *Practical Crime Scene Processing and Investigation*, 2nd ed. Boca Raton, FL: CRC Press, 2012.

Ogle, R. R., Jr., *Crime Scene Investigation and Reconstruction*, 3rd ed. Upper Saddle River, NJ: Prentice Hall, 2011.

Osterburg, James W., and Richard H. Ward, *Criminal Investigation—A Method for Reconstructing the Past*, 6th ed. Cincinnati, OH: Anderson, 2011.

Shaler, R. C., *Crime Scene Forensics: A Scientific Method Approach*. Boca Raton, FL: CRC Press, 2012.

Case Analysis

Investigators looking into the kidnapping and murder of DEA special agent Enrique Camarena and DEA source Alfredo Zavala faced several hurdles that threatened to derail their efforts to collect evidence in the case. These hurdles almost prevented forensics experts from determining the facts of the case and threatened to undermine the investigation of the crime. However, despite these obstacles, use of standard forensic techniques eventually enabled investigators to solve the case. Read about the Camarena case in the following Case Files, then answer the following questions:

1. What were the main challenges facing investigators who were collecting evidence in the case? Give specific examples.

2. Explain how investigators used reference samples to determine that the victims had been held at the residence located at 881 Lope De Vega.

3. Explain how investigators used soil evidence to determine that the victims' bodies had been buried and later moved to the site where they were discovered.

The Enrique Camarena Case: A Forensic Nightmare

On February 7, 1985, US Drug Enforcement Agency (DEA) Special Agent (SA) Enrique Camarena was abducted near the US Consulate in Guadalajara, Mexico. A short time later, Capt. Alfredo Zavala, a DEA source, was also abducted from a car near the Guadalajara Airport. These two abductions would trigger a series of events leading to one of the largest investigations ever conducted by the DEA and would result in one of the most extensive cases ever received by the FBI Laboratory …

Michael P. Malone
Special Agent, Laboratory Division
Federal Bureau of Investigation,
Washington, D.C.

The Abduction

On February 7, 1985, SA Camarena left the DEA resident office to meet his wife for lunch. On this day, a witness observed a man being forced into the rear seat of a light-colored compact car in front of the Camelot Restaurant and provided descriptions of several of the assailants. After some initial reluctance, Primer Comandante Pavon-Reyes of the Mexican Federal Judicial Police (MFJP) was put in charge of the investigation, and Mexican investigators were assigned to the case. Two known drug traffickers, Rafael Caro-Quintero and Ernesto Fonseca, were quickly developed as suspects …

The Investigation

During February 1985, searches of several residences and ranches throughout Mexico proved fruitless, despite the efforts of the DEA task force assigned to investigate this matter and the tremendous pressure being applied by the US government to accelerate the investigation. High-level US government officials, as well as their Mexican counterparts, were becoming directly involved in the case. It is believed that, because of this "heat," the Mexican drug traffickers and certain Mexican law enforcement officials fabricated a plan. According to the plan, the MFJP would receive an anonymous letter indicating that SA Camarena and Captain Zavala were being held at the Bravo drug gang's ranch in La Angostura, Michoacan, approximately 60 miles southeast of Guadalajara. The MFJP was supposed to raid the ranch, eliminate the drug gang, and eventually discover the bodies of SA Camarena and Captain Zavala buried on the ranch. The DEA would then be notified and the case would be closed. Thus, the Bravo gang would make an easy scapegoat.

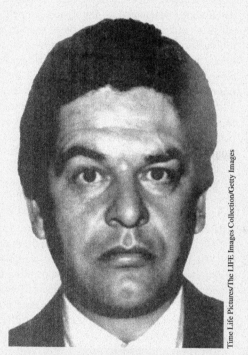

Undated photo of Enrique Camarena.

During early March, MFJP officers raided the Bravo ranch before the DEA agents arrived. In the resulting shootout, all of the gang members, as well as one MFJP officer, were killed. However, due to a mix-up, the bodies of SA Camarena and Captain Zavala were not buried on the Bravo ranch in time to be discovered as planned. Shortly after this shootout, a passerby on a road near the Bravo ranch found two partially decomposed bodies wrapped in plastic bags. The bodies were removed and transported to a local morgue, where they were autopsied. The DEA was then advised of the discovery of the bodies and their subsequent removal to another morgue in Guadalajara, where a second autopsy was performed.

Cadaver number 1 was quickly identified by the fingerprint expert as SA Camarena. Although Mexican officials would not allow the second body to be identified at this time, it was later identified through dental records as Captain Zavala.

The FBI forensic team requested permission to process the clothing, cordage, and burial sheet found with the bodies, but the request was denied. However, they were allowed to cut small, "known" samples from these items and obtain hair samples from both bodies. Soil samples were also removed from the bodies and the clothing items.

In late March 1985, DEA agents located a black Mercury Grand Marquis that they believed was used in the kidnapping or transportation of SA Camarena. The vehicle had been stored in a garage in Guadalajara, and a brick wall had been constructed at the entrance to conceal it. The vehicle was traced to a Ford dealership owned by Caro-Quintero. Under the watchful eye of the MFJP at the Guadalajara Airport, the FBI forensic team processed the vehicle for any hair, fiber, blood, and/or fingerprint evidence it might contain.

During April 1985, the MFJP informed the DEA that they believed they had located the residence where SA Camarena and Captain Zavala had been held. The FBI forensic team was immediately dispatched to Guadalajara; however, they were not allowed to proceed to the residence, located at 881 Lope De Vega, until an MFJP forensic team had processed the residence and had removed all of the obvious evidence.

On the first day after their arrival, the FBI forensic team surveyed and began a crime-scene search of the residence and surrounding grounds (see Figure 1). The residence consisted of a large, two-story structure with a swimming pool, covered patio, aviary, and tennis court surrounded by a common wall. The most logical place to hold a prisoner at this location would be in the small outbuilding located to the rear of the main residence. This outbuilding, designated as the "guest house" by investigators, consisted of a small room with a beige rug and an adjoining bathroom. The entire room and bathroom were processed for hairs, fibers, and latent fingerprints. The single door into this room was made of steel and reinforced by iron bars. It was ultimately determined by means of testimony and forensic evidence that several individuals interrogated and tortured SA Camarena in this room. In addition, a locked bedroom, located on the second floor of the main house, was also processed, and the bed linens were removed from a single bed. Known carpet samples were taken from every room in the residence.

A beige Volkswagen Atlantic parked under a carport at the rear of the residence fit the general description of the smaller vehicle noted by the witness to SA Camarena's abduction. The VW Atlantic was also processed for hairs, fibers, and fingerprints.

On the second day, a thorough grounds search was conducted. As FBI forensic team members were walking around the tennis court, they caught a glimpse of something blue in one of the drains. On closer inspection, there appeared to be a folded license plate at the bottom of the drain. The license plate was retrieved, unfolded, and photographed. The MFJP officers, all of whom were now at the tennis court, became upset at this discovery, and one of them immediately contacted his superior at MFJP headquarters, who ordered them to secure the license plate until the assistant primer comandante arrived on the scene. Upon his arrival approximately 20 minutes later, he seized the license plate and would not allow the Americans to conduct any further searches.

In September 1985, DEA personnel went to La Primavera Park and recovered a soil sample. This sample matched the soil samples from SA Camarena and Captain Zavala's cadavers almost grain for grain, which indicated that this site was almost certainly their burial site before they were relocated to the Bravo ranch.

Later that fall, after further negotiations between the US and the Mexican governments, permission was finally granted for an FBI forensic team to process the evidence seized by the MFJP forensic team from 881 Lope De Vega the previous April. The evidence consisted of small samples the MFJP had taken of SA Camarena's burial sheet, a piece of rope used to bind SA Camarena, a portion of a pillowcase removed from bedroom number 3, a piece of unsoiled rope removed from the covered patio, and a laboratory report prepared by the MFJP Crime Laboratory. The remainder of the evidence had been destroyed for "health reasons."

In January 1986, a drug trafficker named Rene Verdugo, who was considered to be a high-ranking member of the Caro-Quintero gang, was apprehended and taken to San Diego, where he was arrested by the DEA. He was then transported to Washington, D.C., where samples of his hair were taken. He refused to testify before the federal grand jury investigating the Camarena case. Later that year, DEA personnel obtained hair samples in Mexico City from Sergio Espino-Verdin, a former federal comandante who is believed to have been SA Camarena's primary interrogator during his ordeal at 881 Lope De Vega.

The Trial

In July 1988, the main trial for the murder, interrogation, and abduction of SA Camarena began in US District Court in Los Angeles, California. The forensic evidence presented in this trial identified 881 Lope De Vega as the site where SA Camarena had been held. The evidence also strongly associated two Mexican citizens, Rene Verdugo and Sergio Espino-Verdin, with the "guest house" at 881 Lope De Vega. Several types of forensic evidence were used to associate SA Camarena with 881 Lope De Vega: forcibly removed head hairs found in the "guest house" and bedroom number 4, in the VW Atlantic, and in the Mercury Grand Marquis, and two types of polyester rug fibers: a dark, rose-colored fiber and a light-colored fiber (see Figures 2 and 3). Fabric evidence was also presented, which demonstrated the similarities of color, composition, construction, and design between SA Camarena's burial sheet and the two pillowcases recovered from bedrooms number 3 and 5.

Based on this evidence associating SA Camarena and 881 Lope De Vega, the FBI Laboratory examiner was able to testify that SA Camarena was at this residence, as well as in the VW Atlantic and the Mercury Grand Marquis, and that he had been in a position such that his head hairs were forcibly removed. Captain Alfredo Zavala was also found to be associated with the "guest house" at 881 Lope De Vega. Light-colored nylon rug fibers found on samples of his clothing taken at the second autopsy matched the fibers from the "guest house" carpet.

A detailed model of the residence at 881 Lope De Vega was prepared by the Special Projects Section of the FBI Laboratory for the trial (see Figure 4). Over 20 trial charts were also prepared to explain the various types of forensic evidence. These charts proved invaluable in clarifying the complicated techniques and characteristics used in the examination of the hair, fiber, fabric, and cordage evidence (see Figure 5).

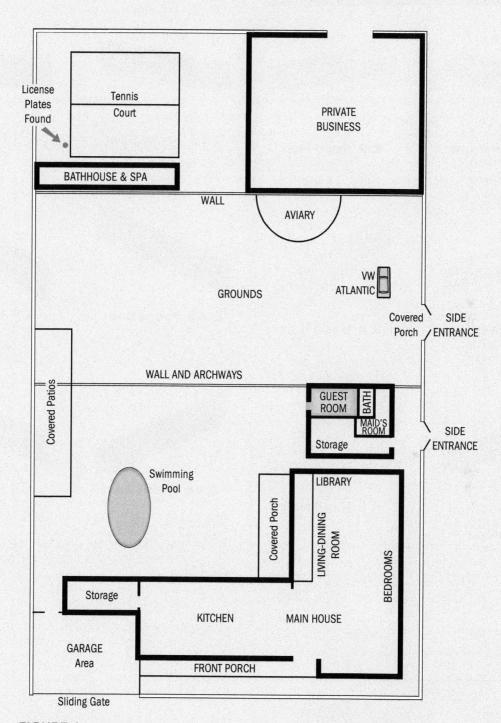

FIGURE 1

A diagram of the 881 Lope De Vega grounds. Camarena was held prisoner in the guest house.

Source: FBI Law Enforcement Bulletin, September, 1989.

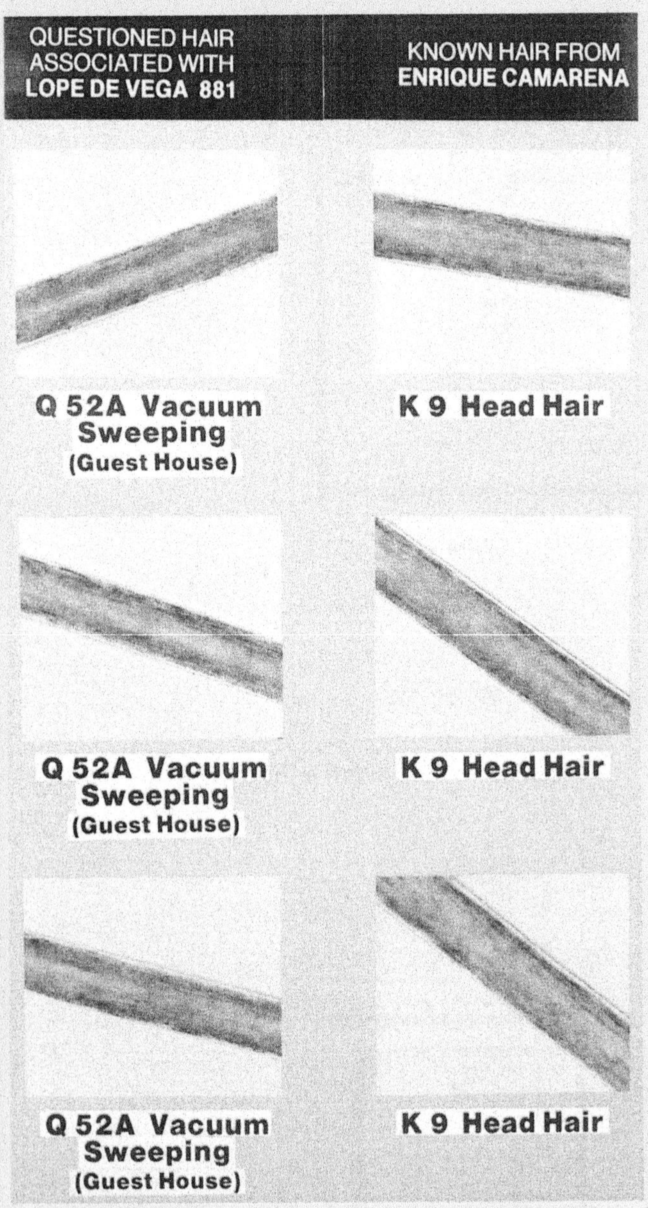

QUESTIONED HAIR ASSOCIATED WITH LOPE DE VEGA 881	KNOWN HAIR FROM ENRIQUE CAMARENA

Q 52A Vacuum Sweeping (Guest House) — **K 9 Head Hair**

Q 52A Vacuum Sweeping (Guest House) — **K 9 Head Hair**

Q 52A Vacuum Sweeping (Guest House) — **K 9 Head Hair**

Federal Bureau of Investigation

FIGURE 2

A trial chart showing hair comparisons between known Camarena hairs and hairs recovered from 881 Lope De Vega.

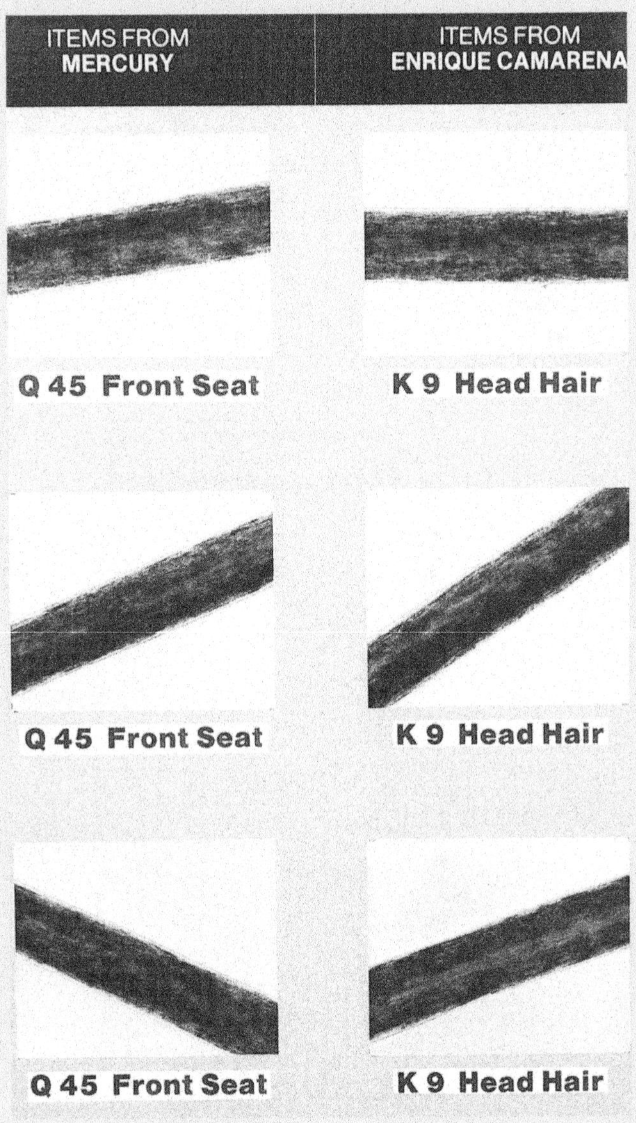

ITEMS FROM MERCURY	ITEMS FROM ENRIQUE CAMARENA

Q 45 Front Seat — **K 9 Head Hair**

Q 45 Front Seat — **K 9 Head Hair**

Q 45 Front Seat — **K 9 Head Hair**

Federal Bureau of Investigation

FIGURE 3

A trial chart showing hair comparisons between known Camarena hairs and hairs recovered from the Mercury Gran Marquis.

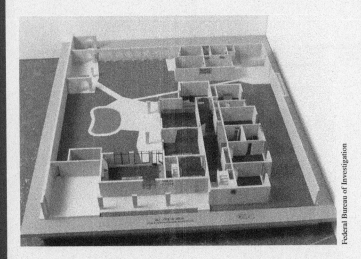

Federal Bureau of Investigation

FIGURE 4

A model of 881 Lope De Vega prepared as a trial exhibit.

CATEGORIES OF FORENSIC EVIDENCE
IN CAMARENA CASE

LOCATION	TYPE OF EVIDENCE					
	Hair	Carpet Fibers	Fabric Match	Cordage Match	Tape Match	Misc.
Mercury	Camarena Head Hair					Blood on Floor Mat
VW Atlantic	Camarena Head Hair					Blood on Tissue
Guest House	Camarena Head Hair	Zavala Clothes Nylon				
Bedroom #3		Camarena Blindfold Polyester	Pillow Case Camarena Burial Sheet			
Bedroom #4	Camarena Head Hair	Camarena Blindfold & Burial Sheet Polyester				
Bedroom #5			Pillow Case Camarena Burial Sheet			
Tennis Court						License Plate VW/Merc.
Camarena Burial Sheet	Camarena Head Hair	Bedroom #4 Polyester	Pillow Case Bedrooms #3 and #5			Soil La Primavera
Source – Blindfold/ Rope	Camarena Head Hair	Bedrooms #3 and #4 Polyester			Camarena Blindfold Tape	
Camarena Burial Cordage				Burial Rope from Covered Patio		
Zavala Clothing	Zavala Head Hair	Guest House Nylon				Soil La Primavera

FIGURE 5

A trial chart used to show the association of Camarena and Zavala with various locations.

Source: Federal Bureau of Investigation.

Conclusion

After an eight-week trial, conducted under tight security and involving hundreds of witnesses, all of the defendants were found guilty and convicted on all counts, and are currently serving lengthy sentences.

Physical Evidence

KEY TERMS

class characteristics
comparison
identification
individual
   characteristics
product rule
rapid DNA

Bruce McArthur: A Mountain of Physical Evidence

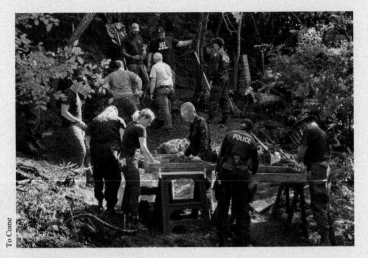
To Come

Over the course of a decade, gay men were vanishing off the streets of Toronto, Canada. The last in the string of unexplained disappearances was Andrew Kinsman, who went missing on January 26, 2017. As part of the investigation, police combed through his belongings for information on his whereabouts the day he went missing. On his calendar, there was just one entry—the name "Bruce." Police were able to pull surveillance footage of Kinsman getting into a red 2004 Dodge Caravan on the day he disappeared. When investigators cross-referenced those pieces of information, there was only one person named "Bruce" who owned a red 2004 Dodge Caravan.

Police began to monitor Bruce McArthur, a 66-year-old landscaper from Toronto. After weeks of surveillance, officers observed a young man entering McArthur's apartment. Fearing for the man's safety, police decided to make entry. Once inside, they discovered the young man tied up but otherwise unharmed. It was at this time that Bruce McArthur was taken into custody on suspicion of murder. The subsequent search yielded a trove of physical evidence that linked McArthur to the killings of eight men with ties to Toronto's Gay Village. A search of his van yielded blood that matched the DNA profiles of some of his victims. Police found a black duffel bag containing duct tape, a surgical glove, rope, zip ties, a black bungee cord, and syringes in McArthur's bedroom. He shaved his victims' heads and beards before burying them and kept hair from the men in bags. He buried the remains of his dismembered victims in planter pots at the home of a landscaping client.

In the face of the "unprecedented amount of real, forensic, digital and documentary evidence" described by the prosecutor in the case, Bruce McArthur pled guilty to eight counts of murder in a Toronto courtroom on January 29, 2019. During the sentencing hearing, the prosecutor walked through each piece of physical evidence amassed by investigators, stating: "For years, members of the LGBTQ community in Toronto believed they were being targeted by a killer and they were right." McArthur was sentenced to life in prison without the possibility of parole for his crimes.

It would be impossible to list all the objects that could conceivably be of importance to a crime; every crime scene obviously has to be treated on an individual basis, having its own peculiar history, circumstances, and problems. It is practical, however, to list items whose scientific examination is likely to yield significant results in ascertaining the nature and circumstances of a crime. The investigator who is thoroughly familiar with the recognition, collection, and analysis of these items, as well as with laboratory procedures and capabilities, can make logical decisions when the uncommon and unexpected are encountered at the crime scene. Just as important, a qualified evidence collector cannot rely on collection procedures memorized from a pamphlet but must be able to make innovative, on-the-spot decisions at the crime scene.

Common Types of Physical Evidence

1. *Blood, semen, and saliva.* All suspected blood, semen, or saliva—liquid or dried, animal or human—present in a form to suggest a relation to the offense or the people involved in a crime. This category includes blood or semen dried onto fabrics or other objects, as well as cigarette butts that may contain saliva residues. These substances are subjected to serological and biochemical analysis to determine their identity and possible origin.

2. *Documents.* Any handwriting and typewriting submitted so that authenticity or source can be determined. Related items include paper, ink, indented writings, obliterations, and burned or charred documents.

3. *Drugs.* Any substance seized in violation of laws regulating the sale, manufacture, distribution, and use of drugs.

4. *Explosives.* Any device containing an explosive charge, as well as all objects removed from the scene of an explosion that are suspected to contain the residues of an explosive.

5. *Fibers.* Any natural or synthetic fiber whose transfer may be useful in establishing a relationship between objects and/or people.

6. *Fingerprints.* All prints of this nature, latent and visible.

7. *Firearms and ammunition.* Any firearm, as well as discharged or intact ammunition, suspected of being involved in a criminal offense.

8. *Glass.* Any glass particle or fragment that may have been transferred to a person or object involved in a crime. Windowpanes containing holes made by a bullet or other projectile are included in this category.

9. *Hair.* Any animal or human hair present that could link a person with a crime.

10. *Impressions.* Tire markings, shoe prints, depressions in soft soils, and all other forms of tracks. Glove and other fabric impressions are also included.

11. *Organs and physiological fluids.* Body organs and fluids are submitted for toxicology to detect the possible existence of drugs and poisons. This category includes blood to be analyzed for the presence of alcohol and other drugs.

12. *Paint.* Any paint, liquid or dried, that may have been transferred from the surface of one object to another during the commission of a crime. A common example is the transfer of paint from one vehicle to another during an automobile collision.

13. *Petroleum products.* Any petroleum product removed from a suspect or recovered from a crime scene. The most common examples are gasoline residues removed from the scene of an arson, or grease and oil stains whose presence may suggest involvement in a crime.

14. *Plastic bags.* A disposable polyethylene bag such as a garbage bag may be evidential in a homicide or drug case. Examinations are conducted to associate a bag with a similar bag in the possession of a suspect.

15. *Plastic, rubber, and other polymers.* Remnants of these manufactured materials recovered at crime scenes may be linked to objects recovered in the possession of a suspect perpetrator.

16. *Powder residues.* Any item suspected of containing firearm discharge residues (see Figure 3–1).

17. *Serial numbers.* This category includes all stolen property submitted to the laboratory for the restoration of erased identification numbers.

18. *Soil and minerals.* All items containing soil or minerals that could link a person or object to a particular location. Common examples are soil embedded in shoes and safe insulation found on garments.

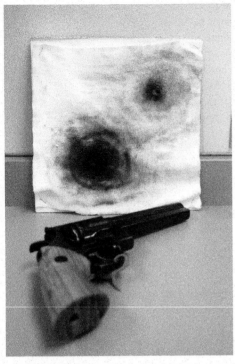

FIGURE 3–1

The gun is fired at a set distance from the target and the gunpowder left on the target is compared to powder stains found on a victim's clothing. The density and shape of the powder stains vary with the distance the gun was fired.

identification

The process of determining a substance's physical or chemical identity. Drug analysis, species determination, and explosive residue analysis are typical examples of this undertaking in a forensic setting.

comparison

The process of ascertaining whether two or more objects have a common origin.

19. ***Tool marks.*** This category includes any object suspected of containing the impression of another object that served as a tool in a crime. For example, a screwdriver or crowbar could produce tool marks by being impressed into or scraped along a surface of a wall.
20. ***Vehicle lights.*** Examination of vehicle headlights and taillights is normally conducted to determine whether a light was on or off at the time of impact.
21. ***Wood and other vegetative matter.*** Any fragments of wood, sawdust, shavings, or vegetative matter discovered on clothing, shoes, or tools that could link a person or object to a crime location.

The Significance of Physical Evidence

The examination of physical evidence by a forensic scientist is usually undertaken for identification or comparison.

Identification

Identification has as its purpose the determination of the physical or chemical identity of a substance with as near absolute certainty as existing analytical techniques will permit. For example, the crime laboratory is frequently asked to identify the chemical composition of an illicit-drug preparation that may contain heroin, cocaine, barbiturates, and so on. It may be asked to identify gasoline in residues recovered from the debris of a fire, or it may have to identify the nature of explosive residues—for example, dynamite or TNT. Also, the identification of blood, semen, hair, or wood would, as a matter of routine, include a determination of species origin. For example, did an evidential bloodstain originate from a human as opposed to a dog or cat? Each of these requests requires the analysis and ultimate identification of a specific physical or chemical substance to the exclusion of all other possible substances.

The process of identification first requires the adoption of testing procedures that give characteristic results for specific standard materials. Once these test results have been established, they may be permanently recorded and used repeatedly to prove the identity of suspect materials. For example, to ascertain that a particular suspect powder is heroin, the test results on the powder must be identical to those that have been previously obtained from a known heroin sample. Second, identification requires that the number and type of tests needed to identify a substance be sufficient to exclude all other substances. This means that the examiner must devise a specific analytical scheme that will eliminate all but one substance from consideration. Hence, if the examiner concludes that a white powder contains heroin, the test results must have been comprehensive enough to have excluded all other drugs—or, for that matter, all other substances—from consideration.

Simple rules cannot be devised for defining what constitutes a thorough and foolproof analytical scheme. Each type of evidence obviously requires different tests, and each test has a different degree of specificity. Thus, one substance could conceivably be identified by one test, whereas another may require a combination of five or six different tests to arrive at an identification. In a science in which the practitioner has little or no control over the quality and quantity of the specimens received, a standard series of tests cannot encompass all possible problems and pitfalls. So, the forensic scientist must determine at what point the analysis can be concluded and the criteria for positive identification satisfied; for this, the forensic scientist must rely on knowledge gained through education and experience. Ultimately, the conclusion will have to be substantiated beyond any reasonable doubt in a court of law.

Comparison

A **comparison** analysis subjects a suspect specimen and a standard/reference specimen to the same tests and examinations for the ultimate purpose of determining whether they have a common origin. For example, the forensic scientist may place a suspect at a particular location by noting the similarities of a hair found at the crime scene to hairs removed from a suspect's head (see Figure 3–2). Or a paint chip found on a hit-and-run victim's garment may be compared with paint removed from

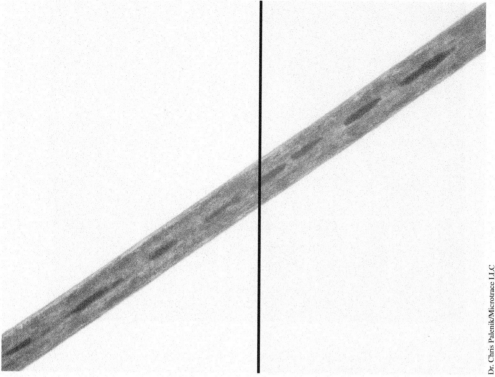

FIGURE 3–2
Side-by-side comparison of hairs.

Dr. Chris Palenik/Microtrace LLC

a vehicle suspected of being involved in the incident. The forensic comparison is actually a two-step procedure. First, combinations of select properties are chosen from the suspect and the standard/reference specimen for comparison. The question of which and how many properties are selected obviously depends on the type of materials being examined. (This subject will receive a good deal of discussion in forthcoming chapters.) The overriding consideration must be the ultimate evidential value of the conclusion. This brings us to the second objective. Once the examination has been completed, the forensic scientist must draw a conclusion about the origins of the specimens. Do they or do they not come from the same source? Certainly, if one or more of the properties selected for comparison do not agree, the analyst will conclude that the specimens are not the same and hence could not have originated from the same source. Suppose, on the other hand, that all the properties do compare and the specimens, as far as the examiner can determine, are indistinguishable. Does it logically follow that they come from the same source? Not necessarily so.

To comprehend the evidential value of a comparison, one must appreciate the role that probability has in ascertaining the origins of two or more specimens. Simply defined, *probability* is the frequency of occurrence of an event. If a coin is flipped one hundred times, in theory we can expect heads to come up 50 times. Hence, the probability of the event (heads) occurring is 50 in 100. In other words, probability defines the odds at which a certain event will occur.

INDIVIDUAL CHARACTERISTICS Evidence that can be associated with a common source with an extremely high degree of probability is said to possess **individual characteristics**. Examples of this are the ridge characteristics of fingerprints, random striation markings on bullets or tool marks, irregular and random wear patterns in tire or footwear impressions, handwriting characteristics, irregular edges of broken objects that can be fitted together like a jigsaw puzzle (see Figure 3–3), or sequentially made plastic bags that can be matched by striation marks running across the bags (see Figure 3–4). In all of these cases, it is not possible to state with mathematical exactness the probability that the specimens are of common origin; it can only be concluded that this probability is so high as to defy mathematical calculations or human comprehension. Furthermore, the conclusion of common origin must be substantiated by the practical experience of the examiner. For example, the French scientist Victor Balthazard has mathematically determined that the probability of two individuals having the same fingerprints is one out of 1×10^{60}, or 1 followed by 60 zeros. This probability is so small as to exclude the possibility of any two

individual characteristics
Properties of evidence that can be attributed to a common source with an extremely high degree of certainty.

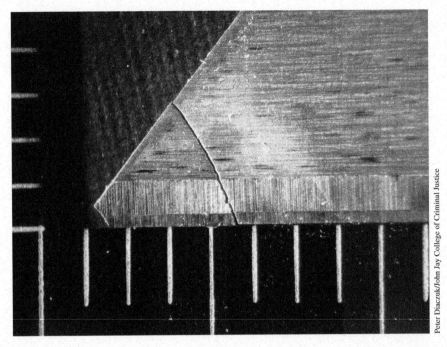

Peter Diacznk/John Jay College of Criminal Justice

FIGURE 3–3

The body of a woman was found with evidence of a stablike wound in the neck. A pathologist found a knife blade tip in the wound in the neck. The knife blade tip was compared with the broken blade of a knife found in the trousers pocket of the accused. A close examination reveals the fit of the indentations on the edges and individual characteristics of stria from the sharpening procedure.

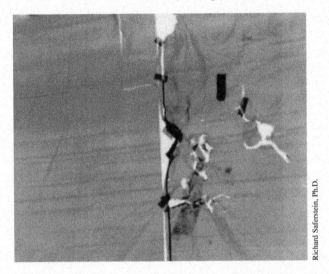

Richard Saferstein, Ph.D.

FIGURE 3–4

The bound body of a young woman was recovered from a river. Her head was covered with a black polyethylene trash bag (shown on the right). Among the items recovered from one of several suspects was a black polyethylene trash bag (shown on the left). A side-by-side comparison of the two bags' extrusion marks and pigment bands showed them to be consecutively manufactured. This information allowed investigators to focus their attention on one suspect, who ultimately was convicted of the homicide.

individuals having the same fingerprints. This contention is also supported by the experience of fingerprint examiners who, after classifying millions of prints over the past hundred years, have never found any two to be exactly alike.

class characteristics
Properties of evidence that can be associated only with a group and never with a single source.

CLASS CHARACTERISTICS   One disappointment awaiting the investigator unfamiliar with the limitations of forensic science is the frequent inability of the laboratory to relate physical evidence to a common origin with a high degree of certainty. Evidence is said to possess **class characteristics**

when it can be associated only with a group and never with a single source. Here again, probability is a determining factor. For example, if we compare two one-layer automobile paint chips of a similar color, their chance of originating from the same car is not nearly as great as when we compare two paint chips having seven similar layers of paint, not all of which were part of the car's original color. The former will have class characteristics and could only be associated at best with one car model (which may number in the thousands), whereas the latter may be judged to have individual characteristics and to have a high probability of originating from one specific car.

Blood offers another good example of evidence that can have class characteristics. For example, suppose that two blood specimens are compared and both are found to be of human origin, type A. The frequency of occurrence in the population of type A blood is 26 percent—hardly offering a basis for establishing the common origin of the stains. However, if other blood factors are also determined and are found to compare, the probability that the two blood samples originated from a common source increases. Thus, if one uses a series of blood factors that occur independently of each other, one can apply the **product rule** to calculate the overall frequency of occurrence of the blood in a population.

For example, in the O. J. Simpson case, a bloodstain located at the crime scene was found to contain a number of factors that compared to O. J.'s blood:

Blood Factors	Frequency
A	26 percent
EsD	85 percent
PGM 2+ 2−	2 percent

The product of all the frequencies shown in the table determines the probability that any one individual possesses such a combination of blood factors. In this instance, applying the product rule, $0.25 \times 0.85 \times 0.02$ equals 0.0044, or 0.44 percent, or about 1 in 200 people who would be expected to have this particular combination of blood factors. These bloodstain factors did not match either of the two victims, Nicole Brown Simpson or Ronald Goldman, thus eliminating them as possible sources of the blood. Although the forensic scientist has still not individualized the bloodstains to one person—in this case, O. J. Simpson—data have been provided that will permit investigators and the courts to better assess the evidential value of the crime-scene stain. As we will learn in Chapter 16, the product rule is used to determine the frequency of occurrence of DNA profiles typically determined from blood and other biological materials. Importantly, modern DNA technology provides enough factors to allow an analyst to individualize blood, semen, and other biological materials to a single person or an identical twin.

product rule
Multiplying together the frequencies of independently occurring genetic markers to obtain an overall frequency of occurrence for a genetic profile.

Assessing the Significance of Physical Evidence

One of the current weaknesses of forensic science is the inability of the examiner to assign exact or even approximate probability values to the comparison of most class physical evidence. For example, what is the probability that a nylon fiber originated from a particular sweater, or that a hair came from a particular person's head, or that a paint chip came from a car suspected to have been involved in a hit-and-run accident? Few statistical data are available from which to derive this information, and in a society that is increasingly dependent on mass-produced products, the gathering of such data is becoming an increasingly elusive goal.

One of the primary endeavors of forensic scientists must be to create and update statistical databases for evaluating the significance of class physical evidence. Of course, when such information—for example, the population frequency of blood factors—is available, it is used; but for the most part, the forensic scientist must rely on personal experience when called on to interpret the significance of class physical evidence.

People who are unfamiliar with the realities of modern criminalistics are often disappointed to learn that most items of physical evidence retrieved at crime scenes cannot be linked definitively to a single person or object. Although investigators always try to uncover physical evidence with individual characteristics—such as fingerprints, tool marks, and bullets—the chances of finding class physical evidence are far greater. To deny or belittle the value of such evidence is to reject the potential role that criminalistics can play in a criminal investigation. In practice, criminal cases are fashioned for the courtroom around a collection of diverse elements, each pointing to the guilt or involvement of a party in a criminal act.

Often, most of the evidence gathered is subjective in nature, prone to human error and bias. The extent to which cognitive biases may influence decision-making in forensic science is an important question with implications for training and practice. There have been a number of studies that support the idea of susceptibility of forensic science practitioners to various types of confirmation bias. As a result, it has been recommended that forensic laboratories implement procedures designed to reduce access to unnecessary information, use of multiple comparison samples rather than a single suspect exemplar, and replication of results by analysts blinded to previous results. The believability of eyewitness accounts, confessions, and informant testimony can all be disputed, maligned, and subjected to severe attack and skepticism in the courtroom. Under these circumstances, errors in human judgment are often magnified to detract from the credibility of the witness.

Assessing the Value of Physical Evidence

The value of class physical evidence lies in its ability to corroborate events with data in a manner that is, as nearly as possible, free of human error and bias. It is the thread that binds together other investigative findings that are more dependent on human judgments and, therefore, more prone to human failings. The fact that scientists have not yet learned to individualize many kinds of physical evidence means that criminal investigators should not abdicate or falter in their pursuit of all investigative leads. However, the ability of scientists to achieve a high degree of success in evaluating class physical evidence means that criminal investigators can pursue their work with a much greater chance of success.

Admittedly, in most situations, trying to define the significance of an item of class evidence in exact mathematical terms is a difficult if not impossible goal. Although class evidence is by its nature not unique, our common experience tells us that meaningful items of physical evidence, such as those listed on pages 63–64, are extremely diverse in our environment. Select, for example, a colored fiber from an article of clothing and try to locate the exact same color on the clothing of random individuals you meet, or select a car color and try to match it to other automobiles you see on local streets. Furthermore, keep in mind that a forensic comparison actually goes beyond a mere color comparison and involves examining and comparing a variety of chemical and/or physical properties (see Figure 3–5). The point is that the chances are low of encountering two

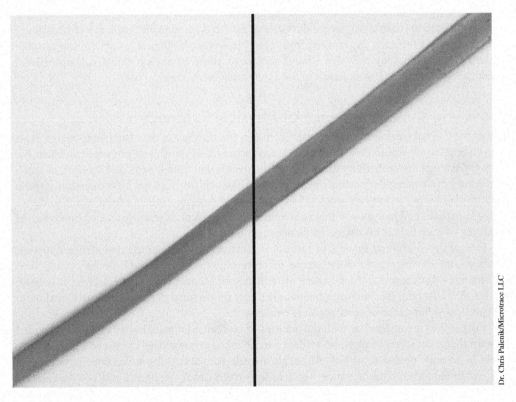

FIGURE 3–5
Side-by-side comparison of fibers.

Dr. Chris Palenik/Microtrace LLC

indistinguishable items of physical evidence at a crime scene that actually originated from different sources. Obviously, given these circumstances, only objects that exhibit a significant amount of diversity in our environment are deemed appropriate for classification as physical evidence.

In the same way, when one is dealing with more than one type of class evidence, their collective presence may lead to an extremely high certainty that they originated from the same source. As the number of different objects linking an individual to a crime increases, the probability of involvement increases—dramatically. A classic example of this situation can be found in the evidence presented at the trial of Wayne Williams. Wayne Williams was charged with the murders of two individuals in the Atlanta, Georgia, metropolitan area; he was also linked to the murders of 10 other adolescent or young males. An essential element of the state's case involved the association of Williams with the victims through a variety of fiber evidence. Twenty-eight different types of fibers linked Williams to the murder victims, evidence that the forensic examiner characterized as "overwhelming." Williams's case is discussed in more detail in Chapter 11.

Before moving beyond the subject of the nature and values that contrast individual and class evidence, one major concern must be addressed. In 2009, the report entitled *Strengthening Forensic Science in the United States: A Path Forward* was issued by the National Research Council (NRC) of the National Academy of Sciences.[1] The report addressed an overarching concern that has permeated the foundation of forensic evidence; that is, whether certain items of class or individual evidence is worthy of admission in a court of law. Putting aside concerns about the lack of a statistical basis to define probabilities to support the comparative significance of many types of physical evidence, the NRC report decries the fact that many forensic determinations involve subjective evaluations, whose correctness is not readily verifiable and whose accuracy is highly dependent on the experience and training of the examiner. While the NRC report encourages research to put forensic science on a more objective footing, this goal will be painstakingly slow. Alternatively, crime laboratories have been encouraged to implement quality assurance measures to measure the competency of their examiners; these include peer review, proficiency testing, analyst certification, and periodic external audits.

Cautions and Limitations in Dealing with Physical Evidence

In further evaluating the contribution of physical evidence, one cannot overlook one important reality in the courtroom: the weight or significance accorded to physical evidence is a determination left entirely to the trier of fact, usually a jury of laypeople. Given the high esteem in which scientists are generally held by society and the infallible image created for forensic science by books and television, it is not hard to understand why scientifically evaluated evidence often takes on an aura of special reliability and trustworthiness in the courtroom. Often physical evidence, whether individual or class, is accorded great weight during jury deliberations and becomes a primary factor in reinforcing or overcoming lingering doubts about guilt or innocence. In fact, a number of jurists have already cautioned against giving carte blanche approval to admitting scientific testimony without first considering its relevance in a case. Given the potential weight of scientific evidence, failure to take proper safeguards may unfairly prejudice a case against the accused.

Physical evidence may also exclude or exonerate a person from suspicion. For instance, if type A blood is linked to the suspect, all individuals who have type B, AB, or O blood can be eliminated from consideration. Because it is not possible to assess at the crime scene what value, if any, the scientist will find in the evidence collected, or what significance such findings will ultimately have to a jury, a thorough collection and scientific evaluation of physical evidence must become a routine part of all criminal investigations.

Just when an item of physical evidence crosses the line that distinguishes class from individual is a difficult question to answer and is often the source of heated debate and honest disagreement among forensic scientists. How many striations are necessary to individualize a mark to a single tool and no other? How many color layers individualize a paint chip to a single car? How many ridge characteristics individualize a fingerprint, and how many handwriting characteristics tie a person to a signature? These questions defy simple answers. The task of the forensic scientist is to find as many characteristics as possible to compare one substance with another. The significance attached to the findings is decided by the quality and composition of the evidence, the case history, and the examiner's experience. Ultimately, the conclusion can range from mere speculation to near certainty.

[1] National Research Council, *Strengthening Forensic Science in the United States: A Path Forward*, Washington, D.C.: National Academies Press, 2009, http://books.nap.edu/openbook.php?record_id=12589&page=R1

There are practical limits to the properties and characteristics the forensic scientist can select for comparison. Carried to the extreme, no two things in this world are alike in every detail. Modern analytical techniques have become so sophisticated and sensitive that the criminalist must be careful to define the limits of natural variation among materials when interpreting the data gathered from a comparative analysis. For example, we will learn in Chapter 10 that two properties, density and refractive index, are best suited for comparing two pieces of glass. But the latest techniques that have been developed to measure these properties are so sensitive that they can even distinguish glass originating from within a single pane of glass. Certainly, this goes beyond the desires of a criminalist trying to determine only whether two glass particles originated from the same window. Similarly, if the surface of a paint chip is magnified 1,600 times with a powerful scanning electron microscope, it is apparent that the fine details that are revealed could not be duplicated in any other paint chip. Under these circumstances, no two paint chips, even those coming from the same surface, could ever compare in the true sense of the word. Therefore, practicality dictates that such examinations be conducted at a less revealing, but more meaningful, magnification (see Figure 3–6).

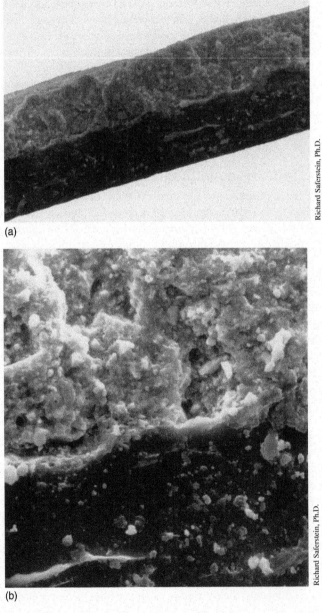

(a)

Richard Saferstein, Ph.D.

(b)

Richard Saferstein, Ph.D.

FIGURE 3–6

(a) Two-layer paint chip magnified 244× with a scanning electron microscope.
(b) The same paint chip viewed at a magnification of 1,600×.

Distinguishing evidential variations from natural variations is not always an easy task. Learning how to use the microscope and all the other modern instruments in a crime laboratory properly is one thing; gaining the proficiency needed to interpret the observations and data is another. As new crime laboratories are created and others expand to meet the requirements of the law enforcement community, many individuals are starting new careers in forensic science. They must be cautioned that merely reading relevant textbooks and journals is no substitute for experience in this most practical of sciences.

Forensic Databases

In a criminal investigation, the ultimate contribution a criminalist can make is to link a suspect to a crime through comparative analyses. This comparison defines the unique role of the criminalist in a criminal investigation. Of course, a one-to-one comparison requires a suspect. Little or nothing of evidential value can be accomplished if crime-scene investigators acquire fingerprints, hairs, fibers, paint, blood, and semen without the ability to link these items to a suspect. In this respect, computer technology has dramatically altered the role of the crime laboratory in the investigative process. No longer is the crime laboratory a passive bystander waiting for investigators to uncover clues about who may have committed a crime. Today, the crime laboratory is on the forefront of the investigation seeking to identify perpetrators. This dramatic reversal of the role of forensic science in criminal investigation has come about through the creation of computerized databases that not only link all 50 states but also tie together police agencies throughout the world.

Fingerprint Databases

The premier model of all forensic database systems is the *Integrated Automated Fingerprint Identification System* (IAFIS), a national fingerprint and criminal history system maintained by the FBI. In 2014, the IAFIS was effectively replaced and integrated into the Next Generation Identification (NGI) system. The expanded capabilities of NGI beyond fingerprints will be discussed in Chapter 7. IAFIS, which first became operational in 1999, contains fingerprints and access to corresponding criminal history information for nearly 75 million subjects (or 750 million fingerprint images), which are submitted voluntarily to the FBI by state, local, and federal law enforcement agencies. In the United States, each state has its own *Automated Fingerprint Identification System* (AFIS), which is linked to the FBI's NGI system. A crime-scene fingerprint or latent fingerprint is a dramatic find for the criminal investigator. Once the quality of the print has been deemed suitable for the NGI system search, the latent-print examiner creates a digital image of the print with either a digital camera or a scanner. Next, the examiner, with the aid of a coder, marks points on the print to guide the computerized search. The print is then electronically submitted to the NGI system, and within minutes the search is completed against all fingerprint images in the NGI system; the examiner may receive a list of potential candidates and their corresponding fingerprints for comparison and verification (see Figure 3–7).

Many countries throughout the world have created national automated fingerprint identification systems that are comparable to the FBI's model. For example, the United Kingdom has also recently created an integrated system that links police and justice agencies called IDENT1. Its primary capabilities include finger and palm print analysis, print search capabilities with access to international databases, verification of the identities of arrested persons, and information sharing capabilities between state, local, and federal agencies throughout England, Scotland, and Wales. IDENT1 provides the basis for future integrated technologies such as biometric or facial imaging.

DNA Databases

In 1998, the FBI's *Combined DNA Index System* (CODIS) became fully operational. CODIS enables federal, state, and local crime laboratories to electronically exchange and compare DNA profiles, thereby linking crimes to each other and to convicted offenders. All 50 states have enacted legislation to establish a data bank containing DNA profiles of individuals convicted of felony sexual offenses (and other crimes, depending on each state's statute). CODIS creates investigative leads from three indexes: the *forensic, offender*, and *arrestee* indices. The forensic index currently contains about 915,000 DNA profiles from unsolved crime-scene evidence. Based on a match, police in multiple jurisdictions can identify serial crimes, allowing coordination of

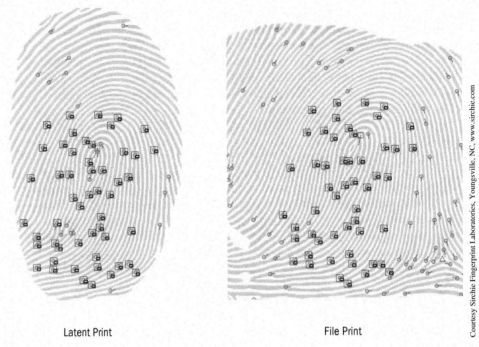

Courtesy Sirchie Fingerprint Laboratories, Youngsville, NC, www.sirchie.com

Latent Print   File Print

FIGURE 3–7

The computerized search of a fingerprint database first requires that selected ridge characteristics be designated by a coder. The positions of these ridge characteristics serve as a basis for comparing the latent print against file fingerprints.

investigations and sharing of leads developed independently. The offender index contains the profiles of more than 13.6 million convicted individuals. The FBI has joined numerous states that collect DNA samples from those awaiting trial and will collect DNA from detained immigrants. This information will be entered into the arrestee index database, presently at 3.4 million.[2] Ultimately, the success of the CODIS program is measured by the crimes it helps to solve. To this end, CODIS has produced more than 451,000 hits assisting in more than 440,000 investigations.

Constitutional issues regarding the appropriateness of collecting DNA from arrestees not convicted of any crime, but who nevertheless were the subject of a CODIS search against DNA collected from unsolved crimes, was decided in the case of *Maryland* v. *King*.[3]

> *When officers make an arrest supported by probable cause to hold for a serious offense and bring the suspect to a station to be detained in custody, taking and analyzing a cheek swab of the arrestee's DNA is, like fingerprinting and photographing, a legitimate police booking procedure that is reasonable under the Fourth Amendment.*

Rapid DNA

A process for developing DNA profiles from a buccal swab in 90 minutes or less that are compatible with a CODIS search.

With the Supreme Court sanctioning the collection of cheek or buccal swabs from arrestees, the necessity for the analysis of a swab as close to the time of arrest as possible becomes apparent. The term **Rapid DNA** has become part of the lingo of forensic science and describes approaches for rapidly obtaining a DNA profile from a buccal swab. A number of compact instruments are already commercially available and others are being developed. These allow for the development of a DNA profile from a buccal swab in less than 90 minutes. Experts envision that rapid DNA devices will take their place alongside fingerprinting units for the routine processing of arrestees. Recently, the FBI permitted profiles collected by Rapid DNA into the CODIS database (see Figure 3–8).

Unfortunately, hundreds of thousands of samples are backlogged, still awaiting DNA analysis and entry into the offender index. Law enforcement agencies search this index against DNA

[2] https://www.fbi.gov/services/laboratory/biometric-analysis/codis/ndis-statistics
[3] 133 S.Ct. 1236 (2013).

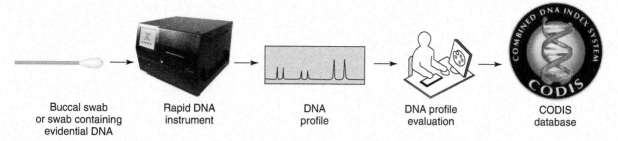

Buccal swab
or swab containing
evidential DNA

Rapid DNA
instrument

DNA
profile

DNA profile
evaluation

CODIS
database

FIGURE 3-8

The process of taking genetic material recovered from a crime scene and entering that information into the CODIS database for comparison.

profiles recovered from biological evidence found at unsolved crime scenes. This approach has proven to be tremendously successful in identifying perpetrators because most crimes involving biological evidence are committed by repeat offenders.

Several countries throughout the world have initiated national DNA data banks. The United Kingdom's *National DNA Database*, established in 1995, was the world's first national database. Currently it holds more than 6 million profiles, and DNA can be taken for entry into the database from anyone arrested for an offense likely to involve a prison term. The National DNA Data Bank, housed in Ottawa, Canada, contains more than 379,000 DNA profiles from convicted individuals and has assisted in more than 54,000 cases, including more than 3,500 murders and more than 5,900 sexual assaults.

Genealogy Databases

An emerging use of forensic DNA profiles from crime scene samples involves searching unknown profiles through genealogy databases, like GEDmatch, to identify close relatives. These databases contain samples that are processed by commercial genealogy companies and uploaded by private citizens. The availability of commercial DNA testing kits, from companies like 23andMe and *Ancestry.com*, is credited with increasing the size and popularity of these genealogy databases.

The primary purpose of these databases is to assist professional and amateur genealogists in identifying potential relatives, but because they contain DNA profiles from a wide cross section of the population, they have proved to be extremely useful in cases where investigators have DNA profiles but have not yet matched it to a source. Searching the databases is akin to a familial search, where a link can be established to a particular family lineage. Once a family lineage has been identified, the family tree can then be further examined to determine if there are individuals that fit the description of the potential person of interest.

Other Databases

The *National Integrated Ballistics Information Network* (NIBIN), maintained by the Bureau of Alcohol, Tobacco, Firearms, and Explosives, allows firearms analysts to acquire, digitize, and compare markings made by a firearm on bullets and cartridge casings recovered from crime scenes. Since the program's inception in 1999, NIBIN partners have processed approximately 99,000 NIBIN leads and 110,000 NIBIN hits. Approximately 16 million images in the network include 3.3 million pieces of evidence. The heart of NIBIN is the *Integrated Ballistic Identification System* (IBIS), comprising a microscope and a computer unit that can capture an image of a bullet or cartridge casing. The images are then forwarded to a regional server, where they are stored and correlated against other images in the regional database. IBIS does not positively match bullets or casings fired from the same weapon; this must be done by a firearms examiner. IBIS does, however, facilitate the work of the firearms examiner by producing a short list of candidates for the examiner to manually compare.

The *International Forensic Automotive Paint Data Query* (PDQ) database contains chemical and color information pertaining to original automotive paints. This database, developed and maintained by the Forensic Laboratory Services of the Royal Canadian Mounted

Police (RCMP), contains information about make, model, year, and assembly plant on more than 21,000 samples corresponding to over 85,000 layers of paint. Contributors to the PDQ include the RCMP and forensic laboratories in Ontario and Quebec, as well as 40 U.S. forensic laboratories and police agencies in 21 other countries. Accredited users of PDQ are required to submit 60 new automotive paint samples per year for addition to the database. The PDQ database has found its greatest utility in the investigation of hit-and-runs by providing police with possible make, model, and year information to aid in the search for the unknown vehicle.

The previously described databases are maintained and controlled by government agencies. There is one exception: a commercially available computer retrieval system for comparing and identifying crime-scene shoe prints known as *SICAR* (shoeprint image capture and retrieval).[4] SICAR's pattern-coding system enables an analyst to create a simple description of a shoe print by assigning codes to individual pattern features (see Figure 3–9). Shoe print images can be entered into SICAR by either a scanner or a digital camera. This product has a comprehensive shoe sole database (Solemate) that includes more than 39,000 footwear entries providing investigators with a means for linking a crime-scene footwear impression to a particular shoe manufacturer. A second database, TreadMate, has been created to house tire tread patterns. Currently, it contains 8,500 records.

Case Files

Gerald Wallace

In 1975, police found Gerald Wallace's body on his living room couch. He had been savagely beaten, his hands bound with an electric cord. Detectives searched his ransacked house, cataloging every piece of evidence they could find. None of it led to the murderer. They had no witnesses. Sixteen years after the fact, a lone fingerprint, lifted from a cigarette pack found in Wallace's house and kept for 16 years in the police files, was entered into the Pennsylvania State Police AFIS database. Within minutes, it hit a match. That print, police say, gave investigators the identity of a man who had been at the house the night of the murder. Police talked to him. He led them to other witnesses, who led them to the man police ultimately charged with the murder of Gerald Wallace.

Case Files

The Center City Rapist

Fort Collins, Colorado, and Philadelphia, Pennsylvania, are separated by nearly 1,800 miles, but in 2001 they were tragically linked through DNA. Troy Graves left the Philadelphia area in 1999, joined the Air Force, and settled down with his wife in Colorado. A frenzied string of eight sexual assaults around the Colorado University campus set off a manhunt that ultimately resulted in the arrest of Graves. However, his DNA profile inextricably identified him as Philadelphia's notorious "Center City rapist." This assailant attacked four women in 1997 and brutally murdered Shannon Schieber, a Wharton School graduate student, in 1998. His last known attack in Philadelphia was the rape of an 18-year-old student in August 1999, shortly before he left the city. In 2002, Graves was returned to Philadelphia, where he was sentenced to life in prison without parole.

[4] Foster & Freeman Limited, http://www.fosterfreeman.co.uk

> > > > > > > > >

Case Files

NIBIN Links Handgun to Suspects

After a series of armed robberies in which suspects fired shots, the sheriff's office of Broward County, Florida, entered the cartridge casings from the crime scenes into NIBIN. Through NIBIN, four of the armed robberies were linked to the same .40-caliber handgun. A short time later, sheriff's deputies noticed suspicious activity around a local business. When they attempted to interview the suspects, the suspects fled in a vehicle. During the chase, the suspects attempted to dispose of a handgun; deputies recovered the gun after making the arrests. The gun was test-fired and the resulting evidence entered into NIBIN, which indicated a possible link between this handgun and the four previous armed robberies. Firearms examiners confirmed the link through examination of the original evidence. The suspects were arrested and charged with four prior armed robbery offenses.

Over 600,000 individuals go missing in the United States every year. Medical examiners and coroners handle approximately 4,000 unidentified human decedent cases, 1,000 of which remain unidentified after one year.

The National Missing and Unidentified Persons System (NamUs) was created in 2007 as a national centralized repository and resource center for missing persons and unidentified decedent records. NamUs is a free online system that can be searched by medical examiners, coroners, law enforcement officials, and the general public from all over the country in hopes of resolving these cases. NamUs comprises three databases, all of which are open to the general public.

The Missing Persons Database contains information about missing persons that can be entered by anyone; however, before a person appears as a case on NamUs, there must be a verification by law enforcement prior to publication in NamUs. When a new missing person is entered into NamUs, the system automatically performs cross-matching with links to state clearinghouses, medical examiners' and coroners' offices, law enforcement agencies, and victim assistance groups to check potential matches between cases.

The Unidentified Persons Database contains information entered by medical examiners and coroners. Unidentified persons are people who have died and whose bodies have not been identified. Anyone can search this database using characteristics such as sex, ancestry, tattoos, and other distinctive body features, as well as dental information. However, sensitive case data is restricted and can be viewed only by select agencies.

The Unclaimed Persons Database contains information about deceased persons who have been identified by name, but for whom no next of kin or family member has been identified or located to claim the body for burial or other disposition. Only medical examiners and coroners may enter cases in this database. However, the database is searchable by the public using a missing person's name and year of birth.

In 2011, the NamUs database was awarded to the University of North Texas Health Science Center for system management and ongoing development.

> > > > > > > > >

Case Files

Aztec Gold Metallic Hit and Run

A 53-year-old man was walking his dog in the early morning hours. He was struck and killed by an unknown vehicle and later found lying in the roadway. No witnesses were present, and the police had no leads regarding the suspect vehicle. A gold metallic painted plastic fragment recovered from the scene and the victim's clothing were submitted to the Virginia Department of Forensic Science for analysis.

The victim's clothing was scraped, and several minute gold metallic paint particles were recovered. Most of these particles contained only topcoats, whereas one minute particle contained two primer layers and a limited amount of colorcoat. The color of the primer surface layer was similar to that typically associated with some Fords. Subsequent spectral searches in the Paint Data Query (PDQ) database indicated that the paint most likely originated from a 1990 or newer Ford.

The most discriminating aspect of this paint was the unusual-looking gold metallic topcoat color. A search of automotive repaint books yielded only one color that closely matched the paint recovered in the case. The color, Aztec Gold Metallic, was determined to have been used only on 1997 Ford Mustangs.

The results of the examination were relayed via telephone to the investigating detective. The investigating detective quickly determined that only 11,000 1997 Ford Mustangs were produced in Aztec Gold Metallic. Only two of these vehicles were registered, and had been previously stopped, in the jurisdiction of the offense. Ninety minutes after the make, model, and year information was relayed to the investigator, he called back to say he had located a suspect vehicle. Molding from the vehicle and known paint samples were submitted for comparison. Subsequent laboratory comparisons showed that the painted plastic piece recovered from the scene could be physically fitted together with the molding, and paint recovered from the victim's clothing was consistent with paint samples taken from the suspect vehicle.

Source: Based on information obtained from Brenda Christy, Virginia Department of Forensic Science.

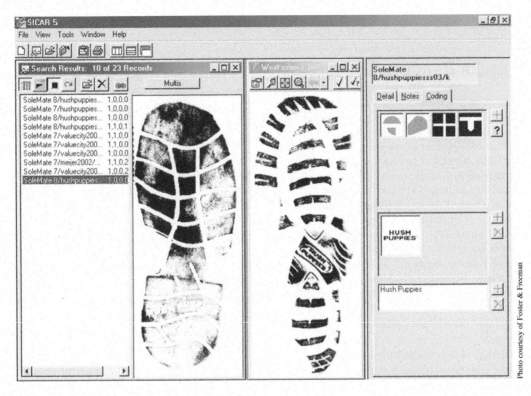

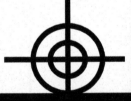

Photo courtesy of Foster & Freeman

FIGURE 3–9
The crime-scene footwear print on the right is being searched against eight thousand sole patterns to determine its make and model.

Chapter Summary > > > > > > > > > > >

Physical evidence is usually examined by a forensic scientist for identification or comparison purposes. The object of identification is to determine the physical or chemical identity with as near absolute certainty as existing analytical techniques will permit. Identification first requires the adoption of testing procedures that give characteristic results for specific standard materials. Once this is done, the examiner uses an appropriate number of tests to identify a substance and exclude all other substances from consideration. The identification process is normally used in crime laboratories to identify drugs, explosives, and petroleum products. Also, evidence such as blood, semen, or hair is routinely identified in a crime laboratory. Normally, these identifications would include a determination for species origin (such as human blood or rabbit hair).

A comparative analysis has the important role of determining whether a suspect specimen and a standard/reference specimen have a common origin. Both the standard/reference specimen and the suspect specimen are subject to the same tests. Evidence that can be associated with a common source with an extremely high degree of probability is said to possess individual characteristics. Evidence associated only with a group is said to have class characteristics. Nevertheless, the high diversity of class evidence in our environment makes their comparison significant in the context of a criminal

investigation. As the number of different objects linking an individual to a crime scene increases, so does the likelihood of that individual's involvement with the crime. Importantly, a person may be exonerated or excluded from suspicion if physical evidence collected at a crime scene is found to be different from standard/reference samples collected from that subject.

A dramatic enhancement of the role of forensic science in criminal investigation has come about through the creation of computerized databases. The Integrated Automated Fingerprint Identification System (IAFIS), a national fingerprint and criminal history system, is maintained by the FBI. The FBI's Combined DNA Index System (CODIS) enables federal, state, and local crime laboratories to electronically exchange and compare DNA profiles, thereby linking crimes to each other and to convicted offenders. The National Integrated Ballistics Information Network (NIBIN), maintained by the Bureau of Alcohol, Tobacco, Firearms and Explosives, allows firearms analysts to acquire, digitize, and compare markings made by a firearm on bullets and cartridge casings recovered from crime scenes. The International Forensic Automotive Paint Data Query (PDQ) database contains chemical and color information pertaining to original automotive paints. SICAR (shoeprint image capture and retrieval) has a comprehensive shoe sole database.

Review Questions

1. The process of _____ determines a substance's physical or chemical identity with as near absolute certainty as existing analytical techniques will permit.

2. The number and type of tests needed to identify a substance must be sufficient to _____ all other substances from consideration.

3. A(n) _____ analysis subjects a suspect specimen and a standard/reference specimen to the same tests and examination in order to determine whether they have a common origin.

4. _____ is the frequency of occurrence of an event.

5. Evidence that can be traced to a common source with an extremely high degree of probability is said to possess _____ characteristics.

6. Evidence associated with a group and not with a single source is said to possess _____ characteristics.

7. True or False: One of the major deficiencies of forensic science is the inability of the examiner to assign exact or approximate probability values to the comparison of most class physical evidence. _____

8. The value of class physical evidence lies in its ability to _____ events with data in a manner that is, as nearly as possible, free of human error and bias.

9. The _____ accorded physical evidence during a trial is left entirely to the trier of fact.

10. Although databases are consistently updated so that scientists can assign probabilities to class evidence, for the most part, forensic scientists must rely on _____ when interpreting the significance of class physical evidence.

11. The believability of _____ accounts, confessions, and informant testimony can all be disputed, maligned, and subjected to severe attack and skepticism in the courtroom.

12. True or False: Physical evidence cannot be used to exclude or exonerate a person from suspicion of committing a crime. _____

13. True or False: The distinction between individual and class evidence is always easy to make. _____

14. True or False: Given the potential weight of scientific evidence in a trial setting, failure to take proper safeguards may unfairly prejudice a case against the suspect. _____

15. Students studying forensic science must be cautioned that merely reading relevant textbooks and journals is no substitute for _____ in this most practical of sciences.

16. Modern analytical techniques have become so sensitive that the forensic examiner must be aware of the _____ among materials when interpreting the significance of comparative data.

17. True or False: A fingerprint can be positively identified through the IAFIS database. _____

18. A database applicable to DNA profiling is _____.

19. The _____ database allows firearm analysts to compare markings made by firearms on bullets that have been recovered from crime scenes.

20. The _____ database contains chemical and color information pertaining to original automotive paints.

Application and Critical Thinking

1. Arrange the following tasks in order from the one that would require the least extensive testing procedure to the one that would require the most extensive. Explain your answer.
   a. Determining whether an unknown substance contains an illicit drug
   b. Determining the composition of an unknown substance
   c. Determining whether an unknown substance contains heroin

2. The following are three possible combinations of DNA characteristics that may be found in an individual's genetic profile. Using the product rule, rank each of these combinations of DNA characteristics from most common to least common. The number after each characteristic indicates its percentage distribution in the population.
   a. FGA 24,24 (3.6%), TH01 6,8 (8.1%), and D16S539 11,12 (8.9%)
   b. vWA 14,19 (6.2%), D21S11 30,30 (3.9%), and D13S317 12,12 (8.5%)
   c. CSF1PO 9,10 (11.2%), D18S51 14,17 (2.8%), and D8S1179 17,18 (6.7%)

3. For each of the following pieces of evidence, indicate whether the item is more likely to possess class or individual characteristics and explain your answers.

   a. An impression from a new automobile tire
   b. A fingerprint
   c. A spent bullet cartridge
   d. A mass-produced synthetic fiber
   e. Pieces of a shredded document
   f. Commercial potting soil
   g. Skin and hair scrapings
   h. Fragments of a multilayer custom automobile paint

4. Which of the forensic databases described in the text contain information that relates primarily to evidence exhibiting class characteristics? Which ones contain information that relates primarily to evidence exhibiting individual characteristics? Explain your answers.

5. An investigator at a murder scene notes signs of a prolonged struggle between the attacker and victim. Name at least three types of physical evidence for which the investigator would probably collect standard/reference samples, and explain why the investigator would collect them.

Further References

Houck, M. M., "Statistics and Trace Evidence: The Tyranny of Numbers," *Forensic Science Communications* 1, no. 3 (1999), https://www.fbi.gov/about-us/lab/forensic-science-communications/fsc/oct1999

Houck, M. M., and J. A. Siegel, *Fundamentals of Forensic Science*, 3rd ed. Burlington, MA: Elsevier Academic Press, 2015.

Osterburg, James W., "The Evaluation of Physical Evidence in Criminalistics: Subjective or Objective Process?" *Journal of Criminal Law, Criminology and Police Science* 60 (1969): 97.

Stoney, D. A., and Paul L. Stoney, "Critical Review of Forensic Trace Evidence Analysis and the Need for a New Approach," *Forensic Science International* 251 (2015): 159.

Chapter 4

Crime-Scene Reconstruction: Bloodstain Pattern Analysis

KEY TERMS

angle of impact
area of convergence
area of origin
backspatter
cast-off
crime-scene
  reconstruction
drip trail pattern
expiration pattern
flows
forward spatter
impact spatter
perimeter stain
projected pattern
satellite stain
spatter pattern
transfer stain
void

Learning Objectives

After studying this chapter, you should be able to:

4.1   Summarize the principles of crime-scene reconstruction and the personnel involved in reconstruction

4.2   Describe the general features of bloodstain formation

4.3   Discuss the methods to determine the area of convergence and area of origin for impact spatter patterns

4.4   Describe how various blood pattern types are created and which features of each pattern can be used to aid in reconstructing events at a crime scene

4.5   Describe the methods for documenting bloodstain patterns at a crime scene

Go to www.pearsonhighered.com/careersresources to access Webextras for this chapter.

The Sam Sheppard Case: A Trail of Blood

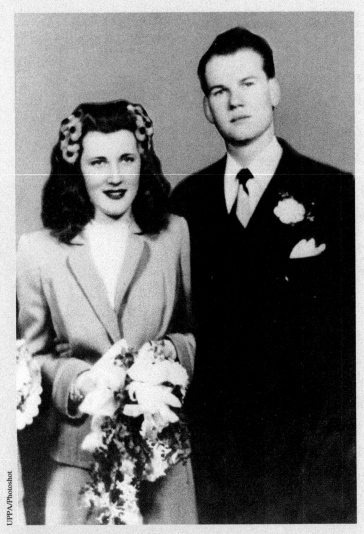

UPPA/Photoshot

Convicted in 1954 of bludgeoning his wife to death,

Dr. Sam Sheppard achieved celebrity status when the storyline of TV's *The Fugitive* was apparently modeled on his efforts to seek vindication for the crime he professed not to have committed. Dr. Sheppard, a physician, claimed he was dozing on his living room couch when his pregnant wife, Marilyn, was attacked. Sheppard's story was that he quickly ran upstairs to stop the carnage but was knocked unconscious briefly by the intruder. The suspicion that fell on Dr. Sheppard was fueled by the revelation that he was having an adulterous affair. At trial, the local coroner testified that a pool of blood on Marilyn's pillow contained the impression of a "surgical instrument." After Sheppard had been imprisoned for 10 years, the U.S. Supreme Court set aside his conviction because of the "massive, pervasive, and prejudicial publicity" that had attended his trial.

In 1966, the second Sheppard trial commenced. This time, the same coroner was forced to back off from his insistence that the bloody outline of a surgical instrument was present on Marilyn's pillow. However, a medical technician from the coroner's office now testified that blood on Dr. Sheppard's watch was from blood spatter, indicating that Dr. Sheppard was wearing the watch in the presence of the battering of his wife. The defense countered with the expert testimony of eminent forensic scientist Dr. Paul Kirk. Dr. Kirk concluded that blood spatter marks in the bedroom showed the killer to be left-handed. Dr. Sheppard was right-handed.

Dr. Kirk further testified that Sheppard stained his watch while attempting to obtain a pulse reading. After less than 12 hours of deliberation, the jury failed to convict Sheppard. But the ordeal had taken its toll. Four years later Sheppard died, a victim of drug and alcohol use.

Crime-Scene Reconstruction

Principles of Crime-Scene Reconstruction

Previous discussions dealing with the processes of identification and comparison have stressed laboratory work routinely performed by forensic scientists. However, there is another dimension to the role that forensic scientists play during the course of a criminal investigation: participating in a team effort to reconstruct events that occurred before, during, and after the commission of a crime.

Law enforcement personnel must take proper action to enhance all aspects of the crime-scene search so as to optimize the crime-scene reconstruction. First, and most important, is securing and protecting the crime scene. Protecting the scene is a continuous endeavor from the beginning to the end of the search. Evidence that can be invaluable to reconstructing the crime can be unknowingly altered or destroyed by people trampling through the scene, rendering the evidence useless. The issue of possible contamination of evidence will certainly be attacked during the litigation process and could make the difference between a guilty and not-guilty verdict.

Before processing the crime scene for physical evidence, the investigator should make a preliminary examination of the scene as it was left by the perpetrator. Each crime scene presents its own set of circumstances. The investigator's experience and the presence or absence of physical evidence become critical factors in reconstructing a crime. The investigator captures the nature of the scene as a whole by performing an initial walk-through of the crime scene. During the walk-through, the investigator's task is to document observations and formulate how the scene should ultimately be processed. As the collection of physical evidence begins, any and all observations should be recorded through photographs, sketches, and notes. By carefully collecting physical evidence and thoroughly documenting the crime scene, the investigator can begin to unravel the sequence of events that took place during the commission of the crime.

Personnel Involved in Reconstruction

Because investigators consider many types of evidence when reconstructing a crime scene, reconstruction is a team effort that involves various professionals putting together many pieces of a puzzle. The team as a whole works to answer the typical "who, what, when, where, why, and how" of a crime scene. Often reconstruction requires the involvement of law enforcement personnel, a medical examiner, and/or a forensic scientist. All of these professionals contribute unique perspectives to develop the crime-scene reconstruction. Was more than one person involved? How was the victim killed? Were actions taken to cover up what took place? The positioning of the victim in a crime scene can often reveal pertinent information for the investigation. Trained medical examiners can examine the victim at a crime scene and determine whether the body has been moved after death by evaluating the livor distribution within the body (see page 114). For example, if livor has developed in areas other than those closest to the ground, the medical examiner can reason that the victim was probably moved after death. Likewise, the examiner can determine whether the victim was clothed after death because livor will not develop in areas of the body that are restricted by clothing.

A forensic scientist or trained crime-scene investigator can also bring special skills to the reconstruction of events that occurred during the commission of a crime. For example, a forensic scientist using a laser beam to plot the approximate bullet path in trajectory analysis can help determine the probable position of the shooter relative to that of the victim (see Figure 4–1). Other skills that a forensic scientist may employ during a crime-scene reconstruction analysis include determining the direction of impact of projectiles penetrating glass objects (see page 243); locating gunshot residues deposited on the victim's clothing for the purpose of estimating the distance of a shooter from a target (see pages 200–202); searching for primer residues deposited on the hands of a suspect shooter (see pages 203–204); and, as we will see from the discussion that follows, analyzing blood spatter patterns.

Crime-scene reconstruction is the method used to support a likely sequence of events at a crime scene by observing and evaluating physical evidence and statements made by individuals involved with the incident. The evidence may also include information obtained from reenactments. Therefore, reconstructions have the best chance of being accurate when investigators use proper documentation and collection methods for all types of evidence.

Physical evidence left behind at a crime scene plays a crucial role in reconstructing the sequence of events surrounding the crime. Although the evidence alone may not describe everything that happened, it can support or contradict accounts given by witnesses and/or suspects.

crime-scene reconstruction
The method used to support a likely sequence of events at a crime scene by the observation and evaluation of physical evidence and statements made by individuals involved with the incident.

FIGURE 4-1

A laser beam is used to determine the search area for the position of a shooter who has fired a bullet through a window and wounded a victim. The bullet path is determined by lining up the victim's bullet wound with the bullet hole present in the glass pane.

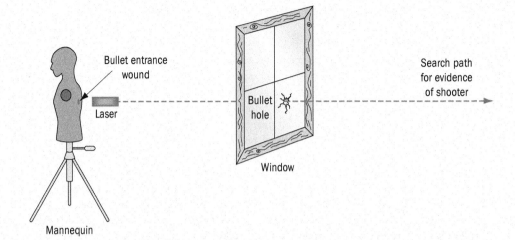

Information obtained from physical evidence can also generate leads and confirm the reconstruction of a crime to a jury. The collection, documentation, and interpretation of physical evidence is the foundation of a reconstruction. Reconstruction develops a likely sequence of events by the observation and evaluation of physical evidence as well as statements made by witnesses and input from those involved with the investigation of the incident. Analysis of all available data will help to create a workable model for reconstruction.

General Features of Bloodstain Formation

Crimes involving violent contact between individuals are frequently accompanied by bleeding and resultant bloodstain patterns. Crime-scene analysts have come to appreciate that bloodstain patterns deposited on floors, walls, ceilings, bedding, and other relevant objects

Case File

Pistorius: A Valentine's Day Murder

Oscar Pistorius overcame leaps and bounds while many others in his position have failed to achieve. Pistorius was a double amputee from the time he was a child; both of his legs had to be removed due to a medical condition he had from birth. Despite his physical disability, Pistorius chased the dream of becoming an Olympic runner. This dream became a reality in 2012, when Pistorius faced able-bodied opponents in the Summer Olympics. Oscar Pistorius has received endless notoriety for his athletic achievement and has been dubbed by the media as the "blade runner."

Pistorius and his super model girlfriend Reeva Steenkamp had been dating for over three months, and according to security logs from Pistorius's gated South African neighborhood, Steenkamp had been staying with him for multiple days. On Valentine's day, 2013, Steenkamp was found lying motionless on the ground, suffering multiple 9 mm pistol wounds to her body and head. Reeva Steenkamp had been shot by Pistorius multiple times through a locked wooden bathroom door. Pistorius claimed that he had fired the shots because he thought there was an intruder in the house. The Olympic runner appeared to be distraught and grieving heavily over his deceased girlfriend. Local South African prosecutors ultimately charged Pistorius with murder due to the circumstances of the event.

During the trial, the prosecution painted a picture of Pistorius as a violent and angry lover. Prosecutors claimed that Steenkamp ran into the bathroom and locked the door to seek protection from a spiteful Pistorius during a heated argument. Detectives placed Steenkamp in a defensive position, crouched behind the bathroom door with her arms and hands crossed in front of her face, as to protect herself from Pistorius. The prosecution also questioned why Pistorius would engage the intruder, rather than grabbing his girlfriend and leaving the residence. The defense called upon the support of Wollie Wolmarans, a ballistics expert, to support Pistorius's account of the incident. According to Wolmarans's reconstruction of the scene, wood splinter marks around Steenkamp's arm proved that she was reaching out to open the door when the incident occurred contrary to the prosecution's account of Steenkamp being crouched and protecting herself in the bathroom.

Oscar Pistorius was found guilty on a charge of culpable homicide, equivalent to manslaughter, after being acquitted of murder in the killing of his girlfriend. The presiding judge ruled that there was not enough evidence to support the contention that Pistorius knew that Steenkamp was behind the toilet door. In 2015, an appeals court overturned the verdict and convicted him of murder. Facing a 15-year jail sentence, Pistorius was sentenced to a jail term of six years.

can provide valuable insights into events that occurred during the commission of a violent crime. The information one may uncover as a result of bloodstain pattern interpretation includes the following:

- The direction from which blood originated
- The angle at which a blood droplet struck a surface
- The location or position of a victim at the time a bloody wound was inflicted
- The movement of a bleeding individual at the crime scene
- The minimum number of blows that struck a bleeding victim
- The approximate location of an individual delivering blows that produced a bloodstain pattern

The crime-scene investigator must not overlook the fact that the location, distribution, and appearance of bloodstains and spatters may be useful for interpreting and reconstructing the events that accompanied the bleeding. A thorough analysis of the significance of the position and shape of blood patterns with respect to their origin and trajectory is exceedingly complex and requires the services of an examiner who is experienced in such determinations. This chapter presents the basic principles and common deductions behind bloodstain pattern analysis to give the reader general knowledge to use at the crime scene.

Surface Texture

Surface texture is of paramount importance in the interpretation of bloodstain patterns; comparisons between standards and unknowns are valid only when identical surfaces are used. In general, harder and nonporous surfaces (such as glass or smooth tile) result in less spatter. Rough surfaces, such as a concrete floor or wood, usually result in irregularly shaped stains with serrated edges, possibly with **satellite stain** (see Figure 4–2).

Direction and Angle of Impact

An investigator may discern the direction of travel of blood that struck an object by studying the stain's shape. As the stain becomes more elliptical in shape, its direction becomes more discernible because the pointed end of a bloodstain faces its direction of travel. The distorted or disrupted edge of an elongated stain indicates the direction of travel of the blood drop. Satellite stain around parent stains will have the pointed end facing against the direction of travel. In Figure 4–3, the bloodstain pattern was produced by several drops of blood that were traveling from left to right before striking a flat, level surface.

It is possible to determine the impact angle of blood on a flat surface by measuring the degree of circular distortion of the stain. A drop deposited at an **angle of impact** of about 90 degrees (directly vertical to the surface) will be approximately circular in shape with no tail or

satellite stain
A smaller bloodstain that originated during the formation of the parent stain as a result of blood impacting a surface.

angle of impact
The angle (alpha), relative to the plane of a target, at which a blood drop strikes the target.

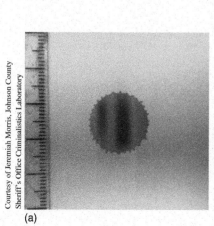

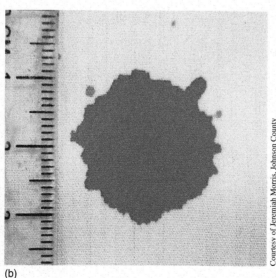

FIGURE 4–2
(a) A bloodstain from a single drop of blood that struck a paper surface after falling.
(b) A bloodstain from a single drop of blood that struck a cotton muslin sheet after falling.

(a)   (b)

FIGURE 4–3
A bloodstain pattern produced by drops of blood that were traveling from right to left.

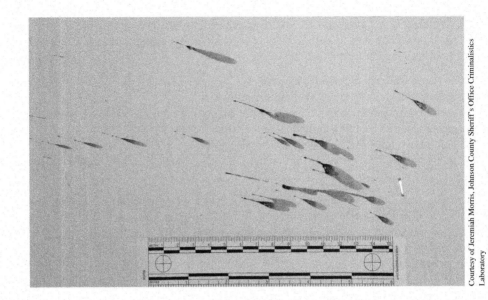

Courtesy of Jeremiah Morris, Johnson County Sheriff's Office Criminalistics Laboratory

WEBEXTRA 4.1
See How Bloodstain Spatter Patterns Are Formed

spatter pattern
A bloodstain resulting from an airborne blood drop created when external force is applied to liquid blood.

impact spatter
A bloodstain pattern resulting from an object striking liquid blood.

forward spatter
A bloodstain pattern resulting from blood drops that can be produced when a projectile creates an exit wound.

backspatter
A bloodstain pattern resulting from blood drops that can be produced when a projectile creates an entrance wound.

buildup of blood. However, as the angle of impact deviates from 90 degrees, the stain becomes elongated in shape. Buildup of blood will occur when the angles are larger, whereas longer and longer tails will appear as the angle of impact becomes smaller (see Figure 4–4).

Bloodstain Spatter Patterns

A **spatter pattern** is a bloodstain resulting from an airborne blood drop created when external force is applied to liquid blood. The most common type of bloodstain pattern found at a crime scene is **impact spatter**. This pattern occurs when an object impacts the source of the blood. Spatter projected outward and away from the source, such as an exit wound, is called **forward spatter**. **Backspatter**, sometimes called *blow-back spatter*, is blood projected backward from a source, such as an entrance wound, and potentially deposited on the object or person who created the impact. Impact spatter patterns consist of many drops radiating in direct lines from the origin of blood to the stained surface (see Figure 4–5).

In general, as the velocity of the force of the impact on the source of blood increases, so does the velocity of the blood drops emanating from the source. It is also generally true that as both the force and velocity of impact increase, the diameter of the resulting blood drops decreases.

FIGURE 4–4
A single drop of human blood that fell and struck hard, smooth cardboard. On this drop the edge characteristics show the direction.

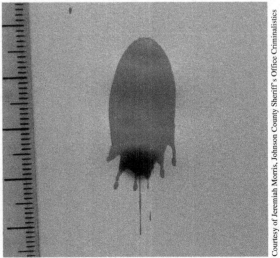

Courtesy of Jeremiah Morris, Johnson County Sheriff's Office Criminalistics Laboratory

FIGURE 4–5
Spatter produced by an automatic weapon.

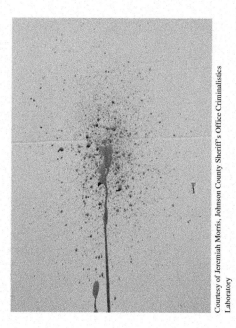

Courtesy of Jeremiah Morris, Johnson County Sheriff's Office Criminalistics Laboratory

Classifying Impact Pattern

In the past, bloodstain analysts used to interpret the droplet size of a bloodstain pattern to classify impact patterns by velocity. Because general principles of fluid dynamics apply to bloodstains, analysts knew generally what type of force was required to create droplets of varying size. However, the classifications of low, medium, and high velocity cannot illuminate the specific events that produced the stain pattern. For example, beatings can produce either high-velocity spatter or stain sizes that look more like low-velocity spatter. The existence of the low, medium, and high classifications only proved problematic for modern bloodstain pattern interpretation because these designations lend themselves, intentionally or unintentionally, to inferences about the type of velocity or mechanism used to create the stain. Forensic scientists have no way of determining the velocity of the object that created the stains or the velocity of the droplets themselves prior to contacting the target surface. As such, these references are no longer recommended by guidance bodies in the field. Proper interpretation for an

Inside the Science

Determining the Angle of Impact of Bloodstains

The distorted or disrupted edge of an elongated stain indicates the direction of travel of the blood drop. One may establish the location or origin of bloodshed by determining the directionality of the stain and the angle at which blood came into contact with the landing surface. To determine the angle of impact, calculate the stain's length-to-width ratio and apply the formula

$$\sin A = \frac{\text{width of blood stain}}{\text{length of blood stain}}$$

where A = the angle of impact.

For example, suppose the width of a stain is 11 mm and the length is 22 mm.

$$\sin A = \frac{11 \text{ mm}}{22 \text{ mm}} = 0.50$$

A scientific calculator with trigonometric functions will calculate that a sine of 0.50 corresponds to a 30-degree angle.

Note: The measurements for length and width should be made with a ruler, micrometer, or photographic loupe.

FIGURE 4–6

The action associated with producing an impact pattern.

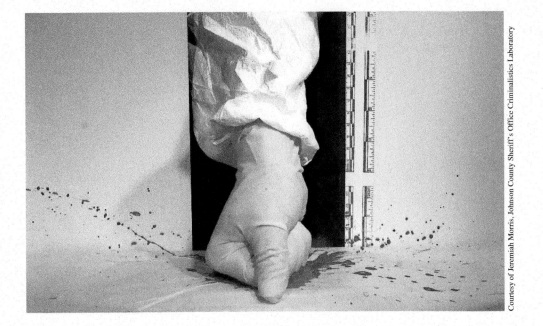

impact pattern should encompass observations of stain size, shape, location, and distribution without any references to the force or mechanism that might have been used to create it.

Blood spatter patterns can arise from a number of distinctly different sources, which will be discussed in this chapter. Illustrations of patterns emanating from impact, cast-off, and projected pattern are shown in Figure 4–6.

FIGURE 4–7

An illustration of stain convergence. Convergence represents the area from which the stains emanated.

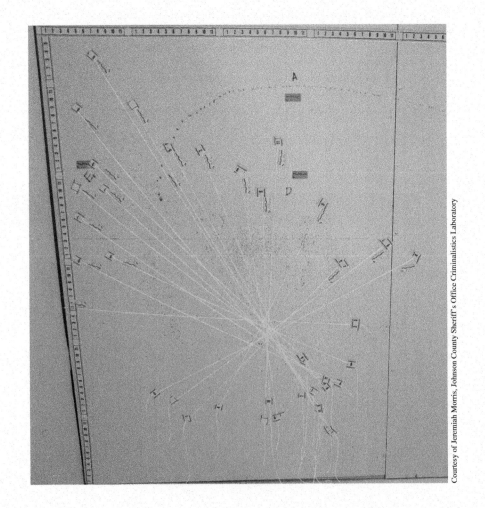

Origin of Impact Patterns

Impact spatter patterns can offer investigators clues about the origin of the blood spatter and, therefore, the position of the victim at the time of the impact.

AREA OF CONVERGENCE   The **area of convergence** is the location on a two-dimensional plane from which the drops originated. This can be established by drawing straight lines through the long axis of several individual bloodstains, following the line of their tails. The intersection of these lines is the area of convergence. Figure 4–7 illustrates how to draw lines to find an area of convergence.

AREA OF ORIGIN   It may also be important to determine the **area of origin** of a bloodstain pattern, the area in a three-dimensional space from which the blood was projected. This will show the position of the individual in space when the stain-producing event took place. Impact patterns produced at a distance close to the surface will appear as clustered stains. As the distance from the surface increases, so do the distribution and distance between drops.

A common method for determining the area of origin at the crime scene is called the *string method*. The steps of the string method are as follows:

1. Find the area of convergence for the stain pattern.
2. Place a pole or stand as an axis coming from the area of convergence.
3. Attach one end of a string next to each droplet. Place a protractor next to each droplet and lift the string until it lines up with the determined angle of impact of the drop. Keeping the string in line with the angle, attach the other end of the string to the axis pole.
4. View the area of origin of the drops where the strings appear to meet. Secure the strings at this area.

area of convergence
The space in two dimensions to which the directionalities of spatter stains can be retraced to determine the location of the spatter-producing event.

area of origin
The space in three dimensions to which the trajectories of spatter can be utilized to determine the location of the spatter-producing event.

WEBEXTRA 4.2
Blood Stain Analysis: Calculating the Area of Convergence and Origin

More Bloodstain Spatter Patterns

Gunshot Spatter

A shooting may leave a distinct gunshot spatter pattern. This may be characterized by both forward spatter from an exit wound and backspatter from an entrance wound. The presence of backspatter on a firearm or a shooter is dependent on the distance, wound location, caliber, and intermediate objects like hair or clothing between the firearm and victim. Forward spatter generally leaves a pattern of very fine drops (see Figure 4–8). Medium- and large-sized drops may also be observed within the spatter pattern.

The location of injury, the size of the wound created, and the distance between the victim and the muzzle of the weapon all affect the amount of backspatter that occurs. Finding spatter

Courtesy of Jeremiah Morris, Johnson County Sheriff's Office Criminalistics Laboratory

FIGURE 4–8
A forward spatter pattern.

from a gunshot wound containing the victim's blood on a suspect can help investigators place the suspect in the vicinity when the gun was discharged. Backspatter created by a gunshot injury generally contains fewer and smaller atomized stains than does forward spatter. Muzzle gases push the blood droplets back toward the wound.

Depending on the distance from the victim at which the gun was discharged, some backspatter may strike the gunman and enter the gun muzzle. This is called the *drawback effect*. Blood within the muzzle of a gun can "place" the weapon in the vicinity of the gunshot wound. The presence of blow-backspatter on a weapon's muzzle is consistent with the weapon's having been close to the victim at the time of firing.

Cast-Off Spatter

cast-off
A bloodstain pattern that is created when blood is flung from a blood-bearing object in motion onto a surface.

A **cast-off** pattern is created when a blood-covered object flings blood in an arc onto a nearby surface. This kind of pattern commonly occurs when a person pulls a bloody fist or weapon back between delivering blows to a victim (see Figure 4–9). The bloodstain tails will point in the direction that the object was moving.

The width of the cast-off pattern created by a bloody object may help suggest the kind of object produced by the pattern. The sizes of the drops are directly related to the size of the point from which they were propelled (Figure 4–9). Drops propelled from a small or pointed surface will be smaller and the pattern more linear; drops propelled from a large or blunt surface will be larger and the pattern wide. The volume of blood deposited on an object from the source also affects the size and number of drops in the cast-off pattern. The less blood on the object, the smaller the stains produced. The pattern may also suggest whether the blow that caused the pattern was directed from right to left or left to right. The pattern will point in the direction of the backward thrust, which will be opposite the direction of the blow. This could suggest which hand the assailant used to deliver the blows.

Cast-off patterns may also show the *minimum* number of blows delivered to a victim. Each blow should be marked by an upward-and-downward or forward-and-backward arc pattern (see Figure 4–9). By counting and pairing the patterns, one can estimate the minimum number of blows. An investigator should take into consideration that the first blow would only cause blood to pool to the area; it would not produce a cast-off pattern. Also, some blows may not come into contact with blood and therefore will not produce a pattern. The medical examiner is in the best position to estimate the number of blows a victim received.

Case Files

Blood-Spatter Evidence

Stephen Scher banged on the door of a cabin in the woods outside Montrose, Pennsylvania. According to Scher, his friend, Marty Dillon, had just shot himself while chasing after a porcupine. The two had been skeet shooting at Scher's cabin, enjoying a friendly sporting weekend, when Dillon spotted a porcupine and took off out of sight. Scher heard a single shot and waited to hear his friend's voice. After a few moments, he chased after Dillon and found him lying on the ground near a tree stump, bleeding from a wound in his chest. Scher administered CPR after locating his dying friend, but he was unable to save Dillon, who later died from his injuries. Police found that Dillon's untied boot had been the cause of his shotgun wound. They determined that he had tripped while running with his loaded gun and shot himself. The grief-stricken Scher aroused no suspicion, so the shooting was ruled an accident.

Shortly thereafter, Scher moved from the area, divorced his wife, and married Dillon's widow. This was too suspicious to be ignored; police reopened the case and decided to reconstruct the crime scene. The reconstruction provided investigators with several pieces of blood evidence that pointed to Scher as Dillon's murderer.

Police noticed that Scher's boots bore the unmistakable spatter stains, evidence that he was standing near Dillon when Dillon was shot. This pattern of bloodstains would not be expected to be created while administering CPR, as Scher claimed had happened. The spatter pattern also clearly refuted Scher's claim that he did not witness the incident. In addition, the tree stump near Dillon's body bore the same type of blood spatter, in a pattern that indicated Dillon was *seated on the stump* and not running when he was shot. Finally, Dillon's ears were free of spatter stains that covered his face, but blood was on his hearing protectors found nearby. This is a clear indication that he was wearing his hearing protectors when he was shot and they were removed before investigators arrived. This and other evidence resulted in Scher's conviction for the murder of his longtime friend, Marty Dillon.

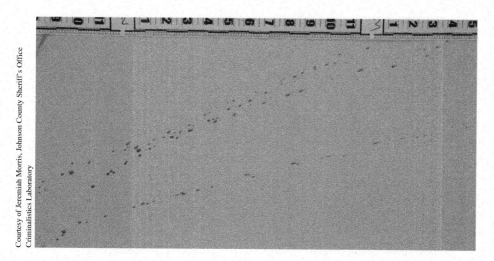

Courtesy of Jeremiah Morris, Johnson County Sheriff's Office Criminalistics Laboratory

FIGURE 4–9
Swing was lower left to upper right. Cast offs depend entirely on the weapon's ability to acquire and hold blood, how the swing is achieved, and where in space the victim is located for the blows to be struck.

Projected Pattern

Projected pattern is created when a victim suffers an injury to a main artery or the heart. The pressure of the continuing pumping of blood causes blood to spurt out of the injured area (see Figure 4–10). Commonly, the pattern shows large spurted stains for each time the heart pumps. Some radial spikes, satellite spatter, or flow patterns may be evident because of the large volume of blood being expelled with each spurt. Drops may also be seen on the surface in fairly uniform size and shape and in parallel arrangement (see Figure 4–10).

The lineup of the stains shows the victim's movement. Any vertical arcs or waves in the line show fluctuations in blood pressure. The site of the initial injury to the artery can be found where the pattern begins with the biggest spurt. Arterial patterns can also be differentiated because the oxygenated blood spurting from the artery tends to be a brighter red color than blood expelled from impact wounds. This may not be seen at crime scenes with dry blood present.

projected pattern
A bloodstain pattern resulting from the ejection of blood under hydraulic pressure, typically from a breach in the circulatory system.

Expiration Patterns

A pattern created by blood that is expelled from the mouth or nose from an internal injury is called an **expiration pattern**. If the blood that creates such a pattern is under great pressure, it produces very fine spatter. Expired blood at very low velocities produces a stain cluster with irregular edges (see Figure 4–11). The presence of bubbles in the drying drops can differentiate a pattern created by expired blood from other types of bloodstains. Expired blood also may be lighter in color than impact spatter as a result of being diluted by saliva. The presence of expirated blood gives an important clue to the injuries suffered and the events that took place at a crime scene.

expiration pattern
A bloodstain pattern resulting from blood forced by airflow out of the nose, mouth, or a wound.

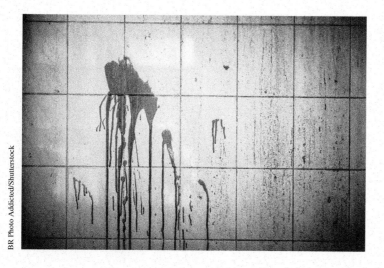

BR Photo Addicted/Shutterstock

FIGURE 4–10
A projected pattern found at a crime scene where a victim suffered injury to an artery.

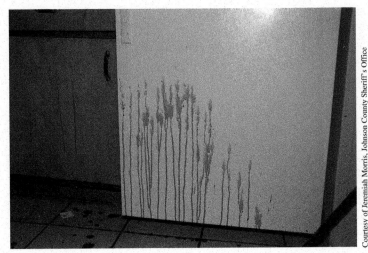

FIGURE 4–11
An example of blood expelled with two wheezes from the mouth.

Void Patterns

void
An absence of blood in an otherwise continuous bloodstain or bloodstain pattern.

A **void** is created when an object blocks the deposition of blood spatter onto a surface or object (see Figure 4–12). It can also be created by limiting angles. The spatter is deposited onto the object or person instead. The blank space on the surface or object may give a clue to the size and shape of the missing object or person. Once the object or person is found, the missing piece of the pattern should fit in, much like a puzzle piece, with the rest of the pattern. Voids may help establish the body position of the victim or assailant at the time of the incident.

Other Bloodstain Patterns

Not all bloodstains at a crime scene appear as spatter patterns. The circumstances of the crime often create other types of stains that can be useful to investigators.

Contact/Transfer Stains

transfer stain
A bloodstain resulting from contact between a blood-bearing surface and another surface.

When an object with blood on it touches another object that did not have blood on it, this produces a contact or **transfer stain**. Examples of transfers with features include fingerprints (see Figure 4–13), handprints, footprints, footwear prints, tool prints, and fabric prints in blood. These may provide further leads by offering individual characteristics.

The size and general shape of a tool may be seen in a simple transfer. This can lead to narrowing the possible tools by class characteristics. A transfer that shows a very individualistic feature may help point to the tool that made the pattern.

Simple transfer stains are produced when the bloody object makes contact with a surface and the object is removed without any further movement. Other transfers known as *wipe patterns* may be

FIGURE 4–12
A void pattern is found behind the door where the surface of the door blocked the deposition of spatter on that area. This void, and the presence of spatter on the door, shows that the door was open when the spatter was deposited.

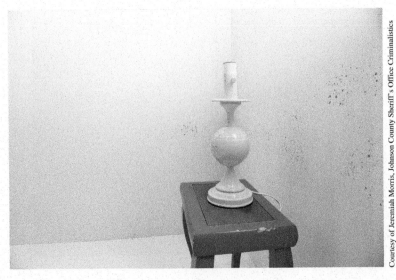

FIGURE 4–13
A transfer stain consisting of bloody fingerprints with apparent ridge detail.

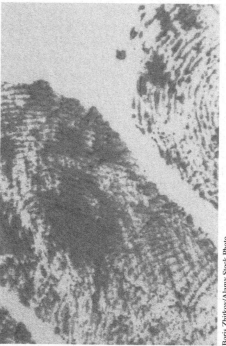

Boris Zhitkov/Alamy Stock Photo

caused by movement of the bloody object across a surface. The pattern may lighten and "feather" as the pattern moves away from the initial contact point (see Figure 4–14). However, because "feathering" is also a function of the amount of pressure being applied to the surface, the analyst must interpret directionality with care. The direction of separate bloody transfers, such as footwear prints in blood, may show the movement of the suspect, victim, or others through the crime scene after the blood was present. The first transfer stain in a series will be dark and heavy with blood, whereas subsequent transfers will be increasingly lighter in color. The transfers get lighter as less and less blood is deposited from the transferring object's surface. Bloody shoe imprints may also suggest whether the wearer was running or walking. Running typically produces imprints with more space between them.

Flows

Patterns made by drops or large amounts of blood flowing with the pull of gravity are called **flows**. Flows may be formed by single drops or large volumes of blood coming from an actively bleeding wound or blood deposited on a surface—from a projected pattern, for example.

flow
A bloodstain resulting from the movement of a volume of blood on a surface due to gravity or movement of the target.

FIGURE 4–14
A wipe pattern.

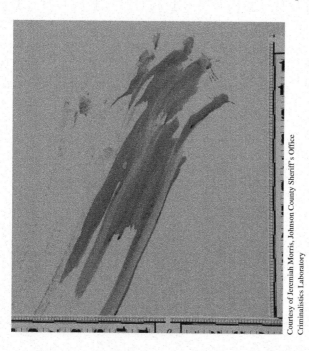

Courtesy of Jeremiah Morris, Johnson County Sheriff's Office Criminalistics Laboratory

The flow direction may show movements of objects or bodies while the flow was still in progress or after the blood had dried. Figure 4–15 illustrates a situation in which movement of the surface while the flow was still in progress led to a specific pattern.

Interruption of a flow pattern may be helpful in assessing the sequence and passage of time between the flow and its interruption. If a flow found on an object or body does not appear to be consistent with the direction of gravity, one may surmise that the object or body was moved after the flow was created.

Pools

A pool of blood occurs when blood collects in a level (not sloped) and undisturbed place. Blood that pools on an absorbent surface may be absorbed throughout the surface and diffuse, creating a pattern larger than the original pool. This often occurs to pools on beds or sofas.

The approximate drying time of a pool of blood is related to the environmental condition of the scene, the surface, and the location of the injury. By experimentation, an analyst may be able to estimate the drying times of stains of different sizes. Small and large pools of blood can be helpful in reconstruction because they can be analyzed to estimate the amount of time that has elapsed since the blood was deposited. Considering the drying time of a blood pool can yield information about the timing of events that accompanied the incident.

perimeter stain
An altered stain consisting of its edge characteristics, the central area having been partially or entirely removed.

The edges of a stain will dry to the surface, producing a **perimeter stain** (see Figure 4–16). This usually occurs within 50 seconds of deposition for drops, and it takes longer for larger volumes of blood. If the central area of the pooled bloodstain is then altered by wiping, the perimeter will be left intact. This can be used to interpret whether movement or activity occurred shortly after the pool was deposited or later, after the perimeter had time to dry first. This may be important for classifying the source of the original stain.

Drip Trail Patterns

drip trail pattern
A bloodstain pattern resulting from a liquid that dripped into another liquid, at least one of which was blood.

A **drip trail pattern** is a series of drops that is separate from other patterns, and it is formed by blood dripping off an object or injury. The stains form a kind of line, usually the path made by the suspect after injuring or killing the victim. It may simply show movement, lead to a discarded weapon, or provide identification of the suspect if it is made from the suspect's own blood. Investigators often see this type of pattern in stabbings during which individuals who commit a crime inadvertently cut themselves as a result of using the force necessary to stab the victim. Figure 4–17 shows a drop trail pattern away from the center of action at a crime scene.

FIGURE 4–15
The image below shows a flow pattern.

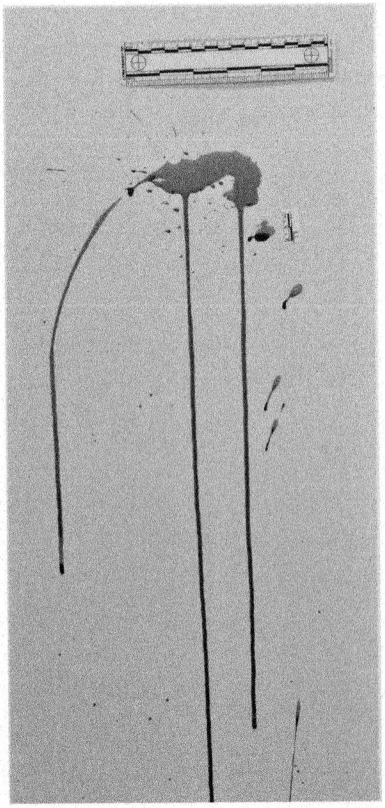

Courtesy of Jeremiah Morris, Johnson County Sheriff's Office Criminalistics Laboratory

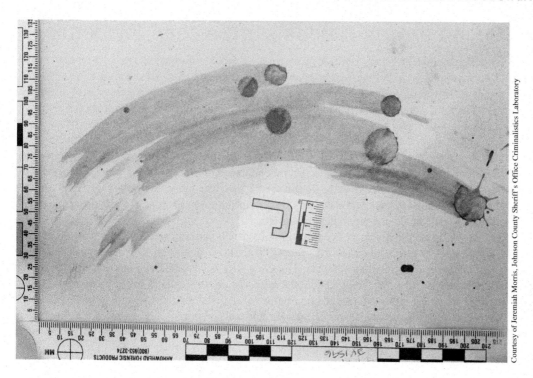

Courtesy of Jeremiah Morris, Johnson County Sheriff's Office Criminalistics Laboratory

FIGURE 4–16
A perimeter stain is shown in a bloodstain that was disturbed after the edges had time to dry.

The shape of the stains in a drip trail pattern can help investigators determine the direction and speed at which a person was moving. The tails of the drops in a trail pattern point in the direction the person was moving. More circular stains are found where the person was moving slowly. This information may be helpful in reconstruction.

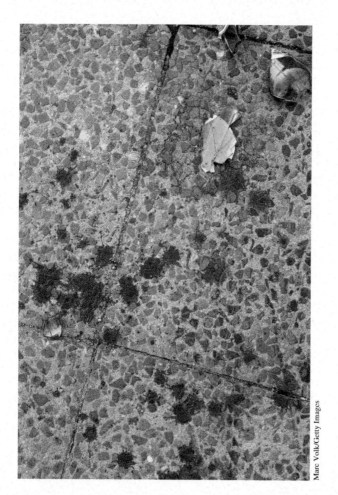

Marc Volk/Getty Images

FIGURE 4–17
This is an example of a drip trail pattern from a crime scene.

Documenting Bloodstain Pattern Evidence

Blood spatter patterns of any kind can provide a great deal of information about the events that took place at a crime scene. For this reason, investigators should note, study, and photograph each pattern and drop. This must be done to accurately record the location of specific patterns and to distinguish the stains from which laboratory samples were taken. The photographs and sketches can also point out specific stains used in determining the direction of force, angle of impact, and area of origin.

Just as in general crime-scene photography, the investigator should create photographs and sketches of the overall pattern to show the orientation of the pattern to the scene. The medium-range documentation should include pictures and sketches of the whole pattern and the relationships between individual stains within the pattern. The close-up photographs and sketches should show the dimensions of each individual stain. Close-up photographs should be taken with a scale of some kind showing in the photograph.

Two common methods of documenting bloodstain patterns place attention on the scale of the patterns. The *grid method* involves setting up a grid of squares of known dimensions over the entire pattern using string and stakes (see Figure 4–18). All overall, medium-range, and close-up photographs are taken with and without the grid. The second method, called the *perimeter ruler method*, involves setting up a rectangular border of rulers around the pattern. In this method, the large rulers show scale in the overall and medium-range photos, whereas the small rulers can be inserted to show scale in the close-up photographs (see Figure 4–19). Some investigation teams use tags in close-up photographs to show evidence numbers or other details.

An area-of-origin determination may be calculated at the discretion of the bloodstain analyst when the circumstances of the case warrant such a determination. All measurements of stains and calculations of angle of impact and point of origin should be recorded in crime-scene notes. Especially important stains can be roughly sketched within the notes.

Only some jurisdictions have a specialist on staff to decipher patterns either at the scene or from photographs at the lab. Therefore, it is important that all personnel be familiar with patterns to properly record and document them for use in reconstruction.

Bloodstain Pattern Analysis: Proceed with Caution

The field of bloodstain pattern analysis has proliferated within the forensic science community, as well as with practitioners who pride themselves as being called crime scene investigators. Within the law enforcement community, there are hundreds of investigators (not necessarily scientists) who are proud to be labeled blood spatter specialists. At this point in time, there is no measurement to judge the uniformity of training in this field within the United States. The closest training criteria stems from the Bloodstain Pattern Analysis Cortication program offered under the auspices of the International Association of Bloodstain Pattern Analysis. The certificate requires a minimum of 40 hours of education in an approved workshop. A minimum of three years of practice within the discipline of bloodstain pattern identification augments the classroom training. Under the best of circumstances, following the successful completion of the certificate requirements, many law enforcement agencies find it appropriate to insert these individuals into the crime-scene investigation process.

The complexity of blood spatter interpretation runs the gamut from the simple to the complex. What should be worrisome to the forensic science community and the judicial system is the apparent absence of uniformity in imposing quality assurance standards on interpreting bloodstain patterns. The forensic science community is already reeling from adverse and embarrassing publicity arising from the misidentification of fingerprints, bullet lead, bite mark impressions, and hair evidence. Warnings are already being clearly and loudly sounded about the error rates associated with bloodstain pattern analysis. In a series of studies sponsored by the National Institute of Justice (NIJ), very high error rates for blunt instrument spatter patterns in the range of 37 percent have been reported:[1] Where a bloodstain pattern classification was required, 13.1 percent of these classifications did not include the correct pattern for rigid surfaces and 23.4 percent for fabric surfaces.[2] Another NIJ study has demonstrated that fabrics

[1]William Ristenpart et al., Quantitative Analysis of High Velocity Bloodstain Patters (2013), available at http://www.ncjrs.gov/pdffiles1/nij/grants/241744.pdf

[2]Terry Laber et al., National Institute of Justice, Final Report, Reliability Assessment of Current Methods in Bloodstain Pattern Analysis (2014), available at http://www.ncjrs.gov/pdffiles1/nij/grants/247180.pdf

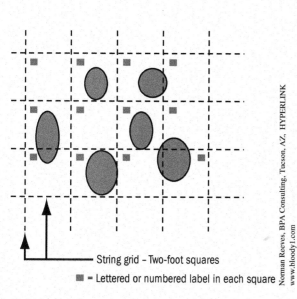

String grid – Two-foot squares

■ = Lettered or numbered label in each square

Norman Reeves, BPA Consulting, Tucson, AZ, HYPERLINK www.bloody1.com

FIGURE 4–18

The grid method may be used for photographing bloodstain pattern evidence.

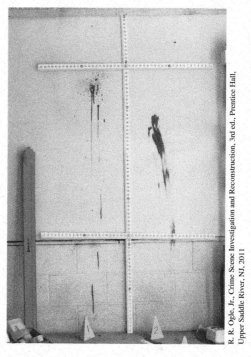

R. R. Ogle, Jr., Crime Scene Investigation and Reconstruction, 3rd ed., Prentice Hall, Upper Saddle River, NJ, 2011

FIGURE 4–19

A drip trail pattern leads away from the center of the mixed bloodstain pattern.

may interact to, distort, and alter a bloodstain pattern in many different and complex ways compared to bloodstains on hard surfaces.[3]

Given the highly subjective nature of bloodstain pattern interpretation and its potential significant error rate, a process of independent assessment of any bloodstain pattern interpretation by two or more examiners at the crime scene and in the laboratory is desirable.[4, 5] The "Analysis, Comparison and Evaluation-Verification" (ACE-V) process utilized by fingerprint examiners (p. 136) may serve as a useful model for general advisory guidance in bloodstain pattern evidence verification.

> > > > > > > > > > >

Case Files

Bloodstain Reconstruction

An older male was found lying dead on his living room floor. He had been beaten about the face and head, and then stabbed in the chest and robbed. The reconstruction of bloodstains found on the interior front door and the adjacent wall documented that the victim was beaten about the face with a fist and struck on the back of the head with his cane. A three-dimensional diagram and photograph illustrating the evidential bloodstain patterns is shown in Figures 1(a) and 1(b).

A detailed photograph of bloodstains next to the interior door is shown in Figure 2. Arrow 1 in Figure 2 points to the cast-off pattern directed left to right as blood was flung from the perpetrator's fist while inflicting blows. Arrow 2 in Figure 2 points to three transfer impression patterns directed left to right as the perpetrator's bloodstained hand contacted the wall and as the fist blows were being inflicted on the victim. Arrow 3 in Figure 2 points to blood flow from the victim's wounds as he slumped against the wall.

Figure 3 contains a series of laboratory test patterns created to evaluate the patterns contained within Figure 2.

(continued)

---

[3]Stephen Michielsen et al., Bloodstain Patterns on Textile Surfaces: A Fundamental Analysis (2015), available at http://www.ncjrs.gov/pdffiles1/nij/grants/248671.pdf

[4]The Forensic Science Regulator, Codes of Practice and Conduct: Bloodstain Pattern Analysis, FSR-C-102. Birmingham: Office (2015), available at https://www.gov.uk/government/uploads/system/uploads/attachment_data/file/484905/C102_Bloodstain_Pattern_Analysis_2015.pdf.

[5]Rachel Zajac et al., "Contextual Bias: What Bloodstain Pattern Analysts Need to Know," *Journal of Bloodstain Pattern Analysis* 31 (2015): 7.

FIGURE 1A
A three-dimensional diagram illustrating blood-stain patterns that were located, documented, and reconstructed.

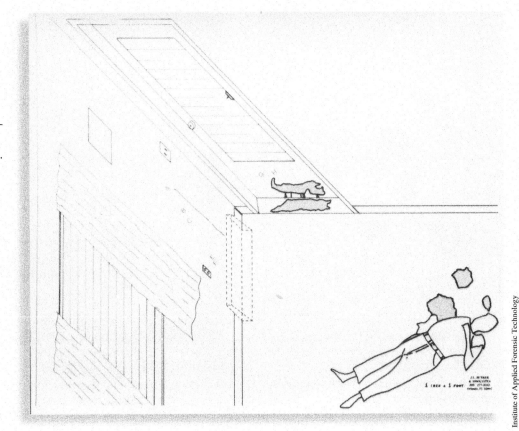

Institute of Applied Forensic Technology

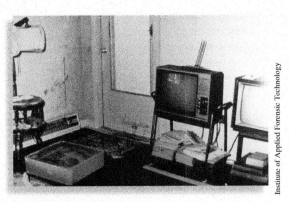

Institute of Applied Forensic Technology

FIGURE 1B
A crime-scene photograph of bloodstained areas.

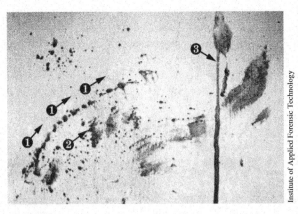

Institute of Applied Forensic Technology

FIGURE 2
Positions of impact spatter from blows that were inflicted on the victim's face.

Figure 4 shows how the origin of individual impact spatter patterns located on the wall and door and emanating from the bleeding victim can be documented by the determination of separate areas of convergence.

A suspect was apprehended three days later, and he was found to have an acute fracture of the right hand. When he was confronted with the bloodstain evidence, the suspect admitted striking the victim, first with his fist, then with a cane, and finally stabbing him with a kitchen knife. The suspect pleaded guilty to three first-degree felonies.

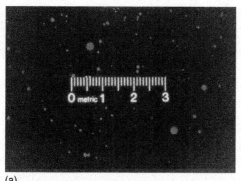

(a)

Institute of Applied Forensic Technology

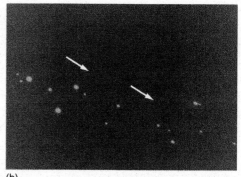

(b)

Institute of Applied Forensic Technology

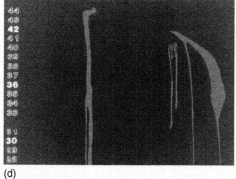

(d)

Institute of Applied Forensic Technology

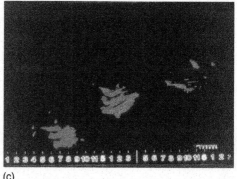

(c)

Institute of Applied Forensic Technology

FIGURE 3

(a) A laboratory test pattern showing an impact spatter. The size and shape of the stains demonstrate a forceful impact 90 degrees to the target. (b) A laboratory test pattern illustrating a cast-off pattern directed left to right from an overhead swing. (c) A laboratory test pattern showing a repetitive transfer impression pattern produced by a bloodstained hand moving left to right across the target. (d) A laboratory test pattern illustrating vertical flow patterns. The left pattern represents a stationary source; the right pattern was produced by left-to-right motion.

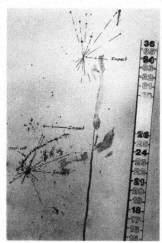

(a) Patterns A, B, C

Institute of Applied Forensic Technology

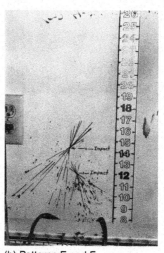

(b) Patterns E and F

Institute of Applied Forensic Technology

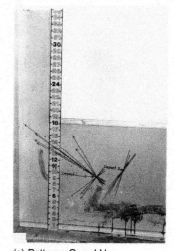

(c) Patterns G and H

Institute of Applied Forensic Technology

FIGURE 4

(a) A convergence of impact spatter patterns associated with beating with a fist. (b) The convergence of impact spatter associated with the victim falling to the floor while bleeding from the nose. (c) The convergence of impact spatter associated with the victim while face down at the door, being struck with a cane.

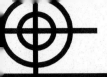

Chapter Summary >>>>>>>>>>>>

Physical evidence left behind at a crime scene, properly handled and preserved, plays a crucial role in reconstructing the events that took place surrounding the crime. Crime-scene reconstruction relies on the combined efforts of medical examiners, forensic scientists, and law enforcement personnel to recover physical evidence and to sort out the events surrounding the occurrence of a crime.

The location, distribution, and appearance of bloodstains and spatters may be useful for interpreting and reconstructing the events that produced the bleeding. An investigator or bloodstain pattern analyst can decipher from individual bloodstains the directionality and angle of impact of the blood when it impacted the surface of deposition. In addition, bloodstain patterns, consisting of many individual bloodstains, may convey to the analyst the location of victims or suspects, the movement of bleeding individuals, and the number of blows delivered.

Surface texture and an individual stain's shape, size, and location must be considered when determining the direction and angle of impact of the bloodstain. Surface texture can greatly affect the shape of a bloodstain. The directionality of an individual bloodstain may be shown by the stain's tail or the accumulation of blood because the tail or accumulation appears on the side opposite the force. The angle of impact of a bloodstain can be approximated by the shape of the bloodstain, or it can be more effectively estimated using the width-to-length ratio of the stain.

An impact spatter pattern occurs when an object impacts a source of blood, producing forward spatter projected forward from the source and backspatter projected backward from the source. The area of convergence of an impact spatter pattern is the area the individual stains emanated from on a two-dimensional plane. The area of origin of a bloodstain pattern in three-dimensional space may represent the position of the victim or suspect when the stain-producing event took place.

Gunshot spatter consists of very fine spatter originating from both forward spatter from an exit wound and backspatter from an entrance wound, or only backspatter if the bullet did not exit the body. Blood cast off from an object, typically a weapon or fist between delivering blows to a victim, may form an arc pattern on a nearby surface. The features of the pattern can suggest the kind of object that created it and the minimum number of blows delivered by the object. The characteristic spurts present in a projected pattern are created by the continuing pumping of blood from an arterial injury. Expired blood expelled from the mouth or nose may at first appear to have very fine droplets or very large droplets. It may feature bubbles of oxygen in the drying drops or possibly be mixed with saliva. A void, where an object (or person) blocks the deposition of blood spatter onto a target surface or object, may give a clue as to the size and shape of the missing object or person.

Transfer stains, created when an object with blood on it makes simple contact with a surface, may reveal the shape or texture characteristics of the object. Because the direction of flows originating from either a single drop or a large amount of blood is caused by gravity, the direction of a pattern may suggest the original position of the surface when the flow was formed. A drip trail pattern shows a path of drops separate from other patterns; it is formed by single blood drops dripping off an object or injury. The presence of the perimeter of a bloodstain suggests that the stain was disturbed after the edges had had sufficient time to dry.

The precise appearance and location of each bloodstain at a crime scene is important. Therefore, each bloodstain pattern located at a crime scene must be properly documented in notes, photographs, and sketches. Medium-range and close-up photographs should be recorded using either the grid method or the perimeter ruler method to show the orientation and relative size of the pattern and individual stains.

Review Questions

1. _____ is the method used to support a likely sequence of events at a crime scene by the observation and evaluation of physical evidence and statements made by individuals involved with the incident.

2. Reconstructing the circumstances of a crime scene is a team effort that may include the help of law enforcement personnel, medical examiners, and _____.

3. Violent contact between individuals at a crime scene frequently produces bleeding and results in the formation of _____.

4. The proper interpretation of bloodstain patterns necessitates carefully planned _____ using surface materials comparable to those found at the crime scene.

5. Bloodstain patterns may convey to the analyst the location and movements of _____ or _____ during the commission of a crime.

6. True or False: Harder and less porous surfaces result in less spatter, whereas rough surfaces result in stains with more spatter and serrated edges. _____

7. Generally, bloodstain diameter (increases, decreases) with height. _____

8. The _____ and _____ of blood striking an object may be discerned by the stain's shape.

9. A drop of blood that strikes a surface at an angle of impact of approximately 90 degrees will be close to (elliptical, circular) in shape. _____

10. The angle of impact of an individual bloodstain can be estimated using the ratio of _____ divided by _____.

11. _____ is the most common type of blood spatter found at a crime scene and is produced when an object forcefully contacts a source of blood.

12. True or False: Forward spatter consists of the blood projected backward from the source, and backspatter is projected outward and away from the source. _____

13. The _____ is the point on a two-dimensional plane from which the drops originated.

14. The _____ of a bloodstain pattern in a three-dimensional space illustrates the position of the victim or suspect when the stain-producing event took place.

15. The _____ method is used at the crime scene to determine the area of origin.

16. A(n) _____ is created by contact between a bloody object and a surface.

17. Movement of a bloody object across a surface, (lightens, darkens) as the pattern moves away from the point of contact. _____

18. True or False: Footwear transfer stains created by an individual who was running typically show imprints with more space between them compared to those of an individual who was walking. _____

19. True or False: The direction of a flow pattern may show movements of objects or bodies while the flow was still in progress or after the blood had dried. _____

20. The approximate drying time of a(n) _____ of blood determined by experimentation is related to the environmental condition of the scene and may suggest how much time has elapsed since its deposition.

21. The edges of a bloodstain generally _____ within 50 seconds of deposition and are left intact even if the central area of a bloodstain is altered by a wiping motion.

22. A(n) _____ pattern commonly originates from repeated strikes from weapons or fists and is characterized by an arc pattern of separate drops showing directionality.

23. True or False: Characteristics of a cast-off pattern arc cannot give clues as to the kind of object that was used to produce the pattern. _____

24. When an injury is suffered to an artery, the pressure of the continuing pumping of blood projects blood out of the injured area in spurts creating a pattern known as _____.

25. If a(n) _____ pattern is found at a scene, it may show movement, lead to a discarded weapon, or provide identification of the suspect by the suspect's own blood.

26. A bloodstain pattern created by _____ features bubbles of oxygen in the drying drops and may be lighter in color when compared to impact spatter.

27. The shape and size of the blank space, or _____, created when an object blocks the deposition of spatter onto a surface and is then removed may give a clue as to the size and shape of the missing object or person.

28. True or False: Each bloodstain pattern found at a crime scene should be noted, studied, and photographed. _____

29. When documenting bloodstain patterns, the _____ involves setting up a grid of squares of known dimensions over the entire pattern and taking overview, medium-range, and close-up photographs with and without the grid.

30. The _____ method of bloodstain documentation involves setting up a border of rulers around the pattern and then placing a small ruler next to each stain to show relative position and size in photographs.

31. True or False: The pointed end of a bloodstain always faces toward its direction of travel. _____

Application and Critical Thinking

1. After looking at the bloodstains in the figure, answer the following questions:

   Which three drops struck the surface closest to a 90-degree angle? Explain your answer.

   Which three drops struck the surface farthest from a 90-degree angle? Explain your answer.

   In what direction were drops 2 and 7 traveling when they struck the surface? Explain your answer.

2. Investigator Priscilla Wright arrives at a murder scene and finds the body of a victim who suffered a gunshot wound, but she sees no blood spatter on the wall or floor behind it. What should she conclude from this observation?

3. Investigator Terry Martin arrives at an assault scene and finds a cast-off pattern consisting of tiny drops of blood in a very narrow linear arc pattern on a wall near the victim. What does this tell him about the weapon used in the crime?

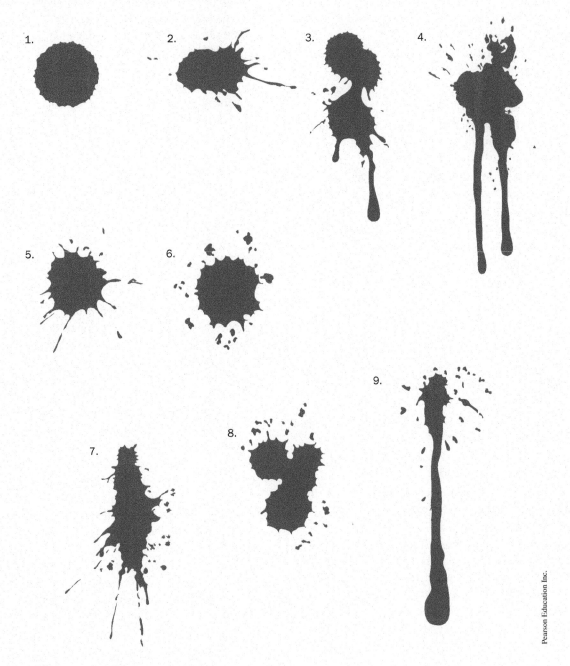

Further References

Bevel, Tom, and Ross Gardner, *Bloodstain Pattern Analysis: With an Introduction to Crime Scene Reconstruction*, 3rd ed. Boca Raton, FL: CRC Press, 2008.

James, Stuart H., Paul E. Kish, and T. P. Sutton, *Principles of Bloodstain Pattern Analysis: Theory and Practice*. Boca Raton, FL: CRC Press, 2005.

Wonder, A. Y., *Blood Dynamics*. Burlington, MA: Elsevier Academic Press, 2001.

Wonder, A. Y., *Bloodstain Pattern Evidence: Objective Approaches and Case Applications*. Burlington, MA: Elsevier Academic Press, 2007.

Wonder, A. Y., and G. M. Yezzo, *Bloodstain Patterns: Identification, Interpretation and Application*. Burlington, MA: Elsevier Academic Press, 2015.

Death Investigation

Learning Objectives

After studying this chapter, you should be able to:

5.1 Describe the role of a forensic pathologist

5.2 Describe autopsy

5.3 Describe common causes of death

5.4 List various categories associated with the manner of death

5.5 Describe chemical and physical changes helpful for estimating time of death

5.6 Discuss the role of the forensic anthropologist in death investigation

5.7 Describe the role of the forensic entomologist in death investigation

KEY TERMS

algor mortis
autopsy
cause of death
forensic anthropology
forensic entomology
forensic pathologist
livor mortis
manner of death
petechiae
postmortem interval
  (PMI)
rigor mortis

Go to www.pearsonhighered.com/careersresources to access Webextras for this chapter.

Freddie Gray: Accident or Murder?

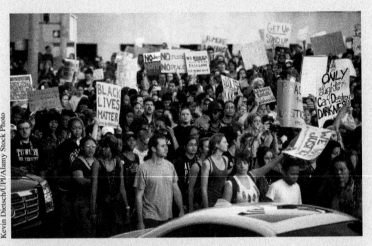

On April 12, 2015, 25-year-old Freddie Gray was handcuffed and placed into the back of a police van. After the arrest, he could be heard yelling and banging around, causing the van to rock. The original plan was that the van was to proceed directly to central booking, but two additional stops were necessary to place restraints on Mr. Gray to prevent him from banging, first leg restraints and then ankle cuffs. After the ankle cuffs were applied, Gray was slid into the van on his belly, head first, reportedly still verbally and physically active.

After a third stop, the driver of the van checks on Gray in the back of the van. When the van stopped a fourth time, the van driver calls for check on Mr. Gray. When he checked, Gray was lying belly down on the floor with his head facing the cabin compartment, asking for help, saying he couldn't breathe, couldn't get up, and needed a medic. At a fifth stop, Gray was found kneeling on the floor, facing the front of the van and slumped over to his right against the bench, lethargic with minimal responses to direct questions. Another arrestee was placed in the van and the vehicle was driven to the Western District headquarters. On arrival at Western Headquarters, Freddie Gray was found in a kneeling position, unresponsive and not breathing.

On examination, it was discovered the Gray suffered a broken neck and a pinched spine. He required spinal surgery and a week after the incident while recovering, Freddie Gray died of sudden cardiac arrest. At autopsy, the medical examiner documented. She reported that based on the sequence of events and the described progressive alteration of mental and physical status, Freddie Gray's neck injury occurred while in custody, in and during transport in the police van. She further found that safety equipment was available but not. Therefore, it was not an accident that a vulnerable individual was injured during operation of the vehicle, and that without prompt medical attention, the injury would prove fatal. Due to the failure of following established safety procedures through acts of omission, the manner of death was best certified as homicide.

Role of the Forensic Pathologist

Few investigations bring with them the intense focus of community interest and news media coverage as that of a suspicious death. Generally, **forensic pathologists** associated with the medical examiner's or coroner's office are responsible for determining the cause of an undetermined or unexpected death. These officers coordinate their response with that of law enforcement in the ensuing investigation. The titles *coroner* and *medical examiner* are often used interchangeably, but there are significant differences in their job descriptions. In the United States, there's a mix of state medical examiner systems, county medical examiner offices, and county coroner systems. The coroner is an elected official and may or may not possess a medical degree. The term *coroner* dates back hundreds of years to the rule of King Richard I of England (1189–1199), who created the office of the coroner to collect money and personal possessions from people who had died. The medical examiner, on the other hand, is almost always an appointed official and is usually a physician who generally is a board-certified forensic pathologist and is responsible for certifying the manner and the cause of a death.

The tasks of examining the case for the cause and manner of death and recording the results on a death certificate are the responsibilities of both offices. However, although both the coroner's office and the medical examiner's office are charged with investigating suspicious deaths, only the pathologist is trained to perform an autopsy. Ideally, the coroner or medical examiner's office should be staffed with physicians who are board certified in forensic pathology and should charge them with determining the cause of death by autopsy. The cause-of-death determination, however, involves not just an autopsy but also the history of death, witness statements, relevant medical records, and any scene investigation, all of which constitute the surrounding circumstances of death.

From a practical point of view, it is often not feasible for the forensic pathologist to personally solicit information regarding the circumstances surrounding a death or to respond in person to every death scene. Thus, the gathering of vital information and the scene investigation can be delegated to trained coroner/medical examiner investigators who, when a crime scene is involved, coordinate their efforts with those of crime-scene and criminal investigators. The forensic pathologist's work is also aided by the skills of specialists, including forensic anthropologists, forensic entomologists, and forensic odontologists.

forensic pathologists
Investigative personnel, typically medical examiners or coroners, who investigate the cause, manner, and time of death of a victim in a crime; can also be a physician who has been trained to conduct autopsies.

Scene Investigation

With regard to any scene investigation, protection of the overall scene and the body are of paramount importance, as is the ultimate removal of the body in a medically acceptable manner. The death investigation involves documenting and photographing the undisturbed scene; collecting relevant physical evidence; attempting to determine time of death, which must be done in a timely fashion at the scene; and, among other things, ascertaining premortem locations of the body and whether any postmortem movement of the body occurred. Examples of observations that can be made of the body at the scene include bruises along the upper lip, which may be evidence of smothering; a black eye limited to the eyelids, which implies an injury from inside the head; or bleeding from the ear, which implies a basal skull fracture.

A critical phase of the death investigation will be a preliminary reconstruction of events that preceded the onset of death, so all significant details of the scene must be recorded. Blood spatter and blood flow patterns must be documented. Blood should be sampled for testing in case some of the blood was cast off by a perpetrator. Any tire marks or shoe prints must be documented. Fingerprints must be processed and collected. Of particular importance is the search for any evidence discarded, dropped, or cast off by a perpetrator. When a weapon is involved, there must be a concerted effort to locate and recover the suspect weapon. In the case of firearm deaths, fired bullets or casings must be found and their locations documented. In such firearm deaths, before the body is moved or clothing is removed, blood spatter directionality and trace evidence (such as hairs) on the hands must be documented. Paper bags then should be placed over the hands and secured around the wrist or arm (paper prevents moisture condensation) to preserve any additional evidence.

Photographs must always be taken before the scene is altered in any way (except from lifesaving efforts). This includes moving the body or anything on the body, such as clothing or jewelry. A particularly violent scene can carry with it a large amount of blood and disorder.

Blood may be found at different locations throughout the scene. This could prove to be important in shaping the events that led to the final outcome; it may be possible to determine the initial location of the injury, as well as victim and assailant movements throughout the course of events. Initially, it may be difficult to properly infer the source of the wounds and the order in which they were received at the scene. Photographs then will play a very large role when reconstructing the events later. As always, photographs should be taken with a scale, always first overall, then at medium range, then close up. The photographer must also be careful not to get caught up in capturing the injuries exclusively. Negative findings can also be significant. This means photographs should also be taken of areas on the body where injuries are not apparent.

Protection of the body and the overall scene is of paramount importance, as is the ultimate removal of the body in a medically acceptable manner. Often the initial phase of the investigation will focus on determining the identity of the deceased, often called the *decedent*. Although this task may be relatively simple to accomplish through a visual examination, complications can arise. Body decomposition and the existence of extensive trauma can complicate the identification. This may necessitate the application of more sophisticated technology, such as DNA, fingerprinting, dental examination, and facial reconstruction.

The Autopsy

autopsy
A surgical procedure performed by a pathologist on a dead body to ascertain—from the body, organs, and bodily fluids—the cause of death.

An **autopsy**, in its broadest definition, is simply the examination of a body after death (i.e., a postmortem examination). The autopsy can be further described as one of two types: a clinical/hospital autopsy or a forensic/medicolegal autopsy. The clinical/hospital autopsy focuses on the internal organ findings and medical conditions. Its purpose is to confirm the clinical diagnoses, the presence and extent of disease, any medical conditions that were overlooked, and the appropriateness and outcome of therapy. In contrast, the goal of a forensic/medicolegal autopsy is to determine the cause of death and confirm the manner of death, often to be used in criminal proceedings. The forensic autopsy usually emphasizes external and internal findings while developing meaningful forensic correlations between sustained injuries and the crime scene (see Figures 5–1 and 5–2).

All the steps of the forensic autopsy must be carefully documented and photographed. The documentation should include date, time, place, by whom the autopsy was performed, and who attended the autopsy. Photographs of the injuries, complete with a scale, and descriptions of each

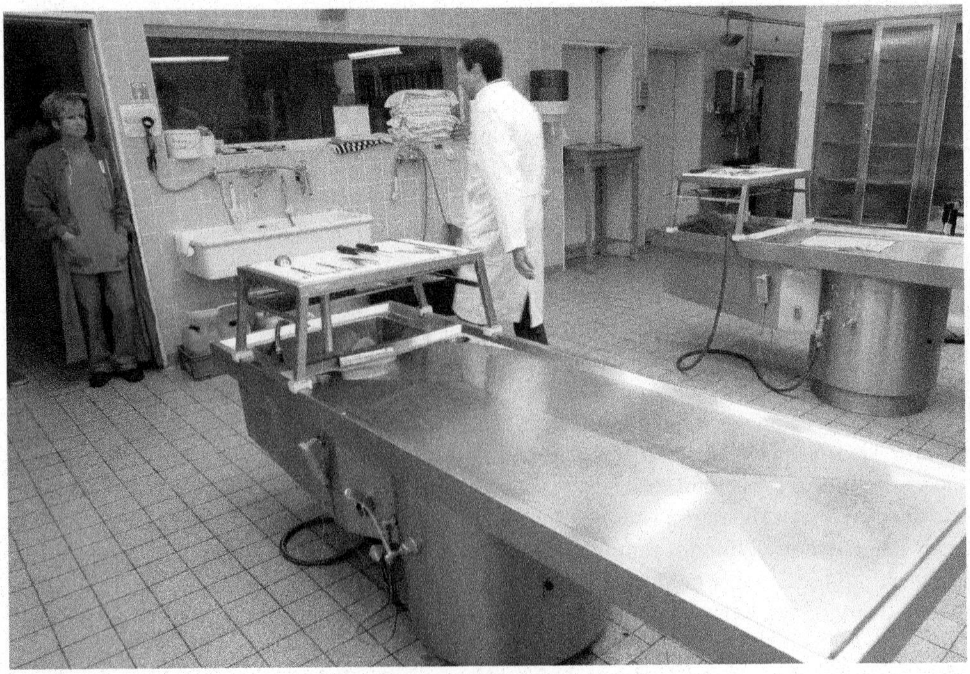

Robert Seeberg/Agencja Fotograficzna Caro/Alamy Stock Photo

FIGURE 5–1
An autopsy suite.

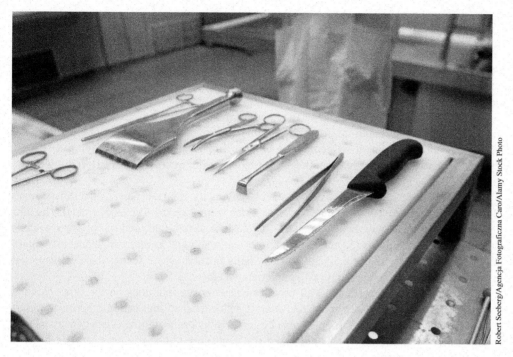

Robert Seeberg/Agencja Fotograficzna Caro/Alamy Stock Photo

FIGURE 5–2
Tools used for an autopsy.

photograph's location are important when correlating external wounds with internal damage. Negative photographs—photographs of uninjured parts of the body—are also important. The autopsy report and photographs are so important because, once the body is buried, no further evidence can be collected and no additional findings can occur.

EVIDENCE FROM THE AUTOPSY The search for physical evidence must extend beyond the crime scene to the autopsy room of a deceased victim. Here, the medical examiner or pathologist carefully examines the victim to establish the cause and manner of death. As a matter of routine, tissues and organs are retained for pathological and toxicological examination. At the same time, arrangements must be made between the examiner and investigator to secure a variety of items that may be obtainable from the body for laboratory examination. The following are among the items to be collected and sent to the forensic laboratory:

- Victim's clothing
- Fingernail scrapings or clippings
- Combings from head and pubic areas
- Buccal swab (for DNA typing purposes)
- Vaginal, anal, and oral swabs (in sex-related crimes)
- Bullets recovered from the body
- Swabs of body areas, such as breasts or penis, suspected of being in contact with DNA arising from touching or saliva
- Hand swabs from shooting victims (for gunshot residue analysis)

These items of evidence should be properly packaged and labeled like all other evidence. Once the body is buried, efforts at obtaining these items may prove difficult or futile. Furthermore, a lengthy time delay in obtaining many of these items will diminish or destroy their forensic value.

EXTERNAL EXAMINATION The forensic autopsy consists of an external examination and an internal examination. The first steps taken for the external examination include a broad overview of the condition of the body and the clothing. Obvious damage to the clothing should be matched up to injuries on the body. General characteristics of the body should be noted, including sex, height, weight, approximate age, color of hair, and physical condition.

The presence of tattoos and scars, as well as puncture and track marks, are noted. All evidence of apparent medical intervention must be carefully noted, described, and photographed because occasionally these may be misinterpreted, especially chest tube insertions and emergency cardiac punctures. The mouth and nose are examined for the presence of vomit and/or blood and trace evidence, and the ears are examined for blood. Any irritations in the nasal cavity can be indicative of drug sniffing.

Often, paper bags are placed over the hands at the crime scene until it is time to examine them. This prevents contamination and possible loss of trace evidence, such as hairs and fibers. This preservation of evidence can play an important role in identifying a suspect. Victims will sometimes have skin and DNA under their fingernails from fighting with the assailant.

The external examination also consists of classifying the injuries. This includes distinguishing between different types of wounds, such as a stab wound versus a gunshot wound. The injuries that are examined may include abrasions, contusions, lacerations, and sharp-injury wounds. Hemorrhages in the eyelids (petechiae) are also essential to note, as they can indicate strangulation. Attention is also paid to the genitalia, especially in cases where sexual abuse is suspected. In these cases, vaginal, oral, and rectal samples are taken.

The discharge from a firearm will produce characteristic markings on the skin. This discharge is a combination of soot and gunpowder. It will leave markings called *stippling* or *tattooing* around the bullet hole. The stippling can be analyzed in terms of its span and density in order to approximate the range of fire. The range of fire may prove to be the most important factor in distinguishing a homicide from a suicide.

X-ray examinations can be very useful in the autopsy process. They are most commonly performed in gunshot wound cases and stab wound cases. Even if the bullet, knife, or other piercing weapon is recovered outside the body, an X-ray will identify any fragments still inside the body. An X-ray will also help determine the path of the projectile or sharp utensil. X-rays can also be very helpful in cases where the victim was beaten, especially situations in which the victim is a child: an X-ray can show past bone fractures and a possible pattern of abuse.

INTERNAL EXAMINATION   The dissection of the human body generally entails the removal of all internal organs through a Y-shaped incision beginning at the top of each shoulder and extending down to the pubic bone. Performing the internal examination entails weighing, dissecting, and sectioning each organ of the body. When required and in accordance with jurisdictional rules, microscopic examination of the sectioned organs is conducted, which can help in determining the cause of death. For example, microscopic examination of lungs and liver can confirm chronic intravenous drug use. Examination of the cranium requires cutting an incision from behind one ear to the other, peeling the scalp upward and backward, and sawing the skull in a circular cut; then the skull cap is removed to reveal the brain, as shown in Figure 5–3.

Special care is taken to identify any preexisting conditions or malformations in the organs that might have contributed to the death of the victim. Pulmonary edema (fluid accumulation in the lungs) is frequently found in victims of chronic cocaine and amphetamine use. Heart malformations may cause suspicious death in an otherwise healthy individual.

Special attention is paid to the digestive tract if poisoning is suspected. The stomach can show partially digested or dissolved pills. Chemical analyses can also be carried out to show signs of poisoning. The amount of pills or tablets in the stomach can aid in the determination of manner of death as well. It is not always a sure sign, but typically it is unlikely that a person will accidentally swallow a large number of pills. This would suggest suicide rather than an accidental overdose. Stomach contents may reveal the deceased's last meal. The extent of digestion can help with determining the time of death.

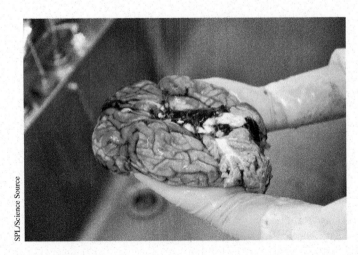

SPL/Science Source

FIGURE 5–3
A brain during autopsy.

TOXICOLOGY   The internal examination is also where toxicological specimens are taken. These include samples of blood, stomach content, bile, and urine. All bile in the gallbladder and all stomach content are collected. In addition to these, brain matter, liver, and vitreous humor are also gathered. These specimens can play especially large roles in cases where poisoning or drug use is suspected.

Blood is often tested to determine the presence and levels of alcohol and drugs. Blood should be taken from areas of the body where there is the least chance of contamination. Blood should never be collected from body cavities, where it may be contaminated from adjacent structures. Many changes occur in the body after death, and these changes can alter the drugs present in the system at the time of death. This can make interpreting how much of a drug was present, if any at all, a very challenging task. Some drugs redistribute or reenter the blood after death and thus may complicate the interpretation of postmortem blood levels of these drugs. This phenomenon is known as *postmortem redistribution*. For this reason, it is best to collect blood at distant areas of the body to allow the toxicologist to compare the agreement of the drug concentrations found. The ideal location to retrieve the blood is internally, directly from the inferior vena cava (the large vein inside the lower abdominal region, which receives its blood from the femoral veins) using a syringe. Where postmortem redistribution of drugs may have occurred, blood should also be collected at autopsy from the superior venous system directly above the heart.

For illicit as well as legal substances, it is necessary to know what levels are indicative of therapeutic use and what levels indicate toxicity of a given substance. Much information regarding therapeutic versus toxic drug levels has been published. This data can help pathologists and toxicologists ascertain the cause of death. Most drug-related deaths are quite apparent from the blood concentrations of alcohol and/or a drug found in the postmortem toxicological report. (Note that depressant drugs will act in concert with alcohol.) However, in some cases of drug-induced death, drug levels may not always provide evidence. Cocaine is a prime example of this. Cocaine-induced sudden death is an event with an incubation period. Structural alterations of the cardiovascular system are required, and such alterations take months, or perhaps years, of chronic cocaine use. In these individuals, death and toxicity may occur after the use of even a trivial amount of the drug.

Unlike drug analyses, general testing for poisons is not a routine procedure carried out by the pathologist. However, if a specific poison is suspected, a particular test must be performed. A body that displays a cherry-red discoloration often leads a pathologist to suspect carbon monoxide poisoning. The pathologist would then perform a toxicological test of the blood. Poisoning by cyanide could also produce a pinkish discoloration. Often, cyanide toxicity will show additional signs, such as a distinct smell of burnt almonds. Corrosion around the lips of a victim may lead to a suspicion of ingesting an acid or alkaline substance.

WEBEXTRA 5.1
See How an Autopsy Is Performed

Cause of Death

A primary objective of the autopsy is to determine the cause of death. The **cause of death** is that which initiates the series of events ending in death. The most important determination in a violent death is the character of the injury that started the chain of events that resulted in death. However, if the sequence of events leading to death is sufficiently prolonged, then the decedent may actually suffer from adverse medical conditions brought about by the initial injury and then die as a result of those conditions. In that case, it will be up to the forensic pathologist to determine that the original injury inflicted on the victim was the underlying cause of death. Some of the more common causes of death are discussed here.

cause of death
Identifies the injury or disease that led to the chain of events resulting in death.

BLUNT-FORCE INJURY   A blunt-force injury is caused by a nonsharpened object such a bat or pipe. A blunt-force injury can abrade, or scrape, tissue. If tissue is crushed by a blunt force to the point of causing skin to overstretch, a laceration will form, characterized by the skin splitting and tearing. Lacerations exhibit abrasions around the open wound, tissue bridging within the open wound, and torn or disturbed tissue beneath the skin surrounding the open portion of the wound. Blunt-force injury can also crush tissue. This will cause bleeding from tiny ruptured blood vessels within and beneath the skin, known as a contusion, or bruise (see Figure 5–4). Much has been written about determining the age of bruises, but forensic pathologists have become keenly

> > > > > > > > > > >

Harold Shipman, Dr. Death

Kathleen Grundy's sudden death in 1998 was shocking news to her daughter, Angela Woodruff. Mrs. Grundy, an 81-year-old widow, was believed to be in good health when her physician, Dr. Harold Shipman, visited her a few hours before her demise. Some hours later, when friends came to her home to check on her whereabouts, they found Mrs. Grundy lying on a sofa fully dressed and dead.

Dr. Shipman pronounced her dead and informed her daughter that an autopsy was not necessary. A few days later, Mrs. Woodruff was surprised to learn that a will had surfaced leaving all of Mrs. Grundy's money to Dr. Shipman. The will was immediately recognized as a forgery and led to the exhumation of Mrs. Grundy's body.

A toxicological analysis of the remains revealed a lethal quantity of morphine.

In retrospect, there was good reason to suspect that Dr. Shipman was capable of foul play. In the 1970s, he was asked to leave a medical practice because of a drug use problem and charges that he obtained drugs by forgery and deception.

However, Dr. Shipman quickly returned to practicing medicine. By 1998, local undertakers became suspicious because of the number of his patients who were dying. What is more, the patients who had died all were older women who were found sitting in a chair or lying fully clothed on a bed. As police investigated, the horror of Dr. Shipman's deeds became apparent. One clinical audit estimated that Dr. Shipman had killed at least 236 of his patients over a 24-year period. Most of the deaths were attributed to fatal doses of heroin or morphine.

Toxicological analysis on seven exhumed bodies clearly showed significant quantities of morphine. Convicted of murder, Dr. Shipman hanged himself in his jail cell in 2004.

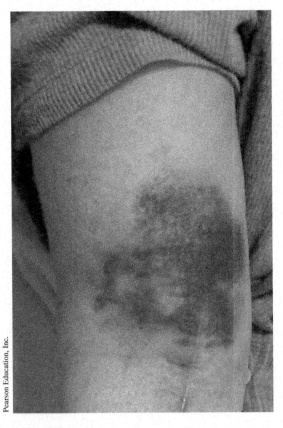

Pearson Education, Inc.

FIGURE 5–4
Bruising (contusions) on the skin.

aware that attempting to "age" bruises based on color and changes in color over time is fraught with difficulty, and contusions must be interpreted with great care and reserve. Some contusions only become visible externally over time, and frequently, bruises will not be visible externally but become eminently visible internally within soft tissues (e.g., in the abdomen and on the back, arms, and legs).

A contusion can sometimes exhibit the pattern of the weapon used. For example, if a person wearing a ring strikes another person, the ring may imprint its pattern onto the skin. A person who stomps on another may leave the impression of their shoe heel. Over time, however, the bruise will lose its original shape and pattern and undergo color changes. Some objects will produce a characteristic bruised perimeter and a white center.

The outward appearance of the injuries does not always coincide with the injuries sustained inside the body. This is something the pathologist must keep in mind when examining blunt-force injuries. A single blow to certain parts of the body can cause instantaneous death with little visible damage. Likewise, a blow to the head can cause a concussion that can be instantly fatal.

SHARP-FORCE INJURIES Sharp-force injuries occur from weapons with sharp edges, such as knives or blades. These weapons are capable of cutting or stabbing. A *cut* is formed when the weapon produces an injury that is longer than it is deep. In contrast, a *stab* is deeper than its length. As shown in Figure 5–5, the tissue associated with these types of wounds is not crushed or torn but sliced.

A scene that involves a sharp-force injury is usually especially bloody and unruly. Blood may be found at different locations throughout the scene. Again, this information may make it possible to determine the initial location of the injury as well as where the body was moved throughout the course of events. Particularly important in sharp-force cases is to examine the victim for defensive wounds. A victim's forearm that exhibits wounds may indicate defense wounds. These occur when the victim attempts to fight off the attacker or block assaults. Though defense wounds are more typical on the outer forearms, they can also be evident on the lower extremities if the victim tries to protect themself by kicking. A lack of any defense wounds can lead a pathologist to conclude that the victim was either unconscious or somehow tied up during the assault.

ASPHYXIA   Asphyxia encompasses a variety of conditions that involve interference with the intake of oxygen. For example, death at a fire scene is caused primarily by the extremely toxic gas carbon monoxide. When carbon monoxide is present, hemoglobin, the protein in red blood cells that transports oxygen, will bind to the carbon monoxide instead of oxygen. This is carbon monoxide poisoning, and this deadly complex of hemoglobin and carbon monoxide is known as carboxyhemoglobin. Bound up with carbon monoxide, the hemoglobin is prevented from transporting oxygen throughout the body, causing asphyxia. High levels of carbon monoxide in the blood will cause death. Low levels of carbon monoxide can cause a victim to become disoriented and lose consciousness.

Carbon monoxide will not continue to build up in the body after death. The levels found in a fire victim then can be used to determine whether the individual was breathing at the time of the fire. The presence of soot is another indicator that the victim was alive during the fire. These black particles are often seen in the airway of fire victims who inhaled smoke before death. During the autopsy, soot can be observed, especially in the larynx and trachea and even in the lungs. Sometimes the victim will actually swallow the soot. In these cases, traces can be found in the esophagus and the lining of the stomach.

The ultimate cause of a death from hanging is typically the cessation of blood flow to or from the brain. Victims of hangings may show signs of petechiae on the eyelids, along with a swollen and a blue/purplish appearance of the face. **Petechiae** are very small and are caused by blood having escaped into the tissues as a result of capillaries bursting (see Figure 5–6). Although petechiae are witnessed in hanging cases, they are more common in strangulation deaths. Typically the hyoid bone (the bone on which the tongue rests) and thyroid cartilage (located below the hyoid) are not fractured in cases of hanging. A break of the thyroid cartilage is common, however, in manual strangulation cases.

In hangings it is vitally important to document exactly how the victim was initially found and the position of the encircling noose, as shown in Figure 5–7. The type of knot used may strongly support the notion that another person was involved in the hanging. This means that the knot should always be preserved for later examination. Either the noose should be slipped off the victim's head intact, or the noose should be cut distant from the knot. Defense wounds are common on strangulation victims. Often the marks found on the neck of a victim are the victim's own, made in the attempt to loosen whatever was constricting their neck. Even in cases of hanging by suicide, there can be defensive wounds on the neck.

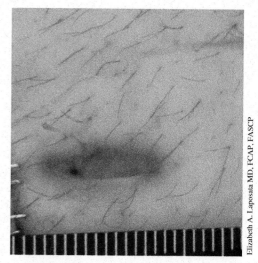

FIGURE 5–5
A stab wound.

petechiae
Pinpoint hemorrhaging often observed in the white area of the victim's eyes; often observed in strangulation cases.

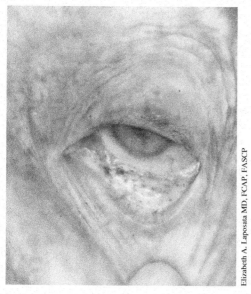

FIGURE 5–6
Petechial hemorrhages in a victim's eye.

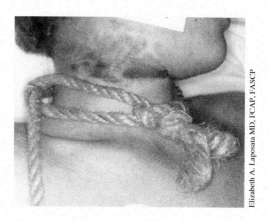

FIGURE 5–7
A ligature pattern on a neck with corresponding ligature.

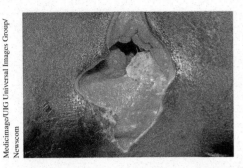

Medicimage/UIG Universal Images Group/ Newscom

FIGURE 5–8
A contact gunshot wound to the temple of a suicide victim.

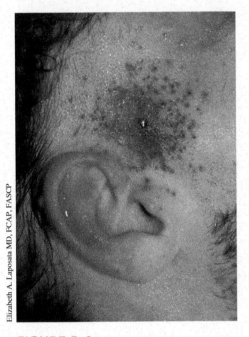

Elizabeth A. Laposata MD, FCAP, FASCP

FIGURE 5–9
A gunshot entrance wound to the head from a weapon fired several inches from the target.

manner of death
A determination made by a forensic pathologist of the cause of death. Five broad categories are homicide, suicide, accidental, natural, and undetermined.

Smothering can occur by various materials that block the mouth, nose, and internal airway. Pillows or a hand can inhibit breathing. Gags that are used to silence a victim can be sucked into the airway and block oxygen flow. Typically a death by smothering is homicidal in nature. Accidental smothering usually occurs only in infants or in cases where a victim is trapped under an obstruction.

GUNSHOT WOUNDS   When evaluating a gunshot wound, the estimated range of fire is one of the most important characteristics to analyze (see Figure 5–8). The appearance of the wound can help in estimating whether the firearm used to inflict the wound was discharged while in contact with the victim's body or from a distance of only inches to many feet away (see Figure 5–9). The investigator will compare powder residue distribution around the wound to test fires collected from the inflicting firearm to make this estimate. Obviously, if the firearm was fired at a distance of several feet, suicide is a highly unlikely cause of death because the wound could not have been self-inflicted. Gunpowder residue on the victim's is a possible indicator of suicide, but this is not always the case. Evidence of contact shots, that is, shots fired with the gun held against the body of the victim, typically indicates that the death was not an accident. The autopsy must include a determination of the path or "wound track" of the projectile. The wound track is determined by observing the wound from the outside of the body, following the track of the projectile through the body, and documenting its terminus. The pathologist will recover any and all projectiles from the body, carefully protecting the forensic markings. The autopsy of gunshot victims should include several facts in addition to the general autopsy facts; scene investigation and the results of toxicological and serological analyses are important. All findings regarding the bullet wounds should be noted, as well as descriptions of the clothing. The police report with a thorough description of the scene is also important.

A gunshot wound may not necessarily explain why a victim died. A person who sustains a gunshot wound can bleed to death in a matter of minutes or up to several hours. Infection can also be a contributory cause of death, especially in cases where the victim was shot in the abdomen; the victim might live several days but eventually succumb to infection. In cases where the victim was shot in the head but survives in a comatose state, pneumonia often develops. These intervening factors are considered contributory causes of death, but the gunshot wound is still considered the underlying cause of death.

SUBSTANCE USE   Drug use continues to be an enormous problem in the United States. Drug enforcement is a multibillion-dollar industry. Many of the drugs in the country that are used by individuals with substance use problems are illegal, but not all are. Deaths as a result of substance use are common cases that a forensic pathologist must face. Because drug use is so common, the forensic pathologist will routinely test for the presence of drugs in nearly all investigations, and routine tests are available for many commonly used drugs. As technology has improved, many drugs can be detected at very low levels. These factors have helped considerably in making substance use testing easier and less expensive.

Drug use can directly cause death, or it can cause complications that can serve as a contributing factor to death. A person with a substance use problem can misuse a drug or a number of drugs for years, accumulating detrimental effects in that time. Death as a result of those effects is typically labeled a natural death by the pathologist. Drugs can also alter a person's judgment and psychomotor skills to the point that a fatal accident occurs. Drugs are also often at the source of acts of violence that result in death.

Manner of Death

The **manner of death** relates to the circumstances that led to the fatal result and is the culmination of the complete investigation, including the determination of cause of death. The certification of the circumstances and manner of death is the responsibility of the coroner's and medical examiner's offices. The manner in which death occurred is classified in death certifications as one of five categories: *homicide, suicide, accidental, natural,* or *undetermined.*

HOMICIDE   Although there is no universal agreement on its definition, generally the term *homicide,* as certified by coroners' and medical examiners' offices, is defined as a nonaccidental death resulting from grossly negligent, reckless, or intentional actions of another person. Both the cause and manner of death, as certified by the coroner's/medical examiner's offices, can become the subject of expert debate during any subsequent judicial proceedings. However, this does not result in a revision of the death certification unless there has been negligence on the part of the certifying offices.

If the pathologist was unable to go to the scene, the pathologist should receive adequate information detailing the conditions of the scene from coroner/medical examiner investigators and law enforcement personnel. This information should include how the body was discovered as well as when and where. It is also an important first step for investigators to make note of the algor mortis, livor mortis, and/or rigor mortis of the body at the scene. These will help determine time of death.

SUICIDE   Suicide is the result of an individual taking their own life with lethal intention. For a determination of suicide, it must be demonstrated that the individual carried out the act alone. If there is any doubt about the intentions of the victim, the death is not classified as a suicide; the death is ruled as an accident or even as undetermined. The most common methods of suicide include self-inflicted gunshot wounds, hanging, and drug overdosing. Although drug use is deliberately committed by a victim, it is not considered suicide unless it was clearly intended as a lethal act.

Various challenges are associated with discriminating suicide from an accident or even homicide. The victim's personal history, including their psychiatric history, becomes relevant. Suicidal threats or past attempts would give obvious evidence of a suicide as opposed to an accident. In all cases of suspected suicide, a thorough search of the victim's possessions should be made to locate a suicide note.

Multiple gunshot wounds might lead one to suspect homicide. However, a person who is committed to ending their own life may take several shots if the wounds are not instantly fatal. It is imperative to confirm that it is physically possible that the victim could inflict the wounds. There are a few areas of the body that strongly point toward homicide. These are areas that are not easily accessible to the victim's own reach. For example, anywhere on the back of a victim is difficult and sometimes impossible for the victim to have shot by their own hand. This is especially true if the wound was made in the back of the head. For suicides, the most common shot is to the temple of the head. The mouth, forehead, and chest are also common.

Also, if the wound was immediately incapacitating, the weapon should be present. Blood spatter analysis should be consistent with the proposed order of events. All victims involved in gunshot cases should have their hands swabbed for gunshot residue.

ACCIDENTAL   In all deaths that are ruled accidental, there must not be intent to cause harm through gross negligence on the part of a perpetrator or the victim. Traffic accidents make up a large percentage of accidental deaths, followed by drug overdoses and drownings. The surviving driver may have vehicular homicide charges brought against them, especially if the driver is determined to have been driving under the influence of drugs or alcohol. In this case, the official manner of death certified on the death certificate in many jurisdictions would be *vehicular homicide.*

All cases that have the possibility of being ruled an accident should have toxicological analyses carried out. The presence of drugs and/or alcohol in the victim's system can potentially affect the determination. Also, the pathologist should be aware that some events might be disguised as accidents to cover up a homicide or suicide. For example, bodies recovered from a house fire might show evidence that the victims were dead before the fire started. This evidence might include a lack of soot in the victims' airways or no indication of elevated levels of carbon monoxide. This scenario, although not common, illustrates how the autopsy and scene can apparently not correlate with each other. No matter how obvious a scene may appear, the two should always correspond with one another. Cases of electrocution are generally ruled as accidents, but this may be difficult to prove. High-voltage electrocutions will usually leave burns on the body.

Low-voltage electrocutions, however, may show few or no signs of trauma. The scene then becomes crucial in ascertaining the events surrounding the death.

The determination of manner of death in drownings (accidental, suicidal, or homicidal), falls (accidental, pushed, or deliberate), and asphyxiations can be exceedingly difficult, and therefore the investigation into all of its components becomes much more important than the autopsy.

NATURAL CAUSES   The differentiation between the categories of manner of death can be difficult to make. The distinction between natural and accidental deaths can pose challenges. The classification of natural death includes disease and continual environmental abuse. This abuse can encompass various events, such as chronic drug and alcohol use or longtime exposure to natural toxins or asbestos. Again, although drug use is deliberately committed by the victim, a death caused by drug use is not considered suicide unless it is clear that drugs were taken as an intentionally lethal act. Acute ethanol intoxication can be ruled as either natural or accidental depending on the circumstances. If the victim suffers from chronic alcoholism, the death is ruled to be natural. If the victim is a teenager experimenting with alcohol for the first time, the death is ruled an accident.

UNDETERMINED   A death is ruled to be undetermined only when a rational classification cannot be established. This can happen when the mechanism that caused the death cannot be determined by a physical finding at the autopsy or because of the absence of meaningful findings in the subsequent toxicological and microscopic examinations.

Case Files

> > > > > > > >

The Sheridans: Murder or Suicide

On September 28, 2014, John Sheridan and his wife Joyce were found dead in the master bedroom of their two-story home in Skillman, New Jersey, a suburban town north of Princeton. John Sheridan was found on the floor at the foot of his bed, with a partly burned armoire that apparently fell over and on top of him. Joyce was found dead on the left side of the bed. The bedroom was set ablaze when gasoline was poured onto the bedroom carpet which was ignited by matches found in the room. A carving knife and a bread knife from the Sheridan kitchen were found on the bed. Nine hundred and fifty dollars was left on John's nightstand. There was no sign of forced entry to the home, though most of the doors of the house were unlocked.

A half empty gas can was found in the bedroom. Subsequent investigation revealed that the gas can in question belonged to the Sheridan family and had been stored in the garage area of the residence. Testing revealed that John Sheridan's DNA was located on the handle of the gas can in question. A flattened box containing wooden matches and individual wooden matches were located on the floor of the master bedroom near the area where John Sheridan was reported by first responders to have been located. The same type of wooden matches was also found in the first floor living room near the fireplace.

John Sheridan spent decades in and around politics, including time as Gov. Thomas H. Kean's transportation secretary and as a member of transition teams for Gov. Christie Whitman and Gov. Christie. He served as the Cooper Health System's CEO since 2008.

In March 2015, six months after the crime, the Prosecutor's Office declared that John Sheridan had killed his wife and himself. The medical examiner determined Joyce's manner of death to be homicide. She suffered first- and second-degree burns and 12 stab wounds. The fatal one was to the chest and perforated her aorta. John's manner of death was determined to be a suicide. He had five knife wounds to his neck and torso. One of those wounds to the neck, however, according to the autopsy report "caused a small perforation to the right jugular vein and would be fatal without medical treatment." Unlike Joyce, he had soot in his mouth, nose, and lungs. Toxicological analysis also showed a significant level of carboxyhemoglobin in his blood, all of which indicated that John was alive when the fire started.

Most troubling, investigators never found the knife that caused John Sheridan's stab wounds, which authorities said were self-inflicted. One of two knives recovered from the bedroom was consistent with Joyce's wounds. However, neither knife caused John Sheridan's injuries because the blades were too wide to cause his narrow wounds.

The murder-suicide ruling was immediately criticized by members of the Sheridan family. The family lambasted the probe as a "bungling," pointing out that a weapon used on John Sheridan was never positively identified and no motive was determined. A renowned forensic pathologist hired by the family was highly critical of the suicide determination, pointing out that Sheridan's five deep wounds were highly unusual for a suicide and deep thrust wounds are indicative of a violent attack. The depth of one of John's wounds was estimated to be at 2.0 inches, with another at 1.5 inches.

The family has formally requested that the state medical examiner's office change the manner of death to undetermined. The matter is still pending.

In January 2017, the state medical examiners office reversed course, reporting the death as "undetermined" rather than a suicide. Their son, Mark Sheridan, thanked the medical examiner's office "for doing the right thing and exercising the courage to admit that a mistake was made."

Estimating Time of Death

A pathologist can never give an exact time of death. However, there are many characteristics that the examiner can analyze in order to arrive at an approximate time of death. Some features can give a very probable time of death, but others are extremely variable. Witnesses can serve to reconstruct the events leading up to the death and the incidents that occurred after the death, along with the times when they occurred, but a single witness's account alone is not enough to make an accurate determination. The chemical and physical changes that occur after death must also be examined.

ALGOR MORTIS   After death, the body undergoes a process in which it continually adjusts to equalize with the environmental temperature. This process is known as **algor mortis**. An algor mortis determination must be performed at the scene as early as possible. The first step is to determine as best as possible what the environmental temperatures may have been prior to discovering the body. Then the environmental temperature and the bilateral axillary and/or ear canal temperatures are recorded at the crime scene (rectal temperatures are usually too disruptive at the scene). The cooling rate of a typical body can be used to estimate the time of death. At average ambient temperatures of 70–72°F, the body loses heat at a rate of approximately of 1–1.5°F per hour until the body reaches the ambient or room temperature. However, the rate of heat loss is influenced by factors such as ambient temperature, the size of the body, and the victim's clothing. Because of such factors, this method can only approximate the amount of time that has elapsed since death.

algor mortis
A process that occurs after death in which the body temperature continually cools until it reaches the ambient or room temperature.

LIVOR MORTIS   Another condition that begins when circulation ceases is **livor mortis**. When the human heart stops pumping, the blood begins to settle in the parts of the body closest to the ground. As shown in Figure 5–10, the skin becomes a bluish-purple color in these areas. The onset of this condition begins 20 minutes to 3 hours after death and under average conditions continues for up to 16 hours after death, at which point all lividity, or coloring, is fixed. Initially, lividity can be pressed out of the vessels when the skin is pressed; that is, lividity can be "blanched." With time, coloring becomes "fixed" in the vessels, beginning in the most dependent (lowest) areas and progressing to the least dependent areas, and then finally no blanching can be elicited anywhere. In any case, levels of lividity are tested at the scene with regard to whether it is completely fixed, blanches when subjected to light pressure, or blanches when subjected to significant pressure. A range of time of death can be estimated if at least some of the lividity is still blanching. However, the environmental temperature and the rate of body temperature decline (i.e., algor mortis) directly affect the rate of fixation of lividity and therefore must be taken into account when attempting to estimate time of death from lividity.

livor mortis
A medical condition that occurs after death and results in the settling of blood in areas of the body closest to the ground.

Different lividity patterns in a body may indicate that the body was moved after death but before livor mortis had fully fixed. The skin does not become discolored in areas where the body is restricted by either clothing or an object pressing against the body. This information can be useful in determining whether the victim's position was changed after death. Livor that is a deep purple is often seen in cases where the victim suffered asphyxia or heart failure.

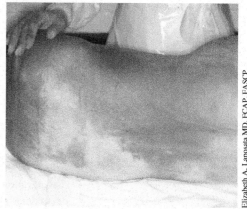

FIGURE 5–10
Livor mortis.

RIGOR MORTIS   Immediately following death, a chemical change occurs in the muscles that causes them to become rigid, as shown in Figure 5–11. This condition, **rigor mortis**, evolves over the first 24 hours under average temperature and body conditions. This rigidity subsides as time goes on, however, and disappears after about 36 hours under average conditions. Rigor will develop in the position that the body was in at the time of death, essentially freezing the body in that pose. Discovering a body in a position that defies gravity is a likely indicator that the body was moved after death.

Although rigor mortis can roughly indicate a time of death, there are factors that can alter this determination. An environment that is hot can speed up the process significantly. Conditions that affected the body before death, such as exercise or physical activity, can also speed up the process. Because rigor mortis occurs as a result of the muscles stiffening, individuals with decreased muscle mass may not develop rigor completely. Examples of these individuals may be infants or older or obese persons.

rigor mortis
A medical condition that occurs after death and results in the stiffening of muscle mass. The rigidity of the body begins within 24 hours of death and disappears within 36 hours of death.

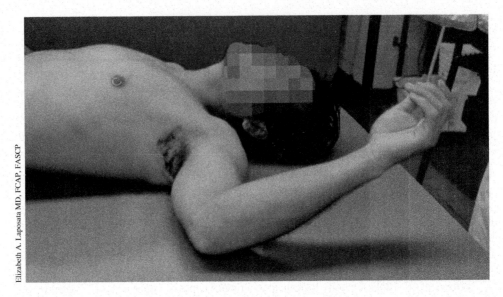

Elizabeth A. Laposata MD, FCAP, FASCP

FIGURE 5–11
Rigor mortis in the arm of a decedent.

POTASSIUM EYE LEVELS   Another approach helpful for estimating the time of death is to determine potassium levels in the decedent's ocular fluid, that is, the fluid within the eye, also known as the *vitreous humor*. It is important to draw a clean, bloodless vitreous sample from one eye with a syringe as soon as possible at the scene, then draw a second sample from the other eye an hour or two later. After death, cells within the inner surface of the eyeball release potassium into the ocular fluid. By analyzing the amount of potassium present at various intervals after death, the forensic pathologist can determine the rate at which potassium is released into the vitreous humor and use it to approximate the time of death. However, the rate of potassium release also is dependent on ambient temperatures.

STOMACH CONTENTS   Special attention must be paid to the digestive tract. The identification of food items in the stomach may help determine the location of the decedent prior to death (during their last meal). The quantity, consistency, and color of bile and the degree of digestion of food in the stomach and its passage into the small intestine can help determine the time of death. The stomach also can contain partially digested or dissolved pills. Chemical analyses can be carried out to identify and analyze substances found in the stomach. These can aid in the determination of cause and manner of death.

DECOMPOSITION   Once decomposition has set in, the preceding methods of determining time of death are no longer of any use. After death, two decomposition processes take place: autolysis and putrefaction. *Autolysis* is fundamentally self-digestion by cells' own enzymes, and its rate varies from organ to organ depending on the mechanism of death, the enzyme content of the respective organs, the position of the body, and environmental factors. *Putrefaction* is decomposition carried out by microorganisms such as bacteria. Putrefaction is accompanied by bloating, discoloration, and a foul smell caused by accumulating gases. Again, the rate of putrefaction is dependent on the mechanism of death (e.g. congestive respiratory versus sudden cardiac death) allowing bacteria to spread from the bowel, presence or absence of infection, environmental temperatures and humidity, degree of obesity, extent of clothing, and so on. Green discoloration often begins in the abdomen. Darker green or purple discoloration follows on the face. The skin begins to blister with gas and then peel (called *slippage*). The skin of the hands and feet can actually detach and come off the body like a glove. This stage is also accompanied by bloating, which causes the eyes to bulge and the tongue to protrude. The chest and extremities will then turn a green/purple discoloration and bloat.

In the postmortem period of decomposition, a waxy substance called *adipocere* may form. Adipocere adds a white or gray waxlike consistency to fatty tissues in the face and extremities that can take on a yellow to tan color. Typically, adipocere takes about three months to develop.

Role of the Forensic Anthropologist

Forensic anthropology is concerned primarily with the identification and examination of human skeletal remains. Skeletal bones are remarkably durable and undergo an extremely slow breakdown process that lasts decades or centuries. Because of their resistance to decomposition, skeletal remains can provide a multitude of individual characteristics long after a victim's death. An examination of bones may reveal a victim's sex, approximate age, ancestry, height, and the nature of a physical injury.

forensic anthropology
The use of anthropological knowledge of humans and skeletal structure to examine and identify human skeletal remains.

Recovering and Processing Remains

Thorough documentation is required throughout the processes of recovery and examination of human remains. A site where human remains are found must be treated as a crime scene (see Figure 5–12). These sites are usually located by civilians who then contact law enforcement personnel. The scene should be secured as soon as possible to prevent any further alteration of the scene. The scene should then be searched to locate all bones, if they are scattered, and any other items of evidence such as footwear impressions or discarded items. Many tools can be useful when searching for evidence at a "tomb" site, including aerial photography, metal detectors, ground-penetrating radar, infrared photography, apparatuses that detect the gases produced by biological decomposition, and so-called cadaver dogs that detect the odors caused by biological decomposition. All items that are found must be tagged, photographed, sketched, and documented in notes. Once all bones and other evidence are found, a scene sketch should be made to show the exact location of each item (preferably using Global Positioning System [GPS] coordinates) and the spatial relationship of all evidence. Once the skeletal remains have been recovered, they can be examined to deduce information about the identity of the decedent.

Determining Victim Characteristics

The sex of the decedent can be determined by the size and shape of various skeletal features, especially those of the pelvis and skull, or cranium. Female pelvic bones tend to form a wider, more circular opening than that in a male pelvis because of a woman's child-bearing capabilities. The female sacrum (flat bone above the tailbone) is wider and shorter (see Figure 5–13[a]) than a male's; the length and width of the male sacrum are roughly equal (see Figure 5–13[b]).

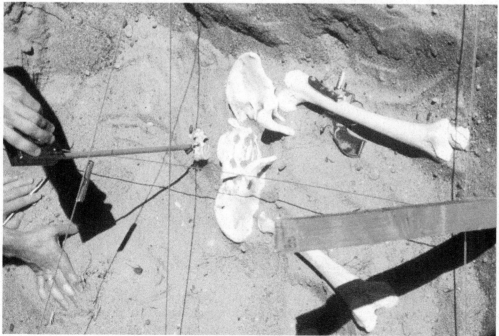

National Transportation Safety Board

FIGURE 5–12
Crime-scene site showing a pelvis partly buried in sand and a femur lying across a revolver.

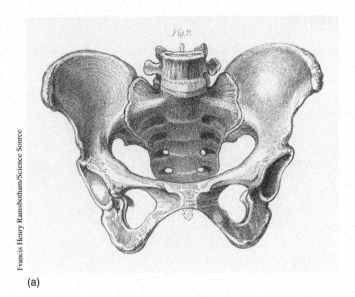

Francis Henry Ramsbotham/Science Source

(a)

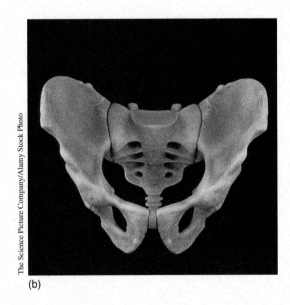

The Science Picture Company/Alamy Stock Photo

(b)

FIGURE 5–13

(a) Frontal shot of female pelvis and hips. This view shows the wide, circular nature of the pelvic opening and the short, wide nature of the sacrum. (b) Human male pelvis. This view shows the narrow pelvic opening and long, narrow sacrum.

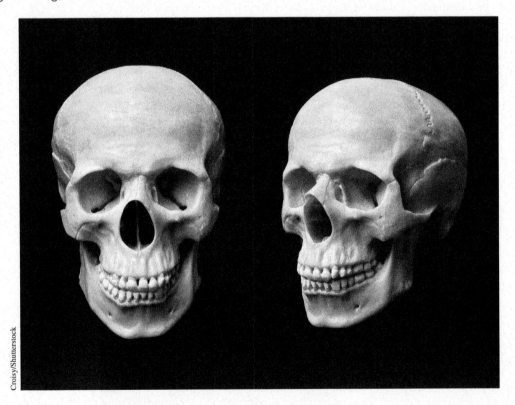

Croisy/Shutterstock

FIGURE 5–14

Male (left) and female (right) human skulls showing male skull's larger size and more pronounced brow bone.

The angle formed at the bottom of the pelvis (i.e., subpubic angle) is approximately a right angle (90 degrees) in females, but it is acute (less than 90 degrees) in males. In general, male craniums are larger in overall size than those of females. A male cranium tends to have a more pronounced brow bone and mastoid process (a bony protrusion behind the jaw) than a female cranium (see Figure 5–14). See Table 5–1 for a summary of the differing features of female and male skeletons from head to toe. These are typical cases; not all skeletons may display the given characteristics to clearly indicate the sex of the decedent.

TABLE 5–1

Summary of Skeletal Features by Sex

	Female	Male
Cranium (skull)	Medium to large in size	Large in size
Forehead	High in height, vaulted, rounded	Low in height, sloped, backward
Brow bone	Diminished	Pronounced
Mastoid process	Diminished or absent	Pronounced
Mandible (jaw) angle	Obtuse (>90 degrees)	Approximately right (90 degrees)
Pelvis opening	Wide, circular	Narrow, noncircular
Sacrum	Short, wide, turned outward	Approximately equal width/length, turned inward
Subpubic angle	Approximately right (90 degrees)	Acute (<90 degrees)
Femur	Narrow, angled inward from pelvis	Thick, relatively straight from pelvis
Overall skeleton	Slender	Robust

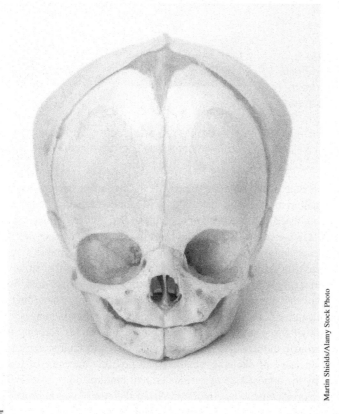

Martin Shields/Alamy Stock Photo

FIGURE 5–15

A lateral view of a fetal skull showing the separated bones of the skull before they have had a chance to fuse.

The method for determining the age of a decedent varies depending on the victim's growth stage. For infants and toddlers, age can be estimated by the length of the long bones (e.g., femur and humerus) when compared to a known growth curve. Different sections of the skull also fuse together at different stages during early development, and the appearance of fused or divided sections can be used to estimate the age of bones still in early developmental stages (see Figure 5–15). In infant skeletons, formation of teeth can be used in age determination; this is based on the fact that permanent teeth start to form at birth. If the skeletal remains belong to a child, the age of the decedent may be determined by observing the fusion or lack of fusion of epiphyseal regions of bones such as those of the mandible (i.e., lower jaw), fingers, wrist, long bones, and clavicle (see Figure 5–16). The average age at which each of these regions fuses is known and can be compared

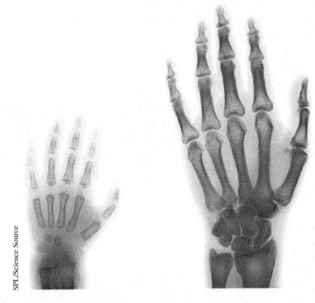

FIGURE 5–16

Colored X-rays of healthy human hands at 3 years (left) and at 20 years. Bones display in red, and flesh is in blue. The child's hand has areas of cartilage in the joints between the finger bones (i.e., epiphyseal areas), where bone growth and fusion will occur. In the adult hand, all the bones are present, and the joints have closed.

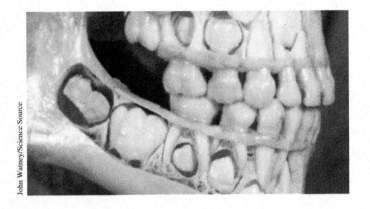

FIGURE 5–17

The skull of an adolescent, with part of the jaw cut away to show the developing teeth.

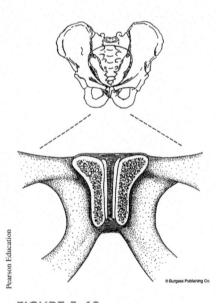

FIGURE 5–18

The symphysis pubis shown magnified beneath human pelvic bones.

against the state of the remains to provide a range of possible ages for the decedent. A child's cranium may also be identified by its smaller size and the presence of developing teeth as contrasted with the skull of an adult showing developing teeth (see Figure 5–17). After age 21, age is estimated by the level of change the surfaces of the bones have undergone, especially in areas of common wear such as the pubic symphysis. The pubic symphyseal face shown in Figure 5–18 is a raised platform that slowly changes over the years from a rough, rugged surface to a smooth, well-defined area. See Table 5–2 for a summary of the skeletal closures by age. It is important to note that these are average ages for closures; not all skeletons display closures at the given ages.

Although the categorization "race" has come under scrutiny and is difficult to define, forensic anthropologists use broad classes to characterize the likely (but not definite) ancestry of skeletal remains. The possible ancestry of the decedent can be assessed by the appearance of various cranial features on the skeletal remains. For example, eye orbits tend to be circular in Asian skeletons, oval in European skeletons, and square in African skeletons. The frontal plane of the cranium may also vary. The frontal plane of Asian craniums may be flat or projected outward, that of European craniums is flat, and that of African craniums is projected outward. The nasal cavity tends to be small and rounded in Asians, long and narrow in Europeans, and wide in Africans. Skeletal remains of decedents of Asian ancestry, including those of Native American descent, also tend to have "scooped-out" or shovel-shaped incisor teeth. See Table 5–3 for a summary of the differing features of skeletons that can indicate ancestry. These are typical cases; not all skeletons may display the given characteristics to indicate the ancestry of the decedent.

The height of the victim when alive can be estimated by measuring the long bones of the skeleton, especially in the lower limbs. Even partial bones can yield useful results. However, meaningful stature calculations from known equations must be based on the determined sex and ancestry of the remains. See Table 5–4 for examples of equations used to calculate the height of the decedent from skeletal remains. These equations should yield estimations within 5 cm of actual height.

TABLE 5–2

Summary of Skeletal Closures by Age

Age (months)	Closure
6–9	Mandible (jaw) fused
4–6	Humerus head bones fused
7–8	Pelvis frontal bones fused
4–16	Femur shaft sections built
9–13	Elbow bones fused
10	Finger bones fused
16–18	Femur head bones fused to shaft bones
18	Wrist bones fused
18–21	Humerus head bones fused to shaft bones
18–24	Sternum fused to clavicle
20–25	Pelvic bones fully formed
21–22	Clavicle fused
21–30	Labodial suture (rear of cranium) fused
24–30	Sacrum bones fused
30–32	Sagittal suture (center of cranium) fused
48–50	Coronal suture (front of cranium) fused

Forensic Anthropology Note
Ancestry assessment represents a major component of forensic anthropological analysis of recovered human remains. Interpretations of ancestry, together with other aspects of the biological profile, can help narrow the search of missing persons and contribute to eventual positive identification. Such information can prove useful to authorities involved in the identification and investigative process since many lists of missing persons have a reference to this parameter. Recent research has strengthened available methodologies involving metric, non-metric morphological as well as chemical and genetic approaches.

TABLE 5–3

Summary of Skeletal Characteristics Indicating Racial Ancestry

	Eye Orbitals	Nasal Cavity	Incisors	Cranium Frontal Plane
European	Oval	Long, narrow	Smooth	Flat
Asian	Circular	Small, rounded	Shoveled interior	Flat or projected outward
African	Square	Wide	Smooth	Projected outward

TABLE 5–4

Equations for Height Calculation from Skeletal Remains

	European	African	Unknown Ancestry
Female	Height (cm) = femur length (cm) × 2.47 + 54.10	Height (cm) = femur length (cm) × 2.28 + 59.76	Height (cm) = femur length (cm) × 3.01 + 32.52
	Height (cm) = humerus length (cm) × 3.36 + 57.97	Height (cm) = humerus length (cm) × 3.08 + 64.67	Height (cm) = humerus length (cm) × 4.62 + 19.00
Male	Height (cm) = femur length (cm) × 2.32 + 65.53	Height (cm) = femur length (cm) × 2.10 + 72.22	Height (cm) = femur length (cm) × 2.71 + 45.86
	Height (cm) = humerus length (cm) × 2.89 + 78.10	Height (cm) = humerus length (cm) × 2.88 + 75.48	Height (cm) = humerus length (cm) × 4.62 + 19.00

Other Contributions of Forensic Anthropology

A forensic anthropologist may create facial reconstructions to help identify skeletal remains. Facial reconstruction clay is placed and shaped over the victim's actual cranium, and it takes into account the decedent's estimated age, ancestry, and sex (see Figure 5–19). With the help of this technique, a composite of the victim can be drawn and advertised in an attempt to identify the victim.

Forensic anthropologists are also helpful in identifying victims of a mass disaster such as a plane crash. When such a tragedy occurs, forensic anthropologists can help identify victims using the collection of bone fragments. Usually, the identification of the remains will depend on

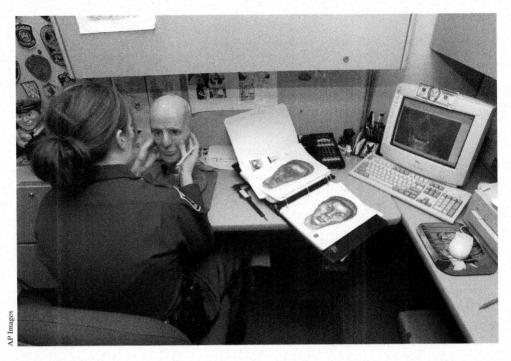

FIGURE 5–19

Trooper Sarah Foster, a Michigan State Police forensic artist, works on a three-dimensional facial reconstruction from an unidentified human skull at Richmond Post in Richmond, MI.

medical records, especially dental records of the individuals. However, definite identification of remains can be made only by analyzing the decedent's DNA profile, fingerprints, or medical records. Recovered remains may still contain some soft tissue material, such as the tissue of the hand, which may yield a DNA profile for identification purposes. If the tissue is dried out, it may be possible to rehydrate it to recover fingerprints also.

Case Files

Identifying a Serial Killer's Victims

The worst serial killer in the United States calmly admitted his guilt as he led investigators to a crawl space under his house. There, John Wayne Gacy had buried 28 young men, after brutally raping and murdering them in cold blood. Because no forms of identification were found with the bodies, the police were forced to examine missing-person reports for leads. However, these boys and men were so alike in age, ancestry, and stature that police were unable to individually identify most of the victims. Clyde Snow, the world-renowned forensic anthropologist from Oklahoma, was asked to help the investigators make these difficult identifications.

Snow began by making a 35-point examination of each skull for comparison to known individuals. By examining each skeleton, he made sure each bone was correctly attributed to an individual. This was crucial to later efforts because some of the victims had been buried on top of older graves, mingling their remains. Once Snow was sure all the bones were sorted properly, he began his in-depth study. Long bones such as the femur (thigh bone) were used to estimate each individual's height. This helped narrow the search

in the attempt to match the victims with the descriptions of missing people.

After narrowing the list of missing people to those fitting the general description, investigators consulted missing persons' hospital and dental records. Evidence of injury, illness, or surgery and other unique skeletal defects of the victims were matched to information in the records to make identifications. Snow also pointed out features that gave useful clues to the victim's behavior and medical history. For example, he discovered that one of Gacy's victims had a healed fracture on his left arm, and that his left scapula (shoulder blade) and arm bore the telltale signs of a left-handed individual. These details were matched to a missing-person report, and another young victim was identified.

For the most difficult cases, Snow called in the help of forensic sculptor and facial reconstructionist Betty Pat Gatliff. She used clay and depth markers to put the "flesh" back on the faces of these forgotten boys in the hopes that someone would recognize them after the photographs of the reconstructed faces were released to the media. Her efforts were successful, but investigators found some families unwilling to accept the idea that their loved one was among Gacy's victims. Even with Gatliff's help, nine of Gacy's victims remain unidentified.

Role of the Forensic Entomologist

The study of insects and their relation to a criminal investigation is known as forensic entomology. In practice, **forensic entomology** is commonly used to estimate the time of death when the circumstances surrounding the crime are unknown. This determination can be carried out by observing the stage of development of maggots or insects' sequence of arrival.

Determining Time of Death

After decomposition begins, necrophilious insects, or insects that feed on dead tissue, are the first to infest the body, usually within 24 hours. The most common and important of these is the blowfly, recognized by its green or blue color. Blowfly eggs are laid in human remains and ultimately hatch into maggots, or fly larvae, that consume human organs and tissues (see Figure 5–20). Typically, a single blowfly can lay up to 2,000 eggs during its lifetime. The resulting larvae gather and feed as a "maggot mass" on the decomposing remains. Forensic entomologists can approximate how long a body has been left exposed by examining the stage of development of the fly larvae. This kind of determination is best for a timeline of hours to approximately one month because the blowfly goes through the stages of its life cycle at a known sequence and in known time intervals that span this period. By determining the most developed stage of fly found on the body, entomologists can approximate the **postmortem interval (PMI)**, or the time that has elapsed since death (see Figure 5–21). Newly emerged flies are of important forensic interest, as they indicate that an entire blowfly cycle has been completed on the decomposing body. Likewise, empty pupal cases indicate that a fly has completed its entire life cycle on the body. Flies known as cheese skippers are primarily found on human corpses in the later stages of decomposition, long after the blowflies have left the corpse.

Time determinations based on the blowfly cycle are not always straightforward, however. The time required for each stage of development is affected by environmental influences such as geographical location, climate, weather conditions, and the presence of drugs. For example, cold temperatures hinder the development of fly eggs into adult flies. The forensic entomologist must consider these conditions when estimating the PMI.

Information about the arrival of other species of insects may also help determine the PMI. The sequence of arrival of these groups depends mostly on the body's natural decomposition process. Predator insects generally arrive and prey on the necrophilious insects. Several kinds of beetles will be found, either feeding directly on the corpse's tissues or as predators feeding on blowfly eggs and maggots present on the corpse. Next, omnivore insects arrive at the body. These insects feed on the body, on other insects, and on any surrounding vegetation. Ants and wasps are an example of omnivore insects. Last comes the arrival of indigenous insects, such as spiders, whose presence on or near the body is coincidental as they move about their environment.

Other Contributions of Forensic Entomology

Entomological evidence can also provide other pertinent information. In general, insects first colonize the body's naturally moist orifices. However, if open wounds are present, they will colonize there first. Although the decomposition processes may conceal wounds, colonization away from natural orifices may indicate the locations of wounds on the body. If maggots are found extensively on the hands and forearms, for example, this suggests the presence of defensive wounds on the victim. Insects that have fed on the body may also have accumulated any drugs present in the flesh, and analyzing these insects can yield the identity of these drugs.

If resources allow, all insect evidence should be carefully collected by a forensic entomology expert. When this is not possible, collection should be carried out by an investigator with experience in death investigation. The entire body and the area where insect evidence was found must be photographed and documented before collection. Insect specimens should be taken from each area on the body where they are found and labeled to show where they were collected from.

forensic entomology
The study of insect matter, growth patterns, and succession of arrival at a crime scene to determine the time since death.

postmortem interval (PMI)
The length of time that has elapsed since a person has died. If the time is not known, a number of medical or scientific techniques may be used to estimate it.

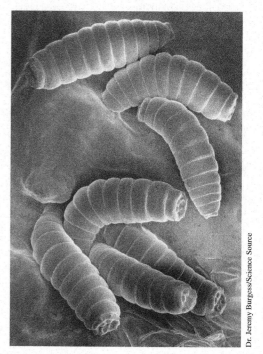

Dr. Jeremy Burgess/Science Source

FIGURE 5–20

A scanning electron micrograph of two-hour-old blowfly maggots.

Richard Saferstein, *Criminalistics: An Introduction to Forensic Science*, 12e, © 2018. Pearson Education, Inc., New York, NY.

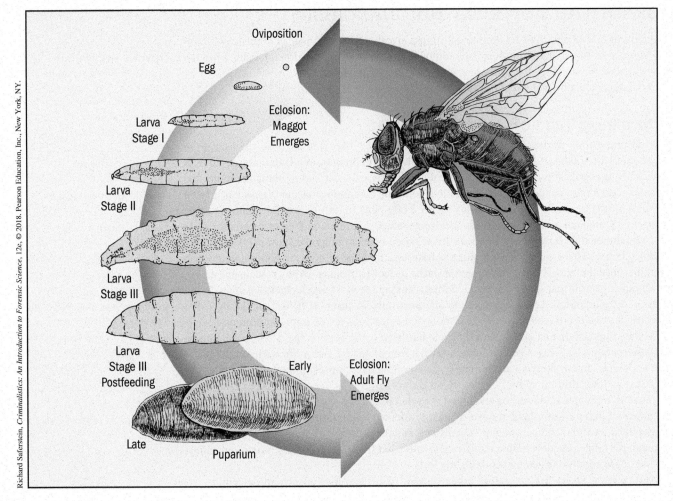

FIGURE 5–21

Typical blowfly life cycle from egg deposition to adult fly emergence. This cycle is representative of any 1 of nearly 90 species of blowflies in North America.

Case Files

The Danielle Van Dam Murder Case

Sometime during the night of February 1, 2002, 7-year-old Danielle Van Dam disappeared from her bedroom in the Sabre Springs suburb of San Diego, California. On February 27, three and a half weeks later, searchers found her naked body in a trash-covered lot about 25 miles from her home. Because of the high degree of decomposition of the girl's remains, the medical examiner could not pinpoint the exact time of the girl's death. Her neighbor, 50-year-old engineer David Westerfield, was accused of kidnapping Danielle, killing her, and dumping her body in the desert. During the subsequent investigation, Danielle's blood was found on Westerfield's clothes, her fingerprints and blood were found in his RV, and child pornography was found on his home computer.

The actual time of the 7-year-old's death became a central issue during the murder trial. Westerfield had been under constant police surveillance since February 4. Any suggestion that Danielle was placed at the dump site after that date would have eliminated him as a suspect. Conflicting expert testimony was elicited from forensic entomologists who were called on to estimate when the body was dumped. The forensic entomologist who went to the dump site, witnessed the autopsy, and collected and analyzed insects from both locations estimated that Danielle died between February 16 and 18. A forensic entomologist and a forensic anthropologist both called to testify on behalf of the prosecution noted that the very hot, very dry weather at the dump site might have mummified Danielle's body almost immediately, thus causing a delay in the flies colonizing the body.

The jurors convicted Westerfield of the kidnapping and murder of Danielle Van Dam, and a San Diego judge sentenced David Westerfield to death. Danielle Van Dam's parents filed and settled a wrongful death suit against Westerfield, requiring his automotive and homeowner's insurance carriers to pay the Van Dams an undisclosed amount, reported to be between $400,000 and $1 million.

Forensic pathologists associated with the medical examiner's or coroner's office are responsible for determining the cause of an undetermined or unexpected death. Although both the coroner's office and the medical examiner's office are charged with investigating suspicious deaths, only the pathologist is trained to perform an autopsy. The tasks of examining the body for cause and manner of death and recording the results in the death certificate are all responsibilities of both offices. Protection of the body and the overall scene is of paramount importance, as is the ultimate removal of the body in a medically acceptable manner. A primary objective of the autopsy is to determine the cause of death. The cause of death is defined as that which initiates the series of events ending in death. The most important determination in a violent death is the character of the injury that started the chain of events that resulted in death. Some of the more common causes of death are blunt-force injury, sharp-force injury, asphyxia, gunshot wounds, and substance use.

An autopsy, in its broadest definition, is simply the examination of a body after death. The forensic autopsy consists of an external examination and an internal examination of the condition of the body and the clothing. The dissection of the human body generally entails the removal of all internal organs through a Y-shaped incision beginning at the top of each shoulder and extending down to the pubic bone.

The internal examination entails weighing, dissecting, and sectioning each organ of the body. Blood is often tested to determine the presence and levels of alcohol and drugs. The manner in which death occurred is classified in death certifications as one of five categories: homicide, suicide, accidental, natural, or undetermined.

After death, the body undergoes a process known as algor mortis in which it will continually adjust to equalize with the environmental temperature. Another condition beginning when circulation ceases is livor mortis. When the human heart stops pumping, the blood begins to settle in the parts of the body closest to the ground. The skin appears bluish-purple in these areas. Immediately following death, a chemical change known as rigor mortis occurs in the muscles, causing them to become rigid.

Forensic anthropology is concerned primarily with the identification and examination of human skeletal remains. The sex of the decedent can be determined by the size and shape of various skeletal features, especially those in the pelvis and skull, or cranium. The height of the victim when alive can be estimated by measuring the long bones of the skeleton, especially those in the lower limbs. Forensic entomologists can approximate how long a body has been left exposed by examining the stage of development of the fly larvae on the body.

Review Questions

1. The titles of _____ and _____ are often used interchangeably, but there are significant differences in their job descriptions.

2. True or False: The medical examiner is an elected official and is not required to possess a medical degree. _____

3. Although both a coroner and a forensic pathologist are charged with investigating a suspicious death, only the _____ is trained to perform an autopsy.

4. True or False: If it appears that a victim did not shoot themself or anyone else, the victim's hands should not be swabbed. _____

5. The primary objective of the autopsy is to determine the _____.

6. True or False: The manner of death is defined as that which initiates the series of events ending in death. _____

7. A(n) _____-force injury can abrade and crush tissue.

8. True or False: The outward appearance of the injuries will always match the injuries sustained inside the body. _____

9. Wounds on a victim's forearm may be _____ wounds.

10. True or False: A lack of any defense wounds can lead a pathologist to believe that the victim was either unconscious or somehow tied up during the assault. _____

11. Asphyxia encompasses a variety of conditions that involve interference with the intake of _____.

12. True or False: Death at a fire scene is primarily caused by the extremely toxic gas carbon monoxide. _____

13. The protein in red blood cells that transports oxygen is known as _____.

14. True or False: High levels of carbon monoxide must be present for a victim to become disoriented and lose consciousness. _____

15. True or False: Carbon monoxide will continue to build up in the body after death. _____

16. Carbon monoxide levels and the presence of soot can be used to determine whether the individual was ____ at the time of the fire.

17. Victims of hangings often show signs of ____ on the eyelids, cheeks, and forehead.

18. Petechiae are caused by the escaping of blood into the tissue as a result of ____ bursting.

19. True or False: Petechiae are more common in hangings than strangulation deaths. ____

20. True or False: Typically the hyoid bone and thyroid cartilage are not fractured in hanging cases. ____

21. True or False: For gunshot victims, the cause of death can be listed as a gunshot wound. ____

22. True or False: Because drug use is so common, the forensic pathologist will routinely test for the presence of drugs in nearly all investigations. ____

23. A(n) ____ in its broadest definition is simply the examination of a body after death.

24. True or False: There are two types of autopsies: a forensic/medicolegal autopsy and a clinical/hospital autopsy. ____

25. The autopsy consists of a(n) ____ examination and a(n) ____ examination.

26. The discharge from a firearm will produce characteristic markings on the skin known as ____.

27. True or False: X-ray examinations are most commonly performed in gunshot wound cases and stab wound cases. ____

28. Pulmonary ____, or fluid accumulation in the lungs, is frequently found in victims of chronic cocaine and amphetamine use.

29. True or False: The liver can contain partially digested or dissolved pills. ____

30. True or False: The ideal location to take a blood sample is from the heart. ____

31. ____ is the redistribution of drugs after death.

32. True or False: General testing for poisons is not a routine procedure carried out by the pathologist. ____

33. A body that displays a cherry-red discoloration often leads a pathologist to suspect poisoning by ____.

34. True or False: A pathologist can often give an exact time of death. ____

35. The process of the body's continually decreasing in temperature after death until it reaches the environmental temperature is known as ____.

36. The process of the blood settling in parts of the body closest to the ground after death is known as ____.

37. True or False: Different lividity patterns on a body may indicate that the body was moved after death but before livor mortis had fully fixed. ____

38. Levels of ____ in the ocular fluid can help indicate the time of death.

39. After death, two decomposition processes take place: ____ and ____.

40. The female bone structure differs from the male structure within the ____ area because of a woman's childbearing capabilities.

41. True or False: A definite identification of remains cannot be made through the analysis of the decedent's DNA profile, fingerprints, or medical records. ____

42. True or False: A site where human remains are found must be treated as a crime scene, and the site and surrounding area should be secured, searched, and carefully processed. ____

43. The field of ____ takes advantage of the durable nature of bones over a long period of time to examine and identify human skeletal remains through a multitude of individual characteristics.

44. The study of insects and their relation to a criminal investigation, known as ____, is commonly used to estimate the time of death when the circumstances surrounding the crime are unknown.

45. By determining the oldest stage of fly found on the body and taking environmental factors into consideration, entomologists can approximate the ____ interval.

46. True or False: Another method to determine PMI is by observing the schedule of arrival of different insect species on the body. ____

Application and Critical Thinking

1. Rigor mortis, livor mortis, and algor mortis are all used to help determine time of death. However, each method has its limitations. For each method, describe at least one condition that would render that method unsuitable or inaccurate for determining the time of death.

2. What kind of forensic expert would most likely be asked to help identify human remains in each of the following conditions?

   a. A body that has been decomposing for a day or two

   b. Fragmentary remains of a few arm bones and part of a jaw

   c. A skeleton that is missing its skull

3. Identify a reasonable manner of death for each of the following situations:

   a. A contact wound to the back of the head

   b. An elevated carboxyhemoglobin blood level in a fire victim

   c. A fractured hyoid bone

   d. Death by overdose of a first-time user of alcohol

   e. A gunshot wound to the chest from a distance of 3 feet

   f. Sudden death of a young chronic user of cocaine

4. In cooperation with the medical examiner or coroner, evidence retrieved from a deceased victim and sent to the crime lab should include which items?

5. **Creating a Forensic Anthropology Victim Profile** A nearly complete human skeleton has been found. The skeleton has the features shown in the accompanying table and image. Approximate the sex, ancestry, age range, and height of the individual based on this information.

6. **Sequence of Insect Arrival in Forensic Entomology** The following images depict the sequence of events at the site of a decomposing body. Place the arrival events in order of occurrence from earliest to latest.

Cranium	
Size	Medium
Forehead	Rounded, projected outward
Mastoid process	Absent
Jaw	Angle = 110 degrees
Teeth	All permanent
Sagittal suture	Not fused
Coronal suture	Not fused
Eye orbits	Squared
Nasal cavity	Large, wide
Incisors	Smooth
Pelvis	
Opening	*See figure*
Sacrum	*See figure*
Subpubic angle	90–100 degrees
Long Bones	
Femur	Fully fused, 44.1 cm long
Clavicle	Fully fused
Sex ____	Ancestry ____
Age range ____	Height ____

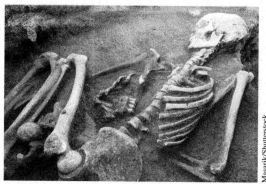

Masarik/Shutterstock

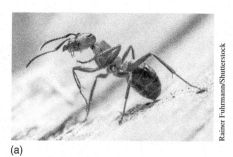

(a)

Rainer Fuhrmann/Shutterstock

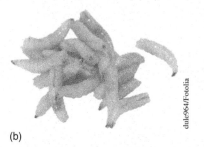

(b)

dule964/Fotolia

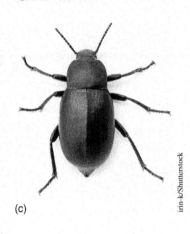

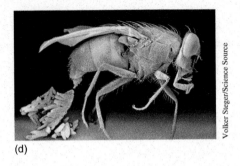

(c)

irin-k/Shutterstock

(d)

Volker Steger/Science Source

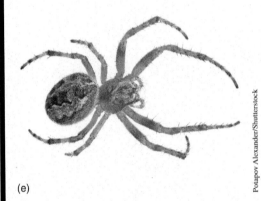

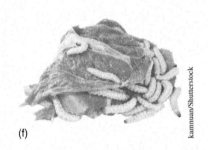

(e)

Potapov Alexander/Shutterstock

(f)

kanmuan/Shutterstock

Further References

DiMaio, V. J. M., and S. E. Dana, *Handbook of Forensic Pathology*, 2nd ed. Boca Raton, FL: CRC Press, 2006.

James, S. H., J. J. Norby, and S. Bell, eds. *Forensic Science: An Introduction to Scientific and Investigative Techniques*, 4th ed. Boca Raton, FL: CRC Press, 2014.

Spitz, W. U., and D. J. Spitz, eds., *Spitz and Fisher's Medicolegal Investigation of Death: Guidelines for the Application of Pathology to Crime Investigation*, 4th ed. Springfield, IL: Charles C. Thomas, 2006.

Fingerprints

Go to www.pearsonhighered.com/careersresources to access Webextras for this chapter.

Learning Objectives

After studying this chapter, you should be able to:

6.1 Recount the development of fingerprinting as a means of identification

6.2 Summarize the three fundamental principles of fingerprints

6.3 Explain the primary classification system of fingerprints

6.4 Describe the concept of an automated fingerprint identification system (AFIS)

6.5 Describe visible, plastic, and latent fingerprints and the techniques for developing latent fingerprints

6.6 Describe the proper procedures for preserving a developed latent fingerprint

6.7 Discuss the tools involved in fingerprint analysis and enhancement

KEY TERMS

anthropometry
arch
digital imaging
fluoresce
iodine fuming
latent fingerprint
livescan
loop
ninhydrin
Physical Developer
pixel
plastic print
portrait parlé
ridge characteristics
   (minutiae)
sublimation
superglue fuming
visible print
whorl

Killer Twin: Ronald and Donald Smith

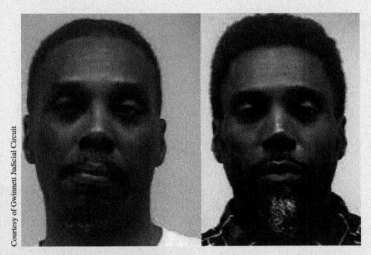

School teacher Genai Coleman had been waiting to pick up her teenage daughter from a transit station in Duluth, Georgia, on July 18, 2008, when someone shot her and stole her car. The car was later found abandoned and processed by police as part of the investigation into her death. Inside, they found a cigarette butt that was later submitted to the Georgia Bureau of Investigation. At the crime lab, DNA analysts recovered a profile from the cigarette and uploaded it to the CODIS database. The profile returned a hit to Donald Smith, who had a prior drug conviction. When investigators reviewed video of Smith from a QuickTrip gas station in the area of the shooting, they were sure they had the evidence they needed to convict him of Genai Coleman's murder.

Donald Smith was arrested and confronted with the DNA and video evidence. Smith insisted it was not him on the surveillance video, it was his identical twin, Ronald. He told police to show the video to show the video footage to his parents and his sister to see if they could identify the twin pictured. The Smith family identified Ronald Smith as the individual on the tape. When DNA and video evidence failed to identify the killer twin, the police turned to the fingerprints collected from the vehicle. After a comparison of the latent prints collected from Coleman's car to the twins, police discovered it was Ronald Smith who had been in the victim's car after all.

When confronted with the fingerprint evidence, Ronald Smith confessed to police that he had killed the victim on accident. Later, he recanted his statements and claimed at trial that he was not the killer, that his twin brother Donald had committed the crime. He claimed his fingerprints were only on the victim's car because he had helped his brother clean it. Donald Smith's fingerprints were not located anywhere on the inside or outside of Genai Coleman's vehicle. Ronald Smith was convicted of the murder of Genai Coleman on October 19, 2012, and sentenced to life in prison plus 25 years.

History of Fingerprinting

Since the beginnings of criminal investigation, police have sought an infallible means of human identification. The first systematic attempt at personal identification was devised and introduced by a French police expert, Alphonse Bertillon, in 1883. The Bertillon system relied on a detailed description (**portrait parlé**) of the subject, combined with full-length and profile photographs and a system of precise body measurements known as **anthropometry**.

The use of anthropometry as a method of identification rested on the premise that the dimensions of the human bone system remained fixed from age 20 until death. Skeleton sizes were thought to be so extremely diverse that no two individuals could have exactly the same measurements. Bertillon recommended routine taking of 11 measurements of the human anatomy. These included height, reach, width of head, and length of the left foot (see Figure 1–3).

For two decades, this system was considered the most accurate method of identification. But in the first years of the new century, police began to appreciate and accept a system of identification based on the classification of finger ridge patterns known as *fingerprints*. Today, the fingerprint is the pillar of modern criminal identification.

Early Use of Fingerprints

Evidence exists that the Chinese used the fingerprint to sign legal documents as far back as 3,000 years ago. However, whether this practice was performed for ceremonial custom or as a means of personal identity remains a point of conjecture lost to history. In any case, the examples of fingerprinting in ancient history are ambiguous, and the few that exist did not contribute to the development of fingerprinting techniques as we know them today.

Several years before Bertillon began work on his system, William Herschel, an English civil servant stationed in India, started the practice of requiring Indian citizens to sign contracts with the imprint of their right hand, which was pressed against a stamp pad for the purpose. The motives for Herschel's requirement remain unclear; he may have envisioned fingerprinting as a means of personal identification or just as a form of the Hindu custom that a trace of bodily contact was more binding than a signature on a contract. In any case, he did not publish anything about his activities until after a Scottish physician, Henry Faulds, working in a hospital in Japan, published his views on the potential application of fingerprinting to personal identification.

In 1880, Faulds suggested that skin ridge patterns could be important for the identification of people who commit crimes. He told about a thief who left his fingerprint on a whitewashed wall, and how in comparing these prints with those of a suspect, he found that they were quite different. A few days later, another suspect was found whose fingerprints compared with those on the wall. When confronted with this evidence, the individual confessed to the crime.

Faulds was convinced that fingerprints furnished infallible proof of identification. He even offered to set up, at his own expense, a fingerprint bureau at Scotland Yard to test the practicality of the method. But his offer was rejected in favor of the Bertillon system. This decision was reversed less than two decades later.

Early Classification of Fingerprints

The extensive research into fingerprinting conducted by another Englishman, Francis Galton, provided the needed impetus that made police agencies aware of its potential application. In 1892, Galton published his classic textbook *Finger Prints*, the first book of its kind on the subject. In his book, he discussed the anatomy of fingerprints and suggested methods for recording them. Galton also proposed assigning fingerprints to three pattern types—loops, arches, and whorls. Most importantly, the book demonstrated that no two prints were identical and that an individual's prints remained unchanged from year to year. At Galton's insistence, the British government adopted fingerprinting as a supplement to the Bertillon system.

The next step in the development of fingerprint technology was the creation of classification systems capable of filing thousands of prints in a logical and searchable sequence. Dr. Juan Vucetich, an Argentinian police officer fascinated by Galton's work, devised a workable concept in 1891. His classification system has been refined over the years and is still widely used today in most Spanish-speaking countries. In 1897, another classification system was proposed by an Englishman, Sir Edward Richard Henry. Four years later, Henry's system was adopted by Scotland Yard. Today, most English-speaking countries, including the United States, use some version of Henry's classification system to file fingerprints.

portrait parlé
A verbal description of a perpetrator's physical characteristics and dress provided by an eyewitness.

anthropometry
A system of identification of individuals by measurement of parts of the body, developed by Alphonse Bertillon.

Adoption of Fingerprinting

Early in the 20th century, Bertillon's measurement system began to fall into disfavor. Its results were highly susceptible to error, particularly when the measurements were taken by people who were not thoroughly trained. The method was dealt its most severe and notable setback in 1903 when a convict, Will West, arrived at Fort Leavenworth prison. A routine check of the prison files startlingly revealed that a William West, already in the prison, could not be distinguished from the new prisoner by body measurements or even by photographs. In fact, the two men looked just like twins, and their measurements were practically the same. Subsequently, fingerprints of the prisoners clearly distinguished them.

In the United States, the first systematic and official use of fingerprints for personal identification was adopted by the New York City Civil Service Commission in 1901. The method was used for certifying all civil service applications. Several American police officials received instruction in fingerprint identification at the 1904 World's Fair in St. Louis from representatives of Scotland Yard. After the fair and the Will West incident, fingerprinting began to be used in earnest in all major cities of the United States. In 1924, the fingerprint records of the Bureau of Investigation and Leavenworth were merged to form the nucleus of the identification records of the new Federal Bureau of Investigation. The FBI has the largest collection of fingerprints in the world. By the beginning of World War I, England and practically all of Europe had adopted fingerprinting as their primary method of identifying people who commit crimes.

In 1999, the admissibility of fingerprint evidence was challenged in the case of *United States* v. *Byron C. Mitchell* in the Eastern District of Pennsylvania. The defendant's attorneys argued that fingerprints could not be proven unique under the guidelines cited in *Daubert* (see pages 18–19). Government experts vigorously disputed this claim. After a four-and-a-half-day *Daubert* hearing, the judge upheld the admissibility of fingerprints as scientific evidence and ruled that (1) human friction ridges are unique and permanent and (2) human friction ridge skin arrangements are unique and permanent.

Fundamental Principles of Fingerprints

First Principle: A Fingerprint Is an Individual Characteristic; No Two Fingers Have yet Been Found to Possess Identical Ridge Characteristics

The acceptance of fingerprint evidence by the courts has always been predicated on the assumption that no two individuals have identical fingerprints. Early fingerprint experts consistently referred to Galton's calculation, showing the possible existence of 64 billion different fingerprints, to support this contention. Later, researchers questioned the validity of Galton's figures and attempted to devise mathematical models to better approximate this value. However, no matter what mathematical model one refers to, the conclusions are always the same: the probability for the existence of two identical fingerprint patterns in the world's population is extremely small.

Not only is this principle supported by theoretical calculations, but just as important, it is verified by the millions of individuals who have had their prints classified during the past 120 years—no two have ever been found to be identical. The FBI has nearly 101 million fingerprint records in its computer database and has yet to find an identical image belonging to two different people.

ridge characteristics (minutiae)
Ridge endings, bifurcations, enclosures, and other ridge details, which must match in two fingerprints in order for their common origin to be established.

RIDGE CHARACTERISTICS   The individuality of a fingerprint is not determined by its general shape or pattern but by a careful study of its **ridge characteristics** (also known as **minutiae**). The identity, number, and relative location of characteristics such as those illustrated in Figure 6–1 impart individuality to a fingerprint. If two prints are to match, they must reveal characteristics that not only are identical but have the same relative location to one another in a print. In a judicial proceeding, a point-by-point comparison must be demonstrated by the expert, using charts similar to the one shown in Figure 6–2, in order to prove the identity of an individual.

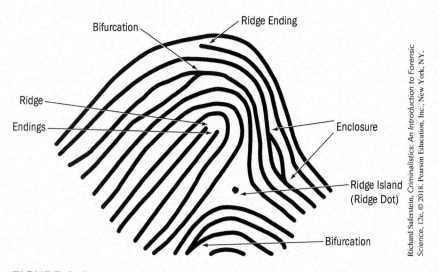

FIGURE 6–1

Fingerprint ridge characteristics.

If an expert were asked to compare the characteristics of the complete fingerprint, no difficulty would be encountered in completing such an assignment; the average fingerprint has as many as 150 individual ridge characteristics. However, most prints recovered at crime scenes are partial impressions, showing only a segment of the entire print. Under these circumstances, the expert can compare only a small number of ridge characteristics from the recovered print to a known recorded print.

RIDGE COMPARISONS   For years, experts have debated how many ridge comparisons are necessary to identify two fingerprints as the same. Numbers that range from 8 to 16 have been suggested as being sufficient to meet the criteria of individuality. However, the difficulty in establishing such a minimum is that no comprehensive statistical study has ever been undertaken to determine the frequency of occurrence of different ridge characteristics and their relative

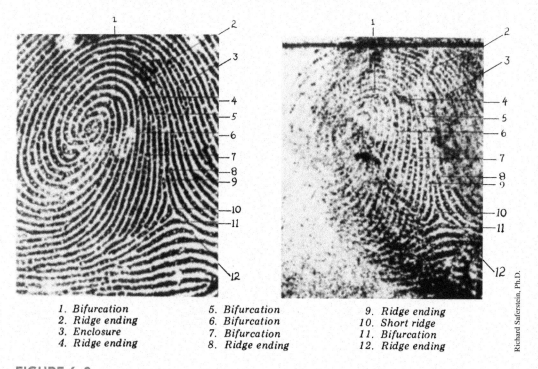

1. Bifurcation	5. Bifurcation	9. Ridge ending
2. Ridge ending	6. Bifurcation	10. Short ridge
3. Enclosure	7. Bifurcation	11. Bifurcation
4. Ridge ending	8. Ridge ending	12. Ridge ending

FIGURE 6–2

A fingerprint exhibit illustrating the matching ridge characteristics between the crime-scene print and an inked impression of one of the suspect's fingers.

locations. Until such a study is undertaken and completed, no meaningful guidelines can be established for defining the uniqueness of a fingerprint.

In 1973, the International Association for Identification, after a three-year study of this question, concluded that "no valid basis exists for requiring a predetermined minimum number of friction ridge characteristics which must be present in two impressions in order to establish positive identification." Hence, the final determination must be based on the experience and knowledge of the expert, with the understanding that others may profess honest differences of opinion on the uniqueness of a fingerprint if the question of minimal number of ridge characteristics exists. In 1995, members of the international fingerprint community at a conference in Israel issued the Ne'urim Declaration, which supported the 1973 International Association for Identification resolution.

Second Principle: A Fingerprint Remains Unchanged During an Individual's Lifetime

Fingerprints are a reproduction of friction skin ridges found on the palm side of the fingers and thumbs. Similar friction skin can also be found on the surface of the palms and soles of the feet. Apparently, these skin surfaces have been designed by nature to provide our bodies with a firmer grasp and a resistance to slippage. A visual inspection of friction skin reveals a series of lines corresponding to hills (ridges) and valleys (grooves). The shape and form of the skin ridges are what one sees as the black lines of an inked fingerprint impression.

STRUCTURE OF THE SKIN   Skin is composed of layers of cells. Those nearest the surface make up the outer portion of the skin known as the *epidermis*, and the inner skin is known as the *dermis*. A cross section of skin (see Figure 6–3) reveals a boundary of cells separating the epidermis and dermis. The shape of this boundary, made up of *dermal papillae*, determines the form and pattern of the ridges on the surface of the skin. Once the dermal papillae develop in the human fetus, the ridge patterns remain unchanged throughout life except to enlarge during growth.

Each skin ridge is populated by a single row of pores that are the openings for ducts leading from the sweat glands. Through these pores, perspiration is discharged and deposited on the surface of the skin. Once the finger touches a surface, perspiration, along with oils that may have been picked up by touching the hairy portions of the body, is transferred onto that surface, thereby leaving an impression of the finger's ridge pattern (a fingerprint). Prints deposited in this manner are invisible to the eye and are commonly referred to as **latent fingerprints**.

latent fingerprint
A fingerprint made by the deposit of oils and/or perspiration; it is invisible to the naked eye.

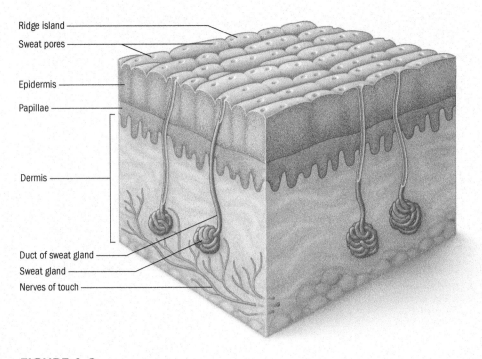

Ridge island
Sweat pores
Epidermis
Papillae
Dermis
Duct of sweat gland
Sweat gland
Nerves of touch

Pearson Education, Inc.

FIGURE 6–3
Cross-section of human skin.

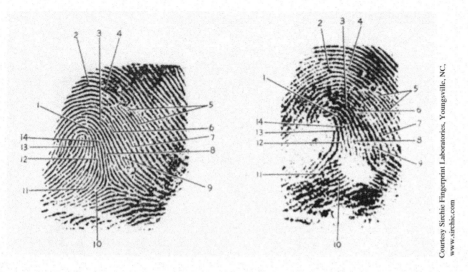

FIGURE 6–4

The right index finger impression of John Dillinger, before scarification on the left and afterward on the right. Comparison is proved by the 14 matching ridge characteristics.

CHANGING FINGERPRINTS   Although it is impossible to change one's fingerprints, there has been no lack of effort on the part of some people who commit crimes to obscure them. If an injury reaches deeply enough into the skin and damages the dermal papillae, a permanent scar will form. However, for this to happen, such a wound would have to penetrate 1 to 2 millimeters beneath the skin's surface. Indeed, efforts at intentionally scarring the skin can only be self-defeating, for it would be totally impossible to obliterate all of the ridge characteristics on the hand, and the presence of permanent scars merely provides new characteristics for identification.

Perhaps the most publicized attempt at obliteration was that of the notorious gangster John Dillinger, who tried to destroy his own fingerprints by applying a corrosive acid to them. Prints taken at the morgue after he was shot to death, compared with fingerprints recorded at the time of a previous arrest, proved that his efforts had been fruitless (see Figure 6–4).

Third Principle: Fingerprints Have General Ridge Patterns That Permit Them to Be Systematically Classified

All fingerprints are divided into three classes on the basis of their general pattern: **loops**, **whorls**, and **arches**. Sixty to 65 percent of the population have loops, 30 to 35 percent have whorls, and about 5 percent have arches. These three classes form the basis for all 10-finger classification systems presently in use.

LOOPS   A typical loop pattern is illustrated in Figure 6–5. A loop must have one or more ridges entering from one side of the print, recurving, and exiting from the same side. If the loop opens toward the little finger, it is called an *ulnar loop*; if it opens toward the thumb, it is a *radial loop*. The pattern area of the loop is surrounded by two diverging ridges known as *type lines*. The ridge point at or nearest the type-line divergence and located at or directly in front of the point of divergence is known as the *delta*. To many, a fingerprint delta resembles the silt formation that builds up as a river flows into the entrance of a lake—hence, the analogy to the geological formation known as a delta. All loops must have one delta. The *core*, as the name suggests, is the approximate center of the pattern.

WHORLS   Whorls are actually divided into four distinct groups, as shown in Figure 6–6: plain, central pocket loop, double loop, and accidental. All whorl patterns must have type lines and at least two deltas. A plain whorl and a central pocket loop have at least one ridge that makes a complete circuit. This ridge may be in the form of a spiral, an oval, or any variant of a circle. If an imaginary line drawn between the two deltas contained within these two patterns touches any one of the spiral ridges, the pattern is a plain whorl. If no such ridge is touched, the pattern is a central pocket loop.

loop
A class of fingerprints characterized by ridge lines that enter from one side of the pattern and curve around to exit from the same side of the pattern.

whorl
A class of fingerprints that includes ridge patterns that are generally rounded or circular in shape and have two deltas.

FIGURE 6–5
Loop pattern.

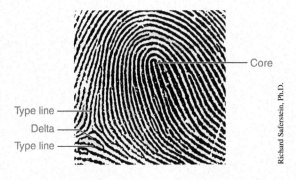

FIGURE 6–6
Whorl patterns.

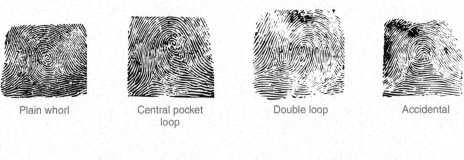

Plain whorl   Central pocket loop   Double loop   Accidental

FIGURE 6–7
Arch patterns.

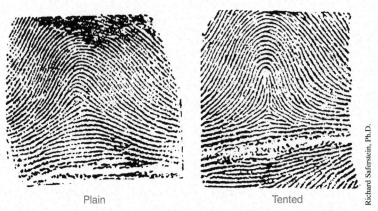

Plain   Tented

As the name implies, the double loop is made up of two loops combined into one fingerprint. Any whorl classified as an accidental either contains two or more patterns (not including the plain arch) or is a pattern not covered by other categories. Hence, an accidental may consist of a combination loop and plain whorl or loop and tented arch.

arch
A class of fingerprints characterized by ridge lines that enter the print from one side and flow out the other side.

ARCHES   Arches, the least common of the three general patterns, are subdivided into two distinct groups: plain arches and tented arches, as shown in Figure 6–7. The plain arch is the simplest of all fingerprint patterns; it is formed by ridges entering from one side of the print and exiting on the opposite side. Generally, these ridges tend to rise in the center of the pattern, forming a wavelike pattern. The tented arch is similar to the plain arch except that instead of rising smoothly at the center, there is a sharp upthrust or spike, or the ridges meet at an angle that is less than 90 degrees.[1] Arches do not have type lines, deltas, or cores.

With a knowledge of basic fingerprint pattern classes, we can now begin to develop an appreciation for fingerprint classification systems. However, the subject is far more complex than can be described in a textbook of this nature. The student seeking a more detailed treatment of the subject would do well to consult the references cited at the end of the chapter.

---

[1] A tented arch is also any pattern that resembles a loop but lacks one of the essential requirements for classification as a loop.

Inside the Science

The ACE-V Process

ACE-V is an acronym for the four-step process—*analysis, comparison, evaluation,* and *verification*—used to identify and individualize a fingerprint. The first step requires the examiner to identify any distortions associated with the friction ridges, as well as any external factors, such as surface or deposition factors or processing techniques, that may impinge on the print's appearance. If the examiner determines the latent print adequate, they will declare the print to be of value for the comparison stage.

The comparison step requires the examiner to compare the questioned print to the known print at three levels. Level 1 looks at the general ridge flow and pattern configuration. Level 2 includes locating and comparing ridge characteristics, or minutiae. Level 2 details can individualize a print. Level 3 includes the examination and location of ridge pores,

breaks, creases, scars, and other permanent minutiae. During the comparison phase, the examiner compares the latent print side by side with an exemplar print in its totality.

The evaluation stage requires one of three decisions to be arrived at. The decisions that can be reported are *identification* (the latent print and exemplar came from the same source); *exclusion* (the latent print and exemplar did not come from the same source); *inconclusive* (one cannot determine that the latent print and exemplar came from the same source, or not, to a sufficiently strong level of certainty).

The final step in the process involves verification of the examiner's result. It requires an independent examination of the questioned and known prints by a second examiner. Ultimately, a consensus between the two examiners must be arrived at before a final conclusion is drawn.

Classification of Fingerprints

The original Henry system, as it was adopted by Scotland Yard in 1901, converted ridge patterns on all 10 fingers into a series of letters and numbers arranged in the form of a fraction. However, the system as it was originally designed could accommodate files of up to only 100,000 sets of prints; thus, as collections grew in size, it became necessary to expand the capacity of the classification system. In the United States, the FBI, faced with the problem of filing ever-increasing numbers of prints, expanded its classification capacity by modifying and extending the original Henry system. These modifications are collectively known as the *FBI system* and are used by most agencies in the United States today.

The Primary Classification

Although we will not discuss all of the different divisions of the FBI system, a description of just one part, the primary classification, will provide an interesting insight into the process of fingerprint classification.

The primary classification is part of the original Henry system and provides the first classification step in the FBI system. Using this classification alone, all of the fingerprint cards in the world could be divided into 1,024 groups. The first step in obtaining the primary classification is to pair up fingers, placing one finger in the numerator of a fraction, the other in the denominator. The fingers are paired in the following sequence:

$$\frac{\text{R. Index}}{\text{R. Thumb}} \qquad \frac{\text{R. Ring}}{\text{R. Middle}} \qquad \frac{\text{L. Thumb}}{\text{R. Little}} \qquad \frac{\text{L. Middle}}{\text{L. Index}} \qquad \frac{\text{L. Little}}{\text{L. Ring}}$$

The presence or absence of the whorl pattern is the basis for determination of the primary classification. If a whorl pattern is found on any finger of the first pair, it is assigned a value of 16; on the second pair, a value of 8; on the third pair, a value of 4; on the fourth pair, a value of 2; and on the last pair, a value of 1. Any finger with an arch or loop pattern is assigned a value of 0.

After values for all 10 fingers are obtained in this manner, they are totaled, and 1 is added to both the numerator and denominator. The fraction thus obtained is the primary classification.

For example, if the right index and right middle fingers are whorls and all the others are loops, the primary classification is

$$\frac{16 + 0 + 0 + 0 + 0 + 1}{0 + 8 + 0 + 0 + 0 + 1} = \frac{17}{9}$$

Approximately 25 percent of the population falls into the 1/1 category; that is, all their fingers have either loops or arches.

A fingerprint classification system cannot in itself unequivocally identify an individual; it merely provides the fingerprint examiner with a number of candidates, all of whom have an indistinguishable set of prints in the system's file. The identification must always be made by a final visual comparison of the suspect print's and file print's ridge characteristics; only these features can impart individuality to a fingerprint. Although ridge patterns impart class characteristics to the print, the type and position of ridge characteristics give it its individual character.

Automated Fingerprint Identification Systems

The Henry system and its subclassifications have proven to be a cumbersome system for storing, retrieving, and searching for fingerprints, particularly as fingerprint collections grow in size. Nevertheless, until the emergence of fingerprint computer technology, this manual approach was the only viable method for the maintenance of fingerprint collections. Since 1970, technological advances have made possible the classification and retrieval of fingerprints by computers. Automated Fingerprint Identification Systems (AFISs) have proliferated throughout the law enforcement community.

In 1999, the FBI initiated full operation of the Integrated Automated Fingerprint Identification System (IAFIS), the largest AFIS in the United States, which links state AFIS computers with the FBI database. In 2014, the IAFIS was effectively replaced and integrated into the Next Generation Identification (NGI) system. The expanded capabilities of NGI beyond fingerprints will be discussed in Chapter 7. This database contains over 100 million fingerprint records. However, an AFIS can come in all sizes ranging from the FBI's to independent systems operated by cities, counties, and other agencies of local government (see Figure 6–8). Unfortunately, these local systems often are not linked to the state's AFIS system because of differences in software configurations.

How AFIS Works

The heart of AFIS technology is the ability of a computer to scan and digitally encode fingerprints so that they can be subject to high-speed computer processing. **The AFIS uses automatic scanning devices that convert the image of a fingerprint into digital minutiae that contain data showing ridges at their points of termination (ridge endings) and the branching of ridges into two ridges (bifurcations). The relative position and orientation of the minutiae are also determined, allowing the computer to store each fingerprint in the form of a digitally recorded geometric pattern.**

The computer's search algorithm determines the degree of correlation between the location and relationship of the minutiae for both the search and file prints. In this manner, a computer can make thousands of fingerprint comparisons in a second; for example, a set of 10 fingerprints can be searched against a file of 500,000 ten-finger prints (ten-prints) in about eight-tenths of a second. During the search for a match, the computer uses a scoring system that assigns prints to each of the criteria set by an operator. When the search is complete, the computer produces a list of file prints that have the closest correlation to the search prints. All of the selected prints are then examined by a trained fingerprint expert, who makes the final verification of the print's identity. Thus, the AFIS makes no final decisions on the identity of a fingerprint, leaving this function to the eyes of a trained examiner.

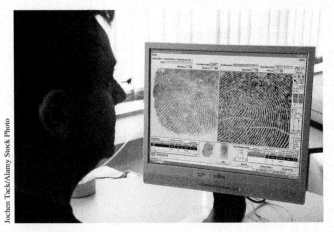

Jochen Tack/Alamy Stock Photo

FIGURE 6–8

An AFIS system designed for use by local law enforcement agencies.

The speed and accuracy of ten-print processing by AFIS have made possible the search of single latent crime-scene fingerprints against an entire file's print collection. Before the AFIS, police were usually restricted to comparing crime-scene fingerprints against those of known suspects. The impact of the AFIS on no-suspect cases has been dramatic. Minutes after California's AFIS network received its first assignment, the computer scored a direct hit by identifying an individual who had committed 15 murders, terrorizing the city of Los Angeles. Police estimate that it would have taken a single technician, manually searching the city's 1.7 million print cards, 67 years to come up with the perpetrator's prints. With the AFIS, the search took approximately 20 minutes. In its first year of operation, San Francisco's AFIS computer conducted 5,514 latent fingerprint searches and achieved 1,001 identifications—a hit rate of 18 percent. This compares to the previous year's average of 8 percent for manual latent-print searches.

As an example of how an AFIS computer operates, one system has been designed to automatically filter out imperfections in a latent print, enhance its image, and create a graphic representation of the fingerprint's ridge endings and bifurcations and their direction. The print is then computer searched against file prints. The image of the latent print and a matching file print are then displayed side by side on a high-resolution video monitor, as shown in Figure 6–9. The matching latent and file prints are then verified and charted by a fingerprint examiner at a video workstation.

The stereotypical image of a booking officer rolling inked fingers onto a standard ten-print card for ultimate transmission to a database has, for the most part, been replaced with digital-capture devices (**livescan**) that eliminate ink and paper. The livescan captures the image on each finger and the palms as they are lightly pressed against a glass platen. These livescan images can then be sent to the AFIS database electronically, so that within minutes the booking agency can enter the fingerprint record into the AFIS database and search the database for previous entries of the same individual (see Figure 6–10).

livescan

An inkless device that captures the digital images of fingerprints and palm prints and electronically transmits the images to an AFIS.

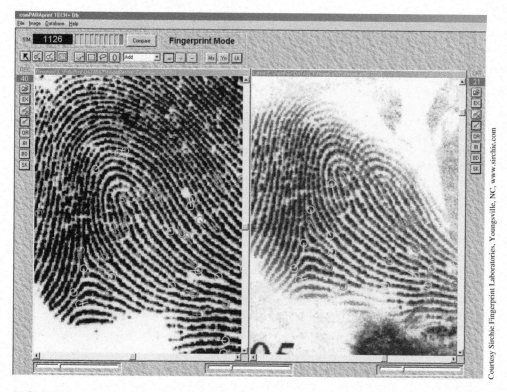

FIGURE 6–9

A side-by-side comparison of a latent print against a file fingerprint is conducted in seconds, and their similarity rating (SIM) is displayed on the upper-left portion of the screen.

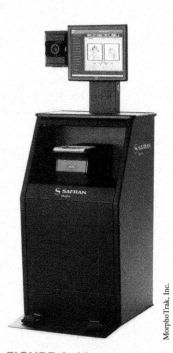

FIGURE 6–10

Livescan technology enables law enforcement to print and compare a subject's fingerprints rapidly, without inking the fingerprints.

Considerations with AFIS

AFIS has fundamentally changed the way criminal investigators operate, allowing them to spend less time developing suspect lists and more time investigating the suspects generated by the computer. However, investigators must be cautioned against overreliance on a computer. Sometimes a latent print does not make a hit because of the poor quality of the file print. To avoid these potential problems, investigators must still print all known suspects in a case and manually search these prints against the crime-scene prints.

AFIS computers are available from several different suppliers. Each system scans fingerprint images and detects and records information about minutiae (ridge endings and bifurcations); however, they do not all incorporate exactly the same features, coordinate systems, or units of measure to record fingerprint information. These software incompatibilities often mean that, although state systems can communicate with the FBI's NGI system, they may not communicate with each other directly. Likewise, local and state systems frequently cannot share information with each other. Many of these technical problems will be resolved as more agencies follow transmission standards developed by the National Institute of Standards and Technology and the FBI.

Methods of Detecting Fingerprints

Through common usage, the term *latent fingerprint* has come to be associated with any fingerprint discovered at a crime scene. Sometimes, however, prints found at the scene of a crime are quite visible to the eye, and the word *latent* is a misnomer. Actually, there are three kinds of

Case Files

The Night Stalker

Richard Ramirez committed his first murder in June 1984. His victim was a 79-year-old woman who was stabbed repeatedly and sexually assaulted and then had her throat slashed. It would be eight months before Ramirez murdered again. In the spring, Ramirez began a murderous rampage that resulted in 13 additional killings and 5 rapes.

His modus operandi was to enter a home through an open window, shoot the male residents, and savagely rape his female victims. He scribed a pentagram on the wall of one of his victims and the words *Jack the Knife* and was reported by another to force her to "swear to Satan" during the assault. His identity still unknown, the news media dubbed him the "Night Stalker." As the body count continued to rise, public hysteria and a media frenzy prevailed.

The break in the case came when the license plate of what seemed to be a suspicious car related to a sighting of the Night Stalker was reported to the police. The police determined that the car had been stolen and eventually located it, abandoned in a parking lot. After processing the car for prints, police found one usable partial fingerprint. This fingerprint was entered into the Los Angeles Police Department's brand-new AFIS computerized fingerprint system.

The Night Stalker was identified as Richard Ramirez, who had been fingerprinted following a traffic violation some years before. Police searching the home of one of his friends found the gun used to commit the murders, and jewelry belonging to his victims was found in the possession of

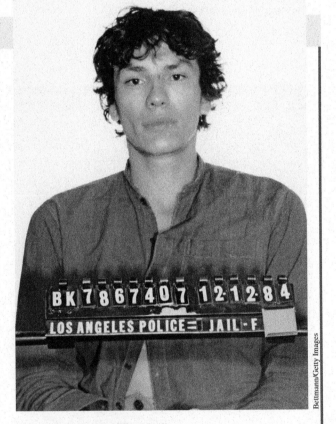

Richard Ramirez, the Night Stalker.

Ramirez's sister. Ramirez was convicted of murder and sentenced to death in 1989, where he died from natural causes in 2013.

> > > > > > > > >

Case Files

The Mayfield Affair

On March 11, 2004, a series of 10 explosions at four sites occurred on commuter trains traveling to or near the Atocha train station in Madrid, Spain. The death toll from these explosions was nearly 200, with more than 1,500 injured. On the day of the attack, a plastic bag was found in a van previously reported as stolen. The bag contained copper detonators like those used on the train bombs. On March 17, the FBI received electronic images of latent fingerprints that were recovered from the plastic bag. A search was initiated on the FBI's IAFIS. A senior fingerprint examiner encoded seven minutiae points from the high-resolution image of one suspect latent fingerprint and initiated an IAFIS search matching the print to Brandon Mayfield.

Mayfield's prints were in the FBI's central database because they had been taken when he joined the military, where he served for eight years before being honorably discharged as a second lieutenant. After a visual comparison of the suspect and file prints, the examiner concluded a "100 percent match." The identification was verified by a retired FBI fingerprint examiner with more than 30 years of experience who was under contract with the bureau, as well as by a court-appointed independent fingerprint examiner (see figure).

Mayfield, age 37, a Muslim convert, was arrested on May 6 on a material witness warrant. The U.S. Attorney's Office came up with a list of Mayfield's potential ties to Muslim terrorists, which they included in the affidavit they presented to the federal judge who ordered his arrest and detention. The document also said that, although no travel records were found for Mayfield, "It is believed that Mayfield may have traveled under a false or fictitious name." On May 24, after the Spaniards had linked the print from the plastic bag to an Algerian national, Mayfield's case was thrown out. The FBI issued him a highly unusual official apology, and his ordeal became a stunning embarrassment to the U.S. government.

The Mayfield incident has also been the subject of an investigation by the Office of the Inspector General (OIG), U.S. Department of Justice (http://www.usdoj.gov/oig/special/s0601/final.pdf). The OIG investigation concluded that a "series of systemic issues" in the FBI laboratory contributed to the Mayfield misidentification. The report noted that the FBI has made significant procedural modifications to help prevent similar errors in the future and strongly supported the FBI's decision to undertake research to develop more objective standards for fingerprint identification.

The impact of the Mayfield affair on fingerprint technology as currently practiced and the weight courts will assign to fingerprint matches remain open questions.

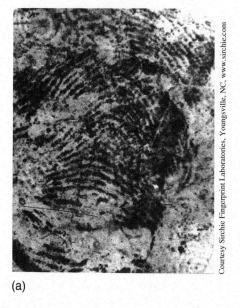

(a)

Courtesy Sirchie Fingerprint Laboratories, Youngsville, NC, www.sirchie.com

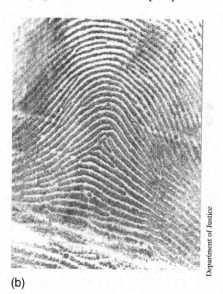

(b)

Department of Justice

(a) Questioned print recovered in connection with the Madrid bombing investigation. (b) File print of Brandon Mayfield.

crime-scene prints: **visible prints** are made by fingers touching a surface after the ridges have been in contact with a colored material such as blood, paint, grease, or ink; **plastic prints** are ridge impressions left on a soft material such as putty, wax, soap, or dust; and *latent* or *invisible prints* are impressions caused by the transfer of body perspiration or oils present on finger ridges to the surface of an object.

Locating Fingerprints

Locating visible or plastic prints at the crime scene normally presents little problem to the investigator because these prints are usually distinct and visible to the eye. Locating latent or invisible

visible print
A fingerprint made when the finger deposits a visible material such as ink, dirt, or blood onto a surface.

plastic print
A fingerprint impressed in a soft surface.

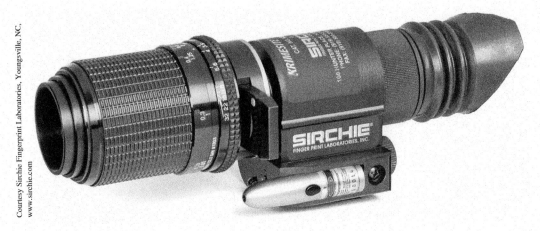

Courtesy Sirchie Fingerprint Laboratories, Youngsville, NC, www.sirchie.com

FIGURE 6–11

A Reflected Ultraviolet Imaging System allows an investigator to directly view surfaces for the presence of untreated latent fingerprints.

prints is obviously much more difficult and requires the use of techniques to make the print visible. Although the investigator can choose from several methods for visualizing a latent print, the choice depends on the type of surface being examined.

Hard and nonabsorbent surfaces (such as glass, mirror, tile, and painted wood) require different development procedures from surfaces that are soft and porous (such as papers, cardboard, and cloth). Prints on the former are preferably developed by the application of a powder or treatment with superglue, whereas prints on the latter generally require treatment with one or more chemicals.

Sometimes the most difficult aspect of fingerprint examination is the location of prints. Recent advances in fingerprint technology have led to the development of an ultraviolet (UV) image converter for the purpose of detecting latent fingerprints. This device, called the Reflected Ultraviolet Imaging System (RUVIS), can locate prints on most nonabsorbent surfaces without the aid of chemical or powder treatments (see Figure 6–11).

RUVIS detects the print in its natural state by aiming UV light at the surface suspected of containing prints. When the UV light strikes the fingerprint, the light is reflected back to the viewer, differentiating the print from its background surface. The transmitted UV light is then converted into visible light by an image intensifier. Once the print is located in this manner, the crime-scene investigator can develop it in the most appropriate fashion (see Figure 6–12).

Developing Latent Prints

FINGERPRINT POWDERS Fingerprint powders are commercially available in a variety of compositions and colors. These powders, when applied lightly to a nonabsorbent surface with a camel's-hair or fiberglass brush, readily adhere to perspiration residues and/or deposits of body oils left on the surface (see Figure 6–13).

Experienced examiners find that gray and black powders are adequate for most latent-print work; the examiner selects the powder that affords the best color contrast with the surface being dusted. Hence, the gray powder, composed of an aluminum dust, is used on dark-colored surfaces. It is also applied to mirrors and metal surfaces that are polished to a mirrorlike finish because these surfaces photograph as black. The black powder, composed basically of black carbon or charcoal, is applied to white or light-colored surfaces.

Other types of powders are available for developing latent prints. A magnetic-sensitive powder can be spread over a surface with a

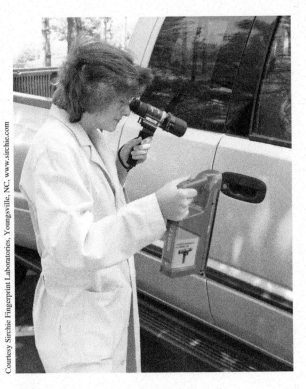

Courtesy Sirchie Fingerprint Laboratories, Youngsville, NC, www.sirchie.com

FIGURE 6–12

Using a Reflected Ultraviolet Imaging System with the aid of a UV lamp to search for latent fingerprints.

magnet in the form of a Magna Brush. A Magna Brush does not have any bristles to come in contact with the surface, so there is less chance that the print will be destroyed or damaged. The magnetic-sensitive powder comes in black and gray and is especially useful on such items as finished leather and rough plastics, where the minute texture of the surface tends to hold particles of ordinary powder. Fluorescent powders are also used to develop latent fingerprints. These powders fluoresce under UV light. By photographing the fluorescence pattern of the developing print under UV light, it is possible to avoid having the color of the surface obscure the print.

IODINE FUMING   Of the several chemical methods used for visualizing latent prints, **iodine fuming** is the oldest. Iodine is a solid crystal that, when heated, is transformed into a vapor without passing through a liquid phase; such a transformation is called **sublimation**. Most often, the suspect material is placed in an enclosed cabinet along with iodine crystals (see Figure 6–14). As the crystals are heated, the resultant vapors fill the chamber and combine with constituents of the latent print to make it visible. The reasons why latent prints are visualized by iodine vapors are not yet fully understood. Many believe that the iodine fumes combine with fatty oils; however, there is also convincing evidence that the iodine may actually interact with residual water left on a print from perspiration.[2]

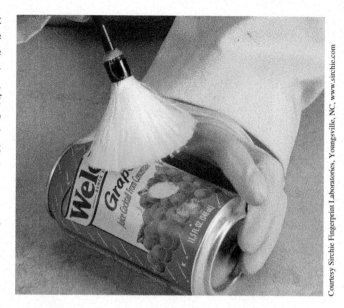

Courtesy Sirchie Fingerprint Laboratories, Youngsville, NC, www.sirchie.com

FIGURE 6–13
Developing a latent fingerprint on a surface by applying a fingerprint powder with a fiberglass brush.

Unfortunately, iodine prints are not permanent and begin to fade once the fuming process is stopped. Therefore, the examiner must photograph the prints immediately on development in order to retain a permanent record. However, if the developed print is simply covered with a clear cellophane tape soon after development, it will be usable for at least several months. Also, iodine-developed prints can be fixed with a 1 percent solution of starch in water, applied by spraying. The print turns blue and lasts for several weeks to several months.

NINHYDRIN   Another chemical used for visualizing latent prints is **ninhydrin**. The development of latent prints with ninhydrin depends on its chemical reaction to form a purple-blue color with amino acids present in trace amounts in perspiration. Ninhydrin (triketohydrindene hydrate) is commonly sprayed onto the porous surface from an aerosol can. A solution is prepared by mixing the ninhydrin powder with a suitable solvent, such as acetone or ethyl alcohol; a 0.6 percent solution appears to be effective for most applications.

Generally, prints begin to appear within an hour or two after ninhydrin application; however, weaker prints may be visualized after 24 to 48 hours. The development can be hastened if the treated specimen is heated in an oven or on a hot plate at a temperature of 80–100°C. The ninhydrin method has developed latent prints on papers as old as 15 years.

PHYSICAL DEVELOPER   **Physical Developer** is a third chemical mixture used for visualizing latent prints. Physical Developer is a silver nitrate–based liquid reagent. The procedure for preparing and using Physical Developer is described in Appendix V. This method has gained wide acceptance by fingerprint examiners, who have found it effective for visualizing latent prints that remain undetected by the previously described methods. Also, this technique is effective for developing latent fingerprints on porous articles that may have been wet at one time.

For most fingerprint examiners, the chemical method of choice is ninhydrin. Its extreme sensitivity and ease of application have all but eliminated the use of iodine for latent-print visualization. However, when ninhydrin fails, development with Physical Developer may provide identifiable results. Application of Physical Developer washes away any traces of proteins from

iodine fuming
A technique for visualizing latent fingerprints by exposing them to iodine vapors.

sublimation
A physical change from the solid directly into the gaseous state.

ninhydrin
A chemical reagent used to develop latent fingerprints on porous materials by reacting with amino acids in perspiration.

Physical Developer
A silver nitrate–based reagent formulated to develop latent fingerprints on porous surfaces.

---

[2] J. Almag, Y. Sasson, and A. Anati, "Chemical Reagents for the Development of Latent Fingerprints II: Controlled Addition of Water Vapor to Iodine Fumes—A Solution to the Aging Problem," *Journal of Forensic Sciences* 24 (1979): 431.

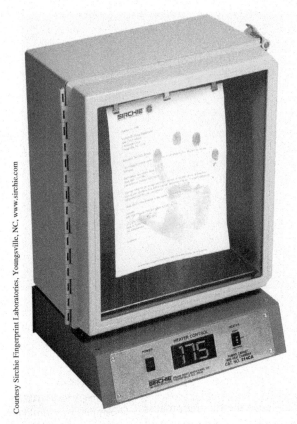

FIGURE 6–14
A heated fuming cabinet.

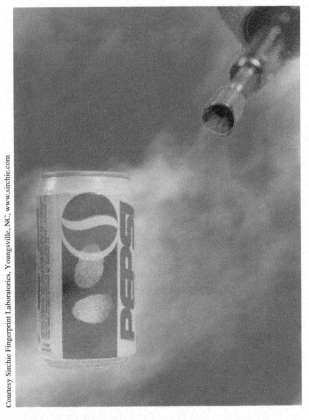

FIGURE 6–15
Superglue fuming a nonporous metallic surface in the search for latent fingerprints.

an object's surface; **hence, if one wishes to use all of the previously mentioned chemical development methods on the same surface, it is necessary to first fume with iodine, follow this treatment with ninhydrin, and then apply Physical Developer to the object.**

superglue fuming
A technique for visualizing latent fingerprints on nonporous surfaces by exposing them to cyanoacrylate vapors; named for the commercial product Super Glue.

SUPERGLUE FUMING   In the past, chemical treatment for fingerprint development was reserved for porous surfaces such as paper and cardboard. However, since 1982, a chemical technique known as **superglue fuming** has gained wide popularity for developing latent prints on nonporous surfaces such as metals, electrical tape, leather, and plastic bags (see Figure 6–15).[3]

Superglue is approximately 98–99 percent cyanoacrylate ester, a chemical that interacts with and visualizes a latent fingerprint. Cyanoacrylate ester fumes can be created when superglue is placed on absorbent cotton treated with sodium hydroxide. The fumes can also be created by heating the glue. The fumes and the evidential object are contained within an enclosed chamber for up to six hours. Development occurs when fumes from the glue adhere to the latent print, usually producing a white-appearing latent print. Interestingly, small enclosed areas, such as the interior of an automobile, have been successfully processed for latent prints with fumes from superglue.

Through the use of a small handheld wand, cyanoacrylate fuming is now easily done at a crime scene or in a laboratory setting. The wand heats a small cartridge containing cyanoacrylate. Once heated, the cyanoacrylate vaporizes, allowing the operator to direct the fumes onto the suspect area (see Figure 6–16).

OTHER TECHNIQUES FOR VISUALIZATION   One of the most exciting and dynamic areas of research in forensic science today is the application of chemical techniques to the visualization of latent fingerprints. Changes are occurring rapidly as researchers uncover a variety of

[3] F. G. Kendall and B. W. Rehn, "Rapid Method of Superglue Fuming Application for the Development of Latent Fingerprints," *Journal of Forensic Sciences* 28 (1983): 777.

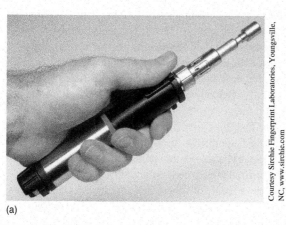

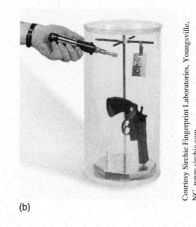

(a) (b)

FIGURE 6–16

(a) A handheld fuming wand uses disposable cartridges containing cyanoacrylate. The wand is used to develop prints at the crime scene and (b) in the laboratory.

processes applicable to the visualization of latent fingerprints. Interestingly, for many years progress in this field was minimal, and fingerprint specialists traditionally relied on three chemical techniques—iodine, ninhydrin, and silver nitrate—to reveal a hidden fingerprint. Then superglue fuming extended chemical development to prints deposited on nonporous surfaces.

fluoresce
To emit visible light when exposed to light of a shorter wavelength.

Inside the Science

Fluorescence

The first hint of things to come was the discovery that latent fingerprints could be visualized by exposure to laser light. This laser method took advantage of the fact that perspiration contains a variety of components that **fluoresce** when illuminated by laser light. Fluorescence occurs when a substance absorbs light and reemits the light in wavelengths longer than the illuminating source. Importantly, substances that emit light or fluoresce are more readily seen with either the naked eye or through photography than are non-light-emitting materials. The high sensitivity of fluorescence serves as the underlying principle of many of the new chemical techniques used to visualize latent fingerprints.

The earliest use of fluorescence to visualize fingerprints came with the direct illumination of a fingerprint with argon-ion lasers. This laser type was chosen because its blue-green light output induced some of the perspiration components of a fingerprint to fluoresce (see figure). The major drawback of this approach is that the perspiration components of a fingerprint are often present in quantities too minute to observe even with the aid of fluorescence. The fingerprint examiner, wearing safety goggles containing optical filters, visually examines the specimen being exposed to the laser light. The filters absorb the laser light and permit the wavelengths at which latent-print residues fluoresce to pass through to the eyes of the wearer. The filter also

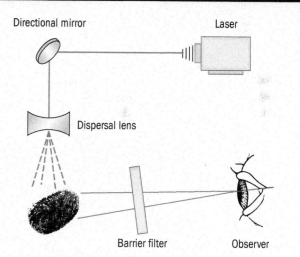

Schematic depicting latent-print detection with the aid of a laser. A fingerprint examiner, wearing safety goggles containing optical filters, examines the specimen being exposed to the laser light. The filter absorbs the laser light and permits the wavelengths at which latent-print residues fluoresce to pass through to the eyes of the wearer.

protects the operator against eye damage from scattered or reflected laser light. Likewise, latent-print residue producing sufficient fluorescence can be photographed by placing this same filter across the lens of the camera. Examination of specimens and photography of the fluorescing latent prints are carried out in a darkened room.

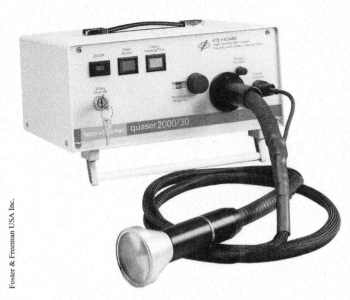

Foster & Freeman USA Inc.

FIGURE 6–17

An alternate light source system incorporating a high-intensity light source.

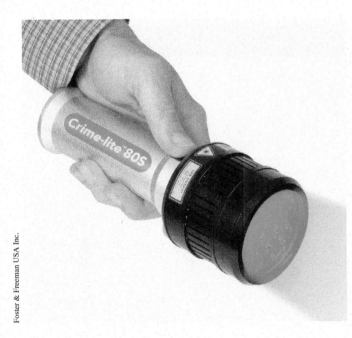

Foster & Freeman USA Inc.

FIGURE 6–18

Lightweight handheld alternate light source that uses an LED light source.

The next advancement in latent-fingerprint development occurred with the discovery that fingerprints could be treated with chemicals that would induce fluorescence when exposed to laser illumination. For example, the application of zinc chloride after ninhydrin treatment or the application of the dye rhodamine 6G after superglue fuming caused fluorescence and increased the sensitivity of detection on exposure to laser illumination. The discovery of numerous chemical developers for visualizing fingerprints through fluorescence quickly followed. This knowledge set the stage for the next advance in latent-fingerprint development—the *alternate light source*.

With the advent of chemically induced fluorescence, lasers were no longer needed to induce fingerprints to fluoresce through their perspiration residues. High-intensity light sources or alternate light sources have proliferated and all but replaced laser lights (see Figure 6–17). High-intensity quartz halogen or xenon-arc light sources can be focused on a suspect area through a fiber-optic cable. This light can be passed through several filters, giving the user more flexibility in selecting the wavelength of light to be aimed at the latent print. Alternatively, lightweight, portable alternate light sources that use light-emitting diodes (LEDs) are also commercially available (see Figure 6–18). In most cases, these light sources have proven to be as effective as laser light in developing latent prints, and they are commercially available at costs significantly less than those of laser illuminators. Furthermore, these light sources are portable and can be readily taken to any crime scene.

NEWER CHEMICAL PROCESSES   A large number of chemical treatment processes are available to the fingerprint examiner, and the field is in a constant state of flux. Selection of an appropriate procedure is best left to technicians who have developed their skills through casework experience.

Newer chemical processes include a substitute for ninhydrin called DFO (1,8-diazafluoren-9-one). This chemical visualizes latent prints on porous materials when exposed to an alternate light source. DFO has been shown to develop 2.5 times as many latent prints on paper as ninhydrin. A chemical called 1,2-indanedione is also emerging as a potential reagent for the development of latent fingerprints on porous surfaces. 1,2-Indanedione gives both good initial color and strong fluorescence when reacted with amino acids derived from prints and thus has the potential to provide in one process what ninhydrin and DFO can do in two different steps.

Dye combinations known as RAM, RAY, and MRM 10, when used in conjunction with superglue fuming, have been effective in visualizing latent fingerprints by fluorescence. A number of chemical formulas useful for latent-print development are listed in Appendix V.

Studies have demonstrated that common fingerprint-developing agents do not interfere with DNA-testing methods used for characterizing bloodstains.[4] Nonetheless, in cases involving items with material adhering to their surfaces and/or items that will require further laboratory

[4] C. Roux et al., "A Further Study to Investigate the Effect of Fingerprint Enhancement Techniques on the DNA Analysis of Bloodstains," *Journal of Forensic Identification* 49 (1999): 357; C. J. Frégeau et al., "Fingerprint Enhancement Revisited and the Effects of Blood Enhancement Chemicals on Subsequent Profiler Plus™ Fluorescent Short Tandem Repeat DNA Analysis of Fresh and Aged Bloody Fingerprints," *Journal of Forensic Sciences* 45 (2000): 354; and P. Grubwieser et al., "Systematic Study on STR Profiling on Blood and Saliva Traces After Visualization of Fingerprints," *Journal of Forensic Sciences* 48 (2003): 733.

examinations, fingerprint processing should not be performed at the crime scene. Rather, the items should be submitted to the laboratory, where they can be processed for fingerprints in conjunction with other necessary examinations.

Preservation of Developed Prints

Once the latent print has been visualized, it must be permanently preserved for future comparison and possible use in court as evidence. A photograph must be taken before any further attempts at preservation. Any camera equipped with a close-up lens will do; however, many investigators prefer to use a camera specially designed for fingerprint photography. Such a camera comes equipped with a fixed focus to take photographs on a 1:1 scale when the camera's open eye is held exactly flush against the print's surface (see Figure 6–19). In addition, photographs must be taken to provide an overall view of the print's location with respect to other evidential items at the crime scene.

Once photographs have been secured, one of two procedures is to be followed. If the object is small enough to be transported without destroying the print, it should be preserved in its entirety; the print should be covered with cellophane so it will be protected from damage. On the other hand, prints on large immovable objects that have been developed with a powder can best be preserved by "lifting." The most popular type of lifter is a broad adhesive tape similar to clear adhesive tape. When the powdered surface is covered with the adhesive side of the tape and pulled up, the powder is transferred to the tape. Then the tape is placed on a properly labeled card that provides a good background contrast with the powder.

A variation of this procedure is the use of an adhesive-backed clear plastic sheet attached to a colored cardboard backing. Before it is applied to the print, a celluloid separator is peeled from the plastic sheet to expose the adhesive lifting surface. The tape is then pressed evenly and firmly over the powdered print and pulled up (see Figure 6–20). The sheet containing the adhering powder is now pressed against the cardboard backing to provide a permanent record of the fingerprint.

Digital Imaging for Fingerprint Enhancement

When fingerprints are lifted from a crime scene, they are not usually in perfect condition, making the analysis much more difficult. Computers have advanced technology in most fields, and fingerprint identification has not been left behind. With the help of digital imaging software, fingerprints can now be enhanced for the most accurate and comprehensive analysis.

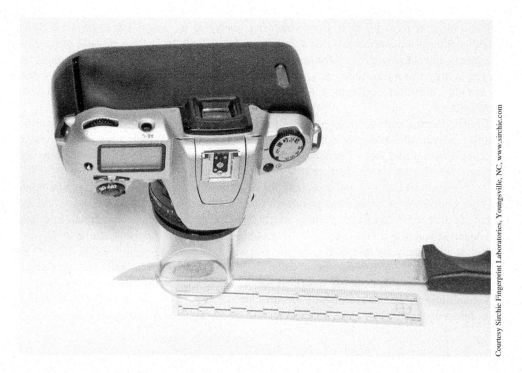

FIGURE 6–19
Camera fitted with an adapter designed to give an approximate 1:1 photograph of a fingerprint.

Courtesy Sirchie Fingerprint Laboratories, Youngsville, NC, www.sirchie.com

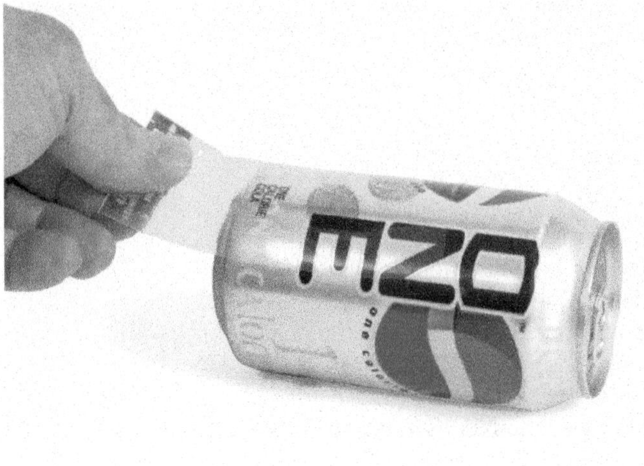

FIGURE 6–20
"Lifting" a fingerprint.

digital imaging
A process through which a picture is converted into a series of square electronic dots known as pixels; the picture is manipulated by computer software that changes the numerical value of each pixel.

pixel
A square electronic dot that is used to compose a digital image.

Creating Digital Images

Digital imaging is the process by which a picture is converted into a digital file. The image produced from this digital file is composed of numerous square electronic dots called **pixels**. Images composed of only black and white elements are referred to as *grayscale images*. Each pixel is assigned a number according to its intensity. The grayscale image is made from the set of numbers to which a pixel may be assigned, ranging from 0 (black) to 255 (white). Once an image is digitally stored, it is manipulated by computer software that changes the numerical value of each pixel, thus altering the image as directed by the user. *Resolution* reveals the degree of detail that can be seen in an image. It is defined in terms of dimensions, such as 800 × 600 pixels. The larger the numbers, the more closely the digital image resembles the real-world image.

The input of pictures into a digital imaging system is usually done through the use of scanners, digital cameras, and video cameras. After the picture is changed to its digital image, several methods can be employed to enhance the image. The overall brightness of an image, as well as the contrast between the image and the background, can be adjusted through contrast-enhancement methods. One approach used to enhance an image is *spatial filtering*. Several types of filters produce various effects. A low-pass filter is used to eliminate harsh edges by reducing the intensity difference between pixels. A second filter, the high-pass filter, operates by modifying a pixel's numerical value to exaggerate its intensity difference from that of its neighbor. The resulting effect increases the contrast of the edges, thus providing a high contrast between the elements and the background.

Analyzing Digital Images

Frequency analysis, also referred to as *frequency Fourier transform* (FFT), is used to identify periodic or repetitive patterns such as lines or dots that interfere with the interpretation of the image. These patterns are diminished or eliminated to enhance the appearance of the image. Interestingly, the spacings between fingerprint ridges are themselves periodic. Therefore, the contribution of the fingerprint can be identified in FFT mode and then enhanced. Likewise, if ridges from overlapping prints are positioned in different directions, their corresponding frequency information is at different locations in FFT mode. The ridges of one latent print can then be enhanced while the ridges of the other are suppressed.

Color interferences also pose a problem when analyzing an image. For example, a latent fingerprint found on paper currency or a check may be difficult to analyze because of the distracting colored background. With the imaging software, the colored background can simply be removed to make the image stand out (see Figure 6–21). If the image itself is a particular color, such as a ninhydrin-developed print, the color can be isolated and enhanced to distinguish it from the background.

Digital imaging software also provides functions in which portions of the image can be examined individually. With a scaling and resizing tool, the user can select a part of an image and resize it for a closer look. This function operates much like a magnifying glass, helping the examiner view fine details of an image.

An important and useful tool, especially for fingerprint identification, is the compare function. This specialized feature places two images side by side and allows the examiner to chart the common features on both images simultaneously (see Figure 6–22). The zoom function is used in conjunction with the compare tool. As the examiner zooms into a portion of one image, the software automatically zooms into the second image for comparison.

Although digital imaging is undoubtedly an effective tool for enhancing and analyzing images, it is only as useful as the images it has to work with. If the details do not exist on the original images, the enhancement procedures are not going to work. The benefits of digital enhancement methods are apparent when weak images are made more distinguishable.

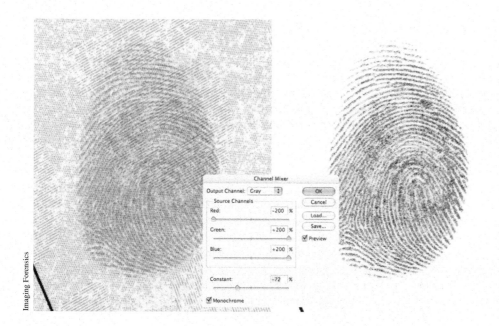

FIGURE 6–21
A fingerprint being enhanced in Adobe Photoshop. In this example, on the left is the original scan of an inked fingerprint on a check. On the right is the same image after using Adobe Photoshop's Channel Mixer to eliminate the green security background.

Case # 05-01234

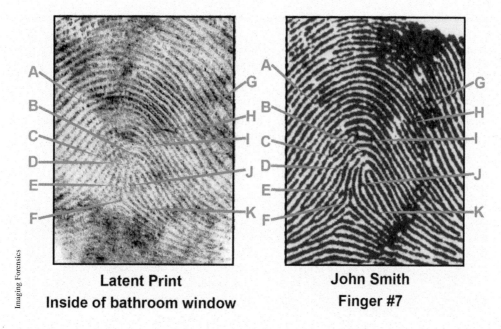

Latent Print
Inside of bathroom window

John Smith
Finger #7

FIGURE 6–22
Current imaging software allows fingerprint analysts to prepare a fingerprint comparison chart. The fingerprint examiner can compare prints side by side and display important features that are consistent between the fingerprints. The time needed to create a display of this sort digitally is about 30 to 60 minutes.

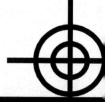

Chapter Summary > > > > > > > > > > >

Fingerprints are a reproduction of friction skin ridges found on the palm side of the fingers and thumbs. The basic principles underlying the use of fingerprints in criminal investigations are that (1) a fingerprint is an individual characteristic because no two fingers have yet been found to possess identical ridge characteristics, (2) a fingerprint remains unchanged during an individual's lifetime, and (3) fingerprints have general ridge patterns that permit them to be systematically classified. All fingerprints are divided into three classes on the basis of their general pattern: loops, whorls, and arches.

Fingerprint classification systems are based on knowledge of fingerprint pattern classes. The individuality of a fingerprint is not determined by its general shape or pattern, but by a careful study of its ridge characteristics. The expert must demonstrate a point-by-point comparison in order to prove the identity of an individual. AFIS aids this process by converting the image of a fingerprint into digital minutiae that contain data showing ridges at their points of termination (ridge endings) and their branching into two ridges (bifurcations). A single fingerprint can be searched against the FBI AFIS digital database of 50 million fingerprint records in a matter of minutes.

Once the finger touches a surface, perspiration, along with oils that may have been picked up by touching the hairy portions of the body, is transferred onto that surface, thereby leaving an impression of the finger's ridge pattern (a fingerprint). Prints deposited in this manner are invisible to the eye and are commonly referred to as latent or invisible fingerprints.

Visible prints are made when fingers touch a surface after the ridges have been in contact with a colored material such as blood, paint, grease, or ink. Plastic prints are ridge impressions left on a soft material, such as putty, wax, soap, or dust. Latent prints deposited on hard and nonabsorbent surfaces (such as glass, mirror, tile, and painted wood) are preferably developed by the application of a powder; prints on porous surfaces (such as paper and cardboard) generally require treatment with a chemical. Examiners use various chemical methods to visualize latent prints, such as iodine fuming, ninhydrin, and Physical Developer. Superglue fuming develops latent prints on nonporous surfaces,

such as metals, electrical tape, leather, and plastic bags. Development occurs when fumes from the glue adhere to the print, usually producing a white latent print.

The high sensitivity of fluorescence serves as the underlying principle of many of the new chemical techniques used to visualize latent fingerprints. Fingerprints are treated with chemicals that induce fluorescence when exposed to a high-intensity light or an alternate light source.

Once the latent print has been visualized, it must be permanently preserved for future comparison and for possible use as court evidence. A photograph must be taken before any further attempts at preservation are made. If the object is small enough to be transported without destroying the print, it should be preserved in its entirety. Prints on large immovable objects that have been developed with a powder are best preserved by "lifting" with a broad adhesive tape.

Some common tools used in the analysis and enhancement of fingerprints are UV and alternate light sources, different types of powders and brushes, chemical treatments like ninhydrin and cyanoacrylate, and tape or latent lifters.

Review Questions

1. The first systematic attempt at personal identification was devised and introduced by _____.

2. A system of identification relying on precise body measurements is known as _____.

3. The fingerprint classification system used in most English-speaking countries was devised by _____.

4. True or False: The first systematic and official use of fingerprints for personal identification in the United States was adopted by the New York City Civil Service Commission. _____

5. The individuality of a fingerprint (is, is not) determined by its pattern.

6. A point-by-point comparison of a fingerprint's _____ must be demonstrated in order to prove identity.

7. _____ are a reproduction of friction skin ridges.

8. The form and pattern of skin ridges are determined by the (epidermis, dermal papillae).

9. A permanent scar forms in the skin only when an injury damages the _____.

10. Fingerprints (can, cannot) be changed during a person's lifetime.

11. The three general patterns into which fingerprints are divided are _____, _____, and _____.

12. The most common fingerprint pattern is the _____.

13. Approximately 5 percent of the population has the _____ fingerprint pattern.

14. A loop pattern that opens toward the thumb is known as a(n) (radial, ulnar) loop.

15. The pattern area of the loop is enclosed by two diverging ridges known as _____.

16. The ridge point nearest the type-line divergence is known as the _____.

17. All loops must have (one, two) delta(s).

18. The approximate center of a loop pattern is called the _____.

19. If an imaginary line drawn between the two deltas of a whorl pattern touches any of the spiral ridges, the pattern is classified as a (plain whorl, central pocket loop).

20. The simplest of all fingerprint patterns is the _____.

21. Arches (have, do not have) type lines, deltas, and cores.

22. ACE-V is an acronym for a four step process: _____, _____, _____, and _____.

23. True or False: Level 2 details cannot individualize a fingerprint. _____

24. The presence or absence of the _____ pattern is used as a basis for determining the primary classification in the Henry system.

25. The largest category (25 percent) in the primary classification system is (1/1, 1/2).

26. A fingerprint classification system (can, cannot) unequivocally identify an individual.

27. True or False: Computerized fingerprint search systems match prints by comparing the position of bifurcations and ridge endings. _____

28. A fingerprint left by a person with soiled or stained fingertips is called a(n) _____.

29. _____ fingerprints are impressions left on a soft material.

30. Fingerprint impressions that are not readily visible are called _____.

31. Fingerprints on hard and nonabsorbent surfaces are best developed by the application of a(n) _____.

32. Fingerprints on porous surfaces are best developed with _____ treatment.

33. _____ vapors chemically combine with fatty oils or residual water to visualize a fingerprint.

34. The chemical _____ visualizes fingerprints by its reaction with amino acids.

35. Chemical treatment with _____ visualizes fingerprints on porous articles that may have been wet at one time.

36. True or False: A latent fingerprint is first treated with Physical Developer followed by ninhydrin. _____

37. A chemical technique known as _____ is used to develop latent prints on nonporous surfaces such as metal and plastic.

38. _____ occurs when a substance absorbs light and reemits the light in wavelengths longer than the illuminating source.

39. High-intensity light sources known as _____ are effective in developing latent fingerprints.

40. Once a fingerprint has been visualized, it must be preserved by _____.

41. The image produced from a digital file is composed of numerous square electronic dots called _____.

42. A (high-pass filter, frequency Fourier transform analysis) is used to identify repetitive patterns such as lines or dots that interfere with the interpretation of a digitized fingerprint image.

Application and Critical Thinking

1. Classify each of the prints shown in the figure as loop, whorl, or arch.

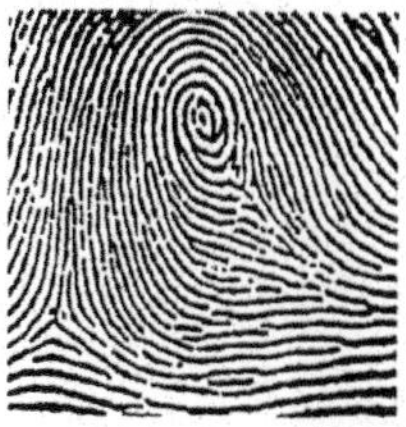

(1). _____

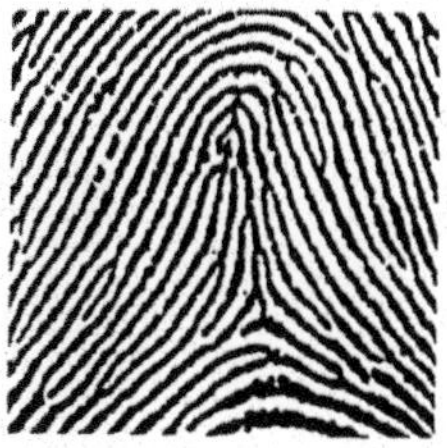

(2). _____

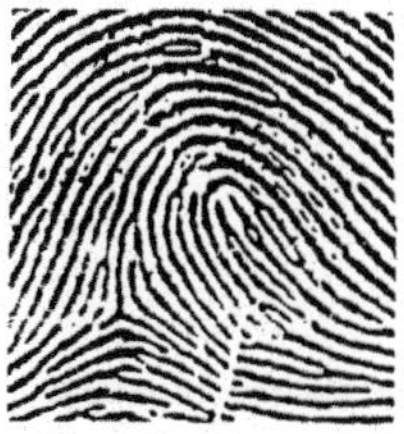

(3). _____

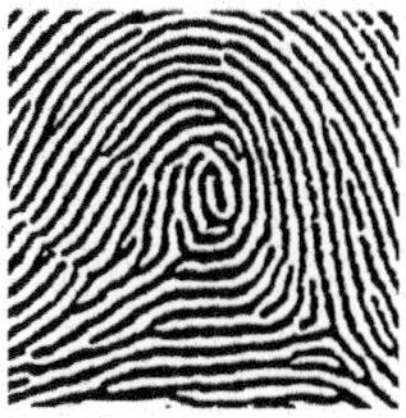

(4). _____

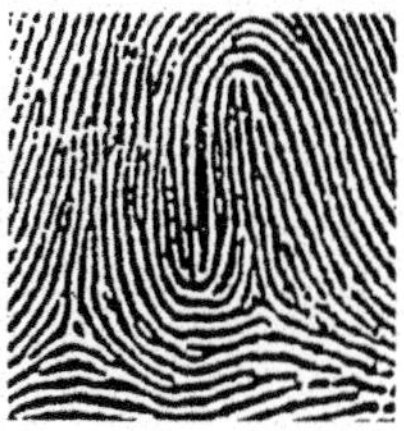

(5). _____

(6). _____

Richard Saferstein, Ph.D.

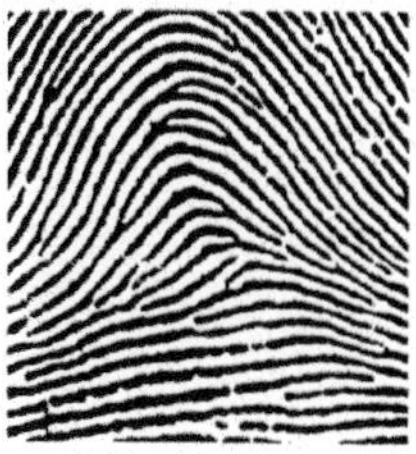

2. A description of the types of prints from the fingers of a criminal suspect appears below. Using the FBI system, determine the primary classification of this individual.

Finger	Right Hand	Left Hand
Thumb	Whorl	Whorl
Index	Loop	Whorl
Middle	Whor	Arch
Ring	Whorl	Whorl
Little	Arch	Whorl

3. While searching a murder scene, you find the following items that you believe may contain latent fingerprints. Indicate whether prints on each item should be developed using fingerprint powder or chemicals.

   a. A leather sofa

   b. A mirror

   c. A painted wooden knife handle

   d. Blood-soaked newspapers

   e. A revolver

4. Criminalist Frank Mortimer is using digital imaging to enhance latent fingerprints. Indicate which features of digital imaging he would most likely use for each of the following tasks:

   a. Isolating part of a print and enlarging it for closer examination

   b. Increasing the contrast between a print and the background surface on which it is located

   c. Examining two prints that overlap one another

5. The following are fingerprint patterns of three males and one female with criminal records for robbery. Identify the following fingerprints according to the three groups and the subgroups of fingerprints.

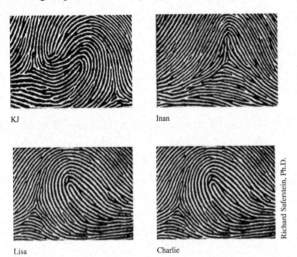

KJ

Inan

Lisa

Charlie

Richard Saferstein, Ph.D.

6. Count the number of bifurcations in the following prints. Choose between 9, 11, and 13 as the number of bifurcations:

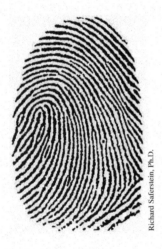

Richard Saferstein, Ph.D.

7. At the Museum of Culture Studies, a diary that belonged to Martin Luther King, Jr., has been stolen and replaced by a fake. The only evidence is a fingerprint impression left by the thief on the fake diary. The police suspects four individuals who have had previous criminal records for similar crimes. Their fingerprints already exist in the police database. KJ, Ivan, Lisa, and Charlie are the four suspects. Carefully examine the fingerprint impression and identify the suspect fingerprint that matches with it.

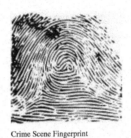

Crime Scene Fingerprint

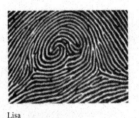

KJ

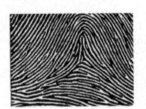

Ivan

Lisa

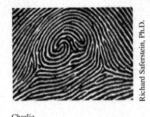

Charlie

Richard Saferstein, Ph.D.

Further References

Komarinski, Peter, *Automated Fingerprint Identification Systems (AFIS)*. Burlington, MA: Elsevier Academic Press, 2004.

Ramotowski, R., ed., *Lee and Gaensleen's Advances in Fingerprint Technology*, 3rd ed. Boca Raton, FL: CRC Press, 2012.

U.S. Department of Justice, *The Fingerprint Sourcebook*, http://www.OJP.usdoj.gov/nij/pubs-sum/225320.htm.

Chapter 7

Forensic Biometrics

Learning Objectives

After studying this chapter, you should be able to:

7.1 List and define the various categories of biometrics

7.2 Distinguish the enrollment process from the extraction process

7.3 Explain how iris details are captured and characterized in a forensic biometric system

7.4 Describe how facial data is captured, verified, and identified in a forensic biometric system

7.5 Explain the scope of the FBI's Next Generation Identification System

KEY TERMS

behavioral biometrics
biometric identification
biometric matching or
    verification
Eigenfaces
enrollment
extraction process
IrisCodes
physiological
    biometrics
template generation
    module

Biometrics and the Boston Marathon Bombing

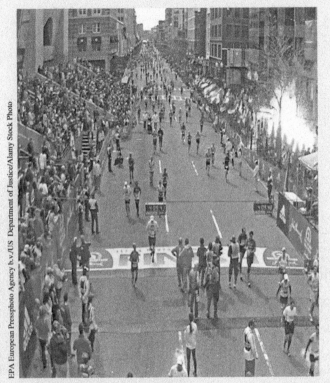

EPA European Pressphoto Agency b.v./US Department of Justice/Alamy Stock Photo

On April 15, 2013, two improvised explosive devices at the annual Boston Marathon killed three people and wounded 264 others. Moments after the vicious Boston Marathon terrorist attack, investigations began in search of possible suspects. Local authorities and the FBI called the support of the public and in no time potential leads started pouring in. Over 2,000 reports and photos of the event were made. Dozens of investigators were tasked with scrutinizing these leads. Among the photographs sent to the FBI, Dzhokhar and Tamerlan Tsarnaev, two radicalized brothers, are seen in plain sight.

The bombs were discovered to be pressure cooker bombs similar to many IEDs found in other extremist terrorist attacks. Dzhokhar and Tamerlan left two bombs placed in a backpack and shopping bag among the onlookers of the Marathon. As they walked away, they remotely triggered the explosions.

The FBI set the task of finding the perpetrators to their most sophisticated facial recognition biometric system. Every image and video that was obtained during the event was scanned by a complex algorithm that would compare suspects against a repository of known terrorists and persons of interest. To the FBI and the public's surprise, the system failed. Out of the many images sent to law enforcement, a few had direct pictures of the Tsarnaev brothers. Both brothers had legally come into this country and had images in American immigration databases. Dzhokhar had a U.S. driver's license with an up-to-date picture. His brother Tamerlan was even the subject of a terrorism investigation and had many images in FBI databases. Despite all of these leads and a wealth of database information, the facial recognition system failed to match the Tsarnaevs' faces to identities.

The problem with facial recognition biometrics in 2013, and what still remains an issue today, is that software has a difficult time analyzing and identifying faces from grainy and low-resolution photographs. Tamerlan also could not be recognized due to the fact that he was wearing sunglasses, which can distort the results of the scan as well. Posture and light exposure can have an effect on this technology, and investigators learned this the hard way after the gruesome attack. Law enforcement eventually identified the Tsarnaev brothers using more conventional methods and apprehended them not long after. Facial recognition technology is evolving and continues to be updated and fine-tuned with the implementation of the Next Generation Information System.

Introduction to Biometrics

In 2013, Apple introduced the iPhone 5s, which contained breakthrough technology. Known as Touch ID, cell phone users could now unlock their phones with a simple fingerprint touch on the home button. Before Touch ID, data was significantly more vulnerable to password attacks, especially when a phone had been stolen or breached. Now with this technology, users can access their music, files, and sensitive information with just a fingerprint on the screen.

Imagine a world where business keys and house keys are rendered obsolete. Every person that belongs to a household can enter and leave freely with just a touch of the doorknob, and those who are not authorized are locked out by a complex security system within the house. Imagine logging on to your favorite websites without ever using a password or access code. You, the user, are able to access the entire Internet by a simple scan of your iris. This is all possible with the implementation of new technologies and techniques known as biometrics.

What Is Biometrics?

Biometrics is a cutting-edge form of access control that accurately and efficiently identifies humans. This system uses an individual's biological and behavioral traits to grant access to an establishment or a computer network. An electronic device will require individuals to use a distinguishable feature of their body to positively identify themselves before they are able to bypass any type of access-control system, such as a security system for a building. Once a match has been made, the person requesting access will be allowed on the premises by a simple electronic pulse that opens the door. If the sensor does not find a positive match within its database, it locks the attempted user out. The military has been using biometrics for an extended period of time to keep sensitive information secure and to prevent espionage and theft in regard to valuable military assets. Law enforcement across the nation implements biometrics for record keeping and on-site access control (i.e., only allowing staff on the premises).

There are two main functions of biometrics. The first function is **biometric matching or verification**. Biometric systems are capable of identifying someone out of a crowd by scanning select biometric characteristics into a database. This is perfectly tailored for law enforcement or government institutions that are seeking a person of interest. Biometric matching will make it harder for wanted individuals to elude the law and hide among the public. The second application of biometrics relates to access control through **biometric identification**. As previously mentioned, the Apple iPhone is capable of identifying an individual for the purpose of entry. Access-control systems will create and store databases of biological traits and compare them to the individual attempting to gain entry into a device of facility. With the use of a facial or retina scan, the system will decide who can gain entry to a facility or device with extreme accuracy.

One of the main causes of stolen accounts and information in computer systems is the use of weak passwords. Hackers are able to crack simple passwords with easily accessible tools, such as Dictionary Attacks. This form of attack generates combinations of every word possible to steal an unsuspecting victim's credentials. Another problem with modern access-control systems is the reliance on physical keys and key cards. Keys are often lost or stolen, which creates a scary situation for someone whose business or home is now vulnerable to an unwanted guest. Biometric systems solve all of these problems by allowing access only to people with a specific biological trait. A key has the potential of being lost or copied, but a human iris is completely unique and almost impossible to duplicate. By implementing fingerprint readers on every computer in the facility, businesses would no longer have to worry about employees sharing passwords and credentials.

Types of Forensic Biometrics

Now that we have established a basic definition of biometrics, let's examine different types of biometric systems that exist. Many forms of biometric technologies are available today, but the majority of them can be split into two different groups. The first group is **physiological biometrics**, which contains fingerprints, hand, iris, retina, and facial scans (see Figure 7–1). The second group is **behavioral biometrics**, which is much less stable and includes handwriting, voice, keystroke, and gait recognition.

PHYSIOLOGICAL BIOMETRICS   Fingerprints have been widely used to identify people for centuries. This form of biometric technology is the most cost-efficient and easy to install. With the addition of a fingerprint scanner on a door, an office can grant specific workers access to a

biometric matching or verification
Biometric systems capable of identifying someone out of a crowd by scanning select biometric characteristics into a database. Law enforcement entities implement this form of biometrics to find wanted fugitives and individuals suspected of terrorism.

biometric identification
A biometric system that can distinguish between subjects by analyzing a biometric trait of one person and compare it against an existing database of enrolled traits.

physiological biometrics
This form of biometrics focuses on identifying humans through their unique physiological traits. Physiological biometrics includes fingerprints, hand, iris, retina, and facial scans.

behavioral biometrics
This form of biometrics focuses on identifying humans through unique behavioral or mental patterns they exhibit. Behavioral biometrics includes handwriting, voice, keystroke, and gait recognition.

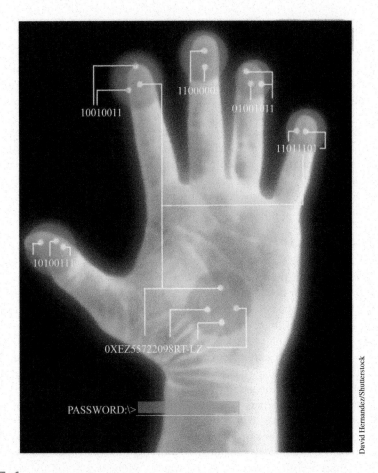

David Hernandez/Shutterstock

FIGURE 7–1

Biometric security scan of a human hand.

sensitive area or a network of computers. Hand and vein scans within the hand work almost the same way. Humans have a unique set of physiological traits pertaining to the hand. When compared, the vein patterns that run through our hands are unique.

Retina and iris scans have been implemented in many government institutions as well as other areas with classified information. This technology is much more secure than the use of fingerprints due to the detailed map of a human eye. Using a tiny camera, a biometric system is able to take a picture of someone's eye and compare all of the intricate muscles and fibers that make it a unique set of characteristics. Eye scanning systems are expensive to install, yet necessary when trying to protect a valuable asset or piece of information.

Facial scans are the least accurate form of biometrics currently available in the physiological category. The human face is just as unique as the eye or hand, but the technology available today has trouble distinguishing subtle traits from still images. This process becomes less accurate when using biometrics for identification purposes, such as picking a face out of a crowd and matching it to a database of wanted persons.

BEHAVIORAL BIOMETRICS   Unlike physiological biometrics, behavioral biometrics is used infrequently and is much more experimental in design and practice. This category of biometrics is more concerned with the way a human performs an action, rather than focusing on a specific physiological trait. Researchers in this field are currently developing technology that can analyze a human's brain wave pattern. As technology and computers evolve on a day-to-day basis, the real-world implementation of behavioral biometrics becomes more of a reality.

Handwriting is the most commonly used type of behavioral biometrics. A sensor can analyze different stroke patterns, curves, and arches of a signature while comparing it to an original document. This type of software can also sense the amount of pressure and force that was used in a questioned signature to determine whether or not it is parallel to the amount of pressure that is exerted on a pen/pencil.

The manner in which an individual types on a keyboard is unique. This can be measured in biometrics using keystroke dynamics. People type at different speeds and also approach pressing each key with their own personal technique. Software is now available that can measure exactly how someone types by using various samples over time to learn unique keystroke dynamics. This can be useful in a computer terminal where many different people may have access to the same device. The software will be able to authenticate exactly who is sitting at the computer at any set time just by analyzing how they are typing. This technology has the ability to sense an intrusion by a hacker trying to operate under the credentials of another user and can potentially protect volumes of information.

We have all seen movies or science fiction shows where someone is magically granted access to a home or facility by saying their name or "Open up." This is now a reality with voice recognition. Many companies are installing voice recognition technology in areas that require clearance, and acceptance of these systems is much greater as they don't require intrusive technologies such as a hand or eye scan. A microphone is used to measure pitch and subtle dynamics in a person's voice to yield a positive or negative match, which is especially useful in access-control systems. Depending on how the software is set up, each person may have to speak their name or a specific phrase to gain positive access. Some cell phone companies are experimenting with this technology as a layer of security when accessing private data on a mobile phone.

The last form of behavioral biometrics is gait recognition. Gait refers to the cycle of walking, which is composed of several stages and is unique for everyone. Every person has a different posture, step length, speed, and foot positioning in regard to the way they walk from one place to another. The system analyzes people from a distance and attempts to find a match based on patterns that are familiar. This type of biometrics is not very accurate and, like many others in the behavioral category, is still experimental. Gait recognition would be useful in practice to pick out a person of interest from a distance.

Enrolling and Extracting Biometric Data

Biometric systems use different algorithms and steps to accomplish what each is designed to do. This varies between physiological and behavioral systems, as well as systems designed to authenticate or identify individuals. The equipment and technology for every biometric system varies greatly as well. For instance, an iris scanner is going to contain a camera as its main component, whereas a voice recognition system will use a sensitive microphone. Regardless of the varied components, biometric systems typically operate using the same series of steps (see Table 7–1).

The first process that each biometric system must perform is known as the **enrollment process**. The enrollment process captures a person's biometric data and stores in a database for later use. It works by collecting data through a sensor and sending it to a data acquisition module. The biometric sensor may consist of various different setups to gather data from the user. Popular equipment includes NIR (near infrared) cameras or digital wavelength cameras to gather data from a human face.

enrollment process
The process of capturing a person's biometric data and storing them in a database for later use. It works by collecting data through a sensor and sending it to a data acquisition module.

TABLE 7–1

Flowchart Depicting the Collection Steps in Gathering Biometric Data

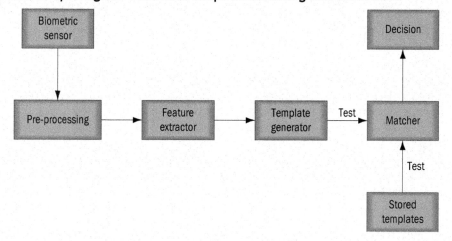

The data preprocessing module collects and enhances only what is needed for each individual system. In the example of a voice recognition system, the data preprocessing module would remove any background noise from a recorded entry. It would enhance the voice of the user and make an effort to isolate it from other noise in the recording. This module also serves the function of normalizing any corrupt or inaccurate data. For an iris scanner, this would include the task of eliminating blur or excessive light in the captured eye image.

Once the information completes its run through a data preprocessing module, feature **extraction** begins. The feature extraction module does most of the heavy lifting for the system. This module is responsible for finding patterns in the traits extracted by the sensor by using mathematical equations. Every system uses different equations and algorithms to judge unique characteristics, and accuracy can vary from system to system. For a retina scan, the feature extraction module may use equations that judge the distance between muscle fibers in the eye. For a fingerprint, this module can determine subtle loop, whorl, and arch changes with almost perfect accuracy. The feature extraction module is debatably one of the most complex and important components of a biometric system.

After select features have been collected, a template is generated of relevant information and is stored in a database. The **template generation module** is responsible for saving all of the raw data produced by feature extraction and putting it into a simple and easy-to-read format for the system. This module compares a user to the rest of the data and makes each individual biometric file smaller, which makes it time efficient. The template generation module saves all files to the database, and it is encrypted to meet the needs of the end user. It is necessary to secure database files to prevent a breach of the biometric system and the possible loss of private biometric data.

extraction
This module is responsible for finding patterns in the traits extracted by the biometric sensor by using mathematical equations. Every system uses different equations and algorithms to judge unique characteristics.

template generation module
Responsible for saving all of the raw data produced by feature extraction and putting it into a simple and easy-to-read format for the system.

The Iris

Introduction

Individuals have been identified by facial characteristics since the dawn of civilization. Among the most common means of identification is the human eye. The iris is the colored section in the eye around the pupil. Muscles in the iris expand and contract to change the size of the pupil, which controls the amount of light that enters the eye. When examined closely, the iris is unique to every human being and consists of tightly grouped muscle patterns that are stained green, blue, brown, and so on. Even without the implementation of biometrics, almost every adult in the United States has been categorized by iris color, as a driver's license contains the eye color of the owner.

A human's eye color has the potential to be genetically linked, but the intricate muscle patterns and iris construction is unique to every person. In other words, someone may possess the same eye color as their father and grandfather, but when examined under a microscope each iris is vastly different. The iris begins to form at the prenatal stage of pregnancy, where muscle fibers start to take shape and construct tight patterns. As the growing fetus nears birth, degeneration of the muscle fibers occurs within the iris and forms the unique patterns used in biometric authentication today.

One of the focal points of the iris system resides in the very nature of the iris itself. The human iris will go physically unchanged for the life of the user, whereas many other physiological attributes can change and become altered over the course of a lifetime. The iris is protected by the cornea and sees little change, as the individual grows older.

Though iris recognition systems are highly effective due to the stable nature of the human iris, these systems are hindered by contact lenses and eyeglasses. They may become ineffective when dealing with people who have injuries or diseases that affect their eyes.

History

The first documented attempt to identify someone using the iris was performed in the 1950s. British ophthalmologist J. H. Doggart wrote several articles comparing the iris to the fingerprint. Doggart noticed that the human iris is capable of forming infinite patterns and is unique for each and every person. Doggart's work was critical as it inspired many scientists and ophthalmologists after him to explore the characteristics of the iris.

In 1985, American ophthalmologists Safir and Flom approached Dr. John Daugman to write a computer system for the analysis and verification of the human iris; in 1994 the groundbreaking technology was complete. Known as "IrisCode," a computer captures and analyzes complex data extracted from an image of an iris and compares the results to a database. Most new applications of iris biometrics still use the infrastructure of Dr. Daugman's algorithm with minor changes to suit each application.

Iris and Retina

Besides examining the iris, biometric systems have also been developed that identifies the retina. The retina is composed of neural cells in the back of the eyeball that provide a "screen" for the cornea and lens to display an image on. The retina is responsible for obtaining a clear picture of what a person is actually seeing. A long series of veins and capillaries is contained within the retina, and just like the muscle fibers in the iris, these veins are unique to every person (Figure 7–2). By shining a light through the pupil, the pattern of veins in a person's retina can be revealed.

One of the main problems with retina biometrics is that viable images can be affected by disease. This is nearly impossible with iris scans as illness will not affect the physiological elements of muscle fibers in the iris.

Usability is also an area in which the iris has advantages over existing retina technology. An iris scan can be acquired with a photograph, with the end user standing a reasonable distance from a camera and a simple picture being taken. Retina scans, however, require the user to have their eyeball within a fraction of an inch of a high-power camera lens. The process may take an extended period of time, and this can be uncomfortable for the average user.

Iris biometrics is replacing retina biometrics because it is an all-around better technology, which is functional for both law enforcement and business security. Retina scanners are largely outdated and considered too intrusive to be practical in real-world applications. Due to the complicated nature of obtaining and analyzing retina scans, this technology is hard to implement and poses problems in the field. Unlike iris and fingerprint biometrics, individuals must be thoroughly trained on how to use retina image-capturing machines. The system and imaging apparatus are complex and will most likely be phased out and replaced by other biometric solutions. Iris systems can be installed relatively easily in a busy marketplace and can be used without human intervention. A retina system would often require an operator to quality check images and run/maintain the machine.

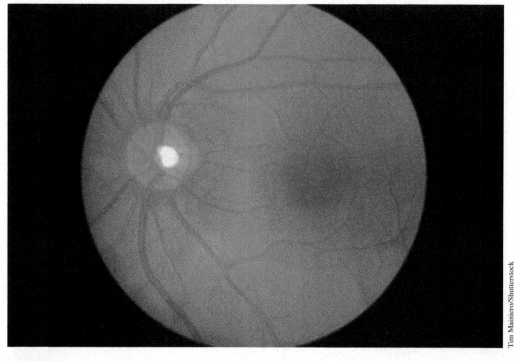

Tim Mainiero/Shutterstock

FIGURE 7–2

View inside human eye showing retina and its optic nerve.

How It Works

All iris capturing systems today use a high-quality digital camera and illuminate the eye using NIR wavelengths along with visible light. The NIR wavelength band is located within 700–900 nm of the electromagnetic spectrum. The use of NIR lighting is due to the rich and detailed results it yields when capturing an image of the iris. In the visible wavelength spectrum, images of the eye appear rich and colorful but lack in depth; on the other hand, an examination with NIR lighting reveals all the subtle craters and nuances that the iris contains.

To isolate the iris from the rest of the eyeball, imaging software uses landmark features. The shape of the iris provides a starting point for isolation and outlines the eye to prepare it for feature extraction. Once the iris has been properly located, the computer system can begin mapping and extracting relevant data from it (see Figure 7–3). A 2D Gabor wavelet filters the iris into multiple partitions known as phasors. These phasors map the orientation and spatial frequency of features found in the iris, as well as the location of where they can be found. The goal of this algorithm is to create a unique template of the iris to be compared against a database of users. This template is known as an **IrisCode**.

IrisCodes use a polar coordinate system to map information found in a particular individual's iris. All characteristics for a single iris can be stored using only 256 bytes of data, which is extremely small considering that a database can potentially be filled with hundreds of thousands of candidates. The entire mapping system is not affected by common problems such as overexposure and contrast. This makes this process reliable and capable of routine use.

Enrollment and Identification

Iris-based biometric systems have one of the easiest enrollment processes that are available today. Applicants that are being entered into the system need only two photographs taken of their eyes. The first high-definition photo that is taken is with normal visible wavelength, like a common picture. The second is taken using the NIR band which picks up all the details that visible wavelengths cannot capture. The digital photographs are then uploaded into a computer that removes unwanted details and scans the images for points of interest. Once the analysis of the two images is complete, the computer creates a simple 512-digit IrisCode for the applicant. The IrisCode is stored with the applicant's name and relevant information within the system's database. The entire process of enrollment takes just a few minutes and is not intrusive.

IrisCodes

IrisCode is a process to analyze and store information on a human iris. This method uses the extracted data from a human iris and processes it through a quantization stage that produces a binary iris code for later comparison.

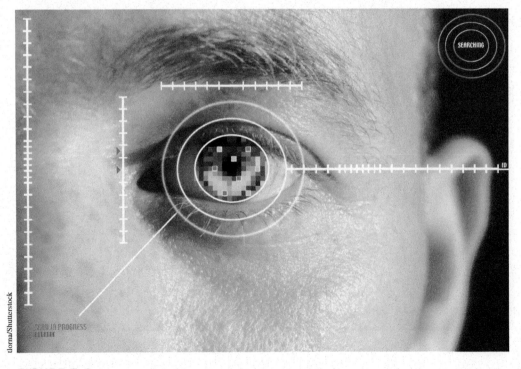

FIGURE 7–3
Iris scan showing eye with scanner and computer interface.

Once a user has been enrolled, they can be identified by access-control systems located within the network of the system. All an individual has to do is stand in front of another camera and get a single picture taken of their eye. One of the key advantages of iris scans (and a shortcoming of retina scans) is that a user can stand a good distance away from the camera and still procure a viable image. The system then analyzes the iris and extracts a unique IrisCode. For identification, this IrisCode is then compared with the computer's database to thousands of stored IrisCodes to find a match. This entire process is performed within the system's CPU (central processing unit) and takes only a couple of seconds to complete.

Current Applications

The Department of Defense and FBI host biometric databases containing thousands of "persons of interest" in regard to terrorists and insurgents. Coinciding with this, American forces and Afghanistan's government have collected biometric data on over 2.5 million citizens. Anyone who is processed through prisons or jails is scanned, along with many workers who perform tasks on U.S. Military installations. This has provided ground forces with a comprehensive list of suspected insurgents, as well as a means to check individuals the Army and Marines come in contact with on a daily basis. Those scanned are compared against a database of persons of interest, and intelligence operatives can obtain a good understanding of who is friend or foe.

During routine patrols, soldiers may order an entire village out of their homes to be scanned and identified. A portable biometric iris scanner is held up to each person's eyes, and within seconds the device lets the soldier know if their subject has been processed through local jails, is a suspected member of the Taliban, or if the individual is just a harmless farm worker. Iris biometrics is also used after a battle on the deceased to identify if any of the dead are high-ranking insurgents or wanted for acts of terrorism. This tool is extremely useful for the military due to its potential to reduce civilian casualties and its ability to provide ground forces with an understanding of who is around them. As it becomes harder to identify enemy forces blending in with civilian population, the need for iris biometrics in military applications will increase dramatically.

The FBI is currently perfecting its data repository and techniques for obtaining iris biometric data for use in its new database: the Next Generation Identification (NGI) system. This is being done through collaborations with law enforcement and corrections agencies across the United States. Prisons and correctional institutions are using iris-based systems to track inmates and efficiently record data that will be shared with members of other various law enforcement communities. For the FBI, iris scans are an effective tool to prevent crime and assist local law enforcement with solving cases and processing suspects who attempt to hide their identity.

Still in its infantile stages, the bureau boasts that the NGI will be the largest repository of IrisCodes in the world. Law enforcement and correctional institutions that implement iris scanners are currently sharing database information with the FBI in hopes of helping them reach this goal. Over 12,000 IrisCodes have been sent to the FBI, as they continue to test the capabilities the NGI system possesses. Funds have been offered to criminal justice organizations on both a state and federal level to assist with acquiring iris-based biometrics systems, and the FBI is confident that this will increase the amount of data they receive.

Facial Recognition

Have you ever seen a missing child's picture placed on the back of a milk carton? How about a "wanted" poster brandishing the mugshot of a person who committed a crime? The simple purpose of these banners is to encourage individuals to identify a person of interest using the features of their face in comparison with the picture distributed. Facial recognition biometrics aims to accomplish this goal in a more efficient manner that does not need the assistance of the public. Instead of having to rely on citizens identifying and reporting suspects that they may or may not come in contact with, a camera and computer system can accomplish the entire process without human intervention.

Along with identifying wanted and missing people, facial recognition biometrics is also a practical and valued tool for user-access control and credential management. Gone are the days of passwords and keys when a face is all that is needed for system access. The capabilities of facial biometrics are plentiful, and real-world applications have already begun.

A significant advantage of automated facial recognition, as compared to other different of biometrics, is that it does not require subjects to participate. For iris and fingerprint systems, the person of interest would have to consent to being photographed or processed. In the case of facial recognition systems, millions of people can walk by a CCTV camera each day without realizing that they are being scanned and identified. This is particularly effective when being used by a government organization that does not want a suspected felon or terrorist to know they are being searched for. People in the United States are used to seeing cameras all over the place, which allows for the perfect opportunity for passive surveillance and monitoring.

Like iris biometrics, facial recognition scans are not intrusive and can gain data in a way that is comfortable and hygienic for its users. This is beneficial for day-to-day access control in institutions that require fast/effective entrance. No part of the system or computer ever has to touch the body, and the entire process is relatively quick.

There exists much contention on whether facial recognition scans can be easily tricked or spoofed, but it is apparent that many variables can throw the results off. First of all, simple obstructions such as glasses, contacts, hats, facial hair, and hooded sweatshirts are able to throw off the results or simply prevent the camera from procuring usable data.

Disadvantages also exist due to the many features that comprise the face. It is much easier for a system to process the similarities in a single iris than it is to categorize and analyze an entire human face. Complex models and graphs need to be stored for every piece of biometric data that is used by the computer. This can slow down processing speeds and ultimately bottleneck an entire operation.

A facial recognition system can be easily tricked by a 2D picture. This is an extreme pitfall that affects automated programs the most. Consideration must always be practiced to ensure there is some form of human over-watch to prevent spoofing or hacking of the camera/computer.

History

Eigenfaces
The Eigenface technique creates matrices of human faces and uses complex mathematical equations to generate templates for individual features that are digitally stored. The library of Eigenfaces can be superimposed over raw facial images when searching for a facial identification.

Modern techniques of facial recognition can be attributed largely to the work of researchers Matthew Turk and Alex Pentland in the 1990s. These researchers used **Eigenfaces** to automate facial recognition in an attempt to identify and authenticate individuals from a series of faces. The Eigenface technique creates matrices of human faces and uses complex mathematical equations to generate templates for individual features. These features are analyzed, and algorithms determine similarities such as symmetry and size.

The significance of Pentland and Turk's research is the fact that they created a fully automated way of categorizing faces. With the Eigenfaces technique, a computer can cycle through thousands of faces in a day without error or human intervention. Facial recognition biometric technologies available today are built on similar principles that are used in the Eigenfaces technique. For companies and scientists developing cutting-edge biometric solutions, automation and accuracy are key ingredients for success. Government institutions evaluate facial recognition software by its ability to yield positive matches with low rates of error and processing time.

How It Works

Biometric facial recognition poses many complex problems and hurdles that are not present in many other biometric options. Due to the ever-changing nature and variety of features present in the human face, researchers must create software that analyzes multiple variables. Facial recognition systems that are used today analyze cheekbones, mouth edges, chin, ridges between the eyebrows, the contour of the jawline, distance between eyes, widow's peak, and many other data points. Unlike iris biometrics, facial recognition focuses on a part of human body that changes dramatically over time and can be manipulated or disguised easily to spoof the automated computer.

To start the process, a clear image must be acquired of the candidate who is being processed. The easiest way this can be done is through the cooperation of the individual (identification), or alternatively through surveillance such as CCTV cameras (matching/verification). With the identification method, an individual would be asked to stand a set distance from a digital camera and a high-definition photo is taken of the face. Using the matching and verification process, CCTV cameras in public places can be used to covertly acquire data of any face that comes in view.

Once the data is obtained, the system normalizes the pictures and makes them uniform for comparison. This normalizing process can consist of changes in light levels, cropping the face to be centered in each picture, and size adjustments that help minimize error and unwanted variables. A template is then created and stored in the computer's database for further analysis and comparison.

Verification and Identification: Techniques

The most intricate step to this biometric process is the verification/identification phase, in which the raw data from the captured image is compared against a database of other participants.

To combat the obstacles that hinder facial recognition software, various techniques have been developed to create an accurate verification and identification process. All of these techniques can be placed under two categories: appearance-based and model-based facial recognition. Appearance-based programs deal with the differences and similarities in the basic features of the face. Model-based facial recognition programs develop a repetition computer-generated model of the participant's face and can map complex features such as eye socket depth.

Facial recognition biometrics has a multitude of different approaches available to analyze facial data. Multiple techniques are required to create a viable reconstruction and analysis of a human face. Among these techniques, the most widely accepted are known today as principal component analysis (PCA), linear discriminant analysis (LDA), and Elastic Bunch Graph Matching (EBGM).

Principal component analysis is based on the Eigenfaces method and is classified as appearance based. PCA uses thousands of stored images of faces and places them over the face in question. Precise algorithms analyze the faces and note subtle differences and similarities that come from the overlap of images. Weights can be assigned to different categories and mathematical equations determine whether the picture in question is a match or not. PCA is effective because the data that is used and stored does not occupy much space. Eigenfaces are simple 2D images in which little data is needed for transfer or storage. The only disadvantage that PCA poses is that a full frontal face image is needed to be a viable sample. This means that this technique cannot be implemented for many verification purposes, as a CCTV camera image is often distorted or taken at an angle.

Linear discriminant analysis is also considered an appearance-based technique. With LDA, an individual's face is placed on a vector, and lines from one feature to another are analyzed. The relationship between the lines is analyzed, and variations are recorded. The raw image is called a fisher face. LDA is widely used and accepted due to its fast pace of processing and data acquisition. It can eliminate many negative variables as well, such as lighting differences and a change of facial expression (which would have a negative effect on the PCA technique). A full face image is required. A major disadvantage of this system is that it requires large amounts of data to store facial scans. This creates the possibility of deterring corporations from implementing its use when data concerns are always relevant.

The final technique, EBGM, is a model-based facial recognition program. EBGM uses a sequence of graphs to map the nonlinear relationships of features on the face. This method identifies landmark features on the face, such as edges of the lips, tips of the nose, top, bottom, and center of the eyes, and assigns some characteristics of the image surrounding that landmark, and then compares these characteristics with a new set of landmark characteristics from a new image (see Figure 7–4). Points on the face are calculated, and the EBGM technique allows for partial and off-center facial pictures to be analyzed. The advantages of EBGM technique include its ability to map the human face with extreme precision and accuracy. It doesn't require a full facial image.

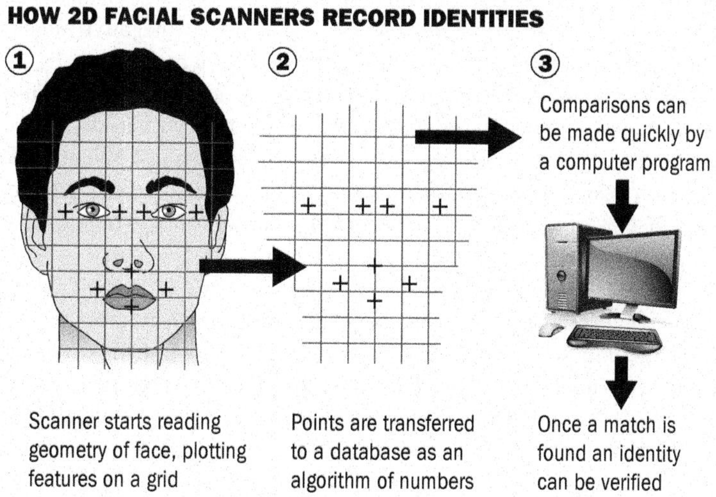

HOW 2D FACIAL SCANNERS RECORD IDENTITIES

① Scanner starts reading geometry of face, plotting features on a grid

② Points are transferred to a database as an algorithm of numbers

③ Comparisons can be made quickly by a computer program

Once a match is found an identity can be verified

FIGURE 7–4

Steps in procuring a facial scan.

> > > > > > > > > >

Living a Double Life

Jose Salvador Lantigua, a Florida businessman took a trip to Venezuela with the intention of faking his death and cheating his insurance company out of large fortunes. With the assistance of his family, Lantigua relocated to North Carolina and assumed a new identity complete with a visual disguise. For months Lantigua went unnoticed under his new alias "Ernest Allen Willis," and he would frequent public areas using a brown toupee and dyed beard.

Lantigua's fatal error came when he applied for a passport under his new alias and identity. When he submitted his passport photo, federal agents matched the picture to the allegedly deceased Lantigua using facial recognition biometrics. Even with his changed appearance the state-of-the-art facial recognition software was able to provide an accurate match. Federal agents approached Lantigua not soon after the match was made and charged him with multiple felonies. Among his possessions, agents found clever disguises and many tools to conceal his identity.

The Next-Generation Identification System

The FBI has begun integrating biometric technology into their new identification system. As of September 2014, the FBI dropped the use of their Integrated Automated Fingerprint Identification System (IAFIS), for a brand new state-of-the-art identification system. The NGI system provides a broader selection of resources and information for law enforcement agencies across the country. A new Tenprint system has been implemented. The FBI has also developed a new latent print search algorithm. This will potentially solve many cold cases and provide new leads for criminal investigations. The NGI is a necessary update for the FBI, as biometrics and new technologies have changed the way we fight crime and process individuals through the criminal justice system. Costing nearly $1.2 billion, the NGI will take a total of seven years before it is completed.

According to the FBI, this new high-tech system will consist of seven identification focal points. The first new NGI increment will be known as the Rap Back service. The Rap Back service sends notifications to agencies throughout the United States pertaining to criminal activity of individuals that have already been processed through the system at one point (arrest, probation, parole). This system will be especially useful for agencies that use any form of criminal supervision, such as a GPS-tracking anklet or a sex offender registry.

The next aspect of the NGI system pertains significantly to biometrics. Facial recognition is now being implemented by the FBI for use in criminal investigations. Images taken of suspects are sent to the FBI and the Bureau compares these images to a large database in the NGI. It is important to note that the NGI does not provide a "positive" or "negative" identification of the suspect; rather it is ranked high or low in probability of being a match.

Scars, marks, and tattoos have been an easy mode of identification throughout the years. This is now being added to the NGI, providing law enforcement with in-depth descriptions of individual's bodily marks. In practice, a law enforcement officer will be able to look up a suspect's distinctive tattoo to possibly establish identification. This can also be used in corrections, where tattoos provide a history of a felon's affiliations and criminal background.

The Interstate Photo System

The NGI system contains many new applications and programs to conduct thorough inquiries of people suspected of committing a crime, as well as generate new investigative leads. Much of the information contained within the NGI has been compiled by the FBI for many years, and new information is being provided to the FBI by criminal justice organizations throughout the United States. This expansive set of information is crucial for solving crimes and apprehending fugitives, especially due to the vast amount of law enforcement agencies that exist. The Interstate Photo System (IPS) has a database containing more than 30 million front-facing mugshot photos of individuals with tenprints on file. To be enrolled in IPS, all face photos must include a tenprint submission of the individual (submission of all 10 fingerprints). The IPS database has two categories of photos: criminal identities (photos submitted as part of a lawful detention, an arrest, or incarceration) and civil identities (photos submitted for licensing, employment, security clearances, military service, volunteer service, and immigration benefits). Over 80 percent of the photos in IPS are criminal.

The IPS users include the FBI and selected state and local law enforcement agencies, which can submit search requests to help identify an unknown person using, for example, a photo from a surveillance camera. The IPS is currently being used as an "investigative lead," and results are not to be interpreted as a positive identification of the suspected individual.

In addition to the IPS, the FBI has an internal unit called Facial Analysis, Comparison, and Evaluation (FACE) Services that provides face recognition capabilities, among other things, to support active FBI investigations. FACE Services not only has access to IPS but can also search or request to search databases owned by the Departments of State and Defense and 16 states, which use their own face recognition systems. Unlike IPS, which primarily contains criminal photos, FACE Services contains civil photos from state and federal government databases, such as visa applicant photos and selected states' driver's license photos. The total number of face photos available to FACE Services in all searchable repositories is over 411 million. FBI agents have requested almost 215,000 searches of external partners' databases. Of these requests, about 36,000 have included searches on state driver's license databases. Any results returned as part of a FACE Services request is treated as an investigative lead only and is not to be considered a positive identification.

Additionally, the FBI cannot take any independent law enforcement action based on the photo, meaning the photo is only one part of the full investigation. By utilizing passive surveillance techniques, the FBI plans to find wanted individuals through video camera feeds and CCTV footage. Many biometric experts insist that faces gathered through this technique will be grainy and low resolution, which will not yield enough data to gain a positive match. To combat this, the FBI has altered the system to generate a set of possible matches rather than trying to create a 1:1 match for facial recognition data.

The FBI has contracted the help of MorphoTrust to implement and maintain all facial recognition biometric systems. MorphoTrust is already responsible for biometric systems used in motor vehicle departments and other government establishments throughout the United States.

In April 2015, the FBI announced that facial recognition had become a fully active increment of the NGI system. Facial recognition works in tandem with the FBI's fingerprint system that holds over 100 million records, and the FBI hopes to link facial recognition data with accompanying fingerprints, name, age, weight, and other essential characteristics.

Fingerprint and the National Palm Print System

The NGI makes use of fingerprint impressions with its brand new Tenprint system. All 10 fingerprints are acquired by police and these are added to a federal database of prints. The FBI makes use of a new algorithm that yields better results across its comparisons. With the dated IAFIS system, fingerprints were only 92 percent accurate, but the accuracy has been bumped up to 99 percent with NGI. The time required has also been reduced between acceptance of prints and positive identification.

Along with the addition of a new Tenprint system, the FBI has developed a new Latent print search algorithm. This will potentially solve many cold cases and provide new leads for criminal investigations. The latent print search will be much more accurate in finding matches and is accessible to more than 18,000 law enforcement agencies across the country. The latent print search algorithm goes hand in hand with the FBI's new National Palm Print System (NPPS). This was previously unavailable to law enforcement and provided a major problem as many prints left at crime scenes are the offender's palm impression. With the addition of the NPPS and Tenprint system, many more prospective crimes will be solvable in the coming years.

In 2013, the FBI implemented the NPPS. The NPPS contains a database of millions of palm prints to be used in criminal investigations and processes. This works hand in hand with the AFIT system because now investigators can match fingerprints with any palm prints found at crime scenes. The NPPS will see great improvements in the search of latent fingerprint files from unsolved cold cases. Eighteen thousand law enforcement agencies will have access to this program and will be able to generate new leads for crimes that may have occurred decades ago and gone unsolved. All criminal and civil searches will now include data found in the Universal Latent File, which may generate hits for new fingerprints as they are added to the system. This will serve as a powerful investigative weapon and may provide closure for families of murder victims.

The FBI has also implemented the Repository of Individuals of Special Concern (RISC). RISC allows for officers to fingerprint individuals they come in contact with and quickly detect whether or not they are a threat. The system compares the suspect against a repository of sex offenders, wanted persons, suspected terrorists, and other high-risk individuals. This system may protect many officers from potential danger, as they will now have a better idea of whom they are dealing with. This application is completely mobile and can be accessed from a patrol vehicle or forward outpost using fingerprint data collected from two index fingers. Once a law enforcement officer has the fingerprints of an individual suspect, it can take as little as 10 seconds for the RISC application to compare with all 2.9 million prints contained within the database. Twenty-one states are currently participating in the RISC increment of the NGI, and the FBI hopes to eventually have the cooperation and assistance of all 50 states.

Searches within the Criminal Master File will now include everything found within the Unsolved Latent File. These new searches will lead law enforcement agencies to gain more hits when searching data that relates to unsolved cases. New algorithms and metrics make the infrastructure of the NGI more powerful and accurate. This will be useful for law enforcement agencies across the country.

We opened up our discussion by exemplifying the utilization of fingerprint biometric technology as a means of gaining access to an iPhone. The combination of a mobile device and a fingerprint scanner has become a reality for law enforcement agencies. MorphoTrak, a leading developer of biometric technology, has developed a mobile fingerprints scanner the size of a cell phone (see Figure 7–5). The law enforcement officer will instruct a potential suspect to put a finger on the face of the device, and the print is transmitted to federal and state databases. The results are acquired very quickly and show information about the suspect including active warrants and identity. This can be very crucial, as potential suspects with open warrants may lie about their identity as a means to avoid arrest.

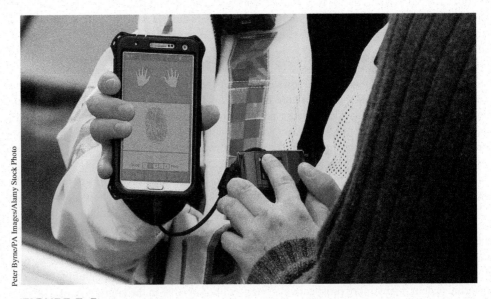

Peter Byrne/PA Images/Alamy Stock Photo

FIGURE 7–5
Mobile fingerprint scanner.

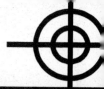
There are two main functions of biometrics. The first function is biometric matching or verification. Biometric systems are capable of identifying someone out of a crowd by scanning select biometric characteristics into a database. The second application of biometrics relates to access control through biometric identification. The first process that each biometric system must perform is known as the *enrollment process*. The enrollment process captures a person's biometric data and stores in a database for later use. Once the information completes its runs through a data preprocessing module, feature extraction begins. This module is responsible for finding patterns in the traits extracted by the sensor by using mathematical equations.

The template generation module is responsible for saving all of the raw data produced by feature extraction and putting it into a simple and easy-to-read format for the system. The FBI has begun integrating biometric technology into their new identification system. The NGI system provides a broader selection of resources and information for law enforcement agencies across the country. A new Tenprint system has been implemented. The FBI has also developed a new latent print search algorithm. Iris biometrics is replacing retina biometrics because it is an all-around better technology and more functional for both law enforcement and business security. The goal is to create a unique template of the iris to be compared against a database in the NGI system. This template is known as an IrisCode. Facial recognition biometrics has a plethora of different approaches available to analyze facial data. Multiple techniques are required to create a viable reconstruction and analysis of a human face. Among these techniques, the most widely accepted are known today as PCA, LDA, and EBGM. Facial recognition had become a fully active increment of the NGI system. Facial recognition works in tandem with the FBI's fingerprint system. The FBI hopes to link facial recognition data with accompanying fingerprints, name, age, weight, and other essential characteristics. The FBI has also implemented the NPPS. The NPPS contains a database of millions of palm prints to be used in criminal investigations and processes.

Review Questions

1. _____ is a cutting-edge type of access control that accurately and efficiently identifies humans.

2. The two main functions of biometrics are _____ and _____.

3. One of the main causes of stolen accounts and information in computer systems is the use of weak _____.

4. Many forms of biometric technology are available today, but the majority of them can be split into two different groups. The first group is _____ biometrics, which contains fingerprints, hand, iris, retina, and facial scans. The second group is _____ biometrics, which is much less stable and includes handwriting, voice, keystroke, and gait recognition.

5. _____ is the most commonly used type of physiological biometric.

6. True or False: The manner in which an individual types on a keyboard is unique. _____

7. Which biometric refers to an individual's different posture, step length, speed, and foot positioning in regard to the way they walk from one place to another? _____

8. _____ is the most commonly used type of behavioral biometrics.

9. _____ have been widely used to identify people for a century.

10. True or False: A data preprocessing module is where extraction begins for a biometric system. _____

11. A second process known as the _____ module compares all collected files to the system's database.

12. The first process that each biometric system must perform is _____.

13. True or False: The human iris will undergo significant changes during one's lifetime. _____

14. True or False: Due to the complicated nature of obtaining and analyzing retina scans, this technology is not easy to implement in the field _____.

15. The acronym NGI stands for _____.

16. The NGI system has replaced the _____ fingerprint system.

17. The NGI's _____ service sends notifications to agencies throughout the United States pertaining to criminal activity of individuals that have already been processed through the system at one point.

18. Facial scans are (more or less) accurate than iris scans.

19. Which government agency created and maintains the NGI system? _____

20. The _____ is the colored section in the eye around the pupil.

21. The iris begins to form at the _____ stage of pregnancy, where muscle fibers start to take shape and construct tight patterns.

22. The _____ is composed of neural cells in the back of the eyeball that provide a "screen" for the cornea and lens to display an image on. The _____ is responsible for obtaining a clear picture of what a person is actually seeing.

23. The near infrared wavelength band is located within the _____ nm range of the electromagnetic spectrum.

24. Iris images are taken with normal visible wavelength pictures, as well as pictures in the _____ band.

25. The _____ program was developed by Dr. John Daugman for the analysis and verification of the human iris.

26. Currently, the number of IrisCodes being shared by law enforcement institutions with the FBI is _____.

27. The first documented attempt to identify someone using the iris was performed in the 1950s by British ophthalmologist _____.

28. A 2D Gabor wavelet filters the iris into multiple partitions known as _____.

29. The U.S. Marines and Army use _____ iris biometric system to identify friend or foe on the battlefield.

30. Matthew Turk and Alex Pentland used _____ to automate facial recognition in attempts to identify and authenticate individuals from a series of faces.

31. A significant advantage of automated facial recognition, as compared to the other different forms of biometrics, is that it does not require subjects to participate. Millions of people can be walking by a _____ each day without realizing that they are being scanned and identified.

32. Hats, glasses, and facial hair can obstruct a _____ biometrics scan.

33. A facial recognition scan can be tricked by a simple _____.

34. With the _____ method, an individual would be asked to stand a set distance from a normal digital camera and a high-definition photo is taken of the face.

35. To combat the obstacles that conflict with facial recognition software, various techniques have been developed to create an accurate verification/matching and identification process. All of these techniques can be placed under two categories: _____ and _____.

36. Elastic Bunch Graph Matching is a _____ facial recognition program.

37. True or False: Over 16 states are participating in the FBI's facial recognition program. _____

38. The _____ system was implemented in 2014 to replace the existing fingerprint IAFIS database.

39. The _____ is a NGI database containing 30 million front-facing photos of individuals with tenprints on file.

40. The _____ contains a NGI database of millions of palm prints to be used in criminal investigations and processes.

41. The NGI system utilized complex matching algorithms that changed the fingerprint accuracy rating from _____ to _____ percent.

42. The FBI has implemented the _____ system to quickly search a fingerprint database containing terrorists and other high-risk individuals.

Application and Critical Thinking

1. Terror suspects take advantage of large crowds and chaotic situations to blend in and become anonymous. How can law enforcement and government agencies use biometrics to gather investigative leads and find suspects? How can biometrics prevent known terrorists from entering a heavily populated event?

2. Computers and sensitive data networks are most sensitive to breaches due to the problems that exist with existing access-control systems. Passwords can be easily cracked by hacking software, and keycards can be shared among multiple people. Keys are about as obsolete as the locks that they are matched too. How can biometrics solve these problems?

Further References

Das, R., *Biometric Technology: Authentication, Biocryptography, and Cloud-Based Architecture*. Boca Raton, FL: CRC Press, 2015.

Du, E. Y., *Biometrics: From Fiction to Practice*. Singapore: Pan Stanford, 2013.

Labati, R. D., V. Pluri, and F. Scotti, *Touchless Fingerprint Biometrics*. Boca Raton, FL: CRC Press, 2015.

The Microscope

KEY TERMS

binocular
condenser
depth of focus
eyepiece lens
field of view
microspectrophotometer
monocular
objective lens
parfocal
plane-polarized light
polarizer
real image
transmitted illumination
vertical or reflected
   illumination
virtual image

Go to www.pearsonhighered.com/careersresources to access Webextras for this chapter.

Baby Doe

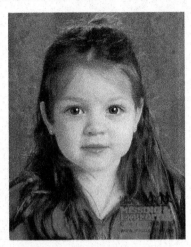

Information Wanted

The Suffolk County District Attorney, Massachusetts State Police, and Winthrop Police are seeking the public's help in identifying a female toddler whose body was found on the western shore of Deer Island on June 25, 2015. This computer-generated composite image depicts her as she may have appeared in life.

The child was approximately four years old at the time of her death, had brown eyes and brown hair, weighed about 30 pounds, and stood about 3½ feet tall.

Suffolk County State Police Detective Unit	Mass State Police Communication Section	Winthrop Police Tip Line

On July 25, 2015, a woman was walking her dog along the beach on Deer Island outside Boston, Massachusetts. The dog stopped to sniff a contractor-style garbage bag and inside that bag the woman discovered the remains of a young girl, approximately 2–4 years old. The child, whom investigators believed to have been deceased for 1–2 days prior to discovery, was wrapped in two blankets and wearing a pair of white pants with black polka dots. An investigation into the identity of the toddler ensued and authorities distributed a composite sketch of her face and a description the clothing she was wearing to the news media. The media dubbed the child, "Baby Doe," and the case garnered national attention.

Weeks went by, and though tips poured in, investigators were still unable to positively identify the girl. Detectives at the Massachusetts State Police began to pursue lesser known forensic methods that could indicate whether the child was local to the Boston area or whether her killers brought her body there in an effort to conceal the crime. They submitted, through the National Center for Missing and Exploited Children, two blankets used to wrap the body, the child's pants, and a sample of the child's hair, to the Laboratories and Scientific Services section of the U.S. Customs and Border Patrol in Houston for pollen analysis.

There, analysts determined that based on the recovered pollen and high quantities of soot, all of the analyzed samples suggest that the child was most likely from a suburban area in the Northeastern United States. They identified spores of oak and pine along with other species typically found in the deciduous forest of North America. Most telling, though, was the recovery of two different types of cedar pollen. The analyst determined that because cedar trees are not native to the Northeast, the only two places in that region where multiple species of cedar are known to grow together are the Arnold Arboretum of Harvard University in Boston and the Morris Arboretum of the University of Pennsylvania in Philadelphia. Although the analyst could not distinguish between the greater Philadelphia and Boston areas, it was determined that the Boston area may be the more likely candidate since the child was found there. This information helped investigators to focus their search in greater Boston and ultimately identify the child and the individuals responsible for her death. Read more about the case evidence in the Forensic Palynology section of this chapter.

Basics of the Microscope

A microscope is an optical instrument that uses a lens or a combination of lenses to magnify and resolve the fine details of an object. The earliest methods for examining physical evidence in crime laboratories relied almost solely on the microscope to study the structure and composition of matter. Even the advent of modern analytical instrumentation and techniques has done little to diminish the usefulness of the microscope for forensic analysis. If anything, the development of the powerful scanning electron microscope (SEM) promises to add a new dimension to forensic science heretofore unattainable within the limits of the ordinary light microscope.

The earliest and simplest microscope was the single lens commonly referred to as a *magnifying glass*. The handheld magnifying glass makes things appear larger than they are because of the way light rays are refracted, or bent, in passing from the air into the glass and back into the air. The magnified image is observed by looking through the lens, as shown in Figure 8–1. Such an image is known as a **virtual image**; it can be seen only by looking through a lens and cannot be viewed directly. This is distinguished from a **real image**, which can be seen directly, like the image that is projected onto a motion picture screen.

The ordinary magnifying glass can achieve a magnification of about 5 to 10 times. Higher magnifying power is obtainable only with a *compound microscope*, constructed of two lenses mounted at each end of a hollow tube. The object to be magnified is placed under the lower lens, called the **objective lens**, and the magnified image is viewed through the upper lens, known as the **eyepiece lens**. As shown in Figure 8–2, the objective lens forms a real, inverted, magnified image of the object. The eyepiece, acting just like a simple magnifying glass, further magnifies this image into a virtual image, which is what is seen by the eye. The combined magnifying power of both lenses can produce an image magnified up to 1,500 times.

The optical principles of the compound microscope are incorporated into the basic design of different types of light microscopes. The microscopes most applicable for examining forensic specimens are as follows:

1. The compound microscope
2. The comparison microscope
3. The stereoscopic microscope
4. The polarizing microscope
5. The microspectrophotometer

After describing these five microscopes, we will talk about a completely different approach to microscopy, the SEM. This instrument focuses a beam of electrons, instead of visible light, onto the specimen to produce a magnified image. The principle and design of this microscope permit magnifying powers as high as 100,000 times.

virtual image
An image that cannot be seen directly. It can be seen only by a viewer looking through a lens.

real image
An image formed by the actual convergence of light rays on a screen.

objective lens
The lower lens of a microscope, which is positioned directly over the specimen.

eyepiece lens
The lens of a microscope into which the viewer looks; same as the ocular lens.

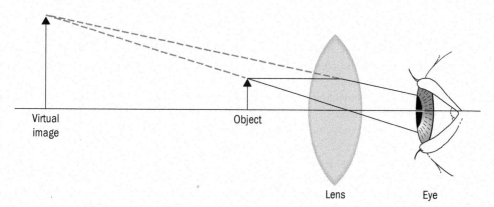

FIGURE 8–1

The passage of light through a lens, showing how magnification is obtained.

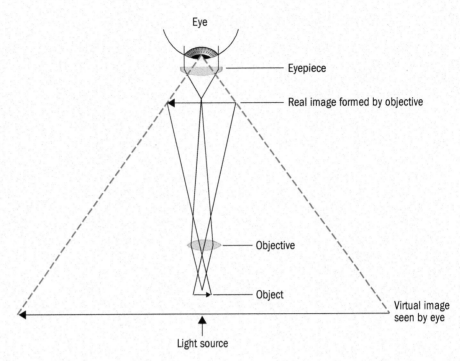

FIGURE 8–2

The principle of the compound microscope. The passage of light through two lenses forms the virtual image of the object seen by the eye.

The Compound Microscope

The parts of the compound microscope are illustrated in Figure 8–3. Basically, this microscope consists of a mechanical system, which supports the microscope, and an optical system. The optical system illuminates the object under investigation and passes the light through a series of lenses to form an image of the specimen on the retina of the eye. The optical path of light through a compound microscope is shown in Figure 8–4.

Parts of the Compound Microscope

The mechanical system of the compound microscope is composed of six parts:

Base (1).   The support on which the instrument rests.

Arm (2).   A C-shaped upright structure, hinged to the base, that supports the microscope and acts as a handle for carrying.

Stage (3).   The horizontal plate on which the specimens are placed for study. The specimens are normally mounted on glass slides that are held firmly in place on the stage by spring clips.

Body tube (4).   A cylindrical hollow tube on which the objective and eyepiece lenses are mounted at opposite ends. This tube merely serves as a corridor through which light passes from one lens to another.

Coarse adjustment (5).   This knob focuses the microscope lenses on the specimen by raising and lowering the body tube.

Fine adjustment (6).   The movements effected by this knob are similar to those of the coarse adjustment but are of a much smaller magnitude.

The optical system is made up of four parts:

Illuminator (7).   Most modern microscopes use artificial light supplied by a lightbulb to illuminate the specimen being examined. If the specimen is transparent, the light is directed up toward and through the specimen stage from an illuminator built into the base of the microscope. This is known as **transmitted illumination**. When the object is opaque—that is, not transparent—the light source must be placed above the specimen so that it can reflect off the specimen's surface and into the lens system of the microscope. This type of illumination is known as **vertical or reflected illumination**.

transmitted illumination
Light that passes up from the condenser and through the specimen.

vertical or reflected illumination
Illumination of a specimen from above; in microscopy it is used to examine opaque specimens.

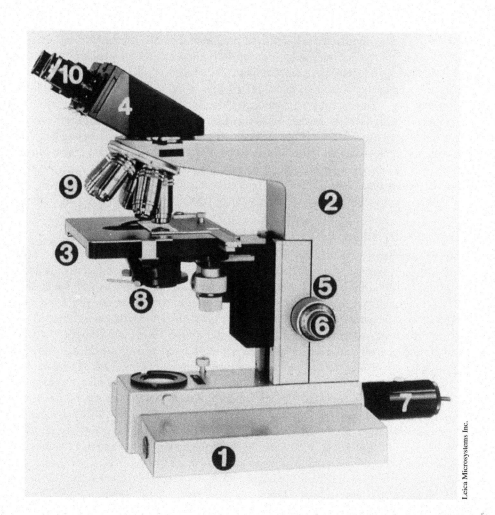

FIGURE 8–3

Parts of the compound microscope: (1) base, (2) arm, (3) stage, (4) body tube, (5) coarse adjust, (6) fine adjust, (7) illuminator, (8) condenser, (9) objective lens, and (10) eyepiece lens.

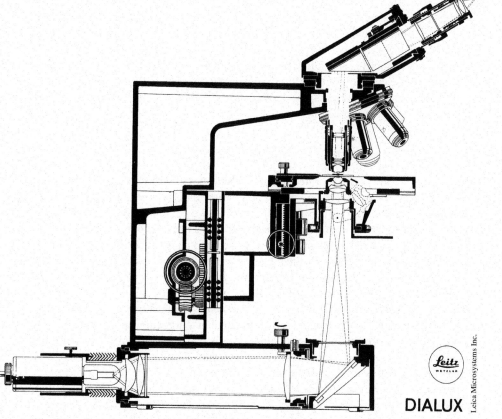

DIALUX

FIGURE 8–4

Optics of the compound microscope.

condenser
The lens system under the microscope stage that focuses light onto
the specimen.

parfocal
Describes a microscope such that
when an image is focused with one
objective in position, the other
objective can be rotated into place
and the field will remain in focus.

monocular
Describes a microscope with one
eyepiece.

binocular
Describes a microscope with two
eyepieces.

Condenser (8).   The **condenser** collects light rays from the base illuminator and concentrates
them on the specimen. The simplest condenser is known as the *Abbé condenser*. It consists
of two lenses held together in a metal mount. The condenser also includes an iris diaphragm
that can be opened or closed to control the amount of light passing into the condenser.

Objective lens (9).   This is the lens positioned closest to the specimen. To facilitate changing
from one objective lens to another, several objectives are mounted on a revolving nosepiece
or turret located above the specimen. Most microscopes are **parfocal**, meaning that when the
microscope is focused with one objective in position, the other objective can be rotated into
place by revolving the nosepiece while the specimen remains very nearly in correct focus.

Eyepiece or ocular lens (10).   This is the lens closest to the eye. A microscope with only one
eyepiece is **monocular**; one constructed with two eyepieces (one for each eye) is **binocular**.

Properties of the Compound Microscope

Each microscope lens is inscribed with a number signifying its magnifying power. The image
viewed by the microscopist will have a total magnification equal to the product of the magnifying
power of the objective and eyepiece lenses. For example, an eyepiece lens with a magnification
of 10× used in combination with an objective lens of 10× has a total magnification power of
100×. Most forensic work requires a 10× eyepiece in combination with either a 4×, 10×, 20×,
or 45× objective. The respective magnifications will be 40×, 100×, 200×, and 450×.

In addition, each objective lens is inscribed with its numerical aperture (N.A.). The ability of
an objective lens to resolve details into separate images instead of one blurred image is directly
proportional to the numerical aperture value of the objective lens. For example, an objective lens
of N.A. 1.30 can separate details at half the distance of a lens with an N.A. of 0.65. The maximum useful magnification of a compound microscope is approximately 1,000 times the N.A. of
the objective being used. This magnification is sufficient to permit the eye to see all the detail
that can be resolved. Any effort to increase the total magnification beyond this figure will yield
no additional detail and is referred to as *empty magnification*.

Although a new student of the microscope may be tempted to immediately choose the highest
magnifying power available to view a specimen, the experienced microscopist weighs a number
of important factors before choosing a magnifying power. A first consideration must be the size
of the specimen area, or the **field of view**, that the examiner wishes to study. As magnifying
power increases, the field of view decreases. Thus, it is best to first select a low magnification in
which a good general overall view of the specimen is seen and to switch later to a higher power
in which a smaller portion of the specimen can be viewed in more detail.

field of view
The area of the specimen that can
be seen after it is magnified.

depth of focus
The thickness of a specimen
that is entirely in focus under a
microscope.

The **depth of focus** is also a function of magnifying power. After a focus has been achieved
on a specimen, the depth of focus defines the thickness of that specimen. Areas above and below
this region will be blurred and can be viewed only when the focus is readjusted. Depth of focus
decreases as magnifying power increases.

WEBEXTRA 8.1
Explore the Concept of
Magnification with a Compound
Microscope

WEBEXTRA 8.2
Scan a Sample Under the Compound
Microscope

WEBEXTRA 8.3
Observe the Concept of Depth of
Focus

The Comparison Microscope

Forensic microscopy often requires a side-by-side comparison of specimens. This kind of
examination can best be performed with a comparison microscope, such as the one pictured in
Figure 8–5. Basically, the comparison microscope is two compound microscopes combined into
one unit. The unique feature of its design is that it uses a bridge incorporating a series of mirrors
and lenses to join two independent objective lenses into a single binocular unit. When a viewer
looks through the eyepiece lenses of the comparison microscope, a circular field, equally divided
into two parts by a fine line, is observed. The specimen mounted under the left-hand objective is
seen in the left half of the field, and the specimen under the right-hand objective is observed in the
right half of the field. It is important to closely match the optical characteristics of the objective
lenses to ensure that both specimens are seen at equal magnification and with minimal but identical lens distortions. Comparison microscopes designed to compare bullets, cartridges, and other
opaque objects are equipped with vertical or reflected illumination. Comparison microscopes
used to compare hairs or fibers use transmitted illumination.

WEBEXTRA 8.4
Practice Matching Bullets with the
Aid of a 3-D Interactive Illustration

Figure 8–6 shows the striation markings on two bullets that have been placed under the
objective lenses of a comparison microscope. Modern firearms examination began with the
introduction of the comparison microscope, with its ability to give the firearms examiner a

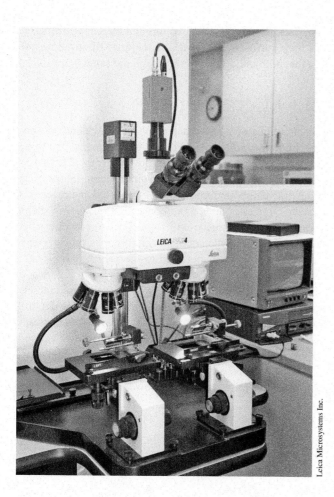

FIGURE 8–5
The comparison microscope—two independent objective lenses joined together by an optical bridge.

Leica Microsystems Inc.

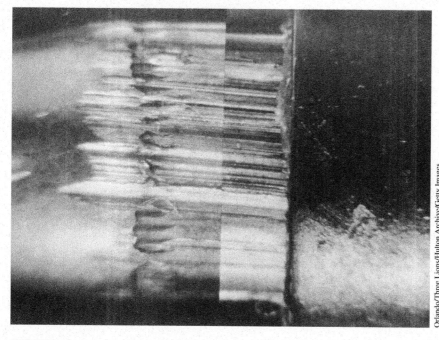

Orlando/Three Lions/Hulton Archive/Getty Images

FIGURE 8–6

Photomicrograph taken through a comparison microscope. On the right are the striation markings on the test-fired bullet, fired through the suspect weapon. On the left are the markings of the crime-scene bullet.

side-by-side magnified view of bullets. Bullets that are fired through the same rifle barrel display comparable rifling markings on their surfaces. Matching the majority of striations present on each bullet justifies a conclusion that both bullets traveled through the same barrel.

The Stereoscopic Microscope

The details that characterize the structures of many types of physical evidence do not always require examination under very high magnifications. For such specimens, the stereoscopic microscope has proven quite adequate, providing magnifying powers from 10× to 125×. This microscope has the advantage of presenting a distinctive three-dimensional image of an object. Also, whereas the image formed by the compound microscope is inverted and reversed (upside-down and backward), the stereoscopic microscope is more convenient because of the prisms in its light path that permit the formation of a right-side-up image. The stereoscopic microscope, shown in Figure 8–7, is actually two monocular compound microscopes properly spaced and aligned to present a three-dimensional image of a specimen to the viewer, who looks through both eyepiece lenses. The light path of a stereoscopic microscope is shown in Figure 8–8.

The stereoscopic microscope is undoubtedly the most frequently used and versatile microscope found in the crime laboratory. Its wide field of view and great depth of focus make it an ideal instrument for locating trace evidence in debris, garments, weapons, or tools. Furthermore, its potentially large *working distance* (the distance between the objective lens and the specimen) makes it quite applicable for the microscopic examination of big, bulky items. When fitted with vertical illumination, the stereoscopic microscope becomes the primary tool for characterizing physical evidence as diverse as paint, soil, gunpowder residues, and marijuana.

WEBEXTRA 8.5
Explore the Stereoscopic
Microscope

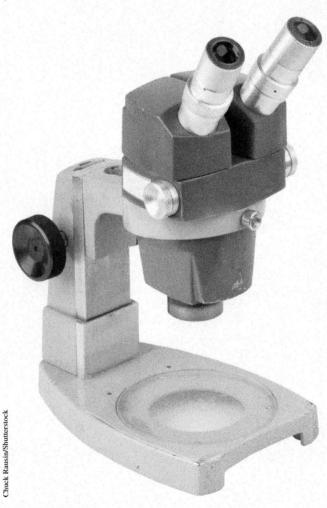

Chuck Rausin/Shutterstock

FIGURE 8–7
A stereoscopic microscope.

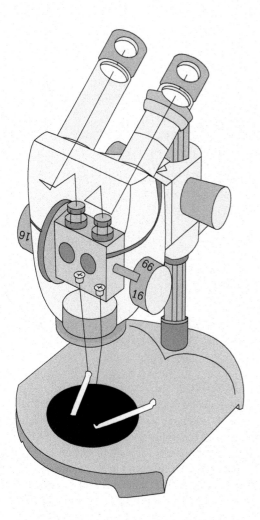

FIGURE 8–8
Schematic diagram of a stereoscopic microscope. This microscope is actually two separate monocular microscopes, each with its own set of lenses except for the lowest objective lens, which is common to both microscopes.

The Polarizing Microscope

Light's wavelike motion in space can be invoked to explain many facets of its behavior. The polarizing microscope takes advantage of one of these facts—the fact that light vibrates.

Polarization

The waves that compose a beam of light can be pictured as vibrating in all directions perpendicular to the direction in which the light is traveling. However, when a beam of light passes through certain types of specially fabricated crystalline substances, it emerges vibrating in only one plane. Light that is confined to a single plane of vibration is said to be **plane-polarized**. The device that polarizes light in this manner is called a **polarizer**. A common example of this phenomenon is the passage of sunlight through polarized sunglasses. By transmitting light vibrating in the vertical plane only, these sunglasses eliminate or reduce light glare. Most glare consists of partially polarized light that has been reflected off horizontal surfaces and thus is vibrating in a horizontal plane.

Because polarized light appears no different to the eye from ordinary light, special means must be devised for detecting it. This is accomplished simply by placing a second polarizing crystal, called an *analyzer*, in the path of the polarized beam. As shown in Figure 8–9, if the polarizer and analyzer are aligned parallel to each other, the polarized light passes through and is seen by the eye. If, on the other hand, the polarizer and analyzer are set perpendicular to one another, or are "crossed," no light penetrates, and the result is total darkness or *extinction*.

In this manner, a compound or stereoscopic microscope can be outfitted with a polarizer and analyzer to allow the viewer to detect polarized light. Such a microscope is known as a *polarizing microscope*. Essentially, the polarizer is placed between the light source and the sample stage to polarize the light before it passes through the specimen. The polarized light penetrating the specimen must then pass through an analyzer before it reaches the eyepiece and finally the eye. Normally, the polarizer and analyzer are "crossed" so that when no specimen is in place, the field

plane-polarized light
Light confined to a single plane of vibration.

polarizer
A device that permits the passage of light waves vibrating in only one plane.

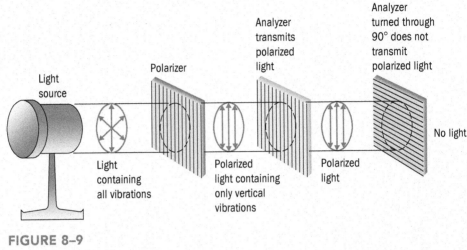

FIGURE 8-9
Polarization of light.

appears dark. However, introducing a specimen that polarizes light reorients the polarized light, allowing it to pass through the analyzer. This result produces vivid colors and intensity contrasts that make the specimen readily distinguishable.

Applications of the Polarized Microscope

WEBEXTRA 8.6
Explore the Polarizing
Microscope—I

WEBEXTRA 8.7
Explore the Polarizing
Microscope—II

The most obvious and important applications of this microscope relate to studying materials that polarize light. For example, as we will learn in Chapter 10 (see page 214), many crystalline substances are birefringent; that is, they split a beam of light into two light-ray components of different refractive index values. What makes this observation particularly relevant to our discussion of the polarizing microscope is that the light beams are polarized at right angles to each other. Thus, polarizing microscopy has found wide application for the examination of birefringent minerals present in soil. By using the immersion method and selecting the proper immersion liquids, a refractive index corresponding to each plane of polarized light can be determined. Thus, when a mineral is viewed under polarized light in a liquid that matches one of its refractive indices, the bright halo that is observed near the border of the particle, known as the Becke line, will no longer be visible. This information, plus observations on crystal color, form, and so on, makes it possible for the microscopist to identify the mineral. Similarly, criminalists use the fact that many synthetic fibers are birefringent to characterize them with a polarizing microscope.

The Microspectrophotometer

From a practical point of view, few instruments in a crime laboratory can match the versatility of the microscope. The microscope's magnifying power is indispensable for finding minute traces of physical evidence. Many items of physical evidence can be characterized by a microscopic examination of their morphological features. Likewise, the microscope can be used to study how light interacts with the material under investigation, or it can be used to observe the effects that other chemical substances have on such evidence. Each of these features allows an examiner to better characterize and identify physical evidence. Recently, linking the microscope to a computerized spectrophotometer has added a new dimension to its capability. This combination has given rise to a new instrument called the **microspectrophotometer**.

microspectrophotometer
An instrument that links a microscope to a spectrophotometer.

In many respects, this is an ideal marriage from the forensic scientist's viewpoint. In Chapter 12, we will see how a chemist can use selective absorption of light by materials to characterize them. In particular, light in the ultraviolet, visible, and infrared regions of the electromagnetic spectrum is most helpful for this purpose. Unfortunately, in the past, forensic chemists were unable to take full advantage of the capabilities of spectrophotometry for examining trace evidence because most spectrophotometers are not well suited for examining the very small particles frequently encountered as evidence. However, with the development of the microspectrophotometer, a forensic analyst can now view a particle under a microscope while a beam of light is directed at the particle

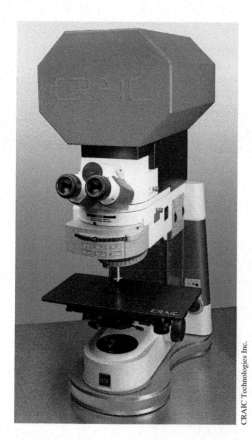

CRAIC Technologies Inc.

FIGURE 8–10
A visible-light microspectrophotometer.

in order to obtain its absorption spectrum. Depending on the type of light employed, an examiner can acquire either a visible or an infrared (IR) spectral pattern of the substance being viewed under the microscope. The obvious advantage of this approach is to provide the forensic scientist with added information that will characterize trace quantities of evidence. A microspectrophotometer designed to measure the uptake of visible light by materials is shown in Figure 8–10.

Visual comparison of color is usually one of the first steps in examining paint, fiber, and ink evidence. Such comparisons are easily obtained using a comparison microscope. Now, with the use of the microspectrophotometer, not only can the color of materials be compared visually but, at the same time, an absorption spectrum can be plotted for each item under examination to display the exact wavelengths at which it absorbs in the visible-light spectrum. Occasionally colors that appear similar by visual examination show significant differences in their absorption spectra. An example of this approach is shown in Figure 8–11, in which the microspectrophotometer is used to distinguish counterfeit and authentic currency by comparing the spectral patterns of inked lines on currency.

Another emerging technique in forensic science is the use of the infrared microspectrophotometer to examine fibers and paints. The "fingerprint" IR spectrum (see discussion in Chapter 12) is unique for each chemical substance. Therefore, obtaining such a spectrum from either a fiber or a paint chip allows the analyst to better identify and compare the type of chemicals from which these materials are manufactured. With a microspectrophotometer, a forensic analyst can view a substance through the microscope and at the same time have the instrument plot the infrared absorption spectrum for that material.

The Scanning Electron Microscope

All the microscopes described thus far use light coming off the specimen to produce a magnified image. The SEM is, however, a special case in the family of microscopes (see Figure 8–12). The image is formed by aiming a beam of electrons onto the specimen and studying electron emissions on a closed TV circuit. The beam of electrons is emitted from a hot tungsten filament and is focused by electromagnets onto the surface of the specimen. This primary electron beam causes the emission of electrons, known as secondary electrons, from the elements that make up the upper layers of

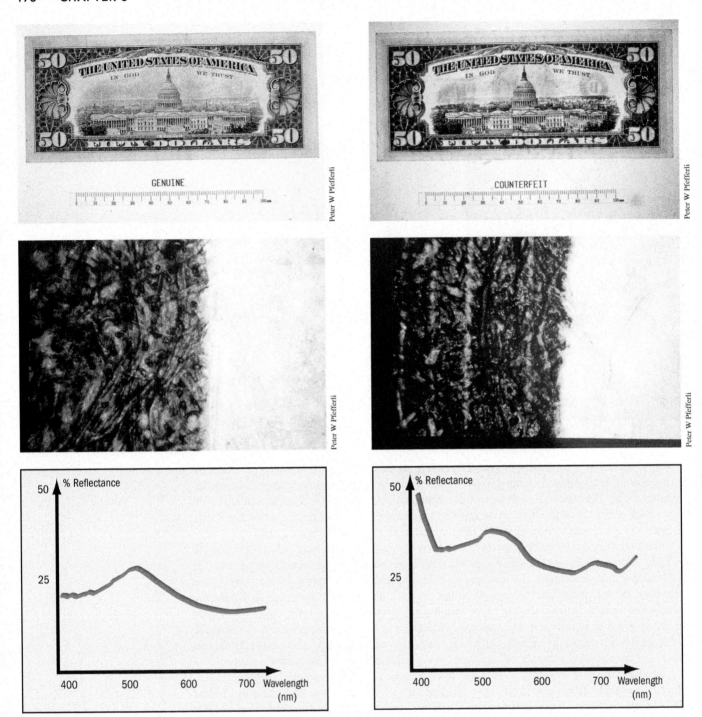

FIGURE 8–11

Two $50 bills are shown at top; one is genuine and the other is counterfeit. Below each bill is a microphotograph of an inked line present on each bill. Each line was examined under a visible-light microspectrophotometer. As shown, the visible absorption spectrum of each line is readily differentiated, thus allowing the examiner to distinguish a counterfeit bill from genuine currency.

the specimen. Also, 20–30 percent of the primary electrons rebound off the surface. These electrons are known as *backscattered electrons*. The emitted electrons (both secondary and backscattered) are collected and the amplified signal is displayed on a monitor. By scanning the primary electron beam across the specimen's surface in synchronization with the cathode-ray tube, it is possible to convert the emitted electrons into an image of the specimen for display on the cathode-ray tube.

The major attractions of the SEM image are its high magnification, high resolution, and great depth of focus. In its usual mode, the SEM has a magnification that ranges from 10× to

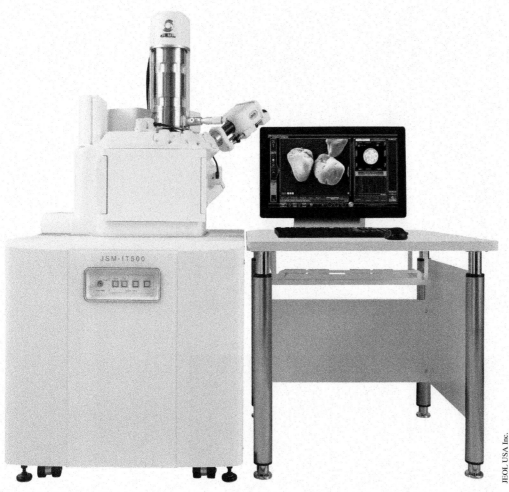

JEOL USA Inc.

FIGURE 8–12

A scanning electron microscope.

100,000×. Its depth of focus is some 300 times better than optical systems at similar magnifications, and the resultant picture is almost stereoscopic in appearance. Its great depth of field and magnification are exemplified by the magnification of cystolithic hair on the marijuana leaf, as shown in Figure 8–13. A SEM image of a vehicle's headlight filaments may reveal whether the headlights were on or off at the time of a collision (see Figures 8–14 and 8–15).

Another facet of scanning electron microscopy has been the use of X-ray production to determine the elemental composition of a specimen. X-rays are generated when the electron beam of the SEM strikes a target. When the SEM is coupled to an X-ray analyzer, the emitted X-rays can be sorted according to their energy values and used to build a picture of the elemental distribution in the specimen. Because each element emits X-rays of characteristic energy values, the X-ray analyzer can identify the elements present in a specimen. Furthermore, the element's concentration can be determined by measuring the intensity of the X-ray emission.

WEBEXTRA 8.8
Explore the Scanning Electron Microscope

Forensic Palynology: Pollen and Spores as Evidence

Of the many plant species on earth, more than half a million produce pollen or spores. The pollen or spores produced by each species has a unique type of ornamentation and morphology. This means that pollen or spores can be identified and used to link a crime scene and a person or object if examined by a trained analyst. This technique is called *forensic palynology* and includes the collection and examination of pollen and spores connected with crime scenes, illegal activities, or terrorism. Microscopy is the principal tool used in the field of forensic palynology.

FIGURE 8–13

The cystolithic hairs of the marijuana leaf, as viewed with a scanning electron microscope (800×).

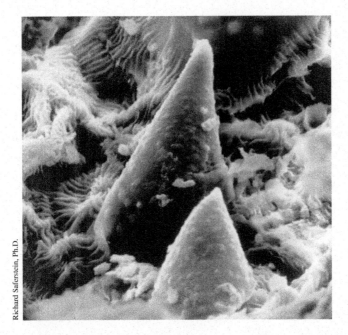

Richard Saferstein, Ph.D.

FIGURE 8–14

The melted ends of a hot filament break indicate that the headlights were on when an accident occurred.

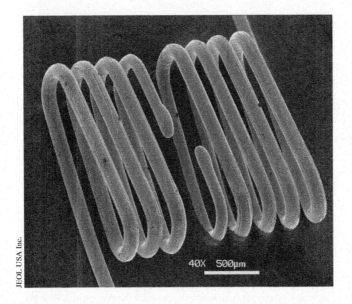

JEOL USA Inc.

FIGURE 8–15

The sharp ends of a cold filament break indicate that the headlights were off when an accident occurred.

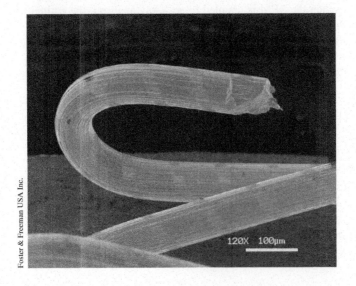

Foster & Freeman USA Inc.

Inside the Science

Detecting Gunshot Residue

One application of scanning electron microscopy has been to determine whether a suspect has recently fired a gun. In this case, an attempt is made to remove any gunshot particles that remain on a shooter's hands by lifting them off with a piece of adhesive tape. The tape is then examined under the SEM for the presence of particles that may have originated from the bullet primer. These particles can be characterized by their size, shape, and elemental composition. As shown in the figure, when the sample of gunshot residue is exposed to a beam of electrons from the SEM, X-rays are emitted. These X-rays are passed into a detector, where they are converted into electrical signals. These signals are sorted and displayed according to the energies of the emitted X-rays. Through the use of this technique, the elements lead, antimony, and barium, frequently found in most primers, can be rapidly detected and identified.

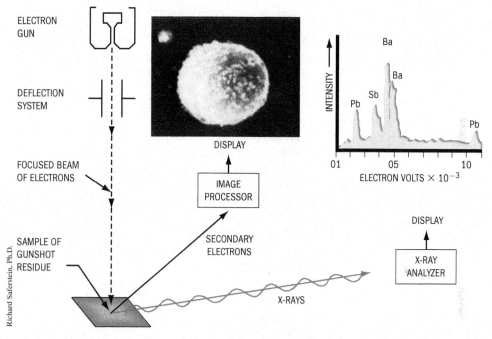

A schematic diagram of a scanning electron microscope displaying the image of a gunshot residue particle. Simultaneously, an X-ray analyzer detects and displays X-ray emissions from the elements lead (Pb), antimony (Sb), and barium (Ba) present in the particle.

Characteristics of Spores and Pollen

In nature, pollen grains are the single-celled male gametophytes (reproductive cells) of seed-bearing plants. The pollen grain wall (*exine*) is durable because it protects and carries the "sperms" needed for plant reproduction. Spores consist of both the male and female gametes of plants such as algae, fungi, mosses, and ferns. Pollen-producing plants are either *anemophilous* (their pollen is dispersed by wind) or *entomophilous* (their pollen is carried and dispersed by insects or small animals). Fairly precise geographical locations can often be identified by the presence of different mixtures of airborne pollens produced by anemophilous plants. For example, it may be possible to identify a geographical origin using a profile of the pollen samples retrieved from a suspect's clothing by analyzing the type and percentages of airborne pollen grains. Entomophilous plants usually produce a small amount of pollen that is very sticky in nature. Therefore, this type of pollen is rarely deposited on clothing or other objects except by direct contact with the plant. This information is useful when reconstructing the events of a crime because it may indicate that the clothing, a vehicle, or other objects on which this pollen is found came into direct contact with plant types found at a crime scene.

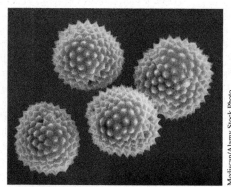

FIGURE 8–16

Scanning electron micrograph of ragweed pollen at a magnification of 1,170× if the image is printed 10 cm wide.

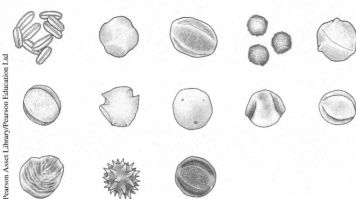

FIGURE 8–17
Diagrams of pollen grains from some plants.

Pearson Asset Library/Pearson Education Ltd

Analysis of Spores and Pollen

Both spores and pollen are microscopic in size and are produced by adult plants and then dispersed by the millions, and both can be analyzed using similar methods that use a variety of microscopic techniques. Using a compound light microscope with magnification capabilities up to 1,000×, analysts usually can identify pollen and spores as having come from a specific plant family or genus, and sometime even the unique species. However, often the pollen or spores of related species may look so similar that identification of the species is possible only by careful analysis using a SEM (see Figure 8–16).

Unique shapes, aperture type, and surface ornamentation are typically used to identify spore samples. Useful features for characterizing pollen grains include shape, apertures, and wall and surface sculpturing. Shapes of pollen grains include spheres, triangles, ellipses, hexagons, pentagons, and many other geometric variations (see Figure 8–17). *Apertures* are the openings on pollen grains from which the pollen tube grows and carries the sperms to the egg to complete fertilization. *Sculpturing* of the pollen refers to the pattern of the pollen grain surface.

To avoid destruction or contamination of pollen evidence, early collection of forensic pollen samples for analysis is important and should be completed as soon as possible at a crime scene by a trained palynologist. This expert's first task is to calculate the estimated production and dispersal patterns of spores and pollen (called the *pollen rain*) for the crime scene or area of interest and, using that information, to produce a kind of "pollen fingerprint" of that location.

The information gained from the analysis of pollen and spore evidence has many possible uses. It can link a suspect or object to the crime scene or the victim, prove or disprove a suspect's alibi, include or exclude suspects, track the previous whereabouts of some item or suspect, or indicate the geographical origin of some item. In the past, pollen and spore evidence has been used to locate human remains and concealed burial sites, establish the season or time of death of a victim, locate the source areas of illegal drugs and fake pharmaceuticals, identify terrorists, and prove the perpetration of illegal poaching and the adulteration of commercial foods.

Case Files

Identifying Baby Doe

The body of a young girl was found on the shore of Deer Island outside Boston by a woman walking her dog (Figure 8–18). The child soon came to be known as "Baby Doe" by the local news media.

Two weeks later, police released a computer-generated composite image of the girl along with photos of the polka-dot leggings and zebra-print blanket that were discovered with her body. In the days after the images were released, tips poured in as millions viewed the photos. Baby Doe's image was placed on billboards in 50 locations throughout the state. In the next three months, investigators followed up 210 leads but were unsuccessful in identifying her.

Investigators began considering the possibility that she washed up on the shore of Deer Island from a boat, or was transported to the area from somewhere else. In order to determine if they were focusing their search in the right place, they explored two forensic examination types which have the

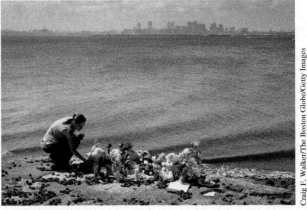

FIGURE 8–18
The beach on Deer Island where the child's body was discovered.

Craig F. Walker/The Boston Globe/Getty Images

potential to indicate geographic origin; Palynology and Stable Isotope Analysis.

To perform the pollen analysis, investigators took vacuum samples from the blanket and pants, and forensic scientists were able to retrieve enough pollen to complete a standard pollen count (Figure 8–19). The pollen taxa encountered were expected to be found in the broad-leafed forests of the Northeastern United States.

The Massachusetts State Police also sent samples to IsoForensics, a lab in Salt Lake City, Utah. Using stable isotopes in the girl's hair and teeth, analysts could examine the chemical characteristics she encountered throughout her life. "What you're eating, what you're drinking, that's recorded in your tissues immediately," IsoForensics President Lesley Chesson said. "You're recording the isotopes of your drinking water into your hair, into your bones." Researchers use that information to paint a general picture of the person's life; where they lived, where they have been recently. An isotope analysis showed the girl spent time in New England before her death.

Efforts of law enforcement paid off when a tip led to the identity of Baby Doe in September 2015. The girl was positively identified as Bella Bond, 2½ years old, from Dorchester,

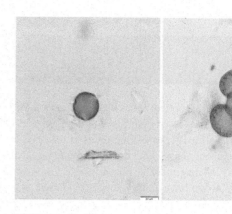

FIGURE 8–19

The pollen spores from the child's clothes were dominated by oak (Quercus), *left*, and pine (Pinus), *right*. *Daniel Herman, Massachusetts State Police.*

MA. As a result of the tip, police subsequently charged Michael P. McCarthy, the child's mother's boyfriend, with her murder. He was convicted and sentenced to life in prison.

Clues from the Cornfield

A case exemplifying the application of forensic palynology to a criminal investigation occurred when a victim was kidnapped, robbed, and then murdered in the eastern part of the American Midwest. The victim's car was stolen but later abandoned when it got stuck in mud near a busy highway. The next night, a drifter was arrested in a nearby town for breaking into a closed store. While in jail awaiting trial, the drifter told a fellow inmate about his car being stuck in the mud and that he would not be in jail but for that mishap. The other prisoner, hoping to work a deal for a lighter sentence, told this story to the sheriff.

During the investigation of the crime scene, one of the law enforcement agents noticed that there was a large field of mature corn (maize, *Zea mays*) growing between the dirt road where the stolen car had been abandoned in the mud and the nearby highway leading to the next town. The investigator wondered if traces of torn maize leaves on the suspect's clothing might link him to the crime scene. Fortunately, the drifter's shirt and pants had been removed and stored in sterile paper bags when he was arrested. As with all prisoners in that region, he had been given a pair of orange overalls to wear while in jail.

The shirt and pants were sent to a botanist who was asked to search for traces of maize leaves on the clothing. The botanist was also a palynologist and thus also collected samples and searched for traces of pollen. The pollen samples provided the best results. The samples collected from the suspect's shirt revealed that the neck and shoulder region of the shirt had high concentrations of fresh maize pollen. The forensic sample collected from the pants also contained maize pollen, but in a lower percentage. The forensic pollen data indicated that the drifter had recently walked through a maize field similar to the one between the abandoned car and the highway. As he walked through the field, he had brushed against blooming male tassels on the corn plants that were about head high. This accounted for the high amount of maize pollen found on the shoulder and neck area of the shirt. Lesser amounts of maize pollen also fell on his pants as he walked through the field. While the suspect awaited trial, additional evidence and several fingerprints from the victim's farm also linked him to the murder.

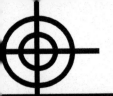

Chapter Summary > > > > > > > > > >

A microscope is an optical instrument that uses a lens or a combination of lenses to magnify and resolve the fine details of an object. Various types of microscopes are used to analyze forensic specimens. In the basic compound microscope, the object to be magnified is placed under the lower lens, called the objective lens, and the magnified image is viewed through the upper lens, known as the eyepiece lens. Forensic microscopy often requires side-by-side comparison of specimens. The comparison microscope consists of two independent objective lenses joined together by an optical bridge to a common eyepiece lens. When a viewer looks through the eyepiece lens of the comparison microscope, the objects under investigation are observed side by side in a circular field that is equally divided into two parts. Modern firearms examination began with the introduction of the comparison microscope, with its ability to give the firearms examiner a side-by-side magnified view of bullets. The stereoscopic microscope is actually two monocular compound microscopes properly spaced and aligned to present a three-dimensional image of a specimen to the viewer, who looks through both eyepiece lenses. Its large working distance makes it quite applicable for the microscopic examination of big, bulky items.

Light that is confined to a single plane of vibration is said to be plane-polarized. The examination of the interaction of plane-polarized light with matter is made possible with the polarizing microscope. Polarizing microscopy has found wide applications for the study of birefringent materials, that is, materials that have a double refraction. These refractive index data help identify minerals present in a soil sample or the identity of a manufactured fiber. The microspectrophotometer is a spectrophotometer coupled with a light microscope. The examiner studying a specimen under a microscope can simultaneously obtain the visible absorption spectrum or IR spectrum of the material being observed.

Finally, the SEM bombards a specimen with a beam of electrons instead of light to produce a highly magnified image from 10× to 100,000×. The bombardment of the specimen's surface with electrons normally produces X-ray emissions that can be used to characterize elements present in the material under investigation.

Forensic palynology involves the collection and examination of pollen and spores connected with crime scenes, illegal activities, or terrorism. The microscope is the principal tool used in the field of forensic palynology.

Review Questions

1. A microscope uses a combination of _____ to magnify an image.

2. A type of image that cannot be viewed directly is called a(n) _____ image.

3. A(n) _____ microscope consists of two lenses mounted at each end of a hollow tube.

4. The lens closest to the specimen is called the _____ .

5. The lens nearest the viewer's eye is called the _____.

6. The image seen through a compound microscope is (virtual, real).

7. True or False: The coarse and fine adjustments are part of the microscope's mechanical system. _____

8. A transparent specimen is viewed through a microscope using _____ light.

9. An opaque object requires _____ illumination for viewing with a microscope.

10. A(n) _____ collects light rays from the base-illuminator and concentrates them on the specimen.

11. A microscope that remains in focus regardless of which objective lens is rotated into place is _____.

12. A microscope with only one eyepiece is _____; one with two eyepieces is _____.

13. Each microscope lens is inscribed with a number signifying its _____.

14. An eyepiece lens of 10× used in combination with an objective lens of 20× has a total magnification power of _____.

15. The ability of an objective lens to resolve details into separate images is directly proportional to its _____.

16. The size of the specimen area in view is known as the _____.

17. As magnification increases, the field of view (increases, decreases).

18. The thickness of a specimen in view is known as the _____.

19. The depth of focus (increases, decreases) with increasing magnification.

20. A side-by-side view of two specimens is best obtained with the _____ microscope.

21. True or False: A bridge is used to join two independent objective lenses into a single binocular unit to form a comparison microscope. _____

22. Two monocular compound microscopes properly spaced and aligned describe the _____ microscope.

23. True or False: The stereoscopic microscope is the least frequently used microscope in a typical crime laboratory. _____

24. The stereoscopic microscope offers a large _____ between the objective lens and the specimen.

25. Light confined to a single plane of vibration is said to be _____.

26. If a polarizer and analyzer are placed (perpendicular, parallel) to each other, no light penetrates.

27. The _____ microscope allows a viewer to detect polarized light.

28. Crystals that are _____ produce two planes of polarized light, each perpendicular to the other.

29. By using the _____, one can view a particle under a microscope while a beam of light is directed at the particle in order to obtain its absorption spectrum.

30. The _____ microscope focuses a beam of electrons on a specimen to produce an image.

31. When a beam of electrons strikes a specimen, _____ are emitted whose energies correspond to elements present in the specimen.

32. True or False: Both spores and pollen can be identified and used to link a crime scene to an individual. _____

33. True or False: Spores can be characterized by shape and surface characteristics through a simple visual examination. _____

Application and Critical Thinking

1. A forensic biologist must examine the outside of a small leaf and a thin slice of the leaf one cell thick. She has at her disposal a transmitted light microscope and a stereomicroscope (vertical illumination). What instrument should she use for the analysis of each object and why?

2. A trace evidence analyst places crystals of an unidentified white powder onto the stage of a polarizing microscope and observes the crystals through the eyepiece. Under correct focus, some of the crystals show bright colors while others appear very dark and hardly distinguishable. What can be concluded about the contents of the white powder?

3. Numerous red-colored fibers from a sexual assault crime scene are delivered to the crime lab along with red fibers from the suspect's clothing. What instrument should the trace analyst use to view the fibers and obtain chemical information that could be used to compare the crime-scene and clothing samples?

4. Upon arriving at the crime scene of an attempted homicide, police officers observe a man fleeing the scene and apprehend him. He is suspected to be the shooter in the attempted homicide, and the police wish to test his hands for the presence of compounds consistent with gunshot residue. How should they proceed?

Further References

Bartick, E. G., "Infrared Microscopy and Its Forensic Applications," in R. Saferstein, ed., *Forensic Science Handbook*, vol. 3, 2nd ed. Upper Saddle River, NJ: Prentice Hall, 2010.

"Basic Concepts in Optical Microscopy," http://micro.magnet.fsu.edu/primer/anatomy/anatomy.html

De Forest, P. R., "Foundations of Forensic Microscopy," in R. Saferstein, ed., *Forensic Science Handbook*, vol. 1, 2nd ed. Upper Saddle River, N J: Prentice Hall, 2002.

Eyring, M. B., "Visible Microscopical Spectrophotometry in the Forensic Sciences," in R. Saferstein, ed., *Forensic Science Handbook*, vol. 1, 2nd ed. Upper Saddle River, NJ: Prentice Hall, 2002.

Palenik, S., and C. Palenik, "Microscopy and Microchemistry of Physical Evidence," in R. Saferstein, ed., *Forensic Science Handbook*, vol. 2, 2nd ed. Upper Saddle River, NJ: Prentice Hall, 2005.

Petraco, N., and T. Kubic, *Basic Concepts in Optical Microscopy for Criminalists, Chemists, and Conservators*. Boca Raton, FL: CRC Press, 2004.

Firearms, Tool Marks, and Other Impressions

Learning Objectives

After studying this chapter, you should be able to:

9.1 Describe the types of firearms and the techniques for rifling a barrel

9.2 Recognize the class and individual characteristics of bullets and cartridge cases

9.3 Discuss the various search systems developed for the FBI and ATF

9.4 Explain the procedure for determining how far a weapon was fired from a target

9.5 Identify the laboratory tests for determining whether an individual has fired a weapon

9.6 Discuss the procedures for collecting and preserving firearms evidence and restoring serial numbers

9.7 Explain the forensic significance of class and individual characteristics to the comparison of tool mark, footwear, and tire impressions

9.8 Discuss the preservation, lifting, casting, and comparison of impressions left at a crime scene

Go to www.pearsonhighered.com/careersresources to access Webextras for this chapter.

The Case Against Aaron Hernandez

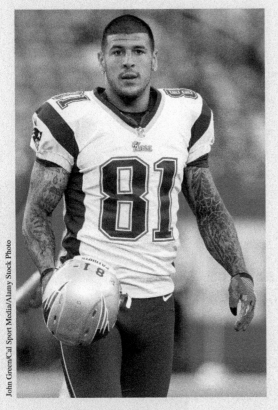

John Green/Cal Sport Media/Alamy Stock Photo

New England Patriots Tight End, Aaron Hernandez, was arrested and charged with the murder of Odin Lloyd in the 2015 NFL offseason. The trial that followed made headlines, not just because of his status, but also because of what appeared to be overwhelming scientific evidence of his guilt. Two important pieces of the forensic puzzle were the footwear and tire tread impressions left behind at the scene where the victim's body was found shot in an industrial park.

Investigators identified consistency in the pattern, design, size and manufacturer in one important footwear impression. According to the examiner, the impression matched a size 13 pair of Nike Air Jordan Retro 11 sneakers. Prosecutors introduced surveillance video of Hernandez at a gas station less than 90 minutes before the killing and at his home less than 10 minutes after wearing similar shoes. A Nike consultant, testified that in the footage Hernandez was wearing Nike Air Jordan Retro 11 sneakers even though investigators never recovered them.

Prosecutors alleged that Hernandez was driving a rented Nissan Altima when he and two accomplices picked up Lloyd and traveled to the industrial park to kill him. The tire tread examiner described the class characteristic examination performed on the tire impressions at the scene, comparing the "grooves," "sipes," and "wear bars." He first eliminated the Nissan's two front tires as the source of the tracks because the class characteristics didn't match. The two rear tires were of the same design as the one that left the track, so those were linked and the individual characteristics were compared to the evidence impression. Four stones wedged into the rear passenger-side tire helped investigators match it to the tire impression left at the scene.

Just as natural variations in skin ridge patterns and characteristics provide a key to human identification, minute random markings on surfaces can impart individuality to inanimate objects. Structural variations and irregularities caused by scratches, nicks, breaks, and wear permit the criminalist to relate a bullet to a gun; a scratch or abrasion mark to a single tool; or a tire track to a particular automobile. Individualization, so vigorously pursued in all other areas of criminalistics, is frequently attainable in firearms and tool mark examination.

Although a portion of this chapter will be devoted to the comparison of surface features for the purposes of bullet identification, a complete description of the services and capabilities of the modern forensic firearms laboratory cannot be restricted to just this one subject, important as it may be. The high frequency of shooting cases means that the science of **firearms identification** must extend beyond mere comparison of bullets to include knowledge of the operation of all types of weapons, restoration of obliterated serial numbers on weapons, detection and characterization of gunpowder residues on garments and around wounds, estimation of muzzle-to-target distances, and in the past the detection of powder residues on hands. Each of these functions will be covered in this chapter.

firearms identification
A discipline mainly concerned with determining whether a bullet or cartridge was fired by a particular weapon; it is not to be confused with ballistics, which is the study of a projectile in motion.

Types of Firearms

Generally, firearms can be divided into two categories: handguns and long guns. *Handguns*, or pistols, are firearms that are designed to be held and fired with one hand. The three most common types of handguns are single-shot handguns, revolvers, and semiautomatic pistols. All handguns can be classified as single-action or double-action firearms. Single-action firearms require the firing component to be manually cocked backward each time before the trigger is pulled in order to fire. Double-action firearms cock the firing component when the trigger is pulled and then reload the firing chamber after the round is fired.

Single-shot pistols can fire only one round, or shot, at a time. Each round must be manually loaded into the chamber before firing.

The revolver features several firing chambers located within a revolving cylinder. As the revolver is fired, the cylinder can rotate clockwise or counterclockwise. Each firing chamber holds one cartridge, which is lined up with the barrel mechanically when the round is fired. The cartridge cases have to be manually ejected to reload the firing chambers. *Swing-out revolvers* feature a cylinder that swings out to the side of the weapon to be loaded (see Figure 9–1). *Break-top revolvers* are hinged so that both the barrel and the cylinder flip downward for loading. *Solid-frame revolvers* have no mechanism to uncover all the firing chambers at once. Instead, a small "gate" at the back of the gun allows one chamber to be loaded at a time; the cylinder is then rotated, and the next chamber is loaded with a cartridge.

Semiautomatic pistols feature a removable magazine that is most often contained within the grip of the firearm. Once the magazine is loaded, the firing component is cocked by pulling the slide on the top of the gun rearward and then releasing it to load the first round. The firing of the cartridge generates gases that are used to eject the cartridge case, cock the firing component, and load the next round. A semiautomatic pistol (see Figure 9–2) fires one shot per trigger pull. An automatic firearm, such as a machine gun, fires as long as the trigger is pressed or until the ammunition is depleted.

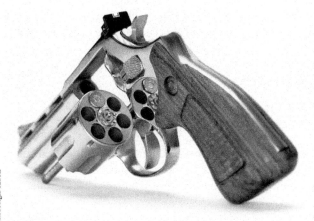

FIGURE 9–1
A swing-out revolver features a cylinder that swings out to the side of the weapon to be loaded.

Ktsdesign/123RF

FIGURE 9–2
A semiautomatic pistol.

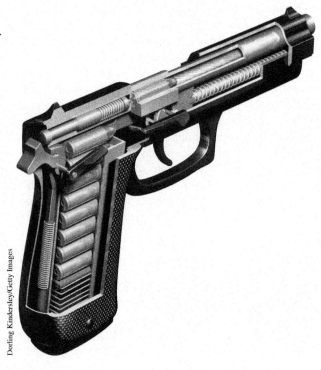

Dorling Kindersley/Getty Images

Long guns are either rifles or shotguns. Rifles and shotguns are designed to be fired while resting on the shoulder. The two principal differences between rifled firearms and shotguns are found in the ammunition and the barrel. Shotgun ammunition, called a shell, contains numerous ball-shaped projectiles, called slug. The barrel of a shotgun is smooth, without the grooves and lands found in rifles. A shotgun barrel can also be narrowed toward the muzzle in order to concentrate shot when fired. This narrowing of the barrel is called the *choke* of the shotgun. A shotgun may be single or double barreled. The two barrels of a double-barreled shotgun may be arranged horizontally (side by side) or vertically (one over another). The barrels may also have different choke diameters.

The various types of rifles and shotguns have different reloading mechanisms. The single-shot gun can chamber and fire only one round at a time. Just as with single-shot pistols, the round has to be loaded manually each time. Repeating long guns use a mechanical instrument of some sort to eject spent cartridge cases, load a new round, and cock the firing component after a round is fired. These include lever-action, pump or slide-action, bolt-action (see Figure 9–3), and semiautomatic (see Figure 9–4) long guns, the names of which refer to the loading mechanism used on each. Semiautomatic rifles use the force of the gas produced during firing to eject the spent cartridge case, load a new round, and cock the firing component. Semiautomatic firearms use a disconnector mechanism to fire one shot per trigger pull, whereas fully automatic firearms do not have such a mechanism and fire multiple consecutive shots with a single pull of the trigger.

Bullet and Cartridge Comparisons

The inner surface of the barrel of a gun leaves its markings on a bullet passing through it. These markings are peculiar to each gun. Hence, if one bullet found at the scene of a crime and another test-fired from a suspect's gun show the same markings, the suspect's gun is linked to the crime. Because these inner surface striations are so important for bullet comparison, it is important to know why and how they originate.

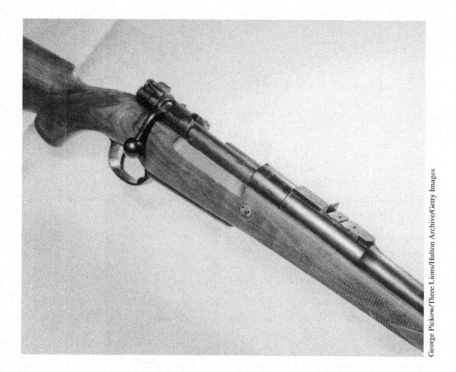

George Pickow/Three Lions/Hulton Archive/Getty Images

FIGURE 9–3

A bolt-action long gun uses the movement of a bolt mechanism to expel the spent cartridge case, load the next round, and cock the firing component.

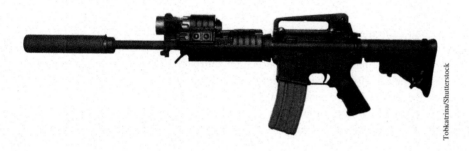

Tobkatrina/Shutterstock

FIGURE 9–4

A semiautomatic long gun uses the energy from the firing reaction to expel the spent cartridge case, load the next round, and cock the firing component.

The Gun Barrel

The gun barrel is produced from a solid bar of steel that has been hollowed out by drilling. The microscopic drill marks left on the barrel's inner surface are randomly irregular and in themselves impart a uniqueness to each barrel. However, the manufacture of a barrel requires the additional step of shaping its inner surface with spiral **grooves**, a step known as **rifling**. The surfaces of the original **bore** remaining between the grooves are called **lands** (see Figure 9–5). As a fired bullet travels through a barrel, it engages the rifling grooves; these grooves then guide the bullet through the barrel, giving it a rapid spin. This is done because a spinning bullet does not tumble end over end on leaving the barrel, but remains instead on a true and accurate course.

The diameter of the gun barrel, sketched in Figure 9–6, measured between opposite lands, is known as the **caliber** of the weapon. In most firearms, the caliber is normally recorded in hundredths of an inch or in millimeters—for example, .22 caliber and 9 mm. Actually, the term *caliber*, as it is commonly applied, is not an exact measurement of the barrel's diameter; for example, a .38-caliber weapon may actually have a bore diameter that ranges from 0.345 to 0.365 inch.

RIFLING METHODS   Before 1940, barrels were rifled by having one or two grooves at a time cut into the surface with steel hook cutters. The cutting tool was rotated as it passed down the barrel, so that the final results were grooves spiraling either to the right or left.

grooves
The cut or low-lying portions between the lands in a rifled bore.

rifling
The spiral grooves formed in the bore of a firearm barrel that impart spin to the projectile when it is fired.

bore
The interior of a firearm barrel.

lands
The raised portion between the grooves in a rifled bore.

caliber
The diameter of the bore of a rifled firearm; the caliber is usually expressed in hundredths of an inch or millimeters—for example, .22 caliber and 9 mm.

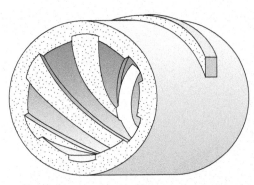

FIGURE 9–5

Interior view of a gun barrel, showing the presence of lands and grooves.

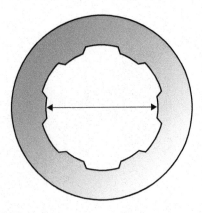

FIGURE 9–6

Cross section of a barrel with six grooves. The diameter of the bore is the caliber.

However, as the need for increased speed in the manufacture of weapons became apparent, newer techniques were developed that were far more suitable for the mass production of weapons.

The broach cutter consists of a series of concentric steel rings, with each ring slightly larger than the preceding one. As the broach passes through the barrel, it simultaneously cuts all grooves into the barrel at the required depth. The broach rotates as it passes through the barrel, giving the grooves their desired direction and rate of twist. A single broach cutter ring is shown in Figure 9–7.

In contrast to the broach, the button process involves no cuttings. A steel plug or "button" impressed with the desired number of grooves is forced under extremely high pressures through the barrel. A single pass of the button down the barrel compresses the metal to create lands and grooves on the barrel walls that are negative forms of those on the button. The button rotates to produce the desired direction and rate of twist (see Figure 9–8).

Like the button process, the mandrel rifling or hummer forging process involves no cutting of metal. A mandrel is a rod of hardened steel machined so its form is the reverse impression of

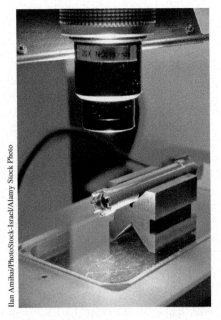

Ilan Amihai/PhotoStock-Israel/Alamy Stock Photo

FIGURE 9–7

A segment of a broach cutter.

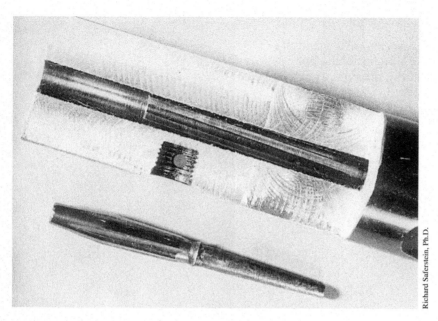

Richard Saferstein, Ph.D.

FIGURE 9–8

(Top) Cross section of a .22-caliber rifled barrel. (Bottom) A button used to produce the lands and grooves in the barrel.

the rifling it is intended to produce. The mandrel is inserted into a slightly oversized bore, and the barrel is compressed with firing componenting or heavy rollers into the mandrel's form.

Every firearms manufacturer chooses a rifling process that is best suited to meet the production standards and requirements of its product. Once the choice is made, however, the class characteristics of the weapon's barrel will remain consistent; each will have the same number of lands and grooves, with the same approximate width and direction of twist. For example, .32-caliber Smith & Wesson revolvers have five lands and grooves twisting to the right. On the other hand, Colt .32-caliber revolvers exhibit six lands and grooves twisting to the left. Although these class characteristics permit the examiner to distinguish one type or brand name of weapon from another, they do not impart individuality to any one barrel; no class characteristic can do this.

If one could cut a barrel open lengthwise, a careful examination of the interior would reveal the existence of fine lines, or *striations*, many running the length of the barrel's lands and grooves. These striations are impressed into the metal as the negatives of minute imperfections found on the rifling cutter's surface, or they are produced by minute chips of steel pushed against the barrel's inner surface by a moving broach cutter. The random distribution and irregularities of these markings are impossible to duplicate exactly in any two barrels. **No two rifled barrels, even those manufactured in succession, have identical striation markings.** These striations form the individual characteristics of the barrel.

COMPARING BULLET MARKINGS   As the bullet passes through the barrel, its surface is scratched by the rifling markings of the barrel. The bullet emerges from the barrel bearing the striations by the bore's interior surface; these impressions reflect both the class and individual characteristics of the barrel (see Figure 9–9). Because there is no practical way of making a direct comparison between the markings on the fired bullet and those found within a barrel, the examiner must obtain test bullets fired through the suspect barrel for comparison. To prevent damage to the test bullet's markings and to facilitate the bullet's recovery, test firings are normally made into a recovery box filled with cotton or into a water tank.

The number of lands and grooves, and their direction of twist, are obvious points of comparison during the initial stages of the examination. Any differences in these class characteristics immediately eliminate the possibility that both bullets traveled through the same barrel. A bullet with five lands and grooves could not possibly have been fired from a weapon of like caliber

FIGURE 9–9
A bullet is impressed with the rifling markings of the barrel when it emerges from the weapon.

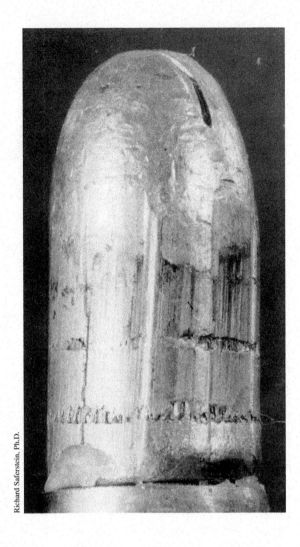

Richard Saferstein, Ph.D.

with six lands and grooves, nor could one having a right twist have come through a barrel impressed with a left twist. If both bullets carry the same class characteristics, the analyst must begin to match the striated markings on both bullets. This can be done only with the assistance of the comparison microscope (see Chapter 8).

Modern firearms identification began with the development and use of the comparison microscope. This instrument is the most important tool at the disposal of the firearms examiner. The test and evidence bullets are mounted on cylindrical adjustable holders beneath the objective lenses of the microscope, each pointing in the same direction (see Figure 9–10). Both bullets are observed simultaneously within the same field of view, and the examiner rotates one bullet until a well-defined land or groove comes into view. Once the striation markings are located, the other bullet is rotated until a matching region is found. Not only must the lands and grooves of the test and evidence bullet have identical widths, but the longitudinal striations on each must coincide. When a matching area is located, the two bullets are simultaneously rotated to obtain additional matching areas around the periphery of the bullets. Figure 9–11 shows a typical photomicrograph of a bullet match as viewed under a comparison microscope.

CONSIDERATIONS IN BULLET COMPARISON Unfortunately, the firearms examiner rarely encounters a perfect match all around the bullet's periphery. The presence of grit and rust can alter the markings on bullets fired through the same barrel. More commonly, recovered evidence bullets may become so mutilated and distorted on impact as to yield only a small area with intact markings.

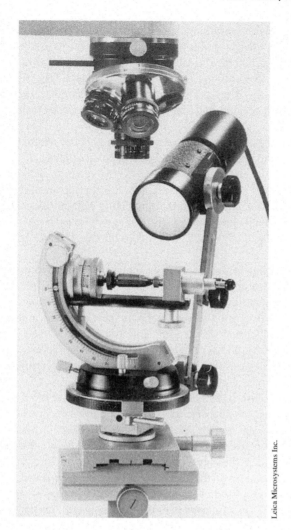

Leica Microsystems Inc.

FIGURE 9–10
A bullet holder beneath the objective lens of a comparison microscope.

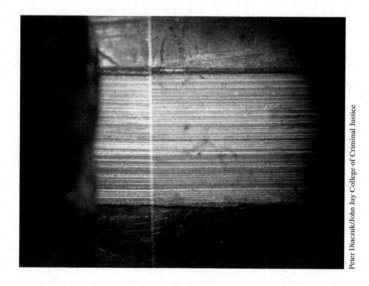

Peter Diaczuk/John Jay College of Criminal Justice

FIGURE 9–11
Photomicrograph of two bullets through a comparison microscope. The test bullet is on the right; the questioned bullet is on the left.

Furthermore, striation markings on a barrel are not permanent structures; they are subject to continuing change and alteration through wear as succeeding bullets traverse the length of the barrel. Fortunately, in most cases, these changes are not dramatic and do not prevent the matching of two bullets fired by the same weapon. As with fingerprint comparison, there are no hard-and-fast rules governing the minimum number of points required for a bullet comparison. The final opinion must be based on the judgment, experience, and knowledge of the expert.

Frequently, the firearms examiner receives a spent bullet without an accompanying suspect weapon and is asked to determine the caliber and possible make of the weapon. If a bullet appears not to have lost its metal, its weight may be one factor in determining its caliber. In some instances, the number of lands and grooves, the direction of twist, and the widths of lands and grooves are useful class characteristics for eliminating certain makes of weapons from consideration. For example, a bullet that has five lands and grooves and twists to the right could not come from a weapon manufactured by Colt if Colt does not manufacture any firearms with these class characteristics.

Sometimes a bullet has rifling marks that set it apart from most other manufactured weapons, as in the case of Marlin rifles. These weapons are rifled by a technique known as *microgrooving* and may have 8 to 24 grooves impressed into their barrels; few other weapons are manufactured in this fashion. In this respect, the FBI maintains a record known as the *General Rifling Characteristics File*. This file contains listings of class characteristics, such as land and groove width dimensions, for known weapons. It is periodically updated and distributed to the law enforcement community to help identify rifled weapons from retrieved bullets.

As previously discussed, unlike rifled firearms, a shotgun has a smooth barrel. It therefore follows that projectiles passing through a shotgun barrel are not impressed with any characteristic markings that can later be related back to the weapon. Shotguns generally fire small lead balls or pellets contained within a shotgun shell (see Figure 9–12). A paper or plastic wad pushes the pellets through the barrel on ignition of the cartridge's powder charge. By weighing and measuring the diameter of the shot recovered at a crime scene, the examiner can usually determine the size of shot used in the shell. The size and shape of the recovered wad may also reveal the gauge of the shotgun used and, in some instances, may indicate the manufacturer of the fired shell.

The diameter of the shotgun barrel is expressed by the term **gauge**.[1] The higher the gauge number, the smaller the barrel's diameter. For example, a 12-gauge shotgun has a bore diameter of 0.730 inch as contrasted to 0.670 inch for a 16-gauge shotgun. The exception to this rule is the .410-gauge shotgun, which refers to a barrel 0.41 inch in diameter.

gauge
Size designation of a shotgun, originally the number of lead balls with the same diameter as the barrel that would make a pound; for example, a 12-gauge shotgun would have a bore diameter of a lead ball 1/12 pound in weight; the only exception is the .410 shotgun, in which bore size is 0.41 inch.

WEBEXTRA 9.1
Practice Matching Bullets with the Aid of a Virtual Comparison Microscope

WEBEXTRA 9.2
Practice Matching Cartridge Cases with the Aid of a Virtual Comparison Microscope

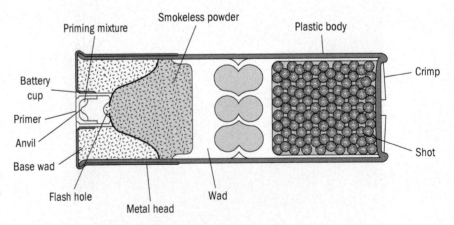

FIGURE 9–12

Cross section of a loaded shotgun shell.

[1] Originally, the number of lead balls with the same diameter as the barrel would make a pound. For example, a 20-gauge shotgun has an inside diameter equal to the diameter of a lead ball that weighs 1/20 of a pound.

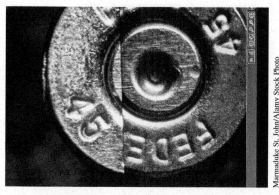
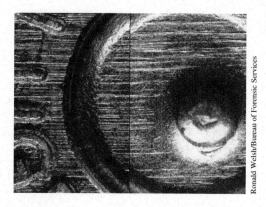

FIGURE 9–13

A comparison microscope photomicrograph showing a match between (a) firing pin impressions and (b) the breech face mark on the two shells.

Cartridge Cases

The act of pulling a trigger releases the weapon's firing pin, causing it to strike the primer, which in turn ignites the powder. The expanding gases generated by the burning gunpowder propel the bullet forward through the barrel, simultaneously pushing the spent cartridge case or shell back with equal force against the **breechface**. As the bullet is marked by its passage through the barrel, the shell is also impressed with markings by its contact with the metal surfaces of the weapon's firing and loading mechanisms. As with bullets, these markings can be reproduced in test-fired cartridges to provide distinctive points of comparison for individualizing a spent shell to a firearm.

The shape of the firing pin is impressed into the relatively soft metal of the primer on the cartridge case, revealing the minute distortions of the firing pin. These imperfections may be sufficiently random to individualize the pin impression to a single weapon. Similarly, the cartridge case, in its rearward thrust, is impressed with the surface markings of the breechface. The breechface, like any machined surface, is populated with random striation markings that become a highly distinctive signature for individualizing its surface. Other distinctive markings that may appear on the shell as a result of metal-to-metal contact are caused by the **extractor** and **ejector** mechanism and the magazine or clip, as well as by imperfections on the fire chamber walls. Photomicrographs in Figure 9–13 reveal a comparison of the firing pin and breechface impressions on evidence and test-fired shells.

Firing pin, breechface, extractor, and ejector marks may also be impressed onto the surface of the brass portion of shells fired by a shotgun. These impressions provide points for individualizing the shell to a weapon that are just as valuable as cartridge cases discharged from a rifled firearm. Furthermore, in the absence of a suspect weapon, the size and shape of a firing pin impression and/or the position of ejector marks in relationship to extractor and other markings may provide some clue to the type or make of the weapon that may have fired the questioned shell, or at least may eliminate a large number of possibilities.

You may wish to test your skills as a forensic firearms examiner by going to the app *CSI: firearmsID Forensic Challenge* available at the Apple store. Compare bullets and cartridge cases recovered from crime scenes to test fired standards.

breechface
The rear part of a firearm barrel.

extractor
The mechanism in a firearm by which a cartridge of a fired case is withdrawn from the chamber.

ejector
The mechanism in a firearm that throws the fired cartridge case from the firearm.

WEBEXTRA 9.3
Ammunition Impact Impressions Animation

Automated Firearms Search Systems

The use of firearms, especially semiautomatic weapons, during the commission of a crime has significantly increased throughout the United States. Because of the expense of such firearms, the likelihood that a specific weapon will be used in multiple crimes has risen. The advent of computerized imaging technology has made possible the storage of bullet and cartridge surface characteristics in a manner analogous to the storage of automated fingerprint files (see pages 137–139). Using this concept, crime laboratories can be networked, allowing them to share information on bullets and cartridge cases retrieved from several jurisdictions.

> > > > > > > >

Sacco and Vanzetti

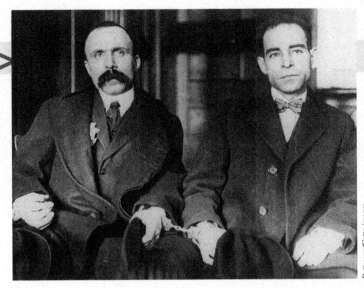

Sacco and Vanzetti.

In 1920, two security guards were viciously gunned down by unidentified assailants. The security guards were transporting shoe factory payroll, nearly $16,000 in cash, at the time of the robbery-murder. Eyewitnesses described the assailants as "Italian-looking," one with a full handlebar mustache. The robbers had used two firearms, leaving behind three different brands of shells.

Two suspects were identified and arrested—Nicola Sacco and his friend, the amply mustachioed Bartolomeo Vanzetti. After denying owning any firearms, each was found to be in possession of a loaded pistol. In fact, Sacco's pistol was .32-caliber, the same caliber as the crime-scene bullets. In Sacco's pockets were found 23 bullets matching the brands of the empty shells found at the murder scene.

This case coincided with the "Red Scare," a politically turbulent time in post–World War I America. Citizens feared socialist zealots, and the media played up these emotions. Political maneuvering and the use of the media muddied the waters surrounding the case, and the fact that both suspects belonged to anarchist political groups that advocated revolutionary violence against the government only incited public animosity toward them. Sympathetic socialist organizations attempted to turn Sacco and Vanzetti into martyrs, calling their prosecution a "witch hunt."

The outcome of the trial ultimately depended on whether the prosecution could prove that Sacco's pistol fired the bullets that killed the two security guards. At trial, the ballistics experts testified that the bullets used were no longer in production and

they could not find similar ammunition to use in test firings—aside from the unused cartridges found in Sacco's pockets. A forensics expert for the prosecution concluded that a visual examination showed that the bullets matched, leading the jury to return a verdict of guilty. Sacco and Vanzetti were sentenced to death.

Because of continued public protests, a committee was appointed in 1927 to review the case. Around this time, Calvin Goddard, at the Bureau of Forensic Ballistics in New York, perfected the comparison microscope for use in forensic firearms investigations. With this instrument, two bullets are viewed side by side to compare the striations imparted to a bullet's surface as it travels through the gun's barrel. The committee asked Goddard to examine the bullets in question. A test-fired bullet from Sacco's weapon was matched conclusively by Goddard to one of the crime-scene bullets. The fates of Sacco and Vanzetti were sealed and they were put to death in 1927.

Search Systems

The effort to build a national computerized database for firearms evidence in the United States had a rather confusing and inefficient start in the early 1990s. Two major federal law enforcement agencies, the FBI and the ATF, offered the law enforcement community competing and incompatible computerized systems.

EARLY SYSTEMS   The automated search system developed for the FBI was known as *DRUGFIRE*. This system emphasized the examination of unique markings on the cartridge casings expended by the weapon. The specimen was analyzed through a microscope attached to a video camera. The magnification allowed for a close-up view to identify individual characteristics. The image was captured by a video camera, digitized, and stored in a database. Although DRUGFIRE emphasized cartridge-case imagery, the images of highly characteristic bullet striations could also be stored in a like manner for comparisons.

The *Integrated Ballistic Identification System (IBIS)*, developed for the Bureau of Alcohol, Tobacco, Firearms and Explosives, processed digital microscopic images of identifying features found on both expended bullets and cartridge casings. IBIS incorporated two software programs: Bulletproof, a bullet-analyzing module, and Brasscatcher, a cartridge-case-analyzing module. A schematic diagram of Bulletproof's operation is depicted in Figure 9–14.

NIBIN   In 1999, members of the FBI and ATF joined forces to introduce the *National Integrated Ballistics Information Network (NIBIN)* program to the discipline of firearms examination.

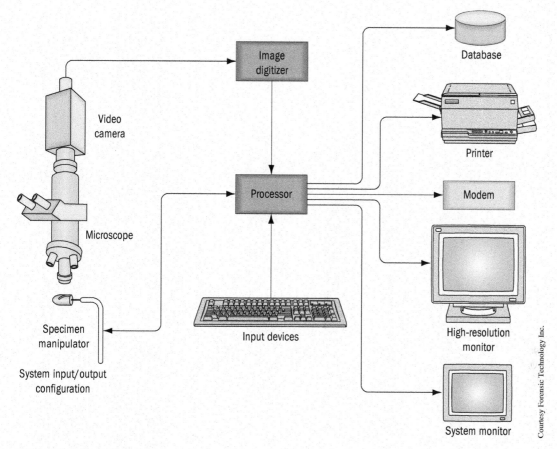

Courtesy Forensic Technology Inc.

FIGURE 9–14

Bulletproof configuration. The sample is mounted on the specimen manipulator and illuminated by the light source from a microscope. The image is captured by a video camera and digitized. This digital image is then stored in a database, available for retrieval and comparison. The search for a match includes analyzing the width of land and groove impressions along with both rifling and individual characteristics. The Brasscatcher software uses the same system configuration but emphasizes the analysis of expended cartridge casings rather than the expended bullets.

NIBIN guides and assists federal, state, and local laboratories interested in housing an automated search system. The new unified system incorporates both DRUGFIRE and IBIS technologies available in prior years. ATF has the overall responsibility for the system sites, whereas the FBI is responsible for the communications network.

Agencies using the new NIBIN technology produce database files from bullets and cartridge casings retrieved from crime scenes or test fires from retrieved firearms. More than 200 law enforcement agencies worldwide have adapted to this technology. The success of the system has been proven with more than 800,000 images compiled; nationwide, law enforcement agencies have connected more than 28,000 bullets and casings to more than one crime (see Figure 9–15).

For example, in a recent case, a Houston security guard was shot and killed during a botched armed robbery. A bullet and .40-caliber Smith & Wesson cartridge casing were recovered and imaged into NIBIN. Earlier that day, a robbery-turned-double-homicide left two store clerks dead. Again, two bullets and two .40-caliber Smith & Wesson cartridge casings were recovered. Once they were processed into NIBIN, a correlation was found with the murder of the security officer and a separate aggravated robbery that occurred two weeks prior. All three crimes were linked with a firearm believed to be a .40-caliber Smith & Wesson pistol.

Further investigation into the use of a victim's credit card aided police in locating two suspects. In the possession of one suspect was a .40-caliber Smith & Wesson pistol. Once retrieved, the gun was test-fired and imaged into NIBIN. The casing from the test-fired weapon matched the evidence obtained in the robbery and the aggravated robbery-homicides. The associations

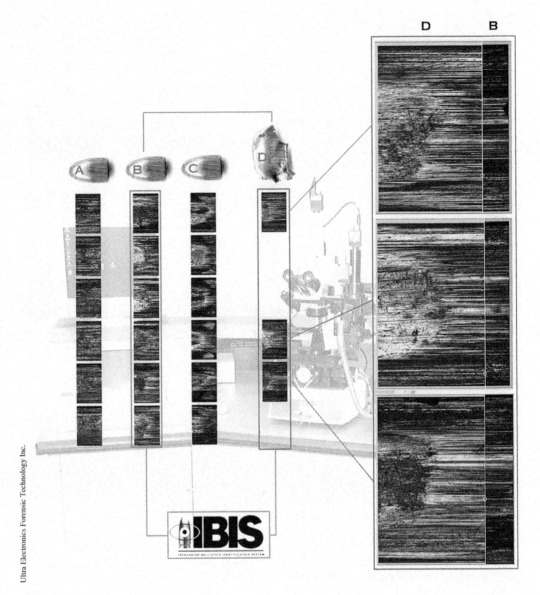

Ultra Electronics Forensic Technology Inc.

FIGURE 9–15

Bullets A, B, C, and D were acquired in the IBIS database at different times from different crime scenes. D is a fragmented bullet that had only three land impressions available for acquisition. Upon the entry of bullet D, IBIS found a potential matching candidate in the database: B. On the far right, bullet D is compared to bullet B using the IBIS imaging software. Finally, a forensic firearms examiner using the actual evidence under a conventional comparison microscope will confirm the match between B and D.

were verified by traditional firearms examination comparisons performed by a firearms examiner. Before this computerized technology was developed, it would have taken years, or may have been impossible, to link all of these shootings to one single firearm.

In another example, the ATF laboratory in Rockville, Maryland, received 1,466 cartridge casings from the Ovcara mass burial site in Bosnia. After processing and imaging profiles for all casings, the examiners determined that 18 different firearms were used at the site. With the help of NIBIN technology and competent examiners, jurists were able to try and convict an individual for war crimes.

NIBIN serves only as a screening tool for firearms evidence. A computerized system does not replace the skills of the firearms examiner. NIBIN can screen hundreds of unsolved firearms cases and may narrow the possibilities to several firearms. However, the final comparison will be made by the forensic examiner through traditional microscopic methods.

WEBEXTRA 9.4
Bullet Standard Helps to Tie Guns to People Who Commit Crimes

Ballistic Fingerprinting

Participating crime laboratories in the United States are building databases of bullet and cartridge cases found at crime scenes and those fired in tests of guns seized from people who commit crimes. As these databases come online and prove their usefulness in solving crimes, law enforcement officials and the political community are scrutinizing the feasibility of scaling this concept up to create a system of *ballistic fingerprinting*. This system would entail the capture and storage of appropriate markings on bullets and cartridges test-fired from handguns and rifles before they are sold to the public. Questions regarding who will be responsible for collecting the images and details of how they will be stored are but two of many issues to be determined. The concept of ballistic fingerprinting is an intriguing one for the law enforcement community and promises to be explored and debated intensely in the future.

Gunpowder Residues

In incidents involving gunshot wounds, it is often necessary to determine the distance from which the weapon was fired. Frequently, in incidents involving a shooting death, the individual apprehended and accused pleads self-defense as the motive for the attack. Such claims are fertile grounds for **distance determinations** because finding the proximity of the parties involved in the incident is necessary to establish the facts of the incident. Similarly, careful examination of the wounds of suicide victims usually reveals characteristics associated with a very close-range gunshot wound. The absence of such characteristics is a strong indication that the wound was not self-inflicted and signals the possibility of foul play.

distance determination
The process of determining the distance between the firearm and a target, usually based on the distribution of powder patterns or the spread of a shot pattern.

Distance Determination

Modern ammunition is propelled toward a target by the expanding gases created by the ignition of smokeless powder or nitrocellulose in a cartridge. Under ideal circumstances, all of the powder would be consumed in the process and converted into the rapidly expanding gases. However, in practice the powder is never totally burned. When a firearm is discharged, unburned and partially burned particles of gunpowder in addition to smoke are propelled out of the barrel along with the bullet toward the target. If the muzzle of the weapon is sufficiently close, these products are deposited onto the target. The distribution of gunpowder particles and other discharge residues around the bullet hole permits an assessment of the distance from which a handgun or rifle was fired.

The accuracy of a distance determination varies according to the circumstances of the case. When the investigator is unable to recover a suspect weapon, the best that the examiner can do is to state whether a shot could have been fired within some distance interval from the target. More exact opinions are possible only when the examiner has the suspect weapon in hand and has knowledge of the type of ammunition used in the shooting.

HANDGUNS AND RIFLES   The precise distance from which a handgun or rifle has been fired must be determined by careful comparison of the powder-residue pattern on the victim's clothing or skin against test patterns made when the suspect weapon is fired at varying distances from a target. A white cloth or a fabric comparable to the victim's clothing may be used as a test target (see Figure 9–16). Because the spread and density of the residue pattern vary widely between weapons and ammunition, such a comparison is significant only when it is made with the suspect weapon and suspect ammunition, or with ammunition of the same type and make. By comparing the test and evidence patterns, the examiner may find enough similarity in shape and density on which to judge the distance from which the shot was fired.

Without the weapon, the examiner is restricted to looking for recognizable characteristics around the bullet hole. Such findings are at best approximations made as a result of general observations and the examiner's experience. However, some noticeable characteristics should be sought. For instance, when the weapon is held in contact with or less than 1 inch from the target, a heavy concentration of smokelike vaporous lead usually surrounds the bullet entrance hole. Often, loose fibers surrounding a contact hole show scorch marks from the flame discharge of the weapon, and some synthetic fibers may show signs of being melted as a result of the heat from the discharge. Furthermore, the blowback of muzzle gases may produce a stellate (star-shaped) tear pattern around the hole. Such a hole is invariably surrounded by a rim of a smokelike deposit of vaporous lead (see Figure 9–17).

WEBEXTRA 9.5
Contact Shot Distance Scale
Animation

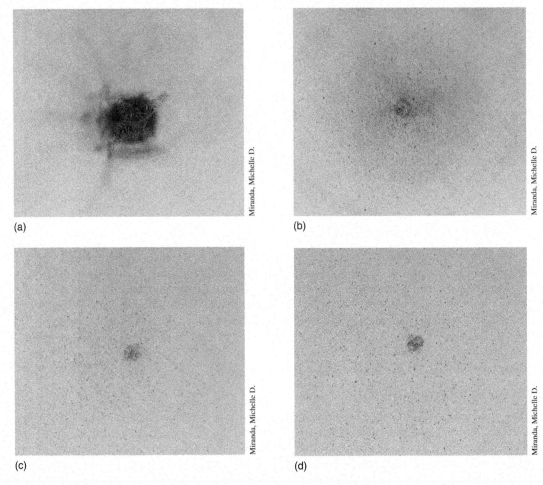

(a)

(b)

(c)

(d)

Miranda, Michelle D.

FIGURE 9–16

Test powder patterns made with a .38 Special Smith & Wesson revolver fired at the following distances from the target: (a) contact, (b) 6 inches, (c) 12 inches, and (d) 18 inches.

A halo of vaporous lead (smoke) deposited around a bullet hole normally indicates a discharge 12 to 18 inches or less from the target. The presence of scattered specks of unburned and partially burned powder grains without any accompanying soot can often be observed at distances up to approximately 25 inches. Occasionally, however, scattered gunpowder particles are noted at a firing distance as far out as 36 inches. With ball powder ammunition, this distance may be extended to 6 to 8 feet.

Finally, a weapon that has been fired more than 3 feet from a target usually does not deposit any powder residues onto the target's surface. In these cases, the only visual indication that the hole was made by a bullet is a dark ring, known as *bullet wipe*, around the perimeter of the entrance hole. Bullet wipe consists of a mixture of carbon, dirt, lubricant, primer residue, and lead wiped off the bullet's surface as it passes through the target. Again, in the absence of a suspect weapon, these observations are general guidelines for estimating target distances. Numerous factors—barrel length, caliber, type of ammunition, and type and condition of the weapon fired—influence the amount of gunpowder residue deposited on a target.

SHOTGUNS   The determination of firing distances involving shotguns must again be related to test firings performed with the suspect weapon, using the same type of ammunition known to be used in the crime. In the absence of a weapon, the muzzle-to-target distance can be estimated by measuring the spread of the discharged shot. With close-range shots varying in distance up to 4 to 5 feet, the shot charge enters the target as a concentrated mass, producing a hole somewhat

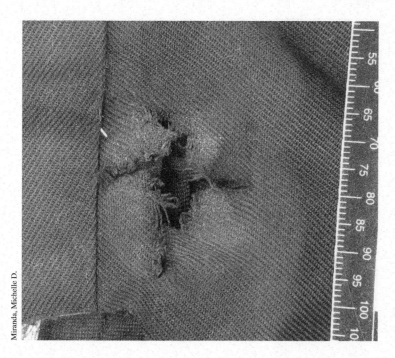

Miranda, Michelle D.

FIGURE 9–17
A contact shot.

larger than the bore of the barrel. As the distance increases, the pellets progressively separate and spread out. Generally speaking, the spread in the pattern made by a 12-gauge shotgun increases 1 inch for each yard of distance. Thus, a 10-inch pattern would be produced at approximately 10 yards. Of course, this is only a rule of thumb; normally, a great number of variables can affect the shot pattern. Other factors to consider include the barrel length, the size and quantity of the pellets fired, the quantity of powder charge used to propel the pellets, and the choke of the gun under examination. **Choke** is the degree of constriction placed at the muzzle end of the barrel. The greater the choke, the narrower the shotgun pattern and the faster and farther the pellets will travel.

choke
An interior constriction placed at or near the muzzle end of a shotgun's barrel to control shot dispersion.

Powder Residues on Garments

When garments or other evidence relevant to a shooting are received in the crime laboratory, the surfaces of all items are first examined microscopically for gunpowder residue. These particles may be identifiable by their characteristic colors, sizes, and shapes. However, the absence of visual indications does not preclude the possibility that gunpowder residue is present. Sometimes the lack of color contrast between the powder and garment or the presence of heavily encrusted deposits of blood can obscure the visual detection of gunpowder. Often, an infrared photograph of the suspect area overcomes the problem. Such a photograph may enhance the contrast, thus revealing vaporous lead and powder particles deposited around the hole (see Figure 9–18). In other situations, this may not help, and the analyst must use chemical tests to detect gunpowder residues.

Nitrites are one type of chemical product that results from the incomplete combustion of smokeless (nitrocellulose) powder. One test method for locating powder residues involves transferring particles embedded on the target surface to chemically treated gelatin-coated photographic paper. This procedure is known as the **Greiss test**. The examiner presses the photographic paper onto the target with a hot iron; once the nitrite particles are on the paper, they are made easily visible by chemical treatment. In addition, comparing the developed nitrite pattern to nitrite patterns obtained from test firings at known distances can be useful in determining the shooting distance from the target. A second chemical test is then performed to detect any trace of lead residue around the bullet hole. The questioned surface is sprayed with a solution of sodium rhodizonate, followed by a series of oversprays with acid solutions. This treatment causes lead particles to exhibit a pink color, followed by a blue-violet color.

Greiss test
A chemical test used to develop patterns of gunpowder residues around bullet holes.

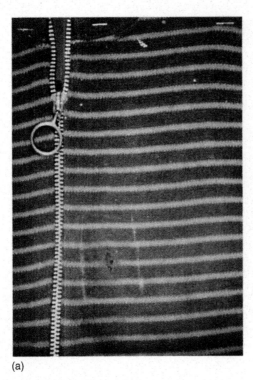
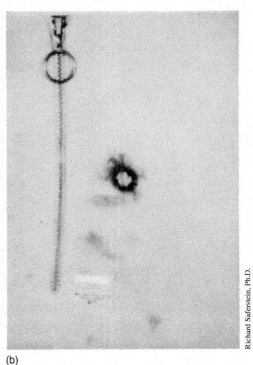

(a)   (b)

FIGURE 9–18

(a) A shirt bearing a powder stain, photographed under normal light. (b) An infrared photograph of the same shirt.

Primer Residues on the Hands

The firing of a weapon not only propels residues toward the target, but also blows gunpowder and primer residues back toward the shooter (see Figure 9–19). As a result, traces of these residues are often deposited on the firing hand of the shooter, and their detection can provide valuable information as to whether an individual has recently fired a weapon.

Detecting Primer Residues

Early efforts at demonstrating powder residues on the hands centered on chemical tests that could detect unburned gunpowder or nitrates. For many years, the *dermal nitrate test* enjoyed popularity. It required the application of hot paraffin or wax to the suspect's hand with a paintbrush. After drying into a solid crust, the paraffin was removed and tested with diphenylamine. A blue color was taken as an indication of a positive reaction for nitrates. However, the dermal nitrate test has fallen into disfavor with law enforcement agencies, owing mainly to its lack of specificity. Common materials such as fertilizers, cosmetics, urine, and tobacco all give positive reactions that are indistinguishable from that obtained for gunpowder by this test.

Efforts to identify a shooter now center on the detection of primer residues deposited on the hand of a shooter at the time of firing. With the exception of most .22-caliber ammunition, primers currently manufactured contain a blend of lead styphnate, barium nitrate, and antimony sulfide. Residues from these materials are most likely to be deposited on the thumb web and the back of the firing hand of a shooter because these areas are closest to gases escaping along the side or back of the gun during discharge. In addition, individuals who handle a gun without firing it may have primer residues deposited on the palm of the hand coming in contact with the weapon.

However, with the handling of a used firearm, the passage of time, and the resumption of normal activities following a shooting, gunshot residues from the back of the hand are frequently redistributed to other areas, including the palms. Therefore, it is not unusual to find higher levels of barium and antimony on the palms than on the backs of the hands of known shooters. Another possibility is the deposition of significant levels of barium and antimony on the hands of an individual who is near a firearm when it is discharged.

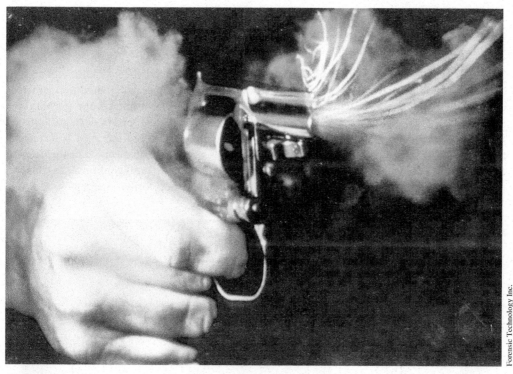

FIGURE 9-19

When a handgun is fired, gunpowder and primer residues are normally blown back toward the hand of the shooter.

Tests for Primer Residues

Determination of whether a person has fired or handled a weapon or has been near a discharged firearm is normally made by measuring the presence and possibly the amount of barium and antimony on the relevant portions of the suspect's hands. A variety of materials and techniques are used for removing these residues. The most popular approach, and certainly the most convenient for the field investigator, requires the application of an adhesive tape or adhesive to the hand's surface in order to remove any adhering residue particles.

SWABBING   Another approach is to remove any residues present by swabbing both the firing and nonfiring hands with cotton that has been moistened with 5 percent nitric acid. The front and back of each hand are separately swabbed. All four swabs, along with a moistened control, are then forwarded to the crime laboratory for analysis (see Appendix III for a detailed description of residue collection procedures).

In any case, once the hands are treated for the collection of barium and antimony, the collection medium must be analyzed for the presence of these elements. High barium and antimony levels on the suspect's hand(s) strongly indicate that the person fired or handled a weapon or was near a firearm when it was discharged. Because these elements are normally present after a firing in small quantities (less than 10 micrograms), only the most sensitive analytical techniques can detect them.

Unfortunately, even though most specimens submitted for this type of analysis have been from individuals strongly suspected of having fired a gun, there has been a low rate of positive findings. The major difficulty appears to be the short time that primer residues remain on the hands. These residues are readily removed by intentional or unintentional washing, rubbing, or wiping of hands. In fact, one study convincingly demonstrated that it is difficult to detect primer residues on cotton hand swabs taken as soon as two hours after firing a weapon.[2] Hence, some laboratories do not accept cotton hand swabs taken from living subjects six or more hours after a firing has occurred.

In cases that involve suicide victims, a higher rate of positives for the presence of gunshot residue is obtained when the hand swabbing is conducted before the person's body is moved or

[2] J. W. Kilty, "Activity After Shooting and Its Effect on the Retention of Primer," *Journal of Forensic Sciences* 29 (1975): 219.

when the hands are protected by paper bags.[3] However, hand swabbing or the application of an adhesive cannot be used to detect firings with most .22-caliber rim-fire ammunition. Such ammunition may contain only barium or neither barium nor antimony in its primer composition.

SEM TESTING   Most laboratories possessing gunshot residue detection capabilities require the application of an adhesive to the shooter's hands. Microscopic primer and gunpowder particles on the adhesive are then located with the aid of a scanning electron microscope (SEM) (see Figure 9–20). These particles have a characteristic size and shape that readily distinguish them from other contaminants present on the hands (see Figure 9–21). When the SEM is linked to an X-ray analyzer (see page 182), an elemental analysis of the particles can be conducted. A finding of a select combination of elements (lead, barium, and antimony) confirms that the particles could be primer residue (see Figure 9–22). A complication to the interpretation of the

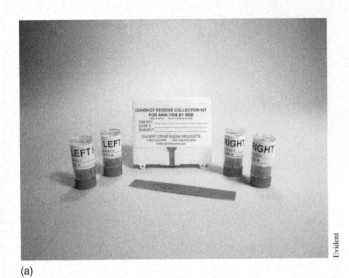

(a)

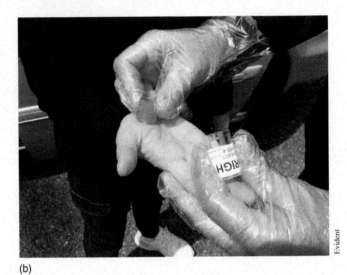

(b)

FIGURE 9–20

(a) Adhesive stubs used to sample a suspect's shooter's hands. (b) Sampling a suspect's hand for gunshot residue with an adhesive stub.

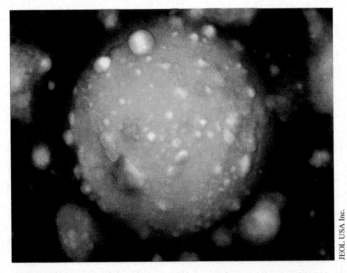

FIGURE 9–21

An SEM view of gunshot residue particles.

[3] G. E. Reed et al., "Analysis of Gunshot Residue Test Results in 112 Suicides," *Journal of Forensic Sciences* 35 (1990): 62.

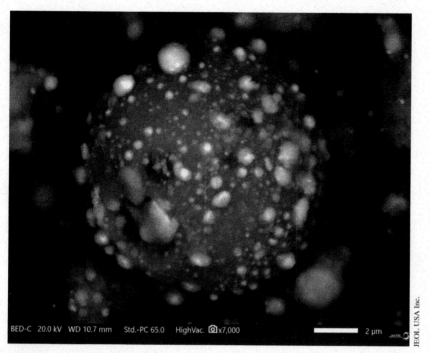

BED-C 20.0 kV WD 10.7 mm   Std.-PC 65.0   HighVac. ⌾x7,000   2 μm

FIGURE 9–22
Spectrum showing the presence of lead, barium, and antimony in gunshot residue.

significance of these findings is that brake linings and fireworks have been reported to yield particles indistinguishable from gunshot residue. Interestingly, bullet manufacturers are moving in the direction of removing lead from bullets, thus further complicating the characterization of primer residue. Appendix II contains a detailed description of the SEM residue collection procedure.

The major advantage of the SEM approach for primer residue detection is its enhanced specificity over hand swabbing. The SEM characterizes primer particles by their size and shape as well as by their chemical composition. Unfortunately, the excessive operator time required to search out and characterize gunshot residue has deterred the use of this technique. The availability of automated particle search and identification systems for use with scanning electron microscopes may overcome this problem. Results of work performed with automated systems show it to be significantly faster than a manual approach for searching out gunshot residue particles.

Serial Number Restoration

Today, many manufactured items, including automobile engine blocks and firearms, are impressed with a serial number for identification. Increasingly, the criminalist is asked to restore such a number when it has been removed or obliterated by grinding, rifling, or punching.

Serial numbers are usually stamped on a metal body or frame, or on a plate, with hard steel dies. These dies strike the metal surface with a force that allows each digit to sink into the metal at a prescribed depth. Serial numbers can be restored because the metal crystals in the stamped zone are placed under a permanent strain that extends a short distance beneath the original numbers. When a suitable etching agent is applied, the strained area dissolves faster than the unaltered metal, thus revealing the etched pattern in the form of the original numbers (see Figure 9–23). However, if the zone of strain has been removed, or if the area has been impressed with a different strain pattern, the number usually cannot be restored.

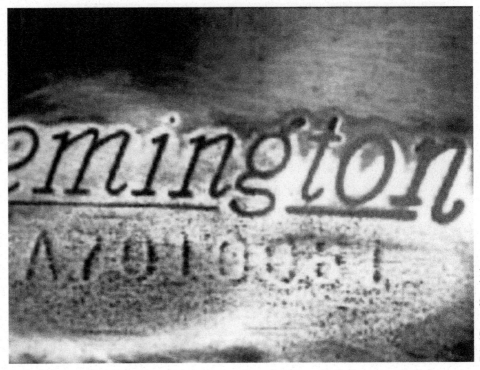

Federal Bureau of Investigation

FIGURE 9–23
Obliterated or altered serial numbers on firearms can be restored by analysts using chemical means.

Before any treatment with the etching reagent, the obliterated surface must be thoroughly cleaned of dirt and oil and polished to a mirrorlike finish. The reagent is swabbed onto the surface with a cotton ball. The choice of etching reagent depends on the type of metal surface being worked on. A solution of hydrochloric acid (120 mL), copper chloride (90 g), and water (100 mL) generally works well for steel surfaces.

Collection and Preservation of Firearms Evidence

Firearms

The Hollywood image of an investigator picking up a weapon by its barrel with a pencil or stick in order to protect fingerprints must be avoided. This practice only disturbs powder deposits, rust, or dirt lodged in the barrel, and consequently may alter the striation markings on test-fired bullets. If recovery of latent fingerprints is a primary concern, hold the weapon by the edge of the trigger guard or by the checkered portion of the grip, which usually does not retain identifiable fingerprints.

The most important consideration in handling a weapon is safety. Before any weapon is sent to the laboratory, all precautions must be taken to prevent an accidental discharge of a loaded weapon in transit. In most cases, it will be necessary to unload the weapon. If this is done, a record should first be made of the weapon's firing component and safety position; likewise, the location of all fired and unfired ammunition in the weapon must be recorded.

When a revolver is recovered, the chamber position in line with the barrel should be indicated by a scratch mark on the cylinder. Each chamber is designated with a number on a diagram, and as each cartridge or casing is removed, it should be marked to correspond to the numbered chambers in the diagram. Knowledge of the cylinder position of a cartridge casing may be useful for later determination of the sequence of events, particularly in shooting cases when more than one shot was fired. Place each round in a separate box or envelope. If the weapon is a pistol, the magazine must be removed and checked for prints and the chamber then emptied.

As with any other type of physical evidence recovered at a crime scene, firearms evidence must be marked for identification and a chain of custody must be established. Therefore, when a firearm is recovered, an identification tag should be attached to the trigger guard. The tag should be marked to show appropriate identifying data, including the weapon's serial number, make, and model and the investigator's initials. Place the unloaded firearm into a ridged box properly labeled for shipment to the examining forensic facility.

When a weapon is recovered from an underwater location, no effort must be made to dry or clean it. Instead, the firearm should be transported to the laboratory in a receptacle containing enough of the same water necessary to keep it submerged. This procedure prevents rust from developing during transport.

Ammunition

Protection of class and individual markings on bullets and cartridge cases must be the primary concern of the field investigator. Thus, extreme caution is needed when removing a lodged bullet from a wall or other object. If the bullet's surface is accidentally scratched during this operation, valuable striation markings could be obliterated. It is best to free bullets from their target by carefully breaking away the surrounding support material while avoiding direct contact with the projectile.

Bullets, cartridge casings, and discharged shells from shotguns should just be placed in a container that is appropriately marked for identification. It is recommended that the investigator not directly mark these items with a scribe. In any case, the investigator must protect the bullet by wrapping it in tissue paper before placing it in a pillbox or an envelope for shipment to the crime laboratory. Minute traces of evidence such as paint and fibers may be adhering to the bullet; the investigator must take care to leave these trace materials intact.

When semiautomatic or automatic weapons have been fired, the ejection pattern of the casings can help establish the relationship of the suspect to their victim. For this reason, the exact location of the place from which a shell casing was recovered is important information that must be noted by the investigator.

In incidents involving shotguns, any wads recovered are to be packaged and sent to the laboratory. An examination of the size and composition of the wad may reveal information about the type of ammunition used and the gauge of the shotgun.

Gunpowder Deposits

The clothing of a firearms victim must be carefully preserved so as to prevent damage or disruption to powder residues deposited around a bullet or shell hole. The cutting or tearing of clothing in the area of the holes must be avoided as the clothing is being removed. All wet clothing should be air-dried out of direct sunlight and then folded carefully so as not to disrupt the area around the bullet hole. Each item should be placed in a separate paper bag.

Tool Marks

A *tool mark* is any impression, cut, gouge, or abrasion caused by a tool coming into contact with another object. Most often, tool marks are encountered at burglary scenes that involve forcible entry into a building or safe. Generally, these marks occur as indented impressions into a softer surface or as abrasion marks caused by the tool cutting or sliding against another object.

Comparing Tool Marks

Typically, an indented impression is left on the frame of a door or window as a result of the prying action of a screwdriver or crowbar. A careful examination of these impressions can reveal important class characteristics—that is, the size and shape of the tool. However, they rarely reveal any significant individual characteristics that could permit the examiner to individualize the mark to a single tool. Such characteristics, when they do exist, usually take the form of discernible random nicks and breaks that the tool has acquired through wear and use (Figure 9–24).

FIGURE 9–24
A comparison of a tool mark with a suspect screwdriver. Note how the presence of nicks and breaks on the tool's edge helps individualize the tool to the mark.

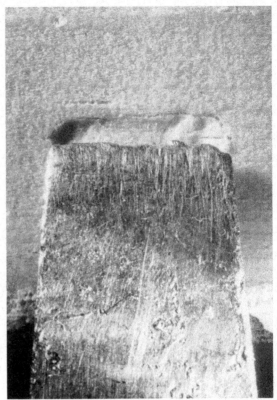

Richard Saferstein, Ph.D.

Just as the machined surfaces of a firearm are impressed with random striations during its manufacture, the edges of a pry bar, chisel, screwdriver, knife, or cutting tool likewise display a series of microscopic irregularities that look like ridges and valleys. Such markings are left as a result of the machining processes used to cut and finish tools. The shape and pattern of such minute imperfections are further modified by damage and wear during the life of the tool. Considering the unending variety of patterns that the hills and valleys can assume, it is highly unlikely that any two tools will be identical. Hence, these minute imperfections impart individuality to each tool.

If the edge of a tool is scraped against a softer surface, it may cut a series of striated lines that reflect that pattern of the tool's edge. Markings left in this manner are compared in the laboratory through a comparison microscope with test tool marks made from the suspect tool. The result can be a positive comparison, and hence a definitive association of the tool with the evidence mark, when a sufficient quantity of striations match between the evidence and test markings.

One of the major problems associated with tool mark comparisons is the difficulty in duplicating in the laboratory the tool mark left at the crime scene. A thorough comparison requires the preparation of a series of test marks obtained by applying the suspect tool at various angles and pressures to a soft metal surface (lead is commonly used). This approach gives the examiner ample opportunity to duplicate many of the details of the original evidence marking. A photomicrograph of a typical tool mark comparison is illustrated in Figure 9–25.

Collecting Tool Mark Evidence

Whenever practical, the entire object or the part of the object bearing a tool mark should be submitted to the crime laboratory for examination. When removal of the tool mark is impractical, the only recourse is to photograph the marked area to scale and make a cast of the mark. Under these circumstances, liquid silicone casting material has been found to be the most satisfactory for reproducing most of the fine details of the mark. See Figure 9–26. However, even under the most optimum conditions, the clarity of many of the tool mark's minute details will be lost or obscured in a photograph or cast. Of course, this will reduce the chance of individualizing the mark to a single tool.

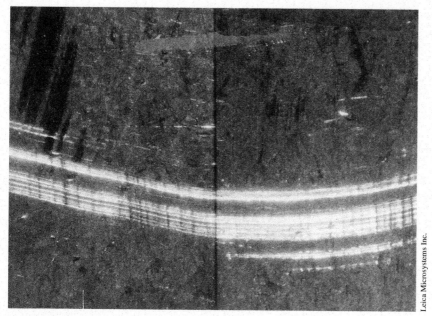

Leica Microsystems Inc.

FIGURE 9–25

A photograph of a tool mark comparison seen under a comparison microscope.

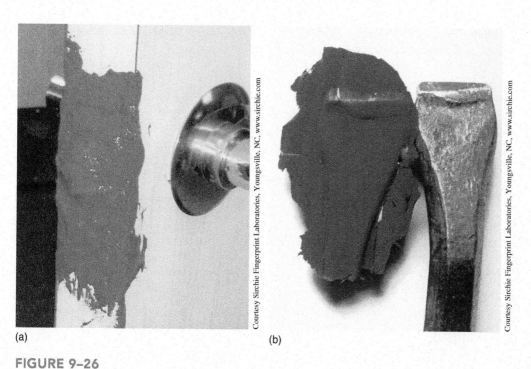

(a) (b)

Courtesy Sirchie Fingerprint Laboratories, Youngsville, NC, www.sirchie.com

FIGURE 9–26

(a) Casting a tool mark impression with a silicone-based putty. (b) Impression alongside suspect tool.

The crime-scene investigator must never attempt to fit the suspect tool into the tool mark. Any contact between the tool and the marked surface may alter the mark and will, at the least, raise serious questions about the integrity of the evidence. The suspect tool and mark must be packaged in separate containers, with every precaution taken to avoid contact between the tool or mark and another hard surface. Failure to properly protect the tool or mark from damage could result in the destruction of its individual characteristics.

Furthermore, the tool or its impression may contain valuable trace evidence. Chips of paint adhering to the mark or tool provide perhaps the best example of how the transfer of trace physical evidence can occur as a result of using a tool to gain forcible entry into a building. Obviously, the presence of trace evidence greatly enhances the evidential value of the tool or its mark and requires special care in handling and packaging the evidence to avoid losing or destroying these items.

Other Impressions

From time to time, impressions of another kind are left at a crime scene. This evidence may take the form of a shoe, tire, or fabric impression and may be as varied as a shoe impression left on a piece of paper at the scene of a burglary (Figure 9–27), or when a hit-and-run victim's garment has come into violent contact with an automobile (Figure 9–28), or an impression of a bloody shoe print left on a carpet and visualized by luminal (see Figure 9–29 a and b).

Preserving Impressions

The primary consideration in collecting impressions at the crime scene is the preservation of the impression or its reproduction for later examination in the crime laboratory. Before any impression is moved or otherwise handled, it must be photographed (a scale should be included in the picture) to show all the observable details of the impression. Several shots should be taken directly over the impression as well as at various angles around the impression. The skillful use of side lighting for illumination will help highlight many ridge details that might otherwise remain obscured. Photographs should also be taken to show the position of the questioned impression in relation to the overall crime scene.

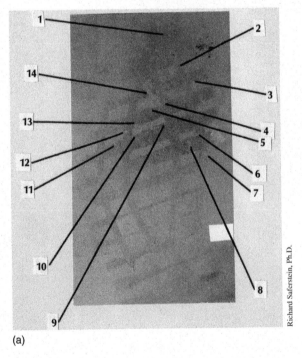

(a)

Richard Saferstein, Ph.D.

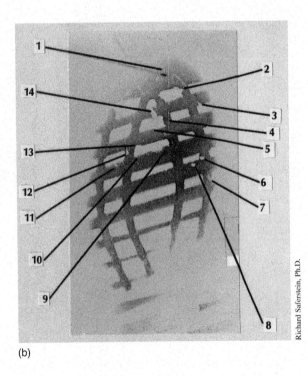

(b)

Richard Saferstein, Ph.D.

FIGURE 9–27

(a) Impression of shoe found at a crime scene. (b) Test impression made with suspect shoe. A sufficient number of points of comparison exist to support the conclusion that the suspect shoe left the impression at the crime scene.

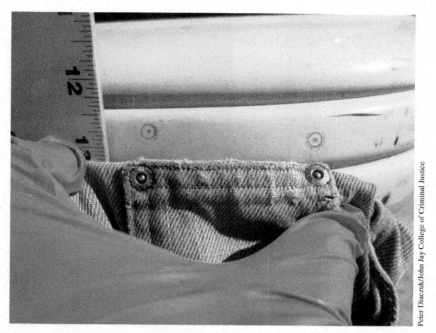

FIGURE 9-28

A pattern impression on a car bumper arising from a hit-and-run. Note rivets from the jeans are present in the impression. The writing from the rivet on the right side of the bumper is visible.

Although photography is an important first step in preserving an impression, it must be considered merely a backup procedure that is available to the examiner if the impression is damaged before reaching the crime laboratory. Naturally, it is preferable for the examiner to receive the original impression for comparison to the suspect shoe, tire, garment, and so forth. In most cases when the impression is on a readily recoverable item, such as glass, paper, or floor tile, little or no difficulty is presented in transporting the evidence intact to the laboratory.

Lifting Impressions

If an impression is encountered on a surface that cannot be submitted to the laboratory, the investigator may be able to preserve the print in a manner that is analogous to lifting a fingerprint. This is especially true of impressions made in light deposits of dust or dirt. A lifting material large enough to lift the entire impression should be used. Carefully place the lifting material over the entire impression. Use a fingerprint roller to eliminate any air pockets before lifting the impression off the surface.

A more exotic approach to lifting and preserving dust impressions involves the use of a portable electrostatic lifting device. The principle employed is similar to that of creating an electrostatic charge on a comb and using the comb to lift small pieces of tissue paper. A sheet of mylar film is placed on top of the dust mark, and the film is pressed against the impression with the aid of a roller. The high-voltage electrode of the electrostatic unit is then placed in contact with the film while the unit's earth electrodes are placed against a metal plate (earth plate) (see Figure 9–30). A charge difference develops between the mylar film and the surface below the dust mark so that the dust is attached to the lifting film. In this manner, dust prints on chairs, walls, floors, and the like, can be transferred to the mylar film. Floor surfaces up to 40 feet long can be covered with a mylar sheet and searched for dust impressions. The electrostatic lifting technique is particularly helpful in recovering barely visible dust prints on colored surfaces. Dust impressions can also be enhanced through chemical development (see Figure 9–31).

(a)

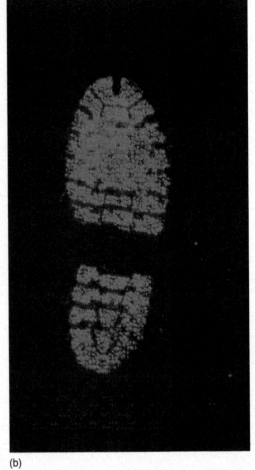

(b)

Sirchie Acquisition Company, LLC (dba Sirchie Fingerprint Laboratories)

FIGURE 9–29

(a) A section of a carpet under normal light showing a faint footprint in blood. (b) Same section of the carpet after spraying with luminal.

FIGURE 9–30
Electrostatic lifting of a dust impression off a floor using an electrostatic unit.

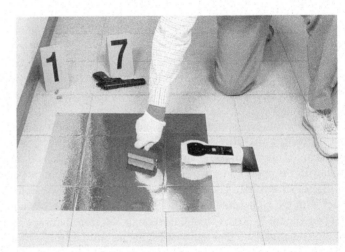

Sirchie Acquisition Company, LLC (dba Sirchie Fingerprint Laboratories)

Casting Impressions

Shoe and tire marks impressed into soft earth at a crime scene are best preserved by photography and casting. Class I dental stone, a form of gypsum, is widely recommended for making casts of shoe and tire impressions. The cast should be allowed to air-dry for 24 to 48 hours before it is shipped to the forensic science laboratory for examination. Figure 9–32 illustrates a cast made from a shoe print in mud. The cast compares to the suspect shoe.

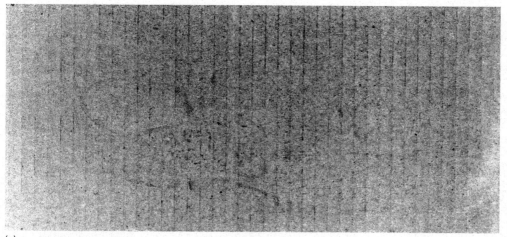

(a)

Israel Police Headquarters

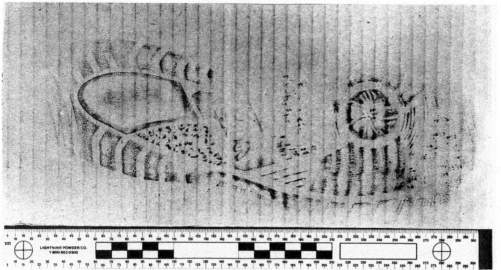

(b)

Israel Police Headquarters

FIGURE 9–31

(a) A dust impression of a shoe print on cardboard before enhancement. (b) Shoe print after chemical enhancement with Bromophenol Blue and exposure to water vapor.

An aerosol product known as Snow Impression Wax is available for casting snow impressions. The recommended procedure is to spray three light coats of the wax at an interval of one to two minutes between layers, and then let it dry for 10 minutes. A viscous mixture of Class I dental stone is then poured into the wax-coated impression. After the casting material has hardened, the cast can be removed.

Several chemicals can be used to develop and enhance footwear impressions made with blood. In areas where a bloody footwear impression is very faint or where a subject has tracked through blood, leaving a trail of bloody impressions, chemical enhancement can visualize latent or nearly invisible footwear impressions. A number of chemical formulas useful for bloody footwear impression analysis are listed in Appendix V.

Several blood enhancement chemicals have been examined for their impact on short tandem repeat (STR) DNA typing. (This particular method of DNA analysis will be discussed in Chapter 16.) None of the chemicals examined had a deleterious effect, on a short-term basis, on the ability to carry out STR DNA typing on the blood.[4]

---

[4] C. J. Frégeau et al., "Fingerprint Enhancement Revisited and the Effects of Blood Enhancement Chemicals on Subsequent Profiler Plus™ Fluorescent Short Tandem Repeat DNA Analysis of Fresh and Aged Bloody Fingerprints," *Journal of Forensic Sciences* 45 (2000): 354.

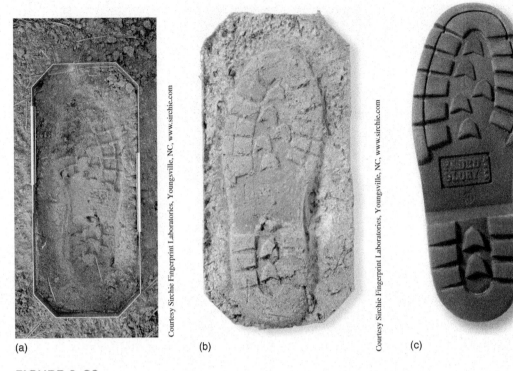

(a)   (b)   (c)

Courtesy Sirchie Fingerprint Laboratories, Youngsville, NC, www.sirchie.com

FIGURE 9–32

(a) Shoe impression in mud. (b) Cast of shoe impression. (c) Shoe suspected of leaving muddy impression.

WEBEXTRA 9.6
Casting a Footwear Impression.

Comparing Impressions

Whatever the circumstances, the laboratory procedures used to examine any type of impression remain the same. Of course, a comparison is possible only when the item suspected of having made the impression is recovered. Test impressions may be necessary to compare the characteristics of the suspect item with the evidence impression.

The evidential value of the impression is determined by the number of class and individual characteristics that the examiner finds. Agreement with respect to size, shape, or design may permit the conclusion that the impression could have been made by a particular shoe, tire, or garment, but one cannot entirely exclude other possible sources from having the same class characteristics. More significant is the existence of individual characteristics arising out of wear, cuts, gouges, or other damage. A sufficient number or the uniqueness of such points of comparison supports a finding that both the evidence and test impressions originated from only one source.

When a tire tread impression is left at a crime scene, the laboratory can examine the design of the impression and possibly determine the style and/or manufacturer of the tire. This may be particularly helpful to investigators when a suspect tire has not yet been located.

New computer software may help the forensic scientist compare shoe prints. For example, an automated shoe print identification system developed in England, called shoeprint image capture and retrieval (SICAR), incorporates multiple databases to search known and unknown footwear files for comparison against footwear specimens. Using the system, an impression from a crime scene can be compared to a reference database to find out what type of shoe caused the imprint. That same impression can also be searched in the suspect and crime databases to reveal whether that shoe print matches the shoes of a person who has been in custody or the shoe prints left behind at another crime scene. When matches are made during the searching process, the images are displayed side by side on the computer screen (see Figure 3–9 in Chapter 3).

Human bite marks on skin and foodstuffs have been important items of evidence for convicting defendants in a number of homicide and rape cases in recent years. If a sufficient number of points of similarity between test and suspect bite marks are present, a forensic odontologist may conclude that a bite mark was made by a particular individual (see Figure 9–33).

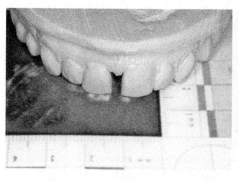
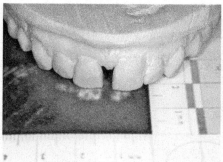
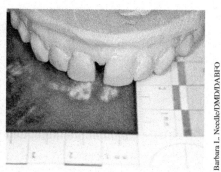

Barbara L. Needle/DMD/DABFO

FIGURE 9–33
Upper dental model from the teeth of the suspect matches the individual teeth characteristics of the bite marks.

Inside the Science

Casting Footwear and Tire Impressions

Footwear and tire impressions may be found at any type of crime scene and can provide a primary means to identify or exclude a suspect. The preferred method of collection for this type of evidence is casting the impression—that is, making a mold and preserving it for analysis in the lab. When a footwear or tire impression is found in dirt at the crime scene, the casting process is as follows:

Materials
Ruler
One small can of aerosol hair spray
1-gallon zip-top bag
Paint stirrer or large, long-handled spoon
Carton of dental stone
Water
Camera
Plastic or metal casting frame (optional)

Procedure
1. Retrieve any fragments or debris that are not imbedded within the impression. Photograph the impression before and after retrieving debris; include a ruler in the photograph. A frame for containing the dental stone may be installed around an impression that is shallow or located on an inclined surface.
2. To solidify the soil, a fixative such as hair spray is used (see Figure (a)). Hold the can of hair spray about 18 inches from the soil within the impression. Very lightly, spray an even layer over the impression, using a sweeping motion and taking care to avoid any damage to the impression.
3. Wait 10 minutes to allow the hair spray to dry.
4. Add an appropriate amount of water to a premeasured amount of dental stone (see Figure (b)). Add water in increments. The usual amount is about 10 to 12 fluid ounces of water to about 1.5 to 2 pounds of dental stone. If using a zip-top bag, seal the bag and mix by working back and

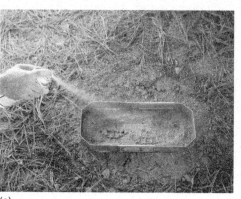

Courtesy Sirchie Fingerprint Laboratories, Youngsville, NC, www.sirchie.com

(a)

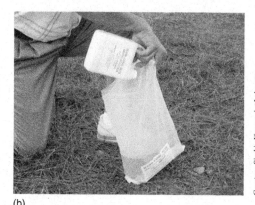

Courtesy Sirchie Fingerprint Laboratories, Youngsville, NC, www.sirchie.com

(b)

(continued)

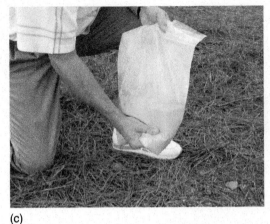

Courtesy Sirchie Fingerprint Laboratories, Youngsville, NC, www.sirchie.com

(c)

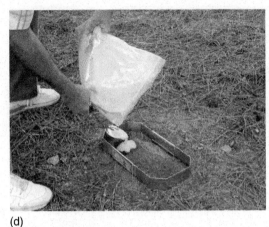

Courtesy Sirchie Fingerprint Laboratories, Youngsville, NC, www.sirchie.com

(d)

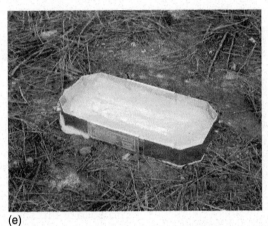

Courtesy Sirchie Fingerprint Laboratories, Youngsville, NC, www.sirchie.com

(e)

forth with your fingers for at least three minutes (see Figure (c)). Mix until a pancake-batter-like consistency is reached.

5. Open one corner of the bag. Pour the dental stone through the opening onto the ground beside the impression and allow it to carefully run into the impression. Use a paint stirrer, a spoon, or a gloved hand as a medium to disperse the stream so it does not destroy the fine details of the impression (see Figure (d)). Continue pouring until the dental stone completely fills the impression (see Figure (e)) and reaches at least ½ inch in thickness. If necessary, additional casting material may be poured over the top of the original cast to add thickness.

6. Label the wet plaster surface with the date, initials, and any other information required for evidence labeling.

7. When the cast no longer adheres to the soil and is relatively dry (usually about one hour), remove the cast. If necessary, the cast can be dug out from the sides.

8. Store the cast for 48 hours to allow it to dry completely. If a cast is not allowed to dry long enough, some ridge details may disappear.

9. Once the cast is dry, rinse any loose soil from it with softly running water. A soft-bristled brush may also be used. Do not scrub or pick off anything. Pat dry with paper towels.

> > > > > > > > > >

Case Files

The O. J. Simpson Trial—Who Left the Impressions at the Crime Scene?

On the night of June 12, 1994, Nicole Brown—ex-wife of football star O. J. Simpson—and her friend Ron Goldman were brutally murdered on the grounds outside her home in Brentwood, California. O. J. Simpson was arrested for their murders but professed his innocence. At the crime scene, investigators found bloody shoe impressions along the concrete walkway leading up to the front door of Brown's condominium. These shoe impressions were of extremely high quality and of intricate detail. The news media broadcast countless images of these bloody shoe prints on television, making it obvious to the killer that those shoes would surely link him to the crime.

Famed FBI shoe print examiner William J. Bodziak investigated the footwear evidence from the scene. His first task was to identify the brand of shoe that made the marks. Because the pattern was clear and distinct, with complete toe-to-heel detail, this seemed a simple task at first. Bodziak compared this pattern to the thousands of sole patterns in the FBI's database. None matched. He then went to his reference collection of books and trade show brochures, again with no success.

Bodziak's experience told him that these were expensive, Italian-made casual dress shoes with a sole made from synthetic material. Using this knowledge, he shopped the high-end stores for a similar tread pattern but still was unable to identify the shoes. He then drew a composite sketch of the sole and faxed the image to law enforcement agencies and shoe manufacturers and distributors worldwide. The owner of the American distributing company for Bruno Magli shoes was the only one to respond.

Further exhaustive investigation revealed that these were extremely rare shoes. There were two styles of shoe bearing this exact sole design. They were available for only two years, and from a mere 40 stores in the United States and Puerto Rico. The Lorenzo style shoe had a bootlike upper that came to the ankle. The Lyon style shoe had the lower, more typical dress shoe cut. The impressions were made by a size 12 shoe, and it was later determined that only 299 pairs of size 12 with this tread pattern were sold in the United States.

Simpson flatly denied ever owning these shoes, adding that he would never wear anything so ugly. However, he was known to wear a size 12, and photographs taken almost nine months before the murders show Simpson wearing a pair of black leather Bruno Magli Lorenzo shoes. These shoes were available in several colors, so this narrows the number of shoes matching Simpson's pair of Lorenzos (this size, color, and style) sold in the United States to 29 pairs.

Proving that Simpson owned a pair of shoes that had the exact pattern found printed in blood at the crime scene was an essential component of the case, but it was not done in time to be used during the criminal prosecution. The photographs of Simpson in his Bruno Magli shoes were released after the culmination of the criminal trial, so the jury never heard the direct evidence that Simpson owned these shoes. However, this proved to be an important link uniting Simpson with the crime scene in the civil trial. Although O. J. Simpson was acquitted of the murders of Nicole Brown and Ron Goldman in the criminal trial, he was judged responsible for their murders in the civil court case.

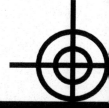

Chapter Summary > > > > > > > > > >

Structural variations and irregularities caused by scratches, nicks, breaks, and wear permit the criminalist to relate a bullet to a gun, a scratch or abrasion mark to a single tool, or a tire track to a particular automobile.

The manufacture of a barrel requires impressing its inner surface with spiral grooves, a step known as rifling. The surfaces of the original bore remaining between the grooves are called lands. No two rifled barrels, even those manufactured in succession, have identical striation markings. These striations form the individual characteristics of the barrel. The inner surface of the barrel of a gun leaves its striation markings on a bullet passing through it. The number of lands and grooves and their direction of twist are obvious points of comparison during the initial stages of an examination. Any differences in these class characteristics immediately eliminate the possibility that both bullets traveled through the same barrel.

The comparison microscope is the most important tool to a firearms examiner. Two bullets can be observed and compared simultaneously within the same field of view. Not only must the lands and grooves of the test and evidence bullet have identical widths, but the longitudinal striations on each must coincide. The firing pin, breechface, and ejector and extractor mechanism also offer a highly distinctive signature for individualization of cartridge cases. The advent of computerized imaging technology has made possible the storage of bullet and cartridge surface characteristics in a manner analogous to automated fingerprint files. However, the final comparison will be made by the forensic examiner through traditional microscopic methods.

The distribution of gunpowder particles and other discharge residues around a bullet hole permits an assessment of the distance from which a handgun or rifle was fired. The firing of a weapon not only propels residues toward the target, but also blows gunpowder and primer residues back toward the shooter. As a result, traces of these residues are often deposited on the firing hand of the shooter, and their detection can provide valuable information as to whether an individual has recently fired a weapon. Examiners measure the amount of barium and antimony on the relevant portion of the suspect's hands or characterize the morphology of particles containing these elements to determine whether a person has fired or handled a weapon, or was near a discharged firearm.

Increasingly, the criminalist is asked to restore a serial number that has been obliterated by grinding, rifling, or punching. Restoration of serial numbers is possible through chemical etching because the metal crystals in the stamped zone are placed under a permanent strain that extends a short distance beneath the original numbers.

The most important consideration for the collection and preservation of a firearm is safety. A trained examiner should always examine the firearm and render it safe before packaging and transport. Firearms are stored in cardboard boxes and labeled clearly with identifying information, as with any other item of evidence. One unique aspect of the collection and preservation of a firearm is that if it is recovered from an underwater location, no effort must be made to dry or clean it. Instead, the firearm should be transported to the laboratory in a receptacle containing enough of the same water necessary to keep it submerged. This procedure prevents rust from developing during transport.

A tool mark is any impression, cut, gouge, or abrasion caused by a tool coming into contact with another object. Hence, any minute imperfections on a tool impart individuality to that tool. The shape and pattern of such imperfections are further modified by damage and wear during the life of the tool. The comparison microscope is used to compare crime-scene tool marks with test impressions made with the suspect tool. When shoe and tire marks are impressed into soft earth at a crime scene, their preservation is best accomplished by photography and casting. In areas where a bloody footwear impression is very faint or where the subject has tracked through blood, leaving a trail of bloody impressions, chemical enhancement can visualize latent or nearly invisible blood impressions. A sufficient number of points of comparison or the uniqueness of such points support a finding that both the questioned and test impressions originated from one and only one source.

Review Questions

1. The _____ is the original part of the bore left after rifling grooves are formed.

2. The diameter of the gun barrel is known as its _____.

3. True or False: The number of lands and grooves is a class characteristic of a barrel. _____

4. The _____ characteristics of a rifled barrel are formed by striations impressed into the barrel's surface.

5. The most important instrument for comparing bullets is the _____.

6. To make a match between a test bullet and a recovered bullet, the lands and grooves of the test and evidence bullet must have identical widths, and the longitudinal _____ on each must coincide.

7. True or False: It is always possible to determine the make of a weapon by examining a bullet it fired. _____

8. A shotgun has a(n) _____ barrel.

9. The diameter of a shotgun barrel is expressed by the term _____.

10. True or False: Shotgun pellets can be individualized to a single weapon. _____

11. True or False: A cartridge case can be individualized to a single weapon. _____

12. The automated firearms search system developed by the FBI and ATF as a unified system incorporating both DRUGFIRE and IBIS technologies available in prior years is known as _____.

13. True or False: The distribution of gunpowder particles and other discharge residues around a bullet hole permits an approximate determination of the distance from which the gun was fired. _____

14. True or False: Without the benefit of a weapon, an examiner can make an exact determination of firing distance. _____

15. A halo of vaporous lead (smoke) deposited around a bullet hole normally indicates a discharge _____ to _____ inches from the target.

16. If a firearm has been fired more than 3 feet from a target, usually no residue is deposited but a dark ring, known as _____, is observed.

17. As a rule of thumb, the spread in the pattern made by a 12-gauge shotgun increases 1 inch for every _____ of distance from the target.

18. A(n) _____ photograph may help visualize gunpowder deposits around a target.

19. True or False: One test method for locating powder residues involves transferring particles embedded on the target surface to chemically treated photographic paper. _____

20. Current methods for identifying a shooter rely on the detection of _____ residues on the hands.

21. Determining whether an individual has fired a weapon is done by measuring the elements _____ and _____ present on the hands.

22. True or False: Firings with all types of ammunition can be detected by hand swabbings with nitric acid. _____

23. Microscopic primer and gunpowder particles on the adhesives applied to a suspected shooter's hand can be found with a(n) _____.

24. True or False: Restoration of serial numbers is possible because in the stamped zone the metal is placed under a(n) permanent strain that extends beneath the original numbers. _____

25. True or False: It is proper to insert a pencil into the barrel when picking up a crime-scene gun. _____

26. Recovered bullets are initialed on either the _____ or _____ of the bullet.

27. True or False: Because minute traces of evidence such as paint and fibers may be adhering to a recovered bullet, the investigator must take care to remove these trace materials immediately. _____

28. True or False: Cartridge cases are best marked at the base of the shell. _____

29. The clothing of the victim of a shooting must be handled so as to prevent disruption of _____ around bullet holes.

30. A(n) _____ is any impression caused by a tool coming into contact with another object.

31. Tool marks compare only when a sufficient number of _____ match between the evidence and test markings.

32. Objects bearing tool marks should be submitted intact to the crime lab or a(n) _____ should be taken of the tool mark.

33. An imprint may be lifted using lifting sheets or a(n) _____.

34. Shoe and tire marks impressed into soft earth at a crime scene are best preserved by _____ and _____.

35. A wear pattern, cut, gouge, or other damage pattern can impart _____ characteristics to a shoe.

Application and Critical Thinking

1. From each of the following descriptions of bullet holes, use general guidelines to estimate the distance from the shooter to the target.
   a. A few widely scattered gunpowder particles with no soot around the entrance hole
   b. A dark ring around the bullet hole, but no soot or gunpowder particles
   c. A halo of soot surrounding the entrance hole along with scattered specks of powder grains
   d. Scorch marks and melted fibers surrounding the entrance hole

2. You are investigating a shooting involving a 12-gauge shotgun with a moderately high choke. The spread of the pattern made by the pellets measures 12 inches. In your opinion, which of the following is probably closest to the distance from the target to the shooter? Explain your answer and explain why the other answers are likely to be incorrect.
   a. 18 yards
   b. 12 yards
   c. 6 yards
   d. 30 yards

3. Criminalist Ben Baldanza is collecting evidence from the scene of a shooting. After locating the revolver suspected of firing the shots, Ben picks the gun up by the grip, unloads it, and places the ammunition in an envelope. He then attaches an identification tag to the grip. Searching the scene, Ben finds a bullet lodged in the wall. He uses pliers to grab the bullet and pull it from the wall, then inscribes the bullet with his initials and places it in an envelope. What mistakes, if any, did Ben make in collecting this evidence?

4. How would you go about collecting impressions in each of the following situations?
   a. You discover a shoe print in dry dirt.
   b. You discover a tool mark on a windowsill.
   c. You discover tire marks in soft earth.
   d. You discover a shoe print on a loose piece of tile.
   e. You discover a very faint shoe print in dust on a colored linoleum floor.

5. Gunshot residue patterns (A) through (D) (contact, 1 inch, 6 inches, and 18 inches) from a 40-caliber pistol are shown in the figures. Match the firing distance to each pattern.

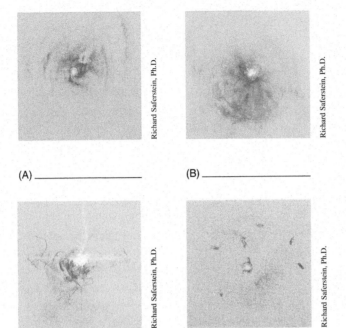

(A) _____

(B) _____

(C) _____

(D) _____

Further References

Bodziak, William J., *Forensic Footwear Evidence*, 3rd ed. Boca Raton, FL: CRC Press, 2016.

Bodziak, William J., *Tire Tread and Tire Track Evidence: Recovery and Forensic Examination.* Boca Raton, FL: CRC Press, 2008.

DiMaio, Vincent J. M., *Gunshot Wounds: Practical Aspects of Firearms, Ballistics, and Forensic Techniques*, 3rd ed. Boca Raton, FL: CRC Press, 2016.

Hilderbrand, Dwane S., *Footwear: The Missed Evidence*, 3rd ed. Wildomar, CA: Staggs, Publishing, 2013.

An Introduction to Forensic Firearm Identification, http://www.firearmsid.com/

Rowe, Walter F., "Firearms Identification," in R. Saferstein, ed., *Forensic Science Handbook*, vol. 2, 2nd ed. Upper Saddle River, NJ: Prentice Hall, 2005.

Schehl, S. A., "Firearms and Toolmarks in the FBI Laboratory," *Forensic Science Communications* 2, no. 2 (2000), https://www2.fbi.gov/hq/lab/fsc/backissu/april2000/index.htm

Matter, Light, and Glass Examination

Learning Objectives

After studying this chapter, you should be able to:

10.1 Discuss the composition of matter

10.2 Explain how density and refractive index of glass is measured and utilized for forensic characterization

10.3 Explain the nature of light as a wave and as a particle

10.4 Explain forensic methods for comparing glass fragments

10.5 Explain how glass fractures reveal information related to the force and direction of an impact

10.6 Describe the proper collection of glass evidence

Mind Hunters: The Ted Bundy Interviews

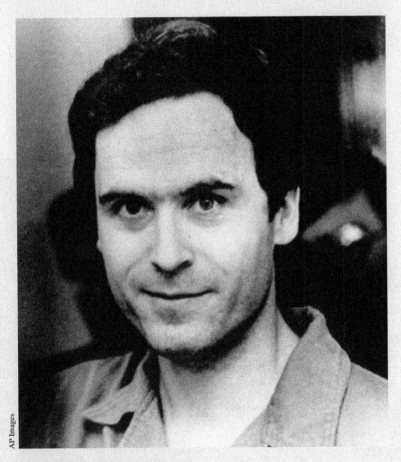

AP Images

The name Ted Bundy is synonymous with the term *serial killer*. This handsome, gregarious, and worldly onetime law student is believed to be responsible for 40 murders between 1964 and 1978. His reign of terror stretched from the Pacific Northwest down into California and into Utah, Idaho, and Colorado, finally ending in Florida. His victims were typically young women, usually murdered with a blunt instrument or by strangulation and sexually assaulted before and after death. First convicted in Utah in 1976 on a charge of kidnapping, Bundy managed to escape after his extradition to Colorado on a murder charge. Ultimately, Bundy found his way to the Tallahassee area of Florida. There he unleashed mayhem, killing two women at a Florida State University sorority house and then murdering a 12-year-old girl three weeks later.

Years later, in the mid-1980s, investigators from King County, Washington, had another serial killer on their hands. This new serial killer was kidnapping, raping, and murdering women and dumping their bodies next to the Green River (see Chapter 14). With no leads to go on, and bodies piling up, investigators traveled to Florida to interview Bundy to see if he could offer any insight into the killer's motivations and behavior. During one interview session, Bundy suggested that the killer was likely returning to the dump sites to engage in sexual intercourse with the bodies. He advised the investigators that if they find a fresh grave, they should stake it out and wait for the killer to return.

This was a helpful piece of information, given that DNA that eventually led to the identification of the man Ted Bundy called, "River Man." Three years after his assistance with the Green River case, Bundy was executed in 1989.

The forensic scientist must constantly determine the properties that impart distinguishing characteristics to matter, giving it a unique identity. The continuing search for distinctive properties ends only when the scientist has completely individualized a substance to one correct source. Properties are the identifying characteristics of substances. In this chapter, we will examine properties that are most useful for characterizing glass and other physical evidence. However, before we begin, we can simplify our understanding of the nature of properties by classifying them into two broad categories: physical and chemical.

Physical properties describe a substance without reference to any other substance. For example, weight, volume, color, boiling point, and melting point are typical physical properties that can be measured for a particular substance without altering the material's composition through a chemical reaction; they are associated only with the physical existence of that substance. **A chemical property describes the behavior of a substance when it reacts or combines with another substance.** For example, when wood burns, it chemically combines with oxygen in the air to form new substances; this transformation describes a chemical property of wood. In the crime laboratory, a routine procedure for determining the presence of heroin in a suspect specimen is to react it with a chemical reagent known as the Marquis reagent, which turns purple in the presence of heroin. This color transformation becomes a chemical property of heroin and provides a convenient test for its identification.

physical property
The behavior of a substance without alteration of the substance's composition through a chemical reaction.

chemical property
The behavior of a substance when it reacts or combines with another substance.

The Nature of Matter

Before we can apply physical properties, as well as chemical properties, to the identification and comparison of evidence, we need to gain an insight into the composition of matter. Beginning with knowledge of the fundamental building block of all substances—the element—we will extend our discussion to compounds.

Elements and Compounds

Matter is anything that has mass and occupies space. As we examine the world that surrounds us and consider the countless variety of materials that we encounter, we must consider one of humankind's most remarkable accomplishments: the discovery of the concept of the atom to explain the composition of all matter. This search had its earliest contribution from the ancient Greek philosophers, who suggested air, water, fire, and earth as matter's fundamental building blocks. It culminated with the development of the atomic theory and the discovery of matter's simplest identity, the **element**.

An element is the simplest substance known and provides the building block from which all matter is composed. At present, 118 elements have been identified (see Table 10–1); of these, 89 occur naturally on the earth, and the remainder have been created in the laboratory. In Figure 10–1, all of the elements are listed by name and symbol in a form that has become known as the **periodic table**. This table is most useful to chemists because it systematically arranges elements with similar chemical properties in the same vertical row or group.

For convenience, chemists have chosen letter symbols to represent the elements. Many of these symbols come from the first letter of the element's English name—for example, carbon (C), hydrogen (H), and oxygen (O). Others are two-letter abbreviations of the English name—for example, calcium (Ca) and zinc (Zn). Some symbols are derived from the first letters of Latin or Greek names. Thus, the symbol for silver, Ag, comes from the Latin name *argentum*; copper, Cu, from the Latin *cuprum*; and helium, He, from the Greek name *helios*.

The smallest particle of an element that can exist and still retain its identity as that element is the atom. When we write the symbol C we mean one atom of carbon; the chemical symbol for carbon dioxide, CO_2, signifies one atom of carbon combined with two atoms of oxygen. When two or more elements are combined to form a substance, as with carbon dioxide,

matter
All things of substance; matter is composed of atoms or molecules.

element
A fundamental particle of matter; an element cannot be broken down into simpler substances by chemical means.

periodic table
A chart of elements arranged in a systematic fashion; vertical rows are called groups or families, and horizontal rows are called series; elements in a given row have similar properties.

TABLE 10–1

List of Elements with Their Symbols and Atomic Masses

Element	Symbol	Atomic Mass[a] (amu)	Element	Symbol	Atomic Mass[a] (amu)
Actinum	Ac	(227)	Lawrencium	Lr	(262)
Aluminum	Al	26.9815	Lead	Pb	207.2
Americium	Am	(243)	Lithium	Li	6.941
Antimony	Sb	121.75	Livermorium	Lv	(293)
Argon	Ar	39.948	Lutetium	Lu	174.97
Arsenic	As	74.9216	Magnesium	Mg	24.305
Astatine	At	(210)	Manganese	Mn	54.9380
Barium	Ba	137.34	Meitnerium	Mt	(278)
Berkelium	Bk	(247)	Mendelevium	Md	(256)
Beryllium	Be	9.01218	Mercury	Hg	200.59
Bismuth	Bi	208.9806	Molybdenum	Mo	95.94
Bohrium	Bh	(270)	Neodymium	Nd	144.24
Boron	B	10.81	Neon	Ne	20.179
Bromine	Br	79.904	Neptunium	Np	237.0482
Cadmium	Cd	112.40	Nickel	Ni	58.71
Calcium	Ca	40.08	Niobium	Nb	92.9064
Californium	Cf	(251)	Nitrogen	N	14.0067
Carbon	C	12.011	Nobelium	No	(254)
Cerium	Ce	140.12	Osmium	Os	190.2
Cesium	Cs	132.9055	Oxygen	O	15.9994
Chlorine	Cl	35.453	Palladium	Pd	106.4
Chromium	Cr	51.996	Phosphorus	P	30.9738
Cobalt	Co	58.9332	Platinum	Pt	195.09
Copernicium	Cn	(285)	Plutonium	Pu	(244)
Copper	Cu	63.546	Polonium	Po	(209)
Curium	Cm	(247)	Potassium	K	39.102
Darmstadtium	Ds	(81)	Praseodymium	Pr	140.9077
Dubnium	Db	(268)	Promethium	Pm	(145)
Dysprosium	Dy	162.50	Protactinium	Pa	231.0359
Einsteinium	Es	(254)	Radium	Ra	226.0254
Erbium	Er	167.26	Radon	Rn	(222)
Europium	Eu	151.96	Rhenium	Re	186.2
Fermium	Fm	(253)	Rhodium	Rh	102.9055
Flerovium	FL	(289)	Roentgenium	Rg	(280)
Fluorine	F	18.998	Rubidium	Rb	85.4678
Francium	Fr	(223)	Ruthenium	Ru	101.07
Gadolinium	Gd	157.25	Rutherfordium	Rf	(265)
Gallium	Ga	69.72	Samarium	Sm	105.4
Germanium	Ge	72.59	Scandium	Sc	44.9559
Gold	Au	196.9665	Seaborgium	Sg	(271)
Hafnium	Hf	178.49	Selenium	Se	78.96
Hassium	Hs	(277)	Silicon	Si	28.086
Helium	He	4.00260	Silver	Ag	107.868
Holmium	Ho	164.9303	Sodium	Na	22.9898
Hydrogen	H	1.0080	Strontium	Sr	87.62
Indium	In	114.82	Sulfur	S	32.06
Iodine	I	126.9045	Tantalum	Ta	180.9479
Iridium	Ir	192.22	Technetium	Tc	98.9062
Iron	Fe	55.847	Tellurium	Te	127.60
Krypton	Kr	83.80	Terbium	Tb	158.9254
Lanthanum	La	138.9055	Thallium	Tl	204.37

Element	Symbol	Atomic Mass[a] (amu)	Element	Symbol	Atomic Mass[a] (amu)
Thorium	Th	232.0381	Ununtrium	Uut	(284)
Thulium	Tm	168.9342	Uranium	U	238.029
Tin	Sn	118.69	Vanadium	V	50.9414
Titanium	Ti	47.90	Xenon	Xe	131.3
Tungsten	W	183.85	Ytterbium	Yb	173.04
Ununoctium	Uuo	(294)	Yttrium	Y	88.9059
Ununpentium	Uup	(288)	Zinc	Zn	65.57
Ununseptium	Uus	(?)	Zirconium	Zr	91.22

[a]Based on the assigned relative atomic mass of C = exactly 12; parentheses denote the mass number of the isotope with the longest half-life.

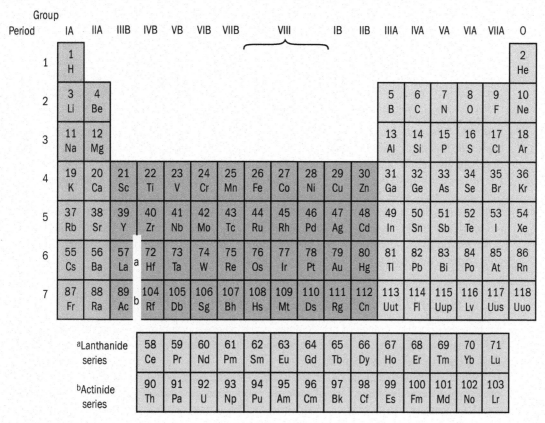

FIGURE 10–1
The periodic table.

a new substance is created, different in its physical and chemical properties from its elemental components. This new material is called a **compound**. Compounds contain at least two elements. Considering that there are 89 natural elements, it is easy to imagine the large number of possible elemental combinations that may form compounds. Not surprisingly, more than 16 million known compounds have already been identified.

    Just as the atom is the basic particle of an element, the molecule is the smallest unit of a compound. Thus, a molecule of carbon dioxide is represented by the symbol CO_2, and a molecule of table salt is symbolized by NaCl, representing the combination of one atom of the element sodium (Na) with one atom of the element chlorine (Cl).

compound
A pure substance composed of two or more elements.

States of Matter

As we look around us and view the materials that make up the earth, it becomes an awesome task even to attempt to estimate the number of different kinds of matter that exist. A much more logical approach is to classify matter according to the physical form it takes. These forms are called **physical states**. There are three such states: **solid**, **liquid**, and **gas (vapor)**. A solid is rigid and therefore has a definite shape and volume. A liquid also occupies a specific volume, but its fluidity causes it to take the shape of the container in which it is residing. A gas has neither a definite shape nor volume, and it will completely fill any container into which it is placed.

CHANGES OF STATE   Substances can change from one state to another. For example, as water is heated, it is converted from a liquid form into a vapor. At a high enough temperature (100°C), water boils and rapidly changes into steam. Similarly, at 0°C, water solidifies or freezes into ice. Under certain conditions, some solids can be converted directly into a gaseous state. For instance, a piece of dry ice (solid carbon dioxide) left standing at room temperature quickly forms carbon dioxide vapor and disappears. This change of state from a solid to a gas is called **sublimation**.

In each of these examples, no new chemical species are formed; matter is simply being changed from one physical state to another. Water, whether in the form of liquid, ice, or steam, remains chemically H_2O. Simply, what has been altered are the attractive forces between the water molecules. In a solid, these forces are very strong, and the molecules are held closely together in a rigid state. In a liquid, the attractive forces are not as strong, and the molecules have more mobility. Finally, in the vapor state, appreciable attractive forces no longer exist among the molecules; thus, they may move in any direction at will.

PHASES   Chemists are forever combining different substances, no matter whether they are in the solid, liquid, or gaseous states, hoping to create new and useful products. Our everyday observations should make it apparent that not all attempts at mixing matter can be productive. For instance, oil spills demonstrate that oil and water do not mix. **Whenever substances can be distinguished by a visible boundary, different phases are said to exist.** Thus, oil floating on water is an example of a two-phase system. The oil and water each constitute a separate liquid phase, clearly distinct from each other. Similarly, when sugar is first added to water, it does not dissolve, and two distinctly different phases exist: the solid sugar and the liquid water. However, after stirring, all the sugar dissolves, leaving just one liquid phase.

Physical Properties of Matter

All materials possess a range of physical properties whose measurement is critical to the work of the forensic scientist. Several of the most important of these for the forensic characterization of glass is density and refractive index.

Which physical and chemical properties the forensic scientist ultimately chooses to observe and measure depends on the type of material that is being examined. Logic requires, however, that if the property can be assigned a numerical value, it must relate to a standard system of measurement accepted throughout the scientific community.

Basic Units of Measurement

The metric system has basic units of measurement for length, mass, and volume: the meter, gram, and liter, respectively. These three basic units can be converted into subunits that are decimal multiples of the basic unit by simply attaching a prefix to the unit name. The following are common prefixes and their equivalent decimal value:

Prefix	Equivalent Value
deci-	1/10 or 0.1
centi-	1/100 or 0.01
milli-	1/1,000 or 0.001
micro-	1/1,000,000 or 0.000001
nano-	1/1,000,000,000 or 0.000000001
kilo-	1,000
mega-	1,000,000

physical state
A condition or stage in the form of matter; a solid, liquid, or gas.

solid
A state of matter in which the molecules are held closely together in a rigid state.

liquid
A state of matter in which molecules are in contact with one another but are not rigidly held in place.

gas (vapor)
A state of matter in which the attractive forces between molecules are small enough to permit them to move with complete freedom.

sublimation
A physical change from the solid state directly into the gaseous state.

phase
A uniform body of matter; different phases are separated by definite visible boundaries.

Inside the Science

The Metric System

Although scientists, including forensic scientists, throughout the world have been using the metric system of measurement for more than a century, the United States still uses the cumbersome "English system" to express length in inches, feet, or yards; weight in ounces or pounds; and volume in pints or quarts. The inherent difficulty of this system is that no simple numerical relationship exists between the various units of measurement. For example, to convert inches to feet one must know that 1 foot equals 12 inches; conversion of ounces to pounds requires the knowledge that 16 ounces equals 1 pound. In 1791, the French Academy of Science devised the simple system of measurement known as the metric system. This system uses a simple decimal relationship so that a unit of length, volume, or mass can be converted into a subunit by simply multiplying or dividing by a multiple of 10—for example, 10, 100, or 1,000.

Even though the United States has not yet adopted the metric system, its system of currency is decimal and, hence, is analogous to the metric system. The basic unit of currency is the dollar. A dollar is divided into 10 equal units called dimes, and each dime is further divided into 10 equal units of cents.

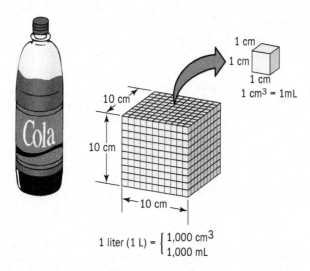

Volume equivalencies in the metric system.

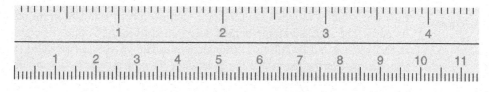

Comparison of the metric and English systems of length measurement; 2.54 centimeters = 1 inch.

Hence, 1/10 or 0.1 gram (g) is the same as a decigram (dg), 1/100 or 0.01 meter is equal to a centimeter (cm), and 1/1,000 liter is a milliliter (mL). A metric conversion is carried out simply by moving the decimal point to the right or left and inserting the proper prefix to show the direction and number of places that the decimal point has been moved. For example, if the weight of a powder is 0.0165 gram, it may be more convenient to multiply this value by 100 and express it as 1.65 centigrams or by 1,000 to show it as its equivalent value of 16.5 milligrams. Similarly, an object that weighs 264,450 grams may be expressed as 264.45 kilograms simply by dividing it by 1,000. It is important to remember that in any of these conversions, the value of the measurement has not changed; 0.0165 gram is still equivalent to 1.65 centigrams, just as one dollar is still equal to 100 cents. We have simply adjusted the position of the decimal and shown the extent of the adjustment with a prefix.

One interesting aspect of the metric system is that volume can be defined in terms of length. A liter by definition is the volume of a cube with sides of length 10 centimeters. One liter is therefore equivalent to a volume of 10 cm $\times$ 10 cm $\times$ 10 cm, or 1,000 cubic centimeters (cc). Thus, 1/1,000 liter or 1 milliliter (mL) is equal to 1 cubic centimeter (cc). Scientists commonly use the subunits mL and cc interchangeably to express volume.

Metric Conversion

At times, it may be necessary to convert units from the metric system into the English system, or vice versa. To accomplish this, we must consult references that list English units and their metric equivalents. Some of the more useful equivalents follow:

1 inch = 2.54 centimeters
1 meter = 39.37 inches
1 pound = 453.6 grams
1 liter = 1.06 quarts
1 kilogram = 2.2 pounds

The general mathematical procedures for converting from one system to another can be illustrated by converting 12 inches into centimeters. To change inches into centimeters, we need to know that there are 2.54 centimeters per inch. Hence, if we multiply 12 inches by 2.54 centimeters per inch (12 in. $\times$ 2.54 cm/in.), the unit of inches will cancel out, leaving the product 30.48 cm. Similarly, applying the conversion of grams to pounds, 227 grams is equivalent to 227 g $\times$ 1 lb/453.6 g or 0.5 lb.

Density

density
A physical property of matter that is equivalent to the mass per unit volume of a substance.

intensive property
A property that is not dependent on the size of an object.

Fahrenheit scale
The temperature scale using the melting point of ice as 32° and the boiling point of water as 212°, with 180 equal divisions or degrees between.

Celsius scale
The temperature scale using the melting point of ice as 0° and the boiling point of water as 100°, with 100 equal divisions or degrees between.

weight
A property of matter that depends on both the mass of a substance and the effects of gravity on that mass.

mass
A constant property of matter that reflects the amount of material present.

An important physical property of matter with respect to the analysis of certain kinds of physical evidence is **density**. **Density is defined as mass per unit volume** [see Equation (10–1)].

$$\text{Density} = \frac{\text{mass}}{\text{volume}} \qquad \textbf{(10–1)}$$

Density is an **intensive property** of matter—that is, it is the same regardless of the size of a substance; thus, it is a characteristic property of a substance and can be used as an aid in identification. Solids tend to be more dense than liquids, and liquids more dense than gases. The densities of some common substances are shown in Table 10–2.

A simple procedure for determining the density of a solid is illustrated in Figure 10–2. First, the solid is weighed on a balance against known standard gram weights to determine its mass. The solid's volume is then determined from the volume of water it displaces. This is easily measured by filling a cylinder with a known volume of water (V_1), adding the object, and measuring the new water level (V_2). The difference $V_2 - V_1$ in milliliters is equal to the volume of the solid. Density can now be calculated from Equation (10–1) in grams per milliliter.

The volumes of gases and liquids vary considerably with temperature; hence, when determining density, it is important to control and record the temperature at which the measurements are made. For example, 1 gram of water occupies a volume of 1 milliliter at 4°C and thus has a density of 1.0 g/mL. However, as the temperature of water increases, its volume expands. Therefore, at 20°C (room temperature) 1 gram of water occupies a volume of 1.002 mL and has a density of 0.998 g/mL.

The observation that a solid object either sinks, floats, or remains suspended when immersed in a liquid can be accounted for by the property of density. For instance, if the density of a solid is greater than that of the liquid in which it is immersed, the object sinks; if the solid's density is less than that of the liquid, it floats; and when the solid and liquid have equal densities, the solid remains suspended in the liquid. As we will shortly see, these observations provide a convenient technique for comparing the densities of solid objects.

Inside the Science

Temperature

Determining the physical properties of any material often requires measuring its temperature. For instance, the temperatures at which a substance melts or boils are readily determinable characteristics that will help identify it. Temperature is a measure of heat intensity, or the amount of heat in a substance.

Temperature is usually measured by causing a thermometer to come into contact with a substance. The familiar mercury-in-glass thermometer functions because mercury expands more than glass when heated and contracts more than glass when cooled. Thus, the length of the mercury column in the glass tube provides a measure of the surrounding environment's temperature.

The construction of a temperature scale requires two reference points and a choice of units. The reference points most conveniently chosen are the freezing point and boiling point of water. The two most common temperature scales used are the Fahrenheit and Celsius (formerly called *centigrade*) scales.

The **Fahrenheit scale** is based on assigning a value of 32°F to the freezing point of water and a value of 212°F to its boiling point. The difference between the two points is evenly divided into 180 units. Thus, a degree Fahrenheit is 1/180 of the temperature change between the freezing point and boiling point of water. The **Celsius scale** is derived by assigning the freezing point of water a value of 0°C and its boiling point a value of 100°C. A degree Celsius is thus 1/100 of the temperature change between the two reference points. Scientists in most countries use the Celsius scale to measure temperature. A comparison of the two scales is shown in the figure.

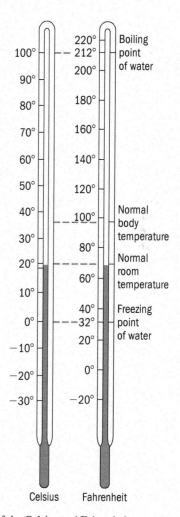

Comparison of the Celsius and Fahrenheit temperature scales.

Inside the Science

Weight and Mass

The force with which gravity attracts a body is called **weight**. If your weight is 180 pounds, this means that the earth's gravity is pulling you down with a force of 180 pounds; on the moon, where the force of gravity is one-sixth that of the earth, your weight would be 30 pounds.

Mass differs from weight because it refers to the amount of matter an object contains and is independent of its location on earth or any other place in the universe. The mathematical relationship between weight (w) and mass (m) is shown in Equation (10–2), where g is the acceleration imparted to a body by the force of gravity.

$$W = mg \qquad (10\text{–}2)$$

(continued)

The weight of a body is directly proportional to its mass; hence, a large mass weighs more than a small mass.

In the metric system, the mass of an object is always specified, rather than its weight. The basic unit of mass is the gram. An object that has a mass of 40 grams on earth will have a mass of 40 grams anywhere else in the universe. Normally, however, the terms *mass* and *weight* are used interchangeably, and we often speak of the weight of an object when we really mean its mass.

The mass of an object is determined by comparing it against the known mass of standard objects. The comparison is confusingly called *weighing*, and the standard objects are called *weights* (*masses* would be a more correct term). The comparison is performed on a balance. The simplest type of balance for weighing is the equal-arm balance shown in the figure. The object to be weighed is placed on the left pan, and the standard weights are placed on the right pan; when the pointer between the two pans is at the center mark, the total mass on the right pan is equal to the mass of the object on the left pan.

The modern laboratory has progressed beyond the simple equal-arm balance, and either the top-loading balance or the single-pan analytical balance as shown in the figures is now likely to be used. The choice depends on the accuracy required and the amount of material being weighed. Each works on the same counterbalancing principle as the simple equal-arm balance. Earlier versions of the single-pan balance had a second pan, the one on which the standard weights were placed. This pan was hidden from view within the balance's housing. Once the object whose weight was to be determined was placed on the visible pan, the operator selected the proper standard weights (also contained within the housing) by manually turning a set of knobs located on the front side of the balance. At the point of balance, the weights selected were automatically recorded on optical readout scales. Modern single-pan balances may employ an electromagnetic field to generate a current to balance the force pressing down on the pan from the sample being weighed. When the scale is properly calibrated, the amount of current needed to keep the pan balanced is used to determine the weight of the sample. The strength of the current is converted to a digitized signal for a readout. Another approach is to employ a bridge circuit incorporating a strain gauge resistor that changes in response to the force applied to it. The top-loading balance can accurately weigh an object to the nearest 1 milligram or 0.001 gram; the analytical balance is even more accurate, weighing to the nearest tenth of a milligram or 0.0001 gram.

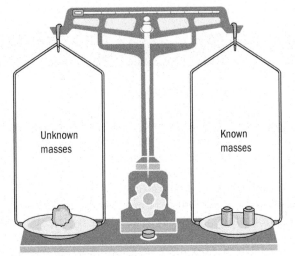

The measurement of mass.

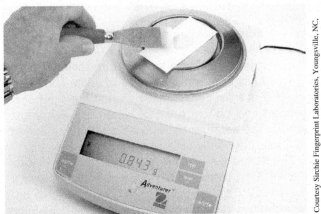

(a)

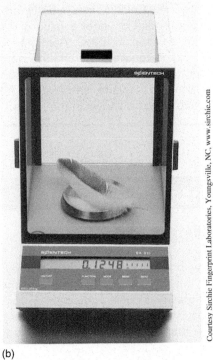

(b)

(a) Top-loading balance. (b) Single-pan analytical balance.

TABLE 10–2

Densities of Select Materials (at 20°C Unless Otherwise Stated)

Substance	Density (g/mL)
Solids	
Silver	10.5
Lead	11.5
Iron	7.8
Aluminum	2.7
Window glass	2.47–2.54
Ice (0°C)	0.92
Liquids	
Mercury	13.6
Benzene	0.88
Ethyl alcohol	0.79
Gasoline	0.69
Water at 4°C	1.00
Water	0.998
Gases	
Air (0°C)	0.0013
Chlorine (0°C)	0.0032
Oxygen (0°C)	0.0014
Carbon dioxide (0°C)	0.0020

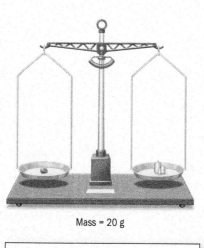

Mass = 20 g

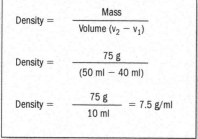

$$\text{Density} = \frac{\text{Mass}}{\text{Volume } (v_2 - v_1)}$$

$$\text{Density} = \frac{75 \text{ g}}{(50 \text{ ml} - 40 \text{ ml})}$$

$$\text{Density} = \frac{75 \text{ g}}{10 \text{ ml}} = 7.5 \text{ g/ml}$$

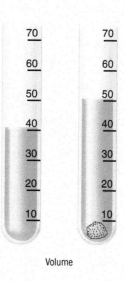

Volume

FIGURE 10–2

A simple procedure for determining the density of a solid is first to measure its mass on a scale and then to measure its volume by noting the volume of water it displaces.

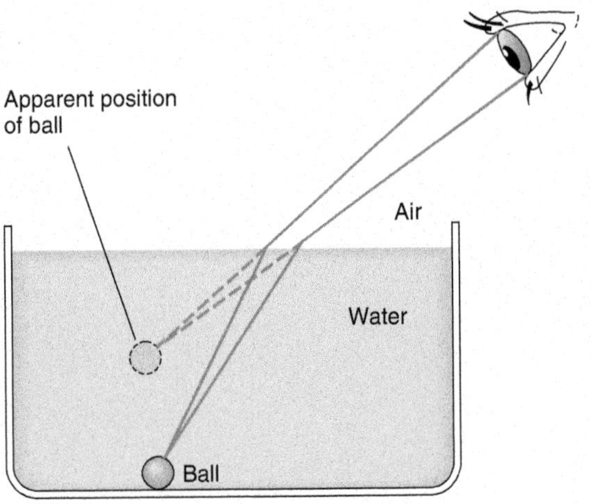

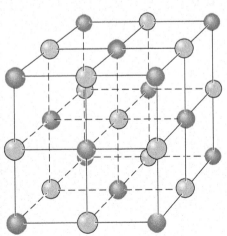

FIGURE 10–3

Light is refracted when it travels obliquely from one medium to another.

refraction

The bending of a light wave as it passes from one medium to another.

refractive index

The ratio of the speed of light in a vacuum to its speed in a given substance.

crystalline solid

A solid in which the constituent atoms have a regular arrangement.

atom

The smallest unit of an element, which is not divisible by ordinary chemical means; atoms are made up of electrons, protons, and neutrons plus other subatomic particles.

Refractive Index

Light, as we will learn in the next section, can have the property of a wave. Light waves travel in air at a constant velocity of nearly 300 million meters per second until they penetrate another medium, such as glass or water, at which point they are suddenly slowed, causing the rays to bend. The bending of a light wave because of a change in velocity is called **refraction**.

The phenomenon of refraction is apparent when we view an object that is immersed in a transparent medium; because we are accustomed to thinking that light travels in a straight line, we often forget to take refraction into account. For instance, suppose a ball is observed at the bottom of a pool of water; the light rays reflected from the ball travel through the water and into the air to reach the eye. As the rays leave the water and enter the air, their velocity suddenly increases, causing them to be refracted. However, because of our assumption that light travels in a straight line, our eyes deceive us and make us think we see an object lying at a higher point than is actually the case. This phenomenon is illustrated in Figure 10–3.

The ratio of the velocity of light in a vacuum to that in any medium determines the **refractive index** of that medium and is expressed as follows:

$$\text{Refractive index} = \frac{\text{velocity of light in vacuum}}{\text{velocity of light in medium}}$$

For example, at 25°C the refractive index of water is 1.333. This means that light travels 1.333 times as fast in a vacuum as it does in water at this temperature.

Like density, the refractive index is an intensive physical property of matter and characterizes a substance. However, any procedure used to determine a substance's refractive index must be performed under carefully controlled temperature and lighting conditions because the refractive index of a substance varies with its temperature and the wavelength of light passing through it. Nearly all tabulated refractive indices are determined at a standard wavelength, usually 589.3 nanometers; this is the predominant wavelength emitted by sodium light and is commonly known as the sodium D light.

COMPARING REFRACTIVE INDICES When a transparent solid is immersed in a liquid with a similar refractive index, light is not refracted as it passes from the liquid into the solid. For this reason, the eye cannot distinguish the liquid–solid boundary, and the solid seems to disappear from view. This observation, as we will see, offers the forensic scientist a simple method for comparing the refractive indices of transparent solids.

Normally, we expect a solid or a liquid to exhibit only one refractive index value for each wavelength of light; however, many crystalline solids have two refractive indices whose values depend in part on the direction in which the light enters the crystal with respect to the crystal axis. **Crystalline solids have definite geometric forms because of the orderly arrangement of the fundamental particle of a solid, the atom.** In any type of crystal, the relative locations and distances between its atoms are repetitive throughout the solid. Figure 10–4 shows the crystalline structure of sodium chloride, or ordinary table salt. Sodium chloride is an example of a cubic crystal in which each sodium atom is surrounded by six chloride atoms and each chloride atom by six sodium atoms, except at the crystal surface. Not all solids are crystalline in nature; some, such as glass, have their atoms arranged randomly throughout the solid; these materials are known as **amorphous solids**.

Most crystals, excluding those that have cubic configurations, refract a beam of light into two different light-ray components. This phenomenon, known as *double refraction*, can be observed by studying the behavior of the crystal calcite. When the calcite is laid on a printed page, the observer sees not one but two images of each word covered. The two light rays that give rise to the double image are refracted at different angles, and each has a different refractive index value. The indices of refraction for calcite are 1.486 and 1.658, and subtracting the two values yields a difference of 0.172; this difference is known as **birefringence**. Thus, the optical properties of crystals provide points of identification that help characterize them.

FIGURE 10–4

Diagram of a sodium chloride crystal. Sodium is represented by the darker spheres, chlorine by the lighter spheres.

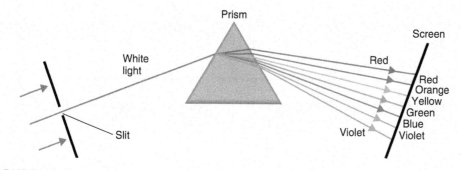

FIGURE 10–5
Representation of the dispersion of light by a glass prism.

DISPERSION   Many of us have held a glass prism up toward the sunlight and watched it transform light into the colors of the rainbow. This observation demonstrates that visible "white light" is not homogeneous but is actually composed of many different colors. The process of separating light into its component colors is called **dispersion**. The ability of a prism to disperse light into its component colors is explained by the property of refraction. Each color component of light, on passing through the glass, is slowed to a speed slightly different from those of the others, causing each component to bend at a different angle as it emerges from the prism. As shown in Figure 10–5, the component colors of visible light extend from red to violet. Dispersion thus separates light into its component wavelengths and demonstrates that glass has a slightly different index of refraction for each wavelength of light passing through it.

We have already seen that when white light passes through a glass prism, it is dispersed into a continuous spectrum of colors. This phenomenon demonstrates that white light is not homogeneous but is actually composed of a range of colors that extends from red through violet. Similarly, the observation that a substance has a color is also consistent with this description of white light. For example, when light passes through a red glass, the glass absorbs all the component colors of light except red, which passes through or is transmitted by the glass. Likewise, one can determine the color of an opaque object by observing its ability to absorb some of the component colors of light while reflecting others back to the eye. Color is thus a visual indication that objects absorb certain portions of **visible light** and transmit or reflect others. Scientists have long recognized this phenomenon and have learned to characterize different chemical substances by the type and quantity of light they absorb.

amorphous solid
A solid in which the constituent atoms or molecules are arranged in random or disordered positions; there is no regular order in amorphous solids.

birefringence
A difference in the two indices of refraction exhibited by most crystalline materials.

dispersion
The separation of light into its component wavelengths.

visible light
Colored light ranging from red to violet in the electromagnetic spectrum.

Theory of Light

To understand why materials absorb light, one must first comprehend the nature of light. Two simple models explain light's behavior. The first model describes light as a continuous wave; the second depicts it as a stream of discrete energy particles. Together, these two very different descriptions explain all of the observed properties of light, but by itself, no one model can explain all the facets of the behavior of light.

LIGHT AS A WAVE   The wave concept depicts light as having an up-and-down motion of a continuous wave, as shown in Figure 10–6. Several terms are used to describe such a wave. The distance between two consecutive crests (or one trough to the next trough) is called the **wavelength**; the Greek letter *lambda* (λ) is used as its symbol, and the unit of nanometers is frequently used to express its value. The number of crests (or troughs) passing any one given point in a unit of time is defined as the **frequency** of the wave. Frequency is normally designated by the letter F and is expressed in cycles per second (cps). The speed of light in a vacuum is a universal constant at 300 million meters per second and is designated by the symbol c. Frequency and wavelength are inversely proportional to one another, as shown by the relationship expressed in Equation (10–3):

wavelength
The distance between crests of adjacent waves.

frequency
The number of waves that pass a given point per second.

$$F = \frac{c}{\lambda}$$

(10–3)

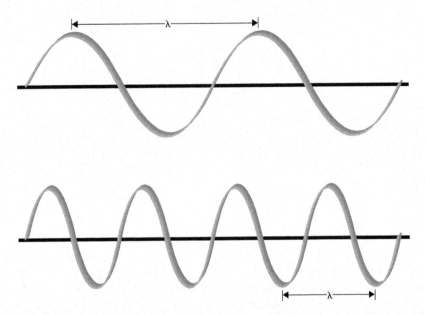

FIGURE 10–6

The frequency of the lower wave is twice that of the upper wave.

electromagnetic spectrum
The entire range of radiation energy from the most energetic cosmic rays to the least energetic radio waves.

X-ray
A high-energy, short-wavelength form of electromagnetic radiation.

laser
An acronym for *light amplification by stimulated emission of radiation*; light that has all its waves pulsating in unison.

THE ELECTROMAGNETIC SPECTRUM Actually, visible light is only a small part of a large family of radiation waves known as the **electromagnetic spectrum**. All electromagnetic waves travel at the speed of light (c) and are distinguishable from one another only by their different wavelengths or frequencies. Figure 10–7 illustrates the various types of electromagnetic waves in order of decreasing frequency. Hence, the only property that distinguishes **X-rays** from radio waves is the different frequencies the two types of waves possess. Similarly, the range of colors that make up the visible spectrum can be correlated with frequency. For instance, the lowest frequencies of visible light are red; waves with a lower frequency fall into the invisible infrared (IR) region. The highest frequencies of visible light are violet; waves with a higher frequency extend into the invisible ultraviolet (UV) region. No definite boundaries exist between any colors or regions of the electromagnetic spectrum; instead, each region is composed of a continuous range of frequencies, each blending into the other.

Ordinarily, light in any region of the electromagnetic spectrum is a collection of waves possessing a range of wavelengths. Under normal circumstances, this light comprises waves that are all out of step with each other (incoherent light). However, scientists can now produce a beam of light that has all of its waves pulsating in unison (see Figure 10–8). This is called *coherent light* or a **laser** (*light amplification by stimulated emission of radiation*) beam. Light in this form is very intense and can be focused on a very small area. Laser beams can be focused to pinpoints that are so intense that they can zap microscopic holes in a diamond.

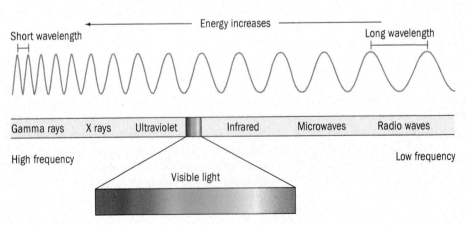

FIGURE 10–7

The electromagnetic spectrum.

LIGHT AS A PARTICLE   As long as electromagnetic radiation is moving through space, its behavior can be described as that of a continuous wave; however, once radiation is absorbed by a substance, the model of light as a stream of discrete particles must be invoked to best describe its behavior. Here, light is depicted as consisting of energy particles that are known as **photons**. Each photon has a definite amount of energy associated with its behavior. This energy is related to the frequency of light, as shown by Equation (10–4):

$$E = hf \qquad (10\text{–}4)$$

where E specifies the energy of the photon, f is the frequency of radiation, and h is a universal constant called Planck's constant. As shown by Equation (10–4), the energy of a photon is directly proportional to its frequency. Therefore, the photons of ultraviolet light will be more energetic than the photons of visible or infrared light, and exposure to the more energetic photons of X-rays presents more danger to human health than exposure to the photons of radio waves.

Now that we have investigated various physical properties of objects, we are ready to apply such properties to the forensic characterization of glass.

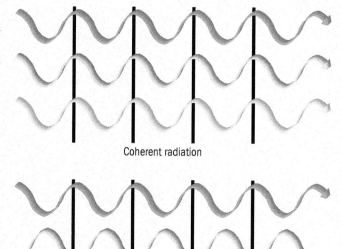

Coherent radiation

Incoherent radiation

FIGURE 10–8
Coherent and incoherent radiation.

Forensic Analysis of Glass

Glass that is broken and shattered into fragments and minute particles during the commission of a crime can be used to place a suspect at the crime scene. For example, chips of broken glass from a window may lodge in a suspect's shoes or garments during a burglary, or particles of headlight glass found at the scene of a hit-and-run accident may offer clues that can confirm the identity of a suspect vehicle. All of these possibilities require the comparison of glass fragments found on the suspect, whether a person or vehicle, with the shattered glass remaining at the crime scene.

Composition of Glass

Glass is a hard, brittle, amorphous substance composed of sand (silicon oxides) mixed with various metal oxides. When sand is mixed with other metal oxides, melted at high temperatures, and then cooled to a rigid condition without crystallization, the product is glass. Soda (sodium carbonate) is normally added to the sand to lower its melting point and make it easier to work with. Another necessary ingredient is lime (calcium oxide), needed to prevent the "soda-lime" glass from dissolving in water. The forensic scientist is often asked to analyze soda-lime glass, which is used for manufacturing most window and bottle glass. Often the molten glass is cooled on a bed of molten tin. This manufacturing process produces flat glass typically used for windows. This type of glass is called *float glass*.

The common metal oxides found in soda-lime glass are sodium, calcium, magnesium, and aluminum. In addition, a wide variety of special glasses can be made by substituting in whole or in part other metal oxides for the silica, sodium, and calcium oxides. For example, automobile headlights and heat-resistant glass, such as Pyrex, are manufactured by adding boron oxide to the oxide mix. These glasses are therefore known as *borosilicates*.

Another type of glass that the reader may be familiar with is **tempered glass**. This glass is made stronger than ordinary window glass by introducing stress through rapid heating and cooling of the glass surfaces. When tempered glass breaks, it does not shatter but rather fragments or "dices" into small squares with little splintering (see Figure 10–9). Because of this safety feature, tempered glass is used in the side and rear windows of automobiles made in the United States, as well as in the windshields of some foreign-made cars. The windshields of all cars manufactured in the United States are constructed from **laminated glass**. This glass derives its strength by sandwiching one layer of plastic between two pieces of ordinary window glass.

photon
A small packet of electromagnetic radiation energy; each photon contains a unit of energy equal to the product of Planck's constant and the frequency of radiation: $E = hf$

tempered glass
Glass that is strengthened by introducing stress through rapid heating and cooling of the glass surfaces.

laminated glass
Two sheets of ordinary glass bonded together with a layer of plastic.

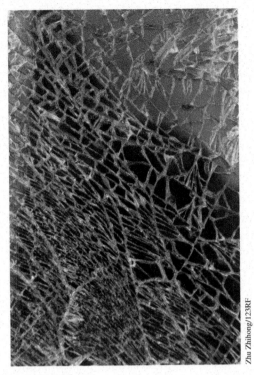

Zhu Zhihong/123RF

FIGURE 10-9
When tempered glass breaks, it usually holds together without splintering.

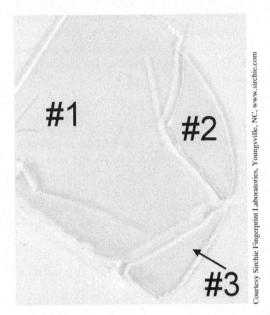

Courtesy Sirchie Fingerprint Laboratories, Youngsville, NC, www.sirchie.com

FIGURE 10-10
Match of broken glass. Note the physical fit of the edges.

Comparing Glass Fragments

For the forensic scientist, comparing glass consists of finding and measuring the properties that will associate one glass fragment with another while minimizing or eliminating the possible existence of other sources. Considering the prevalence of glass in our society, it is easy to appreciate the magnitude of this analytical problem. Obviously, glass possesses its greatest evidential value when it can be individualized to one source. Such a determination, however, can be made only when the suspect and crime-scene fragments are assembled and physically fitted together. Comparisons of this type require piecing together irregular edges of broken glass as well as matching all irregularities and striations on the broken surfaces (see Figure 10–10). The possibility that two pieces of glass originating from different sources will fit together exactly is so unlikely as to exclude all other sources from practical consideration.

Unfortunately, most glass evidence is either too fragmentary or too minute to permit a comparison of this type. In such instances, the search for individual properties has proven fruitless. For example, the general chemical composition of various window glasses within the capability of current analytical methods has so far been found relatively uniform among various manufacturers and thus offers no basis for individualization. However, as discussed in Chapter 14, trace elements present in glass have been shown to be useful for narrowing the origin of a glass specimen. **The physical properties of density and refractive index are most widely used for characterizing glass particles.** However, these properties are class characteristics, which cannot provide the sole criteria for individualizing glass to a common source. They do, however, give the analyst sufficient data to evaluate the significance of a glass comparison, and the absence of comparable density and refractive index values will certainly exclude glass fragments that originate from different sources.

Measuring and Comparing Density

Recall that a solid particle will float, sink, or remain suspended in a liquid, depending on its density relative to the liquid. This knowledge gives the criminalist a rather precise and rapid method for comparing densities of glass. In a method known as *flotation*, a standard/reference glass particle is immersed in a liquid; a mixture of bromoform and bromobenzene may be used. The composition of the liquid is carefully adjusted by the addition of small amounts of bromoform or bromobenzene until the glass chip remains suspended in the liquid medium. At this point, the standard/reference glass and liquid each have the same density. Glass chips of approximately the same size and shape as the standard/reference are now added to the liquid for comparison. If both the unknown and the standard/reference particles remain suspended in the liquid, their densities are equal to each other and to that of the liquid.[1] Particles of different densities either sink or float, depending on whether they are more or less dense than the liquid.

The density of a single sheet of window glass is not completely homogeneous throughout. It has a range of values that can differ by as much as 0.0003 g/mL. Therefore, in order to distinguish between the normal internal density variations of a single sheet of glass and those of glasses of different origins, it is advisable to let the comparative density approach but not exceed a sensitivity value of 0.0003 g/mL. The flotation method meets this requirement and can adequately distinguish glass particles that differ in density by 0.001 g/mL.

Determining and Comparing Refractive Index

Once glass has been distinguished by a density determination, different origins are immediately concluded. Comparable density results, however, require the added comparison of refractive indices. This determination is best accomplished by the *immersion method*. For this, glass particles are immersed in a liquid medium whose refractive index is adjusted until it equals that of the glass particles. At this point, known as the *match point*, the observer notes the disappearance of the **Becke line** and minimum contrast between the glass and liquid medium. The Becke line is a bright halo that is observed near the border of a particle that is immersed in a liquid of a different refractive index. This halo disappears when the medium and fragment have similar refractive indices.

The refractive index of an immersion fluid is best adjusted by changing the temperature of the liquid. Temperature control is, of course, critical to the success of the procedure. One approach to this procedure is to heat the liquid in a special apparatus known as a *hot stage*. The glass is immersed in a liquid, usually a silicone oil, and heated at the rate of 0.2°C per minute until the match point is reached. Increasing the temperature of the liquid has a negligible effect on the refractive index of glass, whereas the liquid's index decreases at the rate of approximately 0.0004 per degree Celsius. The hot stage, as shown in Figure 10–11, is designed to be used in conjunction with a microscope, through which

Becke line
A bright halo that is observed near the border of a particle immersed in a liquid of a different refractive index.

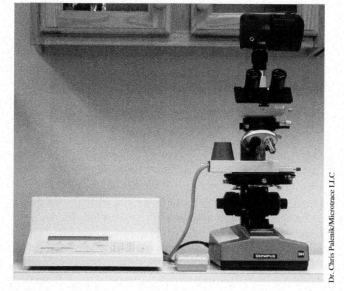

FIGURE 10–11
Hot-stage microscope.

---

[1] As an added step, the analyst can determine the exact numerical density value of the particles of glass by transferring the liquid to a density meter, which will electrically measure and calculate the liquid's density. See A. P. Beveridge and C. Semen, "Glass Density Measurement Using a Calculating Digital Density Meter," *Canadian Society of Forensic Science Journal* 12 (1979): 113.

FIGURE 10–12

Determination of the refractive index of glass. (a) Glass particles are immersed in a liquid of a much higher refractive index at a temperature of 20°C. (b) At 68°C the liquid still has a higher refractive index than the glass. (c) The refractive index of the liquid is closest to that of the glass at 100°C, as shown by the disappearance of the glass and the Becke lines. (d) At the higher temperature of 160°C, the liquid has a much lower index than the glass, resulting in significant edge contrast. The reference glass fragments shown here have a refractive index of 1.529.

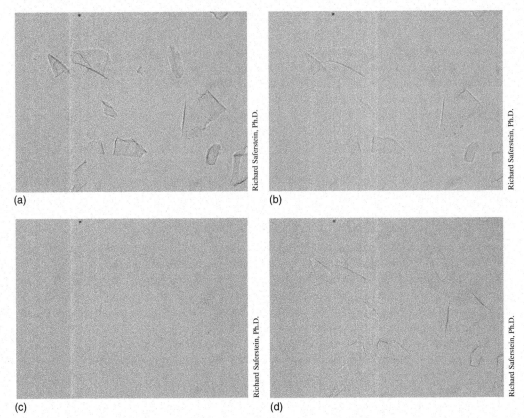

(a)   (b)   (c)   (d)

Richard Saferstein, Ph.D.

the examiner can observe the disappearance of the Becke line on minute glass particles that are illuminated with sodium D light or other wavelengths of light. If all the glass fragments examined have similar match points, it can be concluded that they have comparable refractive indices (see Figure 10–12). Furthermore, the examiner can determine the refractive index value of the immersion fluid as it changes with temperature. With this information, the exact numerical value of the glass refractive index can be calculated at the match point temperature.[2]

As with density, glass fragments removed from a single sheet of plate glass may not have a uniform refractive index value; instead, their values may vary by as much as 0.0002. Hence, for comparison purposes, the difference in refractive index between a standard/reference and questioned glass must exceed this value. This allows the examiner to differentiate between the normal internal variations present in a sheet of glass and those present in glasses that originated from completely different sources.

Classification of Glass Samples

A significant difference in either density or refractive index proves that the glasses examined do not have a common origin. But what if two pieces of glass exhibit comparable densities and comparable refractive indices? How certain can one be that they did, indeed, come from the same source? After all, there are untold millions of windows and other glass objects in this world. To provide a reasonable answer to this question, the FBI Laboratory has collected density and refractive index values from glass submitted to it for examination. What has emerged is a data bank correlating these values to their frequency of occurrence in the glass population of the United States. This collection is available to all forensic laboratories in the United States.

[2] A. R. Cassista and P. M. L. Sandercock, "Precision of Glass Refractive Index Measurements: Temperature Variation and Double Variation Methods, and the Value of Dispersion," *Canadian Society of Forensic Science Journal* 27 (1994): 203.

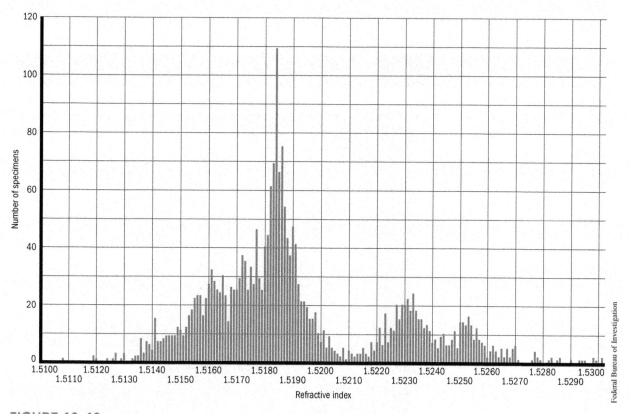

FIGURE 10–13

Frequency of occurrence of refractive index values (measured with sodium D light) for approximately 2,000 flat glass specimens received by the FBI Laboratory.

Once a criminalist has completed a comparison of glass fragments, the criminalist can correlate their density and refractive index values to their frequency of occurrence and assess probability that the fragments came from the same source. Figure 10–13 shows the distribution of refractive index values (measured with sodium D light) for approximately 2,000 glasses analyzed by the FBI. The wide distribution of values clearly demonstrates that the refractive index is a highly distinctive property of glass and is thus useful for defining its frequency of occurrence and hence its evidential value. For example, a glass fragment with a refractive index value of 1.5290 is found in approximately only 1 out of 2,000 specimens, whereas glass with a value of 1.5180 occurs approximately in 22 glasses out of 2,000.

Although refractive index and density have been routinely used for the comparison of glass for some time, forensic scientists have long desired to extract additional information from glass fragments that would make their comparison more meaningful. The trace elemental composition of glass held a longtime attraction to forensic scientists for this purpose. However, until recently, the analytical instrumentation sensitive enough to develop a trace elemental profile from a glass fragment was too costly for most crime laboratories. This handicap has been overcome with the introduction of a technique that aims a high-energy laser pulse to vaporize a microscopic amount of glass, raising its temperature by thousands of degrees. As a result, the elements present in the glass are induced to emit light whose wavelengths correspond to the identity of the elements present (see Figure 10–14).

The distinction between tempered and nontempered glass particles can be made by slowly heating and then cooling the glass (a process known as *annealing*). The change in the refractive index value for tempered glass upon annealing is significantly greater when compared to nontempered glass and thus serves as a point of distinction.[3]

[3] G. Edmondstone, "The Identification of Heat Strengthened Glass in Windshields," *Canadian Society of Forensic Science Journal* 30 (1997): 181.

Inside the Science

GRIM 3

An automated approach for measuring the refractive index of glass fragments by temperature control using the immersion method with a hot stage is with the instrument known as GRIM 3 (glass refractive index measurement) (see the figure). The GRIM 3 is a personal computer/video system designed to automate the measurements of the match temperature and refractive index for glass fragments. This instrument uses a video camera to view the glass fragments as they are being heated. As the immersion oil is heated or cooled, the contrast of the video image is measured continually until a minimum, the match point, is detected (see figure). The match point temperature is then converted to a refractive index using stored calibration data.

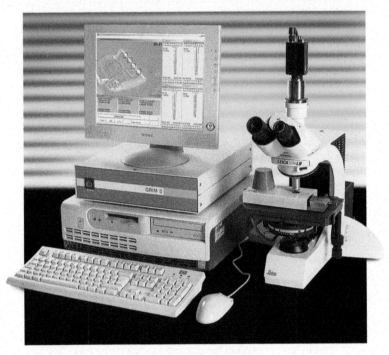

An automated system for glass fragment identification.

GRIM 3 identifies the refraction match point by monitoring a video image of four different areas of the glass fragment immersed in an oil. As the immersion oil is heated or cooled, the contrast of the image is measured continuously until a minimum, the match point, is detected.

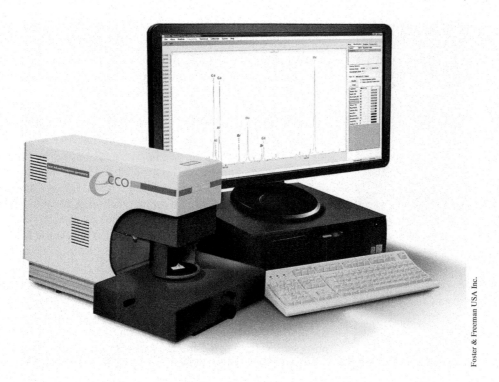

Foster & Freeman USA Inc.

FIGURE 10–14
The elemental profile of a glass fragment is obtained by aiming a high-energy laser beam at a glass particle, inducing the emission of light wavelengths corresponding to the identity of the elements present in the glass.

Glass Fractures

Glass bends in response to any force exerted on any one of its surfaces; when the limit of its elasticity is reached, the glass fractures. Frequently, fractured window glass reveals information that can be related to the force and direction of an impact; such knowledge may be useful for reconstructing events at a crime-scene investigation.

The penetration of ordinary window glass by a projectile, whether a bullet or a stone, produces a familiar fracture pattern in which cracks both radiate outward and encircle the hole, as shown in Figure 10–15. The radiating lines are appropriately known as **radial fractures**, and the circular lines are termed **concentric fractures**.

Often it is difficult to determine just from the size and shape of a hole in glass whether it was made by a bullet or by some other projectile. For instance, a small stone thrown at a comparatively high speed against a pane of glass often produces a hole similar to that produced by a bullet. On the other hand, a large stone can completely shatter a pane of glass in a manner closely resembling the result of a close-range shot. However, in the latter instance, the presence of gunpowder deposits on the shattered glass fragments points to damage caused by a firearm.

When it penetrates glass, a high-velocity projectile such as a bullet often leaves a round, crater-shaped hole surrounded by a nearly symmetrical pattern of radial and concentric cracks. The hole is inevitably wider on the exit side (see Figure 10–16), and hence examining it is an important step in determining the direction of impact. However, as the velocity of the penetrating projectile decreases, the irregularity of the shape of the hole and of its surrounding cracks increases, so that at some point the hole shape will not help determine the direction of impact. At this time, examining the radial and concentric fracture lines may help determine the direction of impact.

When a force pushes on one side of a pane of glass, the elasticity of the glass permits it to bend in the direction of the force applied. Once the elastic limit is exceeded, the glass begins to crack. As shown in Figure 10–17, the first fractures form on the surface opposite that of the penetrating force and develop

radial fracture
A crack in a glass that extends outward like the spoke of a wheel from the point at which the glass was struck.

concentric fracture
A crack in a glass that forms a rough circle around the point of impact.

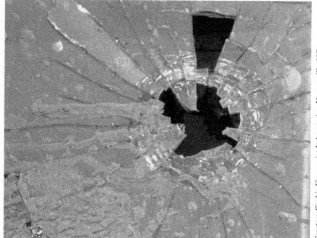

Courtesy Sirchie Fingerprint Laboratories, Youngsville, NC, www.sirchie.com

FIGURE 10–15
Radial and concentric fracture lines in a sheet of glass.

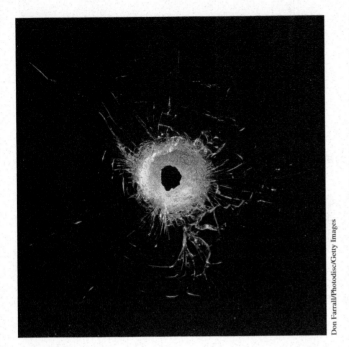

Don Farrall/Photodisc/Getty Images

FIGURE 10–16
Crater-shaped hole made by a bullet passing through glass. The upper surface is the exit side of the projectile.

into radial lines. The continued motion of the force places tension on the front surface of the glass, resulting in the formation of concentric cracks. An examination of the edges of the radial and concentric cracks frequently reveals stress markings (*Wallner lines*) whose shape can be related to the side on which the window first cracked.

Stress marks, shown in Figure 10–18, are shaped like arches that are perpendicular to one glass surface and curved nearly parallel to the opposite surface. The importance of stress marks stems from the observation that the perpendicular edge always faces the surface on which the crack originated. Thus, in examining the stress marks on the edge of a radial crack near the point of impact, the perpendicular end is always found opposite the side from which the force of impact was applied. For a concentric fracture, the perpendicular end always faces the surface on which the force originated. A convenient way for remembering these observations is the 3R rule—**Radial cracks form a *R*ight angle on the *R*everse side of the force.** These facts enable the examiner to determine the side on which a window was broken. Unfortunately, the absence of radial or concentric fracture lines prevents these observations from being applied to broken tempered glass.

When there have been successive penetrations of glass, it is frequently possible to determine the sequence of impact by observing the existing fracture lines and their points of termination. **A fracture always terminates at an existing line of fracture.** In Figure 10–19, the fracture on the left preceded that on the right; we know this because the latter's radial fracture lines terminate at the cracks of the former.

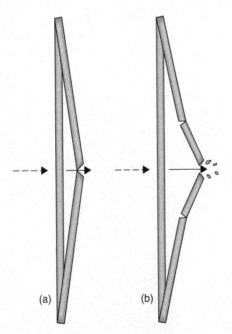

(a)   (b)

FIGURE 10–17
Production of radial and concentric fractures in glass. (a) Radial cracks are formed first, commencing on the side of the glass opposite to the destructive force. (b) Concentric cracks occur afterward, starting on the same side as the force.

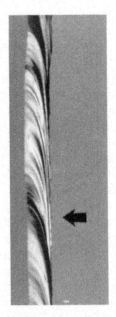

Richard Saferstein, Ph.D.

FIGURE 10–18
Stress marks on the edge of a radial glass fracture. Arrow indicates direction of force.

Collection and Preservation of Glass Evidence

The gathering of glass evidence at the crime scene and from the suspect must be thorough if the examiner is to have any chance of individualizing the fragments to a common source. If even the remotest possibility exists that fragments may be pieced together, every effort must be made to collect all the glass found. For example, evidence collection at hit-and-run scenes must include all the broken parts of the headlight and reflector lenses. This evidence may ultimately prove invaluable in placing a suspect vehicle at the accident scene by matching the fragments with glass remaining in the headlight or reflector shell of the suspect vehicle. In addition, examining the headlight's filaments may reveal whether an automobile's headlights were on or off before the impact (see Figure 10–20).

When an individual fit is improbable, the evidence collector must submit all glass evidence found in the possession of the suspect along with a sample of broken glass remaining at the crime scene. This standard/reference glass should always be taken from any remaining glass in the window or door frames, as close as possible to the point of breakage. About one square inch of sample is usually adequate for this purpose. The glass fragments should be packaged in solid containers to avoid further breakage. If the suspect's shoes and/or clothing are to be examined for the presence of glass fragments, they should be individually wrapped in paper and transmitted to the laboratory. The field investigator should avoid removing such evidence from garments unless absolutely necessary for its preservation.

When a determination of the direction of impact is desired, all broken glass must be recovered and submitted for analysis. Wherever possible, the exterior and interior surfaces of the glass must be indicated. When this is not immediately apparent, the presence of dirt, paint, grease, or putty may indicate the exterior surface of the glass.

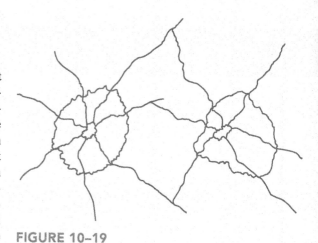

FIGURE 10–19
Two bullet holes in a piece of glass. The left hole preceded the right hole.

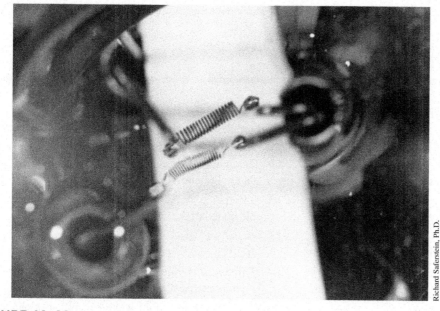

Richard Saferstein, Ph.D.

FIGURE 10–20
Presence of black tungsten oxide on the upper filament indicates that the filament was on when it was exposed to air. The lower filament was off, but its surface was coated with a yellow/white tungsten oxide, which was vaporized from the upper ("on") filament and condensed onto the lower filament.

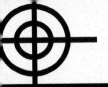
The forensic scientist must constantly determine the properties that impart distinguishing characteristics to matter, giving it a unique identity. Physical properties such as weight, volume, color, boiling point, and melting point describe a substance without reference to any other substance. A chemical property describes the behavior of a substance when it reacts or combines with another substance. Scientists throughout the world use the metric system of measurement. The metric system has basic units of measurement for length, mass, and volume: the meter, gram, and liter, respectively. Temperature is a measure of heat intensity, or the amount of heat in a substance. In science, the most commonly used temperature scale is the Celsius scale. This scale is derived by assigning the freezing point of water a value of 0°C and its boiling point a value of 100°C.

To compare glass fragments, a forensic scientist evaluates two important physical properties: density and refractive index. Density is defined as the mass per unit volume. Refractive index is the ratio of the velocity of light in a vacuum to that in the medium under examination. Crystalline solids have definite geometric forms because of the orderly arrangement of their atoms. These solids refract a beam of light in two different light-ray components. This results in double refraction. Birefringence is the numerical difference between these two refractive indices. Not all solids are crystalline in nature. For example, glass has a random arrangement of atoms that forms an amorphous or noncrystalline solid.

Dispersion is the process of separating light into its component colors. Each component bends, or refracts, at a different angle as it emerges from a prism. The large family of radiation waves is known as the electromagnetic spectrum. Two simple models explain light's behavior. The first model describes light as a continuous wave; the second depicts light as a stream of energy particles.

The flotation and immersion methods are best used to determine a glass fragment's density and refractive index, respectively. In the flotation method, a glass particle is immersed in a liquid. The density of the liquid is carefully adjusted by the addition of small amounts of an appropriate liquid until the glass chip remains suspended in the liquid medium. At this point, the glass will have the same density as the liquid medium and can be compared to other relevant pieces of glass. The immersion method involves immersing a glass particle in a liquid medium whose refractive index is varied until it is equal to that of the glass particle. At this point, known as the match point, minimum contrast between liquid and particle is observed.

By analyzing the radial and concentric fracture patterns in glass, the forensic scientist can determine the direction of impact. This can be accomplished by applying the 3R rule: *R*adial cracks form a *R*ight angle on the *R*everse side of the force.

The glass fragments should be packaged in solid containers to avoid further breakage. If the suspect's shoes and/or clothing are to be examined for the presence of glass fragments, they should be individually wrapped in paper and transmitted to the laboratory. The field investigator should avoid removing such evidence from garments unless absolutely necessary for its preservation.

Review Questions

1. Anything that has mass and occupies space is defined as _____.

2. The basic building blocks of all substances are the _____.

3. The number of elements known today is _____.

4. An arrangement of elements by similar chemical properties is accomplished in the _____ table.

5. A(n) _____ is the smallest particle of an element that can exist.

6. Substances composed of two or more elements are called _____.

7. A(n) _____ is the smallest unit of a compound formed by the union of two or more atoms.

8. The physical state that retains a definite shape and volume is a(n) _____.

9. A gas (has, has no) definite shape or volume.

10. During the process of _____, solids go directly to the gaseous state, bypassing the liquid state.

11. The attraction forces between the molecules of a liquid are (greater, less) than those in a solid.

12. Different _____ are separated by definite visible boundaries.

13. Mass per unit volume defines the property of _____.

14. If an object is immersed in a liquid of greater density, it will (sink, float).

15. The bending of a light wave because of a change in velocity is called _____.

16. The physical property of _____ is determined by the ratio of the velocity of light in a vacuum to light's velocity in a substance.

17. True or False: Solids having an orderly arrangement of their constituent atoms are crystalline. _____

18. Solids that have their atoms randomly arranged are said to be _____.

19. The crystal calcite has two indices of refraction. The difference between these two values is known as _____.

20. The process of separating light into its component colors or frequencies is known as _____.

21. True or False: Color is a usual indication that substances selectively absorb light. _____

22. The distance between two successive identical points on a wave is known as _____.

23. True or False: Frequency and wavelength are directly proportional to one another. _____

24. Light, X-rays, and radio waves are all members of the _____ spectrum.

25. Red light is (higher, lower) in frequency than violet light.

26. A beam of light that has all of its waves pulsating in unison is called a(n) _____.

27. One model of light depicts it as consisting of energy particles known as _____.

28. True or False: The energy of a light particle (photon) is directly proportional to its frequency. _____

29. Red light is (more, less) energetic than violet light.

30. A hard, brittle, amorphous substance composed mainly of silicon oxides is _____.

31. Glass that can be physically pieced together has _____ characteristics.

32. The two most useful physical properties of glass for forensic comparisons are _____ and _____.

33. True or False: Automobile headlights and heat-resistant glass, such as Pyrex, are manufactured with lime oxide added to the oxide mix. _____

34. _____ glass fragments into small squares, or "dices," with little splintering when broken.

35. _____ glass gains added strength from a layer of plastic inserted between two pieces of ordinary window glass; it is used in automobile windshields.

36. Comparing the relative densities of glass fragments is readily accomplished by a method known as _____.

37. When glass is immersed in a liquid of similar refractive index, its _____ disappears and minimum contrast between the glass and liquid is observed.

38. The exact numerical density and refractive indices of glass can be correlated to _____ in order to assess the evidential value of the comparison.

39. The fracture lines radiating outward from a crack in glass are known as _____ fractures.

40. A crater-shaped hole in glass is (narrower, wider) on the side where the projectile entered the glass.

41. True or False: It is easy to determine from the size and shape of a hole in glass whether it was made by a bullet or some other projectile. _____

42. True or False: Stress marks on the edge of a radial crack are always perpendicular to the edge of the surface on which the impact force originated. _____

43. A fracture line (will, will not) terminate at an existing line fracture.

44. Glass fracture lines that encircle the hole in the glass are known as _____ fractures.

45. When glass's elastic limit is exceeded, the first fractures develop into radial lines on the surface of the (same, opposite) side to that of the penetrating force.

46. Collected glass fragment evidence should be packaged in _____ containers to avoid further breakage.

47. Glass-containing shoes and/or clothing should be individually wrapped in _____ and transmitted to the laboratory.

Review Questions for Inside the Science

1. A(n) _____ property describes the behavior of a substance without reference to any other substance.

2. A(n) _____ property describes the behavior of a substance when it reacts or combines with another substance.

3. The _____ system of measurement was devised by the French Academy of Science in 1791.

4. The basic units of measurement for length, mass, and volume in the metric system are the _____, _____, and _____, respectively.

5. A centigram is equivalent to _____ gram(s).

6. A milliliter is equivalent to _____ liter(s).

7. 0.2 gram is equivalent to _____ milligram(s).

8. One cubic centimeter (cc) is equivalent to one _____.

9. True or False: One meter is slightly longer than a yard. _____

10. The equivalent of 1 pound in grams is _____.

11. True or False: A liter is slightly larger than a quart. _____

12. _____ is a measure of a substance's heat intensity.

13. There are _____ degrees Fahrenheit between the freezing and boiling points of water.

14. There are _____ degrees Celsius between the freezing and boiling points of water.

15. The amount of matter an object contains determines its _____.

16. The simplest type of balance for weighing is the _____.

Application and Critical Thinking

1. An accident investigator arrives at the scene of a hit-and-run collision. The driver who remained at the scene reports that the windshield or a side window of the car that struck him shattered on impact. The investigator searches the accident site and collects a large number of fragments of tempered glass. This is the only type of glass recovered from the scene. How can the glass evidence help the investigator locate the vehicle that fled the scene?

2. Indicate the order in which the bullet holes were made in the glass depicted in the accompanying figure. Explain the reason for your answer.

3. The accompanying figure depicts stress marks on the edge of a glass fracture caused by the application of force. If this is a radial fracture, from which side of the glass (left or right) was the force applied? From which side was force applied if it is a concentric fracture? Explain the reason for your answers.

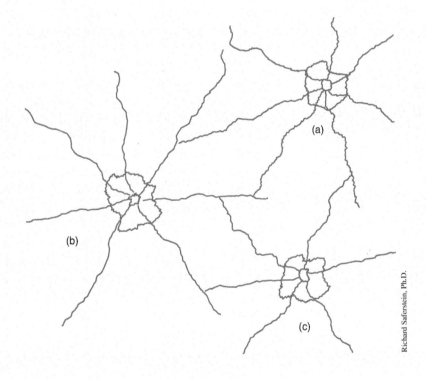

(a)

(b)

(c)

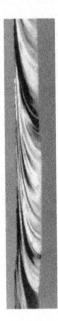

Richard Saferstein, Ph.D.

Further References

Bottrell, M. C., "Forensic Glass Comparison: Background Information Used in Data Interpretation," *Forensic Science Communications* 11, no. 2 (2009), https://www2.fbi.gov/hq/lab/fsc/backissu/april2009/index.htm.

Caddy, B., ed., *Forensic Examination of Glass and Paint.* Boca Raton, FL: CRC Press, 2001.

Koons, R. D., J. Buscaglia, M. Bottrell, and E. T. Miller, "Forensic Glass Comparisons," in R. Saferstein, ed., *Forensic Science Handbook*, vol. 1, 2nd ed. Upper Saddle River, NJ: Prentice Hall, 2002.

Thornton, J. I., "Interpretation of Physical Aspects of Glass Evidence," in B. Caddy, ed., *Forensic Examination of Glass and Paint.* Boca Raton, FL: CRC Press, 2001.

Hairs and Fibers

KEY TERMS

anagen phase
catagen phase
cortex
cuticle
follicular tag
macromolecule
manufactured fibers
medulla
mitochondrial DNA
molecule
monomer
natural fibers
nuclear DNA
polymer
telogen phase

Go to www.pearsonhighered.com/careersresources to access Webextras for this chapter.

Casey Anthony: A Single Hair

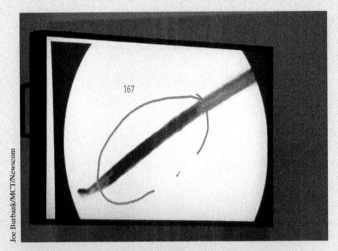

Joe Burbank/MCT/Newscom

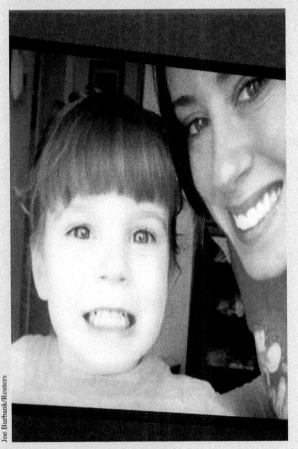

Joe Burbank/Reuters

On July 15, 2008, Caylee Anthony was reported missing by her maternal grandmother, Cindy Anthony, who said she had not seen Caylee for 31 days. After receiving varied explanations as to Caylee's whereabouts, Cindy began searching for the child herself. After retrieving her daughter Casey's car from the impound, she reported to police that it smelled like a dead body had been inside it. Once police were involved, it became clear that Casey Anthony was not being honest about what had happened to the young girl. After a lie about the child being taken by a nanny was quickly unraveled by police, Casey was arrested and charged with giving false statements to law enforcement, child neglect, and obstruction of a criminal investigation.

Caylee Anthony's body was recovered from a wooded area not far from the Anthony family home on December 11, 2008. The investigation into the disappearance of Caylee Anthony quickly turned into a murder investigation. Police examined Casey's car to ascertain whether or not the child had been placed in the trunk before her body had been dumped in the wooded area. They recovered one telling piece of evidence, a single hair was microscopically similar to that of Casey's daughter, Caylee. The hair was microscopically distinguishable from Casey's head hair. Mitochondrial DNA sequence analysis revealed similarity between the trunk hair, Caylee's hair, and Casey's hair, as one would expect from maternally inherited mitochondrial DNA.

An FBI analyst testified that the hair from the truck exhibited *root banding*, a phenomenon consistent with hair from a deceased individual's head. There was only one person who would have the Anthony mitochondrial DNA sequence who was recently deceased and suspected of being present in the trunk: Caylee. This hair was strong evidence that the child was in the trunk of her mother's car for a time before she was left in the wooded area where she was discovered five months later. It was proof that Casey Anthony knew more about the circumstances that led to Caylee's death than she previously led them to believe.

The trace evidence transferred between individuals and objects during the commission of a crime, if recovered, often corroborates other evidence developed during the course of an investigation. Although in most cases physical evidence cannot by itself positively identify a suspect, laboratory examination may narrow the origin of such evidence to a group that includes the suspect. Using many instruments and techniques, the crime laboratory has developed a variety of procedures for comparing and tracing the origins of physical evidence. This chapter and those that follow discuss how to apply these techniques to the analysis of the types of physical evidence most often encountered at crime scenes. We begin with a discussion of hairs and fibers.

Hair is encountered as physical evidence in a wide variety of crimes. However, any review of the forensic aspects of hair examination must start with the observation that it is not yet possible to individualize a human hair to any single head or body through its morphology. Over the years, criminalists have tried to isolate the physical and chemical properties of hair that could serve as individual characteristics of identity. Partial success has finally been achieved by isolating and characterizing the DNA present in hair.

The importance of hair as physical evidence cannot be underemphasized. Its removal from the body often denotes physical contact between a victim and perpetrator and hence a crime of a serious or violent nature. When hair is properly collected at the crime scene and submitted to the laboratory along with enough standard/reference samples, it can provide strong corroborative evidence for placing an individual at a crime site.

The first step in the forensic examination of hair logically starts with its color and structure, or morphology, and, if warranted, progresses to the more detailed DNA extraction, isolation, and characterization.

Morphology of Hair

Hair is an appendage of the skin that grows out of an organ known as the *hair follicle*. The length of a hair extends from its root or bulb embedded in the follicle, continues into the shaft, and terminates at the tip end. The shaft, which is composed of three layers—the **cuticle**, **cortex**, and **medulla**—is subjected to the most intense examination by the forensic scientist (see Figure 11–1).

cuticle
The scale structure covering the exterior of the hair.

cortex
The main body of the hair shaft.

medulla
A cellular column running through the center of the hair.

Cuticle

Two features that make hair a good subject for establishing individual identity are its resistance to chemical decomposition and its ability to retain structural features over a long period of time.

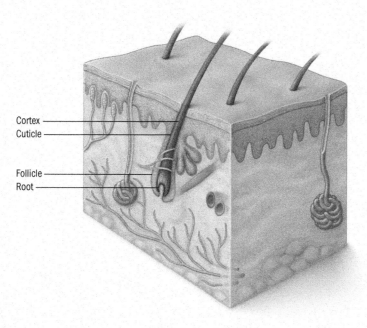

Cortex ——
Cuticle ——

Follicle ——
Root ——

FIGURE 11–1

Cross section of skin showing hair growing out of a tubelike structure called the follicle.

Much of this resistance and stability is attributed to the cuticle, the outside covering of the hair. The cuticle is formed by overlapping scales that always point toward the tip end of each hair. The scales form from specialized cells that have hardened (*keratinized*) and flattened in progressing from the follicle. There are three basic patterns that describe the appearance of the cuticle: coronal, spinous, and imbricate (see Figure 11–2).

The scales of most animal hair can best be described as looking like shingles on a roof. Although the scale pattern is not a useful characteristic for individualizing human hair, the variety of patterns formed by animal hair makes it an important feature for species identification. Figure 11–3 shows the scale patterns of some animal hairs and of a human hair as viewed by the scanning electron microscope. Another method of studying the scale pattern of hair is to make a cast of its surface. This is done by embedding the hair in a soft medium, such as clear nail polish or softened vinyl. When the medium has hardened, the hair is removed, leaving a clear, distinct impression of the hair's cuticle, ideal for examination with a compound microscope.

Cortex

Contained within the protective layer of the cuticle is the cortex. The cortex is made up of spindle-shaped cortical cells aligned in a regular array, parallel to the length of the hair. The cortex derives its major forensic importance from the fact that it is embedded with the pigment granules that give hair its color. The color, shape, and distribution of these granules provide important points of comparison among the hairs of different individuals.

The structural features of the cortex are examined microscopically after the hair has been mounted in a liquid medium with a refractive index close to that of the hair. Under these conditions, the amount of light reflected off the hair's surface is minimized, and the amount of light penetrating the hair is optimized.

Medulla

The medulla is a collection of cells that looks like a central canal running through a hair. In many animals, this canal is a predominant feature, occupying more than half of the hair's diameter. The *medullary index* measures the diameter of the medulla relative to the diameter of the hair shaft and is normally expressed as a fraction. For humans, the index is generally less than one-third; for most other animals, the index is one-half or greater.

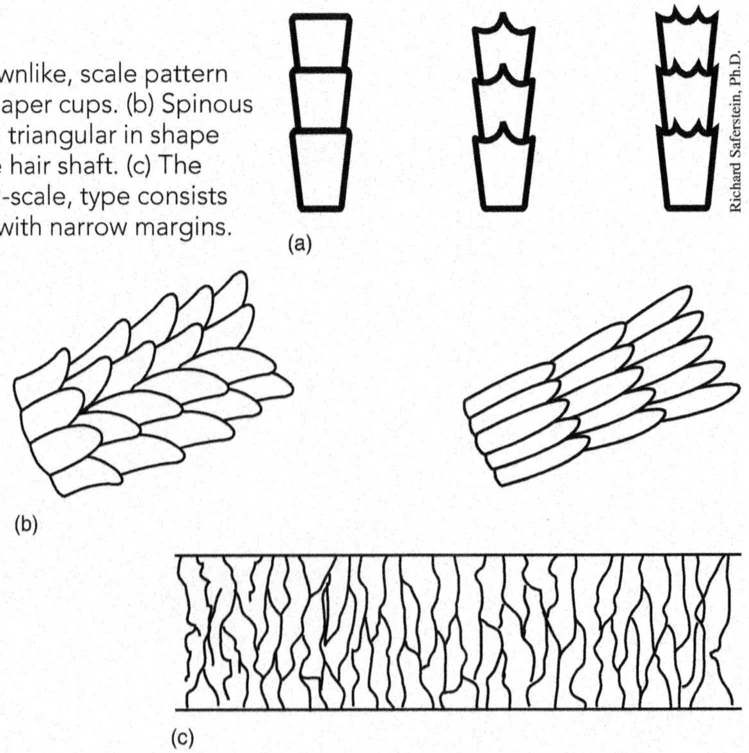

FIGURE 11–2

(a) The coronal, or crownlike, scale pattern resembles a stack of paper cups. (b) Spinous or petal-like scales are triangular in shape and protrude from the hair shaft. (c) The imbricate, or flattened-scale, type consists of overlapping scales with narrow margins.

(a)

(b)

(c)

Richard Saferstein, Ph.D.

FIGURE 11–3

Scale patterns of various types of hair. (a) Human head hair (600×), (b) dog (1250×), (c) deer (120×), (d) rabbit (300×), (e) cat (2000×), and (f) horse (450×).

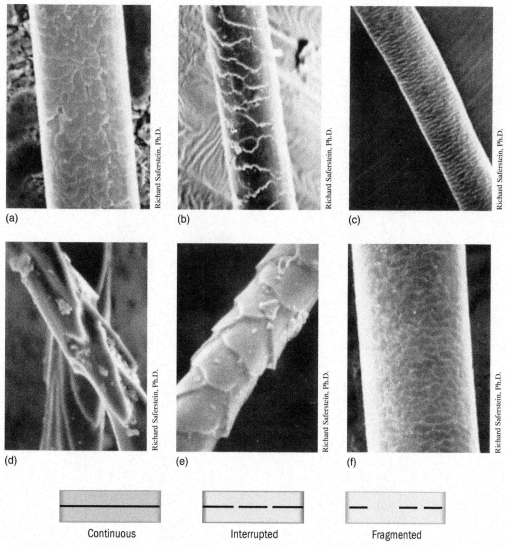

(a)   (b)   (c)

(d)   (e)   (f)

Richard Saferstein, Ph.D.

Continuous   Interrupted   Fragmented

FIGURE 11–4
Medulla patterns.

The presence and appearance of the medulla vary from individual to individual and even among the hairs of a given individual. Not all hairs have medullae, and when they do exist, the degree of medullation can vary. In this respect, medullae may be classified as being continuous, interrupted, fragmented, or absent (see Figure 11–4). Human head hairs generally exhibit no medullae or have fragmented ones; they rarely show continuous medullation. One noted exception is people of Asian ancestry, who usually have head hairs with continuous medullae. Also, most animals have medullae that are either continuous or interrupted.

Another interesting feature of the medulla is its shape. Humans, as well as many animals, have medullae that give a nearly cylindrical appearance. Other animals exhibit medullae that have a patterned shape. For example, the medulla of a cat can best be described as resembling a string of pearls, whereas members of the deer family show a medullary structure consisting of spherical cells occupying the entire hair shaft. Figure 11–5 illustrates medullary sizes and forms for a number of common animal hairs and a human head hair.

A searchable database on CD-ROM of the 35 most common animal hairs encountered in forensic casework is commercially available.[1] This database allows an examiner to rapidly

Hair Analysis Note

There are morphological characteristics of hair that have been linked to individuals with African, Asian, and European ancestry. Microscopic hair analysis is based on the evaluation of these class and individual characteristics. While not dispositive of race or ancestry of the donor, evaluations of the morphology are the basis for any forensic hair comparison..

anagen phase

The initial growth phase during which the hair follicle actively produces hair.

[1] J. D. Baker and D. L. Exline, *Forensic Animal Hair Atlas: A Searchable Database on CD-ROM*. RJ Lee Group, Inc., 350 Hochberg Rd., Monroeville, PA, 15,146.

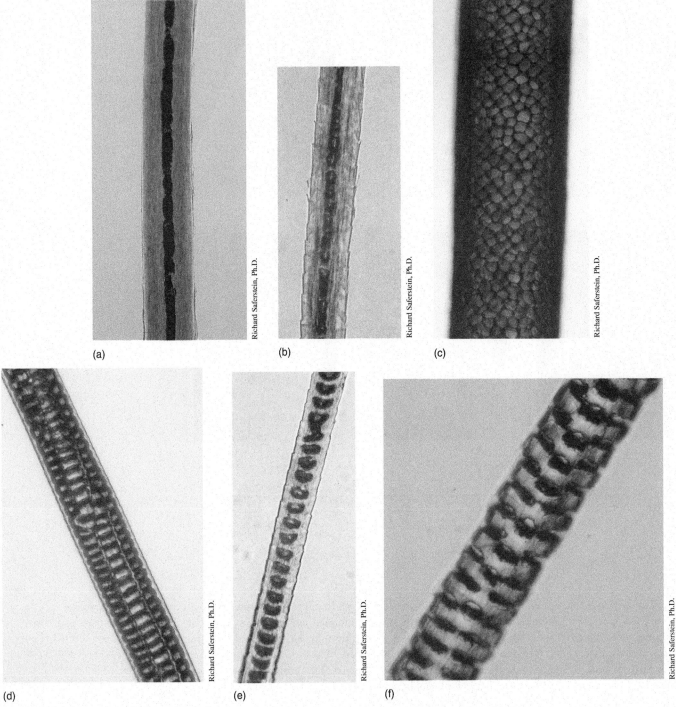

Richard Saferstein, Ph.D.

(a)   (b)   (c)

(d)   (e)   (f)

FIGURE 11–5

Medulla patterns for various types of hair. (a) Human head hair (400×), (b) dog (400×), (c) deer (500×), (d) rabbit (450×), (e) cat (400×), and (f) mouse (500×).

catagen phase

A transition stage between the anagen and telogen phases of hair growth.

telogen phase

The final growth phase in which hair naturally falls out of the skin.

search for animal hairs based on scale patterns and/or medulla type using a PC. A typical screen presentation arising from such a data search is shown in Figure 11–6.

Root

The root and other surrounding cells within the hair follicle provide the tools necessary to produce hair and continue its growth. Human head hair grows in three developmental stages, and the shape and size of the hair root is determined by the growth phase in which the hair happens to be. The three phases of hair growth are the **anagen**, **catagen**, and **telogen** phases.

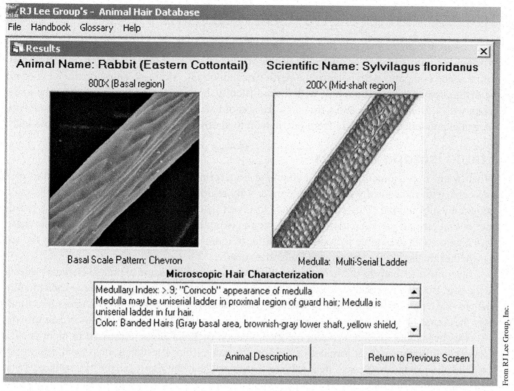

FIGURE 11–6
Information on rabbit hair contained within the Forensic Animal Hair Atlas.

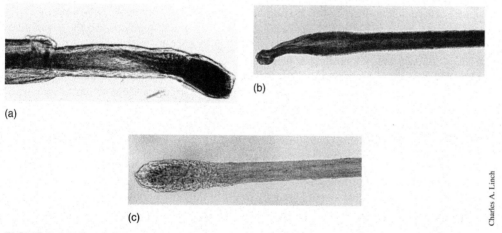

FIGURE 11–7
Hair roots in the (a) anagen phase, (b) catagen phase, and (c) telogen phase (100×).

In the anagen phase, which may last up to six years, the root is attached to the follicle for continued growth, giving the root bulb a flame-shaped appearance (Figure 11–7[a]). When pulled from the root, some hairs in the anagen phase have a **follicular tag**. With the advent of DNA analysis, this follicular tag is important for individualizing hair.

Hair continues to grow, but at a decreasing rate, during the catagen phase, which can last anywhere from two to three weeks. In the catagen phase, roots typically take on an elongated appearance (Figure 11–7[b]) as the root bulb shrinks and is pushed out of the hair follicle.

Once hair growth ends, the telogen phase begins and the root takes on a club-shaped appearance (Figure 11–7[c]). Over two to six months, the hair is pushed out of the follicle, causing the hair to be naturally shed.

follicular tag
A translucent piece of tissue surrounding the hair's shaft near the root; it contains the richest source of DNA associated with hair.

Identification and Comparison of Hair

Most often, the prime purpose for examining hair evidence in a crime laboratory is to establish whether the hair is human or animal in origin or to determine whether human hair retrieved at a crime scene compares with hair from a particular individual. Although animal hair can normally be distinguished from human hair with little difficulty, human hair comparisons must be undertaken with extreme caution and with an awareness of hair's tendency to exhibit variable morphological characteristics, not only from one person to another but also within a single individual.

Stable Isotope Analysis

When water is consumed, it leaves a chemical fingerprint in hair. Because people tend to drink and cook with their local water, which can vary by region, the signature left on the hair will be geographically unique. This can be helpful to investigators when they are faced with a murder victim that has not yet been identified. After exhausting all other avenues to identify the victim, investigators can use stable isotope information to indicate whether a person is local to the area or whether the body was transported there after death.

Scientists can analyze stable isotopes—different forms of the same chemical element—present in the hair. Because hair retains isotopic information, and grows about one centimeter each month, it can provide a personal chronology of where a person has been. If a person moves across the country over the course of a year, that movement will be reflected in the last 12 centimeters of hair growth.

This technology played a role in the identification of Bella Bond, discussed in more detail in Chapter 8. Investigators sent samples of her hair for stable isotope testing to help them determine if the child was local to the Boston area. After tests indicated that she was local, the Massachusetts State Police ramped up efforts to identify her by putting her image on billboards in the Boston metro area.

Considerations in Hair Examination

A careful microscopic examination of hair reveals morphological features that can distinguish human hair from animal hair. The hair of various animals also differs enough in structure that the examiner can often identify the species. Before reaching such a conclusion, however, the examiner must have access to a comprehensive collection of reference standards and the accumulated experience of hundreds of prior hair examinations. Scale structure, medullary index, and medullary shape are particularly important in hair identification.

The most common request when hair is used as forensic evidence is to determine whether hair recovered at the crime scene compares to hair removed from a suspect. In most cases, such a comparison relates to hair obtained from the scalp or pubic area. Ultimately, the evidential value of the comparison depends on the degree of probability with which the examiner can associate the hair in question with a particular individual.

HAIR CHARACTERISTICS   In making a hair comparison, a comparison microscope is an invaluable tool that allows the examiner to view the questioned and known hair together, side by side. Any variations in the microscopic characteristics will thus be readily observed. Because hair from any part of the body exhibits a range of characteristics, it is necessary to have an adequate number of known hairs that are representative of all of its features when making a comparison.

In comparing hair, the criminalist is particularly interested in the color, length, and diameter. Other important features are the presence or absence of a medulla and the distribution, shape, and color intensity of the pigment granules in the cortex. A microscopic examination may also distinguish dyed or bleached hair from natural hair. A dyed color is often present in the cuticle as well as throughout the cortex. Bleaching, on the other hand, tends to remove pigment from the hair and to give it a yellowish tint. If hair has grown since it was last bleached or dyed, the natural-end portion will be quite distinct in color. An estimate of the time since dyeing or bleaching can be made because *hair grows approximately one centimeter per month*. Other significant but less frequent features may be observed in hair. For example, morphological abnormalities may be present because of certain diseases or deficiencies. Also, the presence of fungal and nit infections can further link a hair specimen to a particular individual.

POTENTIAL FOR ERROR   Although microscopic comparison of hairs has long been accepted as an appropriate approach for including and excluding questioned hairs against standard/reference hairs, many forensic scientists have long recognized that this approach is subjective and is highly dependent on the skills and integrity of the analyst as well as the hair morphology being examined. However, until the advent of DNA analysis, the forensic science community had no choice but to rely on the microscope to carry out hair comparisons.

Any lingering doubts about the necessity of augmenting microscopic hair examinations with DNA analysis evaporated with the publication of an FBI study describing significant error rates associated with microscopic comparison of hairs.[2] Hair evidence submitted to the FBI for DNA analysis between 1996 and 2000 was examined both microscopically and by DNA analysis. Approximately 11 percent of the hairs (9 out of 80) in which FBI hair examiners found a positive microscopic "match" between questioned and standard/reference hairs were found to be nonmatches when they were later subjected to DNA analysis. The course of events is clear; microscopic hair comparisons must be regarded by police and courts as presumptive in nature, and all positive microscopic hair comparisons must be confirmed by DNA determinations.

Questions Concerning Hair Examination

A number of questions may be asked to further ascertain the present status of forensic hair examinations.

CAN THE BODY AREA FROM WHICH A HAIR ORIGINATED BE DETERMINED? Normally, it is easy to determine the body area from which a hair came. For example, scalp hairs generally show little diameter variation and have a more uniform distribution of pigment color when

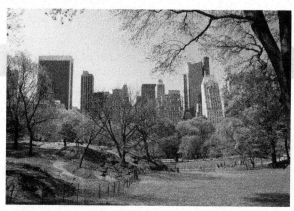

Paolo Omero/Shutterstock

Case Files

The Central Park Jogger Case Revisited

On April 19, 1989, a young woman left her apartment around 9 p.m. to jog in New York's Central Park. Nearly five hours later, she was found comatose lying in a puddle of mud in the park. She had been raped, her skull was fractured, and she had lost 75 percent of her blood. When the woman recovered, she had no memory of what happened to her. The brutality of the crime sent shock waves through the city and seemed to fuel a national perception that crime was running rampant and unchecked through the streets of New York.

Already in custody at the station house of the Central Park Precinct was a group of 14- and 15-year-old boys who had been rounded up leaving the park earlier in the night by police who suspected that they had been involved in a series of random attacks.

Over the next two days, four of the teenagers gave videotaped statements, which they later recanted, admitting to participating in the attack. Ultimately, five of the teenagers were charged with the crime. Interestingly, none of the semen collected from the victim could be linked to any of the defendants. However, according to the testimony of a forensic analyst, two head hairs collected from the clothing of one of the defendants microscopically compared to those of the victim, and a third hair collected from the same defendant's T-shirt microscopically compared to the victim's pubic hair. Besides these three hairs, a fourth hair was found microscopically similar to the victim's. This hair was recovered from the clothing of Steven Lopez, who was originally charged with

rape but not prosecuted for the crime. Hairs were the only pieces of physical evidence offered by the district attorney to directly link any of the teenagers to the crime. The hairs were cited by the district attorney as a way for the jury to know that the videotaped confessions of the teenagers were reliable. The five defendants were convicted and ultimately served from 9 to 13 years.

Matias Reyes was arrested in August 1989, more than three months after the jogger attack. He pleaded guilty to murdering a pregnant woman, raping three others, and committing a robbery. He was sentenced to 33 years to life. In January 2002, Reyes confessed to the Central Park attack. Follow-up tests revealed that Reyes's DNA compared to semen recovered from the jogger's body and her sock. Other DNA tests showed that the hairs offered into evidence at the original trial did not come from the victim, and so could not be used to link the teenagers to the crime as the district attorney had argued.

After an 11-month reinvestigation of the original charges, a New York State Supreme Court judge dismissed all the convictions against the five teenage suspects in the Central Park jogger case.

[2] M. M. Houk and B. Budowle, "Correlation of Microscopic and Mitochondrial DNA Hair Comparisons," *Journal of Forensic Sciences* 47 (2002): 964.

compared to other body hairs. Pubic hairs are short and curly, with wide variations in shaft diameter, and usually have continuous medullae. Beard hairs are coarse, are normally triangular in cross section, and have blunt tips acquired from cutting or shaving.

CAN THE ANCESTRAL ORIGIN OF HAIR BE DETERMINED?   In many instances, the examiner can distinguish hair originating from members of different ancestries; this is especially true of European and African head hair. African hairs are normally kinky, containing dense, unevenly distributed pigments. European hairs are usually straight or wavy, with very fine to coarse pigments that are more evenly distributed when compared to African hair. Sometimes a cross-sectional examination of hair may aid in the identification of ancestry.

Cross sections of hair from Europeans are oval to round in shape, whereas cross sections of African hair are flat to oval in shape. However, all of these observations are general in nature, with many possible exceptions. The criminalist must approach the determination of ancestry from hair with caution and a good deal of experience.

CAN THE AGE AND SEX OF AN INDIVIDUAL BE DETERMINED FROM A HAIR SAMPLE?   The age of an individual cannot be learned from a hair examination with any degree of certainty except with infant hair. Infant hairs are fine, are short in length, have fine pigment, and are rudimentary in character. The recovery of nuclear DNA either from tissue adhering to hair or from the root structure of the hair will allow a determination of whether the hair originated from a male or female (see pages 408–411).

IS IT POSSIBLE TO DETERMINE WHETHER HAIR WAS FORCIBLY REMOVED FROM THE BODY?   A microscopic examination of the hair root may establish whether the hair fell out or was pulled out of the skin. A hair root with follicular tissue (root sheath cells) adhering to it, as shown in Figure 11–8, indicates a hair that has been pulled out either by a person or by brushing or combing. Hair naturally falling off the body has a bulbous-shaped root free of any adhering tissue. However, the absence of sheath cells cannot always be relied on for correctly judging whether hair has been forcibly pulled from the body. In some cases, the root of a hair is devoid of any adhering tissue even when it has been pulled from the body. Apparently, an important consideration is how quickly the hair is pulled out of the head. Hairs pulled quickly from the head are much more likely to have sheath cells compared to hairs that have been removed slowly from the scalp.[3]

ARE EFFORTS BEING MADE TO INDIVIDUALIZE HUMAN HAIR?   As we will learn in Chapter 16, forensic scientists are routinely isolating and characterizing individual variations in DNA. Forensic hair examiners can link human hair to a particular individual by characterizing the **nuclear DNA** in the hair root or in follicular tissue adhering to the root (see Figure 11–8). Recall that the follicular tag is the richest source of DNA associated with hair. In the absence of follicular tissue, an examiner must extract DNA from the hair root. The growth phase of hair (see pages 255–256) is a useful predictor of the likelihood

nuclear DNA
DNA present within the nucleus of a cell; this form of DNA is inherited from both parents.

FIGURE 11–8
Forcibly removed head hair, with follicular tissue attached.

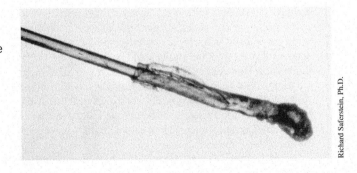

Richard Saferstein, Ph.D.

---

[3] L. A. King, R. Wigmore, and J. M. Twibell, "The Morphology and Occurrence of Human Hair Sheath Cells," *Journal of the Forensic Science Society* 22 (1982): 267.

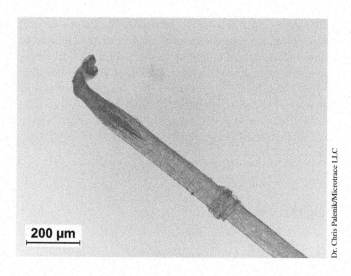

FIGURE 11-9
Hair with a banded root.

200 µm

Dr. Chris Palenik/Microtrace LLC

of successfully typing DNA in human hair.[4] Examiners have a higher rate of success in extracting DNA from hair roots in the anagen phase or from anagen-phase hairs entering the catagen phase of growth. Telogen-phase hairs have an inadequate amount of DNA for successful typing. Because most hairs are naturally shed and are expected to be in the telogen stage, these observations do not portend well for hairs collected at crime scenes. However, some crime scenes are populated with forcibly removed hairs that are expected to be rich sources for nuclear DNA.

When a questioned hair does not have adhering tissue or a root structure amenable to the isolation of nuclear DNA, there is an alternative—**mitochondrial DNA**. Unlike the nuclear DNA described earlier, which is located in the nuclei of practically every cell in our body, mitochondrial DNA is found in cellular material outside the nucleus. Interestingly, unlike nuclear DNA, which is passed down to us from our biological male and female parents, mitochondrial DNA is transmitted only from female parent to offspring. Importantly, many more copies of mitochondrial DNA are located in our cells as compared to nuclear DNA. For this reason, the success rate of finding and typing mitochondrial DNA is much greater from samples, such as hair, that have limited quantities of nuclear DNA. Hairs 1–2 centimeters long can be subjected to mitochondrial analysis with extremely high odds of success. This subject is discussed in greater detail in Chapter 16.

mitochondrial DNA
DNA present in small structures (mitochondria) outside the nucleus of a cell; mitochondria supply energy to the cell; this form of DNA is inherited maternally (from the mother).

IS IT POSSIBLE TO DETERMINE WHETHER HAIR CAME FROM A DECEASED INDIVIDUAL? As exemplified by the Casey Anthony case, a forensic examiner may on occasion be confronted with situations where it's important to know whether hair was deposited after the donor was deceased.

Studies have noted that postmortem decomposition may be accompanied by a darkening or banding around the root area of the hair (see Figure 11–9). Eventually, the hair will break off at the area of the dark hair, leaving a discolored hair end with a point or brushlike appearance.

Recently, it has been confirmed that the onset of postmortem changes to the root portion of hair was observed only in anagenic and catagenic hairs, and specifically within a short area of the root where the hair would have been beneath the scalp. Root banding was slow to occur in cold weather and progressed at a faster rate in warmer temperatures. Significantly, hairs in the telogen stage showed no evidence of postmortem root banding.[5]

[4] C. A. Linch et al., "Evaluation of the Human Hair Root for DNA Typing Subsequent to Microscopic Comparison," *Journal of Forensic Sciences* 43 (1998): 305.

[5] S. L. Koch, A. L. Michaud, and C. Mikell, "Taphonomy of Hair—A Study of Postmortem Root Banding," *Journal of Forensic Sciences* 58 (2013): S52.

CAN DNA INDIVIDUALIZE A HUMAN HAIR?   In some cases, the answer is yes. As we will learn in Chapter 16, nuclear DNA produces frequency of occurrences as low as one in billions or trillions. On the other hand, mitochondrial DNA cannot individualize human hair, but its diversity within the human population often permits exclusion of a significant portion of a population as potential contributors of a hair sample. Ideally, the combination of a positive microscopic comparison and an association through nuclear or mitochondrial DNA analysis provides a strong and meaningful link between a questioned hair and standard/reference hairs. However, a word of caution: mitochondrial DNA cannot distinguish microscopically similar hairs from different individuals who are maternally related.

Collection and Preservation of Hair Evidence

When questioned hairs are submitted to a forensic laboratory for examination, they must always be accompanied by an adequate number of standard/reference samples from the victim of the crime and from individuals suspected of having deposited hair at the crime scene. We have learned that hair from different parts of the body varies significantly in its physical characteristics. Likewise, hair from any one area of the body can also have a wide range of characteristics. For this reason, the questioned and standard/reference hairs must come from the same area of the body; one cannot, for instance, compare head hair to pubic hair. It is also important that the collection of standard/reference hair be carried out in a way to ensure a representative sampling of hair from any one area of the body.

Forensic hair comparisons generally involve either head hair or pubic hair. Collecting 25 full-length hairs from all areas of the scalp normally ensures a representative sampling of head hair. Likewise, a minimum collection of 25 full-length pubic hairs should cover the range of characteristics present in this type of hair. In rape cases, care must first be taken to comb the pubic area with a clean comb to remove all loose foreign hair present before the victim is sampled for standard/reference hair. The comb should then be packaged in a separate envelope.

Because a hair may show variation in color and other morphological features over its entire length, the entire hair length is collected. This requirement is best accomplished by either pulling the hair out of the skin or clipping it at the skin line. During an autopsy, hair samples are collected from a victim of suspicious death as a matter of routine. Because the autopsy may occur early in an investigation, the need for hair standard/reference samples may not always be apparent. However, one should never rule out the possible involvement of hair evidence in subsequent investigative findings. Failure to make this simple collection at an opportune time may result in complicated legal problems at a later date.

Forensic Examination of Fibers

Just as hair left at a crime scene can serve as identification, the same logic can reasonably be extended to the fibers that compose our fabrics and garments. Fibers may become important evidence in incidents that involve personal contact—such as homicide, assault, or sexual offenses—in which cross-transfers may occur between the clothing of suspect and victim. Similarly, the force of impact between a hit-and-run victim and a vehicle often leaves fibers, threads, or even whole pieces of clothing adhering to parts of the vehicle. Fibers may also become fixed in screens or glass broken in the course of a breaking-and-entering attempt.

Regardless of where and under what conditions fibers are recovered, their ultimate value as forensic evidence depends on the criminalist's ability to narrow their origin to a limited number of sources or even to a single source. Unfortunately, mass production of garments and fabrics has limited the value of fiber evidence in this respect, and only under the most unusual circumstances does the recovery of fibers at a crime scene provide individual identification with a high degree of certainty.

> > > > > > > > > >

Case Files

The Ennis Cosby Homicide

The murder of Ennis Cosby, son of entertainer Bill Cosby, at first appeared unsolvable. It was a random act. When his car tire went flat, he pulled off the road and called a friend on his cellular phone to ask for assistance. Shortly thereafter, an assailant demanded money and, when Cosby didn't respond quickly enough, shot him once in the temple. Acting on a tip from a friend of the assailant, police investigators later found a .38 revolver wrapped in a blue cap miles from the crime scene. Mikail Markhasev was arrested and charged with murder. At trial, the district attorney introduced firearms evidence to show that the recovered gun had fired the bullet aimed at Cosby. However, a single hair also recovered from the hat dramatically linked Markhasev to the crime. Los Angeles Police Department forensic analyst Harry Klann identified six DNA markers from the follicular tissue adhering to the hair root that matched Markhasev's

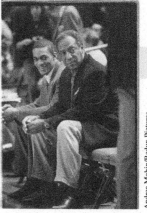

Bill Cosby and his son Ennis Cosby.

DNA. This particular DNA profile is found in one out of 15,500 members of the general population. Upon hearing all the evidence, the jury deliberated and convicted Markhasev of murder. Markhasev maintained his innocence until 2001, when he admitted to committing the murder and asked that appeals in his case stop.

Types of Fibers

For centuries, humans depended on natural sources derived from plants and animals for textile fibers. Early in the 20th century, the first manufactured fiber—rayon—became a practical reality, followed in the 1920s by the introduction of cellulose acetate. Since the late 1930s, scientists have produced dozens of new fibers. In fact, the development of fibers, fabrics, finishes, and other textile-processing techniques has made greater advances since 1900 than in the 5,000 years of recorded history before the 20th century. Today, such varied items as clothing, carpeting, draperies, wigs, and even artificial turf attest to the predominant role that manufactured fibers have come to play in our culture and environment.

For the purpose of discussing the forensic examination of fibers, it is convenient to classify them into two broad groups: *natural* and *manufactured*.

Natural fibers are wholly derived from animal or plant sources. Animal fibers constitute most of the natural fibers encountered in crime laboratory examinations. These include hair coverings from such animals as sheep (wool), goats (mohair, cashmere), camels, llamas, alpacas, and vicuñas; fur fibers include those obtained from animals such as mink, rabbit, beaver, and muskrat.

natural fibers
Fibers derived entirely from animal or plant sources.

Forensic examination of animal fibers uses the same procedures discussed in the previous section for the forensic examination of animal hairs. Identification and comparison of such fibers rely solely on a microscopic examination of color and morphological characteristics. Again, a sufficient number of standard/reference specimens must be examined to establish the range of fiber characteristics of the suspect fabric.

By far the most prevalent plant fiber is cotton. The wide use of undyed white cotton fibers in clothing and other fabrics has made its evidential value almost meaningless, although the presence of dyed cotton in a combination of colors has, in some cases, enhanced its evidential significance. The microscopic view of cotton fiber shown in Figure 11–10 reveals its most distinguishing feature—a ribbon-like shape with twists at irregular intervals.

MANUFACTURED FIBERS   Beginning with the introduction of rayon in 1911 and the development of nylon in 1939, **manufactured fibers** have increasingly replaced natural fibers in garments and fabrics. Today, such fibers are marketed under hundreds of different trade names. To reduce consumer confusion, the U.S. Federal Trade Commission has approved "generic"

manufactured fibers
Fibers derived from either natural or synthetic polymers; the fibers are typically made by forcing the polymeric material through the holes of a spinneret.

FIGURE 11–10
Photomicrograph of cotton fiber (450×).

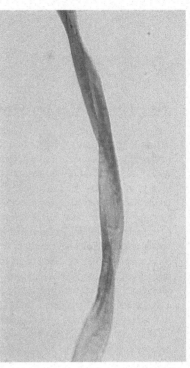

Richard Saferstein, Ph.D.

or family names for the grouping of all manufactured fibers. Many of these generic classes are produced by several manufacturers and are sold under a confusing variety of trade names. For example, in the United States, polyesters are marketed under names that include Dacron, Fortrel, and Kodel. In England, polyesters are called Terylene. Table 11–1 lists major generic fibers, along with common trade names and their characteristics and applications.

TABLE 11–1

Major Generic Fibers

Major Generic Fiber	Description	Common Uses
Acetate Rayon	Acetate Cellulose fiber where 74%–92% of hydroxyl groups are acetylated	*Apparel:* Blouses, dresses, foundation garments, lingerie, linings, shirts, pants, sportswear *Fabrics:* Brocade, crepe, double knits, faille, knitted jerseys, lace, satin, taffeta, tricot *Home Furnishings:* Draperies, upholstery *Other:* Cigarette filters, fiberfill for pillows, quilted products
Acrylic	Fiber comprised of linear macromolecules composed of at least 85% acrylonitrile monomer	*Apparel:* Dresses, infant wear, knitted garments, skiwear, socks, sportswear, sweaters *Fabrics:* Fleece and pile fabrics, facing fabrics in bonded fabrics, simulated furs, jerseys *Home Furnishings:* Blankets, carpets, draperies, upholstery *Other:* Auto tops, awnings, hand-knitting and craft yarns, industrial and geotextile fabrics
Aramid	Aramid fibers are composed of a series of synthetic polymers in which repeating units containing large phenyl rings are linked together by amide groups.	Hot-gas filtration fabrics, protective clothing, military helmets, protective vests, structural composites for aircraft and boats, sailcloth, tires, ropes and cables, mechanical rubber goods, marine and sporting goods

Major Generic Fiber	Description	Common Uses
Bicomponent	A bicomponent fiber is made of two materials, utilizing desired properties of each material. Such fibers can be created by extrusion spinning. One or both materials may remain in the finished product, or one material may be dissolved, leaving only one material remaining.	Uniform distribution of adhesive; fiber remains a part of structure and adds integrity; customized sheath materials to bond various materials; wide range of bonding temperatures; cleaner, environmentally friendly (*no effluent*); recyclable; lamination/molding/densification of composites
Lyocell	Lyocell is a form of rayon that consists of cellulose fiber made from dissolving bleached wood pulp using dry jet-wet spinning.	Dresses, pants, and coats
Rayon	Rayon is made from purified cellulose from wood pulp which is made into a soluble compound. It is then dissolved and forced through a spinneret to produce filaments which are chemically solidified, resulting in fibers of nearly pure cellulose.	*Apparel:* Blouses, coats, dresses, jackets, lingerie, linings, millinery, rainwear, pants, sports shirts, sportswear, suits, ties, work clothes *Home Furnishings:* Bedspreads, blankets, carpets, curtains, draperies, sheets, slipcovers, tablecloths, upholstery *Other:* Industrial products, medical-surgical products, nonwoven products, tire cord
Spandex	Spandex is a lightweight, synthetic fiber that is used to make stretchable clothing such as sportswear. It is made up of a long chain polymer called polyurethane, which is produced by reacting a polyester with a diisocyanate. The polymer is converted into a fiber using a dry spinning technique.	*Apparel* (in which stretch is desired): Athletic apparel, bathing suits, delicate laces, foundation garments, golf jackets, ski pants, pants, support and surgical hose
Melamine	Melamine fiber is a manufactured fiber in which the fiber-forming substance is a synthetic polymer composed of at least 50% by weight of a cross-linked melamine polymer.	*Fire-Blocking Fabrics:* Aircraft seating, fire blockers for upholstered furniture in high-risk occupancies (e.g., to meet California TB 133 requirements) *Protective Clothing:* Firefighters' turnout gear, insulating thermal liners, knit hoods, molten metal splash apparel, heat-resistant gloves *Filter Media:* High-capacity, high-efficiency, high-temperature baghouse air filters
Modacrylic	Modacrylic fibers are manufactured fibers in which the fiber-forming substance is any long-chain synthetic polymer composed of less than 85%, but at least 35% weight acrylonitrile units except when the polymer qualifies as rubber.	*Apparel:* Deep-pile coats, trims, linings, simulated fur, wigs and hairpieces *Fabrics:* Fleece fabrics, industrial fabrics, knit-pile fabric backings, nonwoven fabrics *Home Furnishings:* Awnings, blankets, carpets, flame-resistant draperies and curtains, scatter rugs *Other:* Filters, paint rollers, stuffed toys
Nylon	Nylon is a generic name for a family of synthetic polymers, more specifically, aliphatic or semi-aromatic polyamides in which at least 85% by weight of the amide-linkages ($-CO-NH-$) are attached directly to two aliphatic groups.	*Apparel:* Blouses, dresses, foundation garments, hosiery, lingerie and underwear, raincoats, ski and snow apparel, suits, windbreakers *Home Furnishings:* Bedspreads, carpets, draperies, curtains, upholstery *Other:* Air hoses, conveyor and seat belts, parachutes, racket strings, ropes and nets, sleeping bags, tarpaulins, tents, thread, tire cord, geotextiles
Olefin	Olefin fiber is a manufactured fiber in which the fiber-forming substance is any long-chain synthetic polymer composed of at least 85% by weight of ethylene, propylene, or other olefin units.	*Apparel:* Pantyhose, underwear, knitted sports shirts, men's half-hose, men's knitted sportswear, sweaters *Home Furnishings:* Carpet and carpet backing, slipcovers, upholstery, wall paper *Other:* Dye nets, filter fabrics, laundry and sandbags, geotextiles, automotive interiors, cordage, doll hair, industrial sewing thread

(*continued*)

TABLE 11–1

Major Generic Fibers (*continued*)

Major Generic Fiber	Description	Common Uses
Polyester	Polyester is a synthetic polymer made of purified terephthalic acid (PTA) or its dimethyl ester dimethyl terephthalate (DMT) and monoethylene glycol (MEG). A manufactured fiber in which the fiber forming substance is any long-chain synthetic polymer composed of at least 85% by weight of an ester of a substituted aromatic carboxylic acid.	*Apparel:* Blouses, shirts, career apparel, children's wear, dresses, half-hose, insulated garments, ties, lingerie and underwear, permanent-press garments, pants, suits *Home Furnishings:* Carpets, curtains, draperies, sheets and pillowcases *Other:* Fiberfill for various products, fire hose, power belting, ropes and nets, tire cord, sail, V-belts
PBI	Polybenzimidazole fibers (PBI) are fibers in which the fiber-forming substance is a long-chain aromatic polymer having recurring imidazole groups as one of the main structural repeat units in the polymer backbone. PBI is prepared from an aromatic tetraamine and an aromatic dicarboxylic acid or a derivative of it. The resin is then spun into fibers via a dry spinning process using dimethyl acetamide as a solvent.	Suitable for high-performance protective apparel such as firefighters' turnout coats, astronaut space suits, and applications in which fire resistance is important

Inside the Science

Polymers

The polymer is the basic chemical substance of all synthetic fibers. Indeed, an almost unbelievable array of household, industrial, and recreational products is manufactured from polymers; these include plastics, paints, adhesives, and synthetic rubber. Polymers exist in countless forms and varieties and with the proper treatment can be made to assume different chemical and physical properties.

As we have already observed, chemical substances are composed from basic structural units called **molecules**. The molecules of most materials are composed of just a few atoms; for example, water, H_2O, has two atoms of hydrogen and one atom of oxygen. The heroin molecule, $C_{21}H_{23}O_5N$, contains 21 atoms of

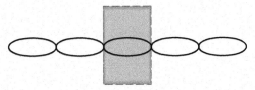

Monomer

The chain-link model of a segment of a polymer molecule. The actual molecule may contain as many as several million monomer units or links.

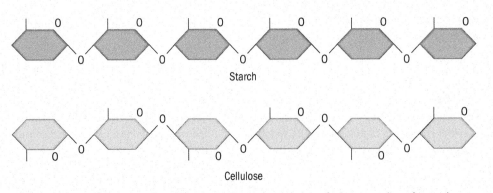

Starch and cellulose are natural carbohydrate polymers consisting of a large number of repeating units or monomers.

carbon, 23 atoms of hydrogen, 5 atoms of oxygen, and 1 atom of nitrogen. Polymers, on the other hand, are formed by linking a large number of molecules, so that it is not unusual for a polymer to contain thousands or even millions of atoms. This is why polymers are often referred to as **macromolecules**, or "big" molecules.

Simply, a polymer can be pictured as resembling a long, repeating chain, with each link representing the basic structure of the polymer (see the figure). The repeating molecular units in the polymer, called **monomers**, are joined end to end, so that thousands are linked to form a long chain. What makes polymer chemistry so fascinating is the countless possibilities for linking different molecules. By simply varying the chemical structure of the basic molecules, or monomers, and by devising numerous ways to weave them together, chemists have created polymers that exhibit different properties. This versatility enables polymer chemists to synthesize glues, plastics, paints, and fibers.

It would be a mistake to give the impression that all polymers are synthesized in the chemical laboratory. Indeed, this is far from true, for nature has produced polymers that humans have not yet been able to copy. For example, the proteins that form the basic structure of animal hairs, as well as of all living matter, are polymers, composed of thousands of amino acids linked in a highly organized arrangement and sequence. Similarly, cellulose, the basic ingredient of wood and cotton, and starch are both natural polymers built by the combination of several thousand carbohydrate monomers, as shown in the figure. Hence, the synthesis of manufactured fibers merely represents an extension of chemical principles that nature has successfully used to produce hair and vegetable fibers.

The first machine-made fibers were manufactured from raw materials derived from cotton or wood pulp. These materials are processed, and pure cellulose is extracted from them. Depending on the type of fiber desired, the cellulose may be chemically treated and dissolved in an appropriate solvent before it is forced through the small holes of a spinning jet or spinneret to produce the fiber. Fibers manufactured from natural raw materials in this manner are classified as *regenerated fibers* and commonly include rayon, acetate, and triacetate, all of which are produced from regenerated cellulose.

Most of the fibers currently manufactured are produced solely from synthetic chemicals and are therefore classified as *synthetic fibers*. These include nylons, polyesters, and acrylics. The creation of synthetic fibers became a reality only when scientists developed a method of synthesizing long-chained molecules called **polymers**.

In 1930, chemists discovered an unusual characteristic of one of the polymers under investigation. When a glass rod in contact with viscous material in a beaker was slowly pulled away, the substance adhered to the rod and formed a fine filament that hardened as soon as it entered the cool air. Furthermore, the cold filaments could be stretched several times their extended length to produce a flexible, strong, and attractive fiber. The first synthetic fiber was improved and then marketed as nylon. Since then, fiber chemists have successfully synthesized new polymers and have developed more efficient methods for manufacturing them. These efforts have produced a multitude of synthetic fibers.

macromolecule
A molecule with a high molecular mass.

molecule
Two or more atoms held together by chemical bonds.

monomer
The basic unit of structure from which a polymer is constructed.

polymer
A substance composed of a large number of atoms; these atoms are usually arranged in repeating units or monomers.

Identification and Comparison of Manufactured Fibers

The evidential value of fibers lies in the criminalist's ability to trace their origin. Obviously, if the examiner is presented with fabrics that can be exactly fitted together at their torn edges, it is a virtual certainty that the fabrics were of common origin. However, more often the criminalist obtains a limited number of fibers for identification and comparison. Generally, in these situations, the possibilities for obtaining a physical match are nonexistent, and the examiner must resort to a side-by-side comparison of the standard/reference and crime-scene fibers.

Microscopic Examination

The first and most important step in the examination is a microscopic comparison for color and diameter using a comparison microscope. Unless these two characteristics agree, there is little reason to suspect a match. Other morphological features that could be present to aid in the comparison are lengthwise striations on the surface of some fibers and the pitting of the fiber's surface with delustering particles (usually titanium dioxide) added in the manufacturing process to reduce shine (Figure 11–11[a] and [b]).

The cross-sectional shape of a fiber may also help characterize the fiber (Figure 11–12).[6] In a serial murder case in the Atlanta, Georgia, area, unusually shaped yellow-green fibers

[6] S. Palenik and C. Fitzsimons, "Fiber Cross-Sections: Part I," *Microscope* 38 (1990): 187.

discovered on a number of the murder victims were ultimately linked to a carpet in the home of the defendant, Wayne Williams. This fiber was a key element in proving Williams's guilt. A photomicrograph of this unusually shaped fiber is shown in Figure 11–13.

Dye Composition

Although two fibers may seem to have the same color when viewed under the microscope, compositional differences may exist in the dyes that were applied to them during their manufacture. In fact, most textile fibers are impregnated with a mixture of dyes selected to obtain a desired shade or color. The significance of a fiber comparison is enhanced when the forensic examiner can show that the questioned and standard/reference fibers have the same dye composition.

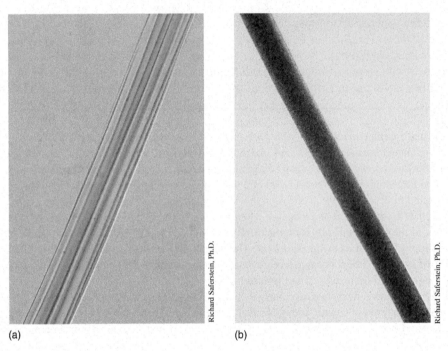

(a)   (b)

FIGURE 11–11

Photomicrographs of synthetic fibers: (a) cellulose triacetate (450×) and (b) olefin fiber embedded with titanium dioxide particles (450×).

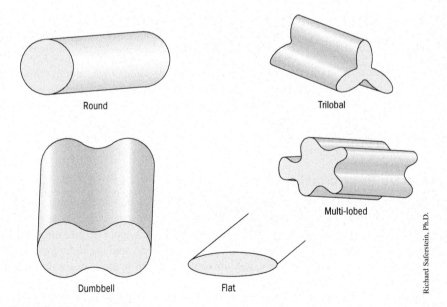

Round   Trilobal

Dumbbell   Flat   Multi-lobed

FIGURE 11–12

Cross-sectional shapes of fibers.

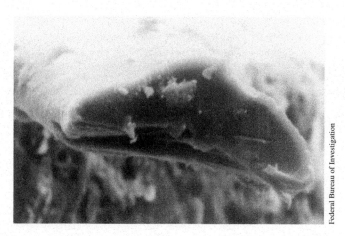

Federal Bureau of Investigation

FIGURE 11–13

A scanning electron photomicrograph of the cross section of a nylon fiber removed from a sheet used to transport the body of a murder victim. The fiber, associated with a carpet in Wayne Williams's home, was manufactured in 1971 in relatively small quantities.

The visible-light microspectrophotometer (pages 177–178) is a convenient way for analysts to compare the colors of fibers through spectral patterns. This technique is not limited by sample size—a fiber as small as one millimeter or less in length can be examined by this type of microscope. The examination is nondestructive and is carried out on fibers simply mounted on a microscope slide.

A more detailed analysis of the fiber's dye composition can be obtained through a chromatographic separation of the dye constituents. To accomplish this, small strands of fibers are compared for dye content by first extracting the dye off each fiber with a suitable solvent and then spotting the dye solution onto a thin-layer chromatography plate. The dye components of the questioned and standard/reference fibers are separated on the thin-layer plate and compared side by side for similarity.[7]

Chemical Composition

Once the microscopic and dye composition phases of the analysis are complete, and before any conclusion can be reached that two or more fibers compare, they must be shown to have the same chemical composition. In this respect, tests are performed to confirm that all of the fibers involved belong to the same broad generic class. Additionally, the comparison will be substantially enhanced if it can be demonstrated that all of the fibers belong to the same subclassification within their generic class. For example, at least four different types of nylon are available in commercial and consumer markets, including nylon 6, nylon 6–10, nylon 11, and nylon 6–6. Although all types of nylon have many properties in common, each may differ in physical shape, appearance, and dyeability because of modifications in basic chemical structure. Similarly, a study of more than 200 different samples of acrylic fibers revealed that they could be divided into 24 distinguishable groups on the basis of their polymeric structure and microscopic characteristics.[8]

Textile chemists have devised numerous tests for determining the class of a fiber. However, unlike the textile chemist, the criminalist frequently does not have the luxury of having a substantial quantity of fabric to work with and must therefore select tests that will yield the most information with the least amount of material. Only a single fiber may be available for analysis, and often this may amount to no more than a minute strand recovered from a fingernail scraping of a homicide or rape victim.

The polymers that compose a manufactured fiber, just as in any other organic substance, selectively absorb infrared light in a characteristic pattern. Infrared spectrophotometry thus provides a rapid and reliable method for identifying the generic class, and in some cases the subclasses, of fibers. The infrared microspectrophotometer combines a microscope with an infrared spectrophotometer (see pages 177–178). Such a combination makes possible the infrared analysis of a small single-strand fiber while it is being viewed under a microscope.[9]

[7] D. K. Laing et al., "The Standardisation of Thin-Layer Chromatographic Systems for Comparisons of Fibre Dyes," *Journal of the Forensic Science Society* 30 (1990): 299.

[8] M. C. Grieve, "Another Look at the Classification of Acrylic Fibres, Using FTIR Microscopy," *Science & Justice* 35 (1995): 179.

[9] M. W. Tungol et al., "Analysis of Single Polymer Fibers by Fourier Transform Infrared Microscopy: The Results of Case Studies," *Journal of Forensic Sciences* 36 (1992): 1027.

Inside the Science

Other Properties for Examination

A most useful physical property of fibers, from the criminalist's point of view, is that many manufactured fibers exhibit double refraction or birefringence (see pages 232–233). Synthetic fibers are manufactured by melting a polymeric substance or dissolving it in a solvent and then forcing it through the fine holes of a spinneret. The polymer emerges as a fine filament, with its molecules aligned parallel to the length of the filament (see figure). Just as the regular arrangement of atoms produces a crystal, so will the regular arrangement of the fiber's polymers cause crystallinity in the finished fiber. This crystallinity makes a fiber stiff and strong and gives it the optical property of double refraction.

Polarized white light passing through a synthetic fiber is split into two rays that are perpendicular to each other, causing the fiber to display polarization or interference colors when viewed under a polarizing microscope (see figure). Depending on the class of fiber, each polarized plane of light has a characteristic index of refraction. This value can be determined by immersing the fiber in a fluid with a comparable refractive index and observing the disappearance of the Becke line under a polarizing microscope. Table 11–2 lists the two refractive indices of some common classes of fibers, along with their birefringence. The virtue of this technique is that a single fiber, microscopic in size, can be analyzed in a nondestructive manner.

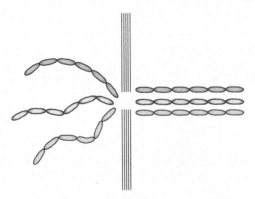

In the production of manufactured fibers, the bulk polymer is forced through small holes to form a filament in which all the polymers are aligned in the same direction.

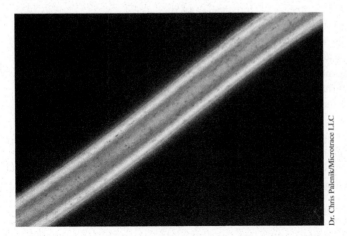

A photomicrograph of a nylon fiber displaying interference colors when observed between the crossed polars of a polarizing microscope (100×).

Dr. Chris Palenik/Microtrace LLC

TABLE 11–2

Refractive Indices of Common Textile Fibers

Fiber	Parallel	Refractive Index	
		Perpendicular	Birefringence
Acetate	1.478	1.477	0.001
Triacetate	1.472	1.471	0.001
Acrylic	1.524	1.520	0.004
Nylon			
Nylon 6	1.568	1.515	0.053
Nylon 6–6	1.582	1.519	0.063
Polyester			
Dacron	1.710	1.535	0.175
Kodel	1.642	1.540	0.102
Modacrylic	1.536	1.531	0.005
Rayon			
Cuprammonium rayon	1.552	1.520	0.032
Viscose rayon	1.544	1.520	0.024

Note: The listed values are for specific fibers, which explains the highly precise values given. In identification work, such precision is not practical; values within 0.02 or 0.03 of those listed will suffice.

Case Files

> > > > > > > > >

Jeffrey MacDonald: Fatal Vision

The grisly murder scene that confronted police on February 17, 1970, is one that cannot be wiped from memory. Summoned to the Fort Bragg residence of Captain Jeffrey MacDonald, a physician, police found the bludgeoned body of MacDonald's wife. She had been repeatedly knifed, and her face was smashed to a pulp. MacDonald's two children, ages 2 and 5, had been brutally and repeatedly knifed and battered to death. Suspicion quickly fell on MacDonald. To the eyes of investigators, the murder scene had a staged appearance. MacDonald described a frantic effort to subdue four intruders who had slashed at him with an ice pick. However, the confrontation left MacDonald with minor wounds and no apparent defense wounds on his arms. MacDonald then described how he had covered his slashed wife with his blue pajama top. Interestingly, when the body was removed, blue threads were observed under the body. In fact, blue threads matching the pajama top turned up throughout the house—19 in one child's bedroom, including one beneath her fingernail, and two in the other child's bedroom. Eight-one blue fibers were recovered from the master bedroom, and two were located on a bloodstained piece of wood outside the house. Later forensic examination showed that the 48 ice pick holes in the pajama top were smooth and cylindrical, a sign that the top was stationary when it was slashed. Also, folding the pajama top demonstrated that the 48 holes actually could have been made by 21 thrusts of an ice pick. This coincided with the number of wounds that MacDonald's

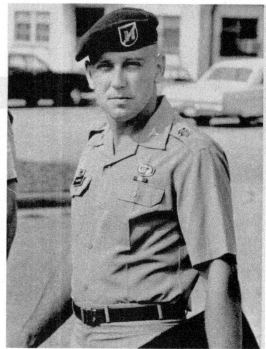

AP Images

wife sustained. As described in the book *Fatal Vision*, which chronicled the murder investigation, when MacDonald was confronted with adulterous conduct, he replied, "You guys are more thorough than I thought." MacDonald is currently serving three consecutive life sentences.

Eleven years after this conviction, MacDonald's attorneys filed a petition for a new trial, claiming the existence of "critical new" evidence. The defense asserted that wig fibers found on a hairbrush in the MacDonald residence were evidence that an intruder dressed in a wig entered the MacDonald home on the day of the murder. Subsequent examination of this claim by the FBI Laboratory focused on a blond wig frequently worn by MacDonald's wife. Fibers removed from the wig were shown to be consistent with fibers on the hairbrush. The examination included the use of infrared microspectrophotometry to demonstrate that the suspect's wig fibers were chemically identical to fibers found in the composition of the MacDonald wig (see the figure). Hence, although wig fibers were found at the crime scene, the source of these fibers could be accounted for—they came from Mrs. MacDonald's wig.

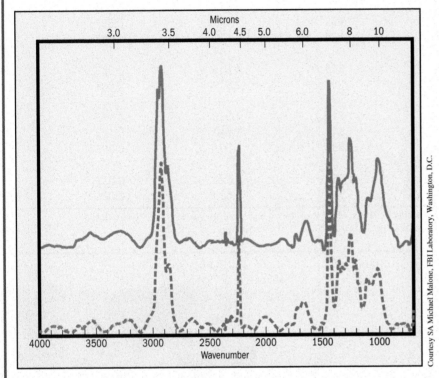

Courtesy SA Michael Malone, FBI Laboratory, Washington, D.C.

A fiber comparison made with an infrared spectrophotometer. The infrared spectrum of a fiber from Mrs. MacDonald's wig compares to a fiber recovered from a hairbrush in the MacDonald home. These fibers were identified as modacrylics, the most common type of synthetic fiber used in the manufacture of human hair goods.

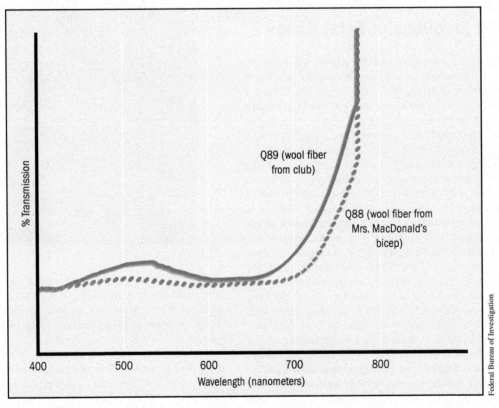

Federal Bureau of Investigation

The visible-light spectrum for the woolen fiber recovered from Mrs. MacDonald's body is clearly different from that of the fiber recovered from the club used to assault her.

Another piece of evidence cited by MacDonald's lawyers was a bluish-black woolen fiber found on the body of Mrs. MacDonald. They claimed that this fiber compared to a bluish-black woolen fiber recovered from the club used to assault her. These wool fibers were central to MacDonald's defense that the "intruders" wore dark-colored clothing. Initial examination showed that the fibers were microscopically indistinguishable. However, the FBI also compared the two wool fibers by visible-light microspectrophotometry. Comparison of their spectra clearly showed that their dye compositions differed, providing no evidence of outside intruders (see the figure). Ultimately, the U.S. Supreme Court denied the merits of MacDonald's petition for a new trial.

Source: Data from B. M. Murtagh and M. P. Malone, "Fatal Vision Revisited," *The Police Chief* (June 1993): 15.

Significance of an Inclusion

Once a fiber has been associated with a textile source, the question of the significance of such a finding is bound to be raised. In reality, no analytical technique permits the criminalist to associate a fiber strand definitively to any single garment. Furthermore, except in the most unusual circumstances, no statistical databases are available for determining the probability of a fiber's origin. Considering the mass distribution of synthetic fibers and the constantly changing fashion tastes of our society, it is highly unlikely that such data will be available in the foreseeable future. Nevertheless, one should not discount or minimize the significance of a fiber association.

An enormous variety of fibers exist in our society. By simply looking at the random individuals we meet every day, we can see how unlikely it is to find two different people wearing identically colored fabrics (with the exception of blue denims or white cottons). There are thousands of different-colored fibers in our environment. Combine this with the fact that forensic scientists compare not only the color of fibers but also their size, shape, microscopic appearance, chemical composition, and dye content, and one can now begin to appreciate how unlikely it is to find two indistinguishable colored fibers emanating from randomly selected sources.

Furthermore, the significance of a fiber association increases dramatically if the analyst can link two or more distinctly different fibers to the same object. Likewise, the associative value of fiber evidence is enhanced if it is accompanied by other types of physical evidence linking a person or object to a crime.

As with most class evidence, the significance of a fiber comparison is dictated by the circumstances of the case; by the location, number, and nature of the fibers examined; and, most important, by the judgment of an experienced examiner.

Collection and Preservation of Fiber Evidence

As criminal investigators have become more aware of the potential contribution of trace physical evidence to the success of their investigations, they have placed greater emphasis on conducting thorough crime-scene searches for evidence of forensic value. Their skill and determination at carrying out these tasks is tested when it comes to the collection of fiber-related evidence. Fiber evidence can be associated with virtually any type of crime. It cannot usually be seen with the naked eye and thus can be easily overlooked by someone not specifically looking for it.

An investigator committed to optimizing the laboratory's chances for locating minute strands of fibers seeks to identify and preserve potential "carriers" of fiber evidence. Relevant articles of clothing should be packaged carefully in paper bags. Each article must be placed in a separate bag to avoid cross-contamination of evidence. Scrupulous care must be taken to prevent articles of clothing from different people or from different locations from coming into contact. Such articles must not even be placed on the same surface before packaging. Likewise, carpets, rugs, and bedding are to be folded carefully to protect areas suspected of containing fibers. Car seats should be carefully covered with polyethylene sheets to protect fiber evidence, and knife blades should be covered to protect adhering fibers. If a body is thought to have been wrapped at one time in a blanket or carpet, adhesive tape lifts of exposed body areas may reveal fiber strands.

Occasionally, the field investigator may need to remove a fiber from an object, particularly if loosely adhering fibrous material may be lost in transit to the laboratory. These fibers must be removed with a clean forceps and placed in a small sheet of paper, which, after folding and

WEBEXTRA 11.1
Step into the Role of the First Officer Responding to a Violent Crime Scene

WEBEXTRA 11.2
Assume the Duties of an Evidence-Collection Technician at a Violent Crime Scene

labeling, can be placed inside another container. Again, scrupulous care must be taken to prevent contact between fibers collected from different objects or from different locations.

In the laboratory, the search for fiber evidence on clothing and other relevant objects, as well as in debris, is time consuming and tedious and will test the skill and patience of the examiner. The crime-scene investigator can reduce this task to manageable proportions by collecting only relevant items for examination. It is essential from the onset of an investigation that the crime-scene investigator pinpoint areas where a likely transfer of fiber evidence occurred and then take necessary measures to ensure proper collection and preservation of these materials.

> > > > > > > > > >

Case Files

Fiber Evidence and the Wayne Williams Trial

On February 26, 1982, a Fulton County, Georgia, Superior Court jury returned a verdict of "guilty as charged" on two counts of murder brought against Wayne Bertram Williams by a Fulton County grand jury in July 1981. Williams had been on trial since December 28, 1981, for the asphyxial murders of Nathaniel Cater and Jimmy Payne in April and May of 1981. During the eight-week trial, evidence linking Williams to those murders and to the murders of 10 other boys or young men was introduced.

An essential part of this case, presented by the Fulton County District Attorney's Office, involved the association of fibrous debris removed from the bodies of 12 murder victims with objects from the everyday environment of Williams.

Fiber evidence has often been an important part of criminal cases, but the Williams trial differed from other cases in several respects. Fiber evidence has not played a significant role in any case involving a large number of murder victims. The victims whose deaths were charged to Williams were 2 of 30 Black children and Black young men who were reported missing or who had died under suspicious circumstances in the Atlanta area over a 22-month period beginning in July 1979. During the trial, fiber evidence was used to associate Williams with 12 of those victims.

Fiber evidence is often used to corroborate other evidence in a case—it is used to support other testimony presented at a trial. This was not the situation in the Williams trial. Other evidence and other aspects of the trial were important but were used to support and complement the fiber evidence, not the usual order of things. The hair and fiber associations between Williams's environment and 11 of the 12 murder victims discussed at the trial were significant links to both the residence and automobiles that were a major part of the world of Wayne Williams.

Another difference between this case and most other cases was the extremely large amount of publicity surrounding both the investigation of the missing and murdered children and the arrest and subsequent trial of Williams. Few other murder trials have received the attention that the Williams case received.

It is often difficult to get an accurate picture from press reports of the physical evidence introduced at a trial and the significance of that evidence. By discussing only the fiber evidence introduced at the trial, many other aspects of the case against Williams are being neglected. Additional evidence dealing with Williams's motivations—his character and behavior, his association with several of the victims by eyewitness accounts, and his link to a victim recovered from a river in Atlanta—[were] also essential to the case.

Development of Williams as a Murder Suspect

Before Wayne Williams became a suspect in the Nathaniel Cater murder case, the Georgia State Crime Laboratory located a number of yellowish-green nylon fibers and some violet acetate fibers on the bodies and clothing of the murder victims whose bodies had been recovered during the period of July 1979 to May 1981. The names of those victims were included on the list of missing and murdered children that was compiled by the Atlanta Task Force (a large group of investigators from law enforcement agencies in the Atlanta area). The yellowish-green nylon fibers were generally similar to each other in appearance and properties. This was also true of the violet acetate fibers. Although there were many other similarities that would link these murders together, the fiber linkage was notable since the possibility existed that a source of these fibers might be located in the future.

Initially, the major concern with these yellowish-green nylon fibers was determining what type of object(s) could have been their source. This information could provide avenues of investigative activity. The fibers were very coarse and had a lobed cross-sectional appearance, tending to indicate that they originated from a carpet or a rug. The lobed cross-sectional shape of these fibers, however, was unique, and initially, the manufacturer of these fibers could not be determined. Photomicrographs of the fibers were prepared for display to contacts within the textile industry. On one occasion, these photomicrographs were distributed among several chemists attending a meeting at the research facilities of a large fiber producer. The chemists concurred that the yellowish-green nylon fiber was very unusual in cross-sectional shape and was consistent with being a carpet fiber, but again, the manufacturer of this fiber could not be determined. Contacts with other textile producers and textile chemists likewise did not result in an identification of the manufacturer.

In February 1981, an Atlanta newspaper article publicized that several different fiber types had been found on two murder victims. Following the publication of this article, bodies recovered from rivers in the Atlanta metropolitan area were either nude or clothed only in undershorts. It appeared possible that the victims were being disposed of in this undressed state and in rivers in order to eliminate fibers from being found on their bodies.[10]

On May 22, 1981, a four-man surveillance team of personnel from the Atlanta Police Department and the Atlanta Office of the FBI was situated under and at both ends of the James Jackson Parkway Bridge over the Chattahoochee River in northwest Atlanta. Around 2 a.m., a loud splash alerted the surveillance team to the presence of an automobile being driven slowly off the bridge. The driver was stopped and identified as Wayne Bertram Williams.

Two days after Williams's presence on the bridge, the nude body of Nathaniel Cater was pulled from the Chattahoochee River, approximately 1 mile downstream from the James Jackson Parkway Bridge. A yellowish-green nylon carpet-type fiber, similar to the nylon fibers discussed above, was recovered from the head hair of Nathaniel Cater. When details of Williams's reason for being on the bridge at 2 a.m. could not be confirmed, search warrants for Williams's home and automobile were obtained and were served on the afternoon of June 3, 1981. During the late evening hours of the same day, the initial associations of fibers from Cater and other murder victims were made with a green carpet in the home of Williams. Associations with a bedspread from Williams's bed and with [Williams's] family dog were also made at that time.

An apparent source of the yellowish-green nylon fibers had been found. It now became important to completely characterize these fibers in order to verify the associations and determine the strength of the associations resulting from the fiber comparisons. Because of the unusual cross-sectional appearance of the nylon fiber and the difficulty in determining the manufacturer, it was believed that this was a relatively rare fiber type, and therefore would not be present in large amounts (or in a large number of carpets).

The Williams Trial

To any experienced forensic fiber examiner, the fiber evidence linking Williams to the murder victims was overwhelming. But regardless of the apparent validity of the fiber findings, it was during the trial that its true weight would be determined. Unless it could be conveyed meaningfully to a jury, its effect would be lost. Because of this, considerable time was spent determining what should be done to convey the full significance of the fiber evidence. Juries are not usually composed of individuals with a scientific background, and therefore, it was necessary to "educate" the jury in what procedures were followed and the significance of the fiber results. In the Williams case, over 40 charts with over 350 photographs were prepared to illustrate exactly what the crime laboratory examiners had observed.

Representatives of the textile fiber industry, including technical representatives from the Wellman and West Point Pepperell Corporations, were involved in educating the jury regarding textile fibers in general and helped lay the foundation for the conclusions of the forensic fiber examiners. The jury also was told about fiber analysis in the crime laboratory.

[10] Prior to the publication of the February 11, 1981, newspaper article, one victim from the task force list, who was fully clothed, had been recovered from a river in the Atlanta area. In the 2½-month period after publication, the nude or nearly nude bodies of seven of the nine victims added to the task force list were recovered from rivers in the Atlanta area.

The trial, as it developed, can be divided into two parts. Initially, testimony was given concerning the murders of Nathaniel Cater and Jimmy Ray Payne, the two victims included in the indictment drawn against Williams in July 1981. Testimony was then given concerning Williams's association with 10 other murder victims.

The fiber associations made between fibers in Williams's environment and fibers from victims Payne and Cater were discussed. Not only is Payne linked to Williams's environment by seven items and Cater linked by six items, but both of the victims are linked strongly to each other based on the fiber associations and circumstances surrounding their deaths. In discussing the significance or strength of an association based on textile fibers, it was emphasized that the more uncommon the fibers, the stronger the association. None of the fiber types from the items in Williams's environment is by definition a "common" fiber type. Several of the fiber types would be termed "uncommon."

One of the fibers linking the body of Jimmy Ray Payne to the carpet in the 1970 station wagon driven by Williams was a small rayon fiber fragment recovered from Payne's shorts. Data were obtained from the station wagon's manufacturer concerning which automobile models produced prior to 1973 contained carpet made of this fiber type. These data were coupled with additional information from Georgia concerning the number of these models registered in the Atlanta metropolitan area during 1981. This allowed a calculation to be made relating to the probability of randomly selecting an automobile having carpet like that in the 1970 Chevrolet station wagon from the 2,373,512 cars registered in the Atlanta metropolitan area. This probability is 1 chance in 3,828, a very low probability representing a significant association.

Another factor to consider when assessing the significance of fiber evidence is the increased strength of the association when multiple fiber links become the basis of the association. This is true if different fiber types from more than one object are found and each fiber type either links two people together or links an individual with a particular environment. As the number of different objects increases, the strength of an association increases dramatically. That is, the chance of randomly finding several particular fiber types in a certain location is much smaller than the chance of finding one particular fiber type.

The following example can be used to illustrate the significance of multiple fibers linking two items together. If one were to throw a single die one time, the chance or probability of throwing a particular number would be one chance in six. The probability of throwing a second die and getting that same number also would be one chance in six. However, the probability of getting 2 of the same numbers on 2 dice thrown simultaneously is only 1 in every 36 double throws—a much smaller chance than with either of the single throws. This number is a result of the product rule of probability theory. That is, the probability of the joint occurrence of a number of mutually independent events equals the product of the individual probabilities of each of the events (in this example—$\frac{1}{6} \times \frac{1}{6} = \frac{1}{36}$). Since numerous fiber types are in existence, the chance of finding one particular fiber type, other than a common type, in a specific randomly selected location is small. The chance then of finding several fiber types together in a specific location is

(continued)

NAME OF VICTIM	Violet-Green Bedspread, Williams' Bedroom	Green Carpet, Williams' Bedroom	Dog Hairs, Williams' Dog	Yellow Blanket, Williams' Bedroom	Blue Rayon Fibers, Debris from Williams' Home	Trunk Liner, 1978 Plymouth	Carpet, 1979 Ford	Carpet, 1970 Chevrolet	ADDITIONAL ITEMS FROM WILLIAMS' HOME, AUTOMOBILES OR PERSON
Alfred Evans	×	×	×			×			
Eric Middlebrooks	×		×		×				YELLOW NYLON — FORD TRUNK LINER
Charles Stephens	×	×	×		×				YELLOW NYLON — WHITE POLYESTER; BACKROOM CARPET — FORD TRUNK LINER
Lubie Geter	×	×	×				×		KITCHEN CARPET
Terry Pue	×	×	×						WHITE POLYESTER BACKROOM CARPET
Patrick Baltazar	×	×	×	×			×		YELLOW NYLON — WHITE POLYESTER — HEAD HAIR; GLOVE — JACKET — PIGMENTED POLYPROPYLENE
Joseph Bell	×			×					
Larry Rogers	×	×	×	×			×		YELLOW NYLON — PORCH BEDSPREAD
John Porter	×	×	×	×	×		×		PORCH BEDSPREAD
Jimmy Payne	×	×	×	×	×		×		BLUE THROW RUG
William Barrett	×	×	×	×	×		×		GLOVE
Nathaniel Cater	×	×	×	×					BACKROOM CARPET — YELLOW-GREEN SYNTHETIC

Fiber findings discussed during the trial and used to associate Williams with the 12 victims.

the product of several small probabilities, resulting in an extremely small chance.

However, no attempt was made to use the product rule and multiply the individual probability numbers together to get an approximation of the probability of finding carpets like Williams's residential carpet and Williams's automobile carpet in the same household. The probability numbers were used only to show that the individual fiber types involved in these associations were very uncommon.[11]

In addition to the two probability numbers already discussed (bedroom and station wagon carpets), each of the other fiber types linking Williams to both Cater and Payne has a probability of being found in a particular location. The chance of finding all of the fiber types indicated on the chart in one location (seven types on Payne's body and six types on Cater's body) would be extremely small. Although an actual probability number for those findings could not be determined, it is believed that the multiple fiber associations shown on this chart are proof that Williams is linked to the bodies of these two victims, even though each fiber by itself does not show a positive association with Williams's environment.

Two crime laboratory examiners testified during the closing stages of the first part of the trial about Williams's association with Payne and Cater. They concluded that it was highly unlikely that any environment other than that present in Wayne Williams's house and car could have resulted in the combination of fibers and hairs found on the victims and that it would be virtually impossible to have linked so many fibers found on

Cater and Payne to items in Williams's house and car unless the victims were in contact with or in some way associated with the environment of Wayne Williams.

After testimony was presented concerning the Payne and Cater cases, the Fulton County District Attorney's Office asked the court to be allowed to introduce evidence in the cases of 10 other victims whose murders were similar in many respects. Georgia law allows evidence of another crime to be introduced "...if some logical connection can be shown between the two from which it can be said that proof of the one tends to establish the other as relevant to some fact other than general bad character."[12] There need be no conviction for the other crime in order for details about that crime to be admissible.

It was ruled that evidence concerning other murders could be introduced in an attempt to prove a "pattern or scheme" of killing that included the two murders with which Williams was charged. The additional evidence in these cases was to be used to help the jury "...decide whether Williams had committed the two murders with which he is charged."[13]

The most important similarities between these additional victims were the fibers that linked 9 of the 10 victims to Williams's environment. The fiber findings discussed during the trial and used to associate Williams to the 12 victims were illustrated during the trial. (See Figure 1.)

The 12 victims were listed in chronological order based on the dates their bodies were recovered. The time period covered by this chart, approximately 22 months, is from July 1979 until May 1981. During that time period, the Williams family had access to a large number of automobiles, including a

[11] Joseph L. Peterson, ed., *Forensic Science* (New York: AMS Press, 1975), pp. 181–225. This collection of articles, dealing with various aspects of forensic science, contains five papers concerned with using statistics to interpret the meaning of physical evidence. It is a good discussion of probability theory and reviews cases where probability theory has been used in trial situations.

[12] *Encyclopedia of Georgia Law*, vol. 11A (The Harrison Company, 1979), p. 70.

[13] *The Atlanta Constitution*, "Williams Jury Told of Other Slayings," Sec. 1-A, 1/26/82, p. 25.

number of rental cars. Three of these automobiles are listed at the top of Figure 1. If one or more of the cars was in the possession of the Williams family at the time a victim was found to be missing, the space under that car(s) and after the particular victim's name is shaded.

Four objects (including the dog) from Williams's residence are listed horizontally across the top of Figure 1, along with objects from three of his automobiles. An "X" on the chart indicates an apparent transfer of textile fibers from the listed object to a victim. Other objects from Williams's environment which were linked to various victims by an apparent fiber transfer are listed on the right side of the chart. Fiber types from objects (never actually located) that were associated with fiber types from one or more victims are also listed either at the top or on the right side of the chart. Fourteen specific objects and five fiber types (probably from five other objects) listed on this chart are linked to one or more of the victims. More than 28 different fiber types, along with the dog hairs, were used to link up to 19 objects from Williams's environment to one or more of the victims. Of the more than 28 fiber types from Williams's environment, 14 of these originated from a rug or carpet.

The combination of more than 28 different fiber types would not be considered so significant if they were primarily common fiber types. In fact, there is only one light green cotton fiber of the 28 that might be considered common. This cotton fiber was blended with acetate fibers in Williams's bedspread. Light green cotton fibers removed from many victims were not considered or compared unless they were physically intermingled with violet acetate fibers which were consistent with originating from the bedspread. It should be noted that a combination of cotton and acetate fibers blended together in a single textile material, as in the bedspread, is in itself uncommon.

The previous discussion concerning the significance of multiple fiber linkages can be applied to the associations made in the cases of all the victims except Bell, but especially to the association of Patrick Baltazar to Williams's environment. Fibers and animal hairs consistent with having originated from 10 sources were removed from Baltazar's body. These 10 sources include the uncommon bedroom carpet and station wagon carpet. In addition to the fiber (and animal hair) linkage, two head hairs of African origin were removed from Baltazar's body that were consistent with originating from the scalp area of Williams. Head hairs similar to Williams' were recovered from Baltazar's body.

Another important aspect of the fiber linkage between Williams and these victims is the correspondence between the fiber findings and the time periods during which Williams had access to the three automobiles listed on the chart. Nine victims are linked to automobiles used by the Williams family. When Williams did not have access to a particular car, no fibers were recovered that were consistent with having originated from that automobile. Trunk liner fibers of the type used in the trunks of many late-model Ford Motor Company automobiles were also recovered from the bodies of two victims.

One final point should be made concerning Williams's bedroom and station wagon carpets where probability numbers had been determined. Fibers consistent with having originated from both of these "unusual" carpets were recovered from Payne's body. Of the nine victims who were killed during the time period when Williams had access to the 1970 station wagon, fibers consistent with having originated from both the station wagon carpet and the bedroom carpet were recovered from six of these victims.

The fact that many of the victims were involved with so many of the same fiber types, all of which linked the victims to Williams's environment, is the basis for arguing conclusively against these fibers originating from a source other than Williams's environment.

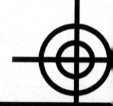

Chapter Summary > > > > > > > > > > >

Hair is an appendage of the skin that grows out of an organ known as the hair follicle. The length of a hair extends from its root or bulb embedded in the follicle, continues into a shaft, and terminates at a tip end. The shaft, which is composed of three layers—the cuticle, cortex, and medulla—is subjected to the most intense examination by the forensic scientist. The comparison microscope is an indispensable tool for comparing these morphological characteristics. When comparing strands of hair, the criminalist is particularly interested in the color, length, and diameter. A careful microscopic examination of hair reveals morphological features that can distinguish human hair from the hair of animals. Scale structure, medullary index,

and medullary shape are particularly important in hair identification. Other important features for comparing hair are the presence or absence of a medulla and the distribution, shape, and color intensity of the pigment granules present in the cortex. However, microscopic hair examinations tend to be subjective and highly dependent on the skills and integrity of the analyst. Recent major breakthroughs in DNA profiling have extended this technology to the individualization of human hair. The probability of detecting DNA in hair roots is more likely for hair being examined in its anagen or early growth phase as opposed to its catagen or telogen phases. Often, when hair is forcibly removed, a follicular tag, a translucent piece of tissue surrounding the hair's shaft near the root, may be present. This has proven to be a rich source of DNA associated with hair. Also, mitochondrial DNA can be extracted from the hair shaft. As a rule, all positive microscopic hair comparisons must be confirmed by DNA analysis.

When questioned hairs are submitted to a forensic laboratory for examination, they must always be accompanied by an adequate number of standard/reference samples from the victim of the crime and from individuals suspected of having deposited hair at the crime scene. Forensic hair comparisons generally involve either head hair or pubic hair. Collecting 25 full-length hairs from all areas of the scalp normally ensures a representative sampling of head hair. Likewise, a minimum collection of 25 full-length pubic hairs should cover the range of characteristics present in this type of hair. In rape cases, care must first be taken to comb the pubic area with a clean comb to remove all loose foreign hair present before the victim is sampled for standard/reference hair. The comb should then be packaged in a separate envelope.

The quality of fiber evidence depends on the ability of the criminalist to identify the origin of the fiber or at least to narrow the possibilities to a limited number of sources. Microscopic comparisons between questioned and standard/reference fibers are initially undertaken for color and diameter characteristics. Other morphological features that could be important in comparing fibers are striations on the surface of the fiber, the presence of de-lustering particles, and the cross-sectional shape of the fiber. The visible-light microspectrophotometer provides a convenient way to compare the colors of fibers through spectral patterns. Infrared spectrophotometry is a rapid and reliable tool for identifying the generic class of fibers, as is the polarizing microscope.

Relevant articles of clothing expected to bear fiber evidence should be packaged carefully in paper bags. Each article must be placed in a separate bag to avoid cross-contamination of evidence. Scrupulous care must be taken to prevent articles of clothing from different people or from different locations from coming into contact. Such articles must not even be placed on the same surface before packaging. Fibers can be packaged in plastic containers or glassine folds placed inside manila coin envelopes.

Review Questions

1. Hair is an appendage of the skin, growing out of an organ known as the _____.
2. The three layers of the hair shaft are the _____, the _____, and the _____.
3. True or False: The scales of most animal hairs can be described as looking like shingles on a roof. _____
4. The scale pattern of hair's _____ can be observed by making a cast of its surface in clear nail polish or softened vinyl.
5. The _____ contains the pigment granules that impart color to hair.
6. The central canal running through many hairs is known as the _____.
7. The diameter of the medulla relative to the diameter of the hair shaft is the _____.
8. Human hair generally has a medullary index of less than _____; the hair of most animals has an index of _____ or greater.
9. True or False: Human head hairs generally exhibit no medullae. _____
10. True or False: If a medulla exhibits a pattern, the hair is animal in origin. _____
11. True or False: Much of a hair's resistance and stability is attributed to the cuticle. _____
12. The three stages of hair growth are the _____, _____, and _____ phases.
13. True or False: Individual hairs can show variable morphological characteristics within a single individual. _____

14. In making hair comparisons, it is best to view the hairs side by side under a(n) _____ microscope.
15. _____ hairs are short and curly, with wide variation in shaft diameter.
16. True or False: It is possible to estimate when hair was last bleached or dyed by microscopic examination. _____
17. True or False: The age and sex of the individual from whom a hair sample has been taken can be determined through an examination of the hair's morphological features. _____
18. Hair forcibly removed from the body (always, often) has follicular tissue adhering to its root.
19. Microscopic hair comparisons must be regarded by police and courts as presumptive in nature, and all positive microscopic hair comparisons must be confirmed by _____ typing.
20. True or False: Currently, DNA typing can individualize a single hair. _____
21. A(n) _____ hair root is a likely candidate for DNA typing.
22. True or False: The onset of postmortem changes to the root portion of hair is only observed in anagenic and catagenic hairs. _____
23. A minimum collection of _____ full-length hairs normally ensures a representative sampling of head hair.
24. A minimum collection of _____ full-length pubic hairs is recommended to cover the range of characteristics present in this region of the body.

25. The ultimate value of fibers as forensic evidence depends on the ability to narrow their _____ to a limited number of sources or even to a single source.

26. _____ fibers are derived totally from animal or plant sources.

27. The most prevalent natural plant fiber is _____.

28. True or False: Regenerated fibers, such as rayon and acetate, are manufactured by chemically treating cellulose and passing it through a spinneret. _____

29. Fibers manufactured solely from synthetic chemicals are classified as _____.

30. True or False: Polyester was the first synthetic fiber. _____

31. True or False: A first step in the forensic examination of fibers is to compare color and diameter. _____

32. The microspectrophotometer employing _____ light is a convenient way for analysts to compare the colors of fibers through spectral patterns.

33. The microspectrophotometer employing _____ light provides a rapid and reliable method for identifying the generic class of a single fiber.

34. Normally, fibers possess (individual, class) characteristics.

35. True or False: Statistical databases are available for determining the probability of a fiber's origin. _____

36. If a body is thought to have been wrapped at one time in a blanket or carpet, _____ of exposed body areas may reveal fiber strands.

Review Questions for Inside the Science

1. _____ are composed of a large number of atoms arranged in repeating units.

2. The basic unit of the polymer is called the _____.

3. _____ are polymers composed of thousands of amino acids linked in a highly organized arrangement and sequence.

4. Synthetic fibers possess the physical property of _____ because they are crystalline.

Application and Critical Thinking

1. Indicate the phase of growth of each of the following hairs:
   a. The root is club shaped
   b. The hair has a follicular tag
   c. The root bulb is flame shaped
   d. The root is elongated

2. A criminalist studying a dyed sample hair notices that the dyed color ends about 1.5 centimeters from the tip of the hair. Approximately how many weeks before the examination was the hair dyed? Explain your answer.

3. Following are descriptions of several hairs; based on these descriptions, indicate the likely ancestry of the person from whom the hair originated:
   a. Evenly distributed, fine pigmentation
   b. Continuous medullation
   c. Dense, uneven pigmentation
   d. Wavy with a round cross-section

4. Criminalist Pete Evett is collecting fiber evidence from a murder scene. He notices fibers on the victim's shirt and trousers, so he places both of these items of clothing in a plastic bag. He also sees fibers on a sheet near the victim, so he balls up the sheet and places it in a separate plastic bag. Noticing fibers adhering to the windowsill from which the attacker gained entrance, Pete carefully removes them with his fingers and places them in a regular envelope. What mistakes, if any, did Pete make while collecting this evidence?

5. For each of the following human hair samples, indicate the medulla pattern present.

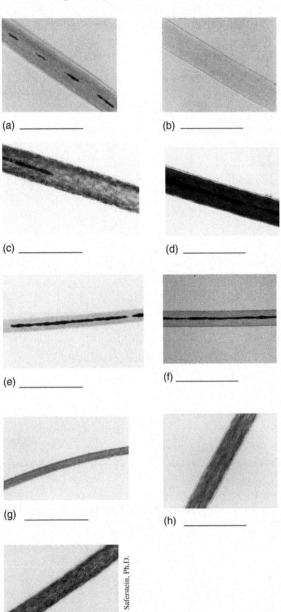

(a) _____

(b) _____

(c) _____

(d) _____

(e) _____

(f) _____

(g) _____

(h) _____

(i) _____

6. The most common scale patterns found on hairs are generally classified as coronal, spinous, and imbricate. Examine the scale casts of animal hairs shown here and indicate the scale pattern of each.

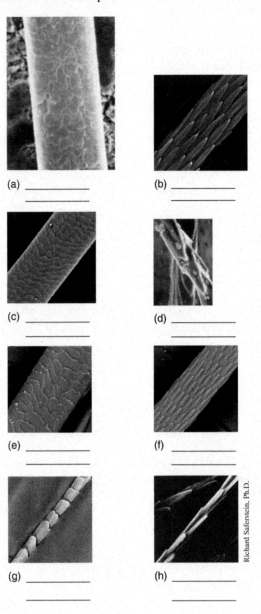

(a) _____
_____

(b) _____

(c) _____
_____

(d) _____

(e) _____

(f) _____

(g) _____
_____

(h) _____
_____

7. A young child is kidnapped from her school playground. Shown below is a reference sample of the kidnapped child's hair. The only cars that left the parking lot before the child was discovered to be missing were those of four cafeteria workers. The car of each worker was searched and hairs collected. These recovered hairs are shown below. Which recovered hair, if any, is consistent with that of the victim and warrants further investigation?

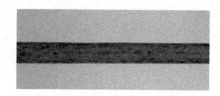

Hair from Car of Worker B.

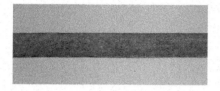

Reference Hair from Victim.

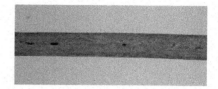

Hair from Car of Worker C.

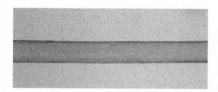

Hair from Car of Worker A.

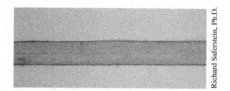

Hair from Car of Worker D.

Richard Saferstein, Ph.D.

Further References

Bisbing, R. E., "The Forensic Identification and Association of Human Hair," in R. Saferstein, ed., *Forensic Science Handbook*, vol. 1, 2nd ed. Upper Saddle River, NJ: Prentice Hall, 2002.

Deedrick, D. W., "Hairs, Fibers, Crime, and Evidence," *Forensic Science Communications* 2, no. 3 (2000), https://www2.fbi.gov/hq/lab/fsc/backissu/july2000/deedrick.htm

Deedrick, D. W., and S. L. Koch, "Microscopy of Hair Part I: A Practical Guide and Manual for Human Hairs," *Forensic Science Communications* 6, no. 1 (2004), https://www2.fbi.gov/hq/lab/fsc/backissu/jan2004/index.htm

Deedrick D. W., and S. L. Koch, "Microscopy of Hair Part II: A Practical Guide and Manual for Animal Hairs," *Forensic Science Communications* 6, no. 3 (2004), https://www2.fbi.gov/hq/lab/fsc/backissu/july2004/index.htm

Eyring M. B., and B. D. Gaudette, "The Forensic Aspects of Textile Fiber Examination," in R. Saferstein, ed., *Forensic Science Handbook*, vol. 2, 2nd ed. Upper Saddle River, NJ: Prentice Hall, 2005.

Ogle R. R., Jr., and M. J. Fox, *Atlas of Human Hair: Microscopic Characteristics*. Boca Raton, FL: CRC Press, 1999.

Oien, C. T., "Forensic Hair Comparison: Background Information for Interpretation," *Forensic Science Communications* 11, no. 2 (2009), https://www2.fbi.gov/hq/lab/fsc/backissu/april2009/index.htm

Petraco N., and P. R. De Forest, "A Guide to the Analysis of Forensic Dust Specimens," in R. Saferstein, ed., *Forensic Science Handbook*, vol. 3, 2nd ed. Upper Saddle River, NJ: Prentice Hall, 2010.

Robertson, J. ed., *Forensic Examination of Hair*. Boca Raton, FL: CRC Press, 1999.

Robertson J., and M. Grieve, eds., *Forensic Examination of Fibres*, 2nd ed. Boca Raton, FL: CRC Press, 1999.

Drugs

Learning Objectives

After studying this chapter, you should be able to:

12.1 Explain psychological and physical dependency on drugs and its impact on society

12.2 Classify the commonly used drugs

12.3 Explain the classification of drugs under the Controlled Substances Act

12.4 Describe the proper collection and preservation of drug evidence

12.5 Describe the laboratory tests normally used to perform a routine drug identification analysis

12.6 Discuss the process of chromatography as well as the difference between thin-layer chromatography and gas chromatography

12.7 Describe the utility of ultraviolet and infrared spectrophotometry for the identification of drugs

12.8 Describe the concept and utility of mass spectrometry for identification analysis

KEY TERMS

anabolic steroids
analgesic
chromatography
confirmation
depressant
fluoresce
hallucinogen
infrared
ion
microcrystalline tests
monochromatic light
monochromator
narcotic
physical dependence
psychological
   dependence
screening test
spectrophotometry
stimulant
ultraviolet

Go to www.pearsonhighered.com/careersresources to access Webextras for this chapter.

El Chapo: Joaquin Guzmán

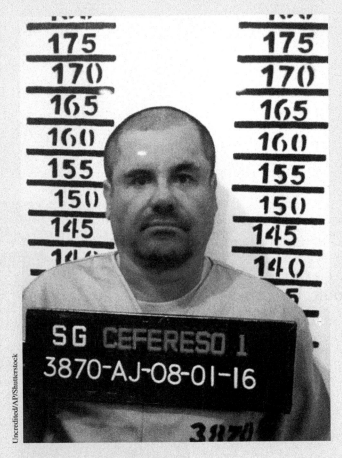

In 2016, the U.S. government filed charges against Joaquin "El Chapo" Guzmán seeking $14 billion dollars in estimated wealth he earned from trafficking drugs for the Sinaloa Cartel. As the leader of the Cartel, Guzmán oversaw drug smuggling operations throughout the United States and Europe. Through the use of distribution cells in the United States and long-range tunnels near borders, Guzmán was able to export more drugs to the United States than any other trafficker in history. His leadership of the Cartel also brought immense wealth and power; Guzmán was ranked by Forbes as one of the most powerful people in the world between 2009 and 2013, while the Drug Enforcement Administration (DEA) estimated that he matched the influence and wealth of Pablo Escobar.

Guzmán was born in Sinaloa and raised in a poor farming family. He entered the drug trade, helping him grow marijuana for local dealers during his early adulthood. In the 1970s, Guzmán began working with Hector Luis Palma Salazar, one of the nation's rising drug lords, whom he helped map routes to move drugs through Sinaloa, and into the United States. He later supervised logistics for Miguel Angel Felix Gallardo, one of the Mexico's leading kingpins. During the 1980s, increased scrutiny on the South American Cartels allowed the Mexican Cartels to flourish. When Gallardo was finally arrested in 1989, Guzmán broke off on his own and started his own Cartel.

Guzmán was first captured in 1993 in Guatemala and was extradited to Mexico to face drug charges. There he was sentenced to 20 years in prison for murder and drug trafficking. He bribed prison guards and escaped from a federal maximum-security prison in 2001. The U.S. and Mexico offered a combined reward of $8.8 million dollars for information leading to his capture, and he was re-arrested in Mexico in 2014. He escaped prior to formal sentencing in 2015, through a tunnel nearly a mile long under his jail cell. He was recaptured by Mexican authorities following a shoot-out in 2016, and was extradited to the United States a year later, where he was tried and convicted of 10 counts, including drug trafficking, weapons charges, and money laundering. He was sentenced in July 2019to a life term of imprisonment plus 30 years to run consecutive to the life sentence for being a principal leader of a continuing criminal enterprise. He was also ordered to pay $12.6 billion in forfeiture.

A *drug* can be defined as a natural or synthetic substance that is used to produce physiological or psychological effects in humans or other higher-order animals. However, this colorless clinical definition does not really tell us what drugs are; in their modern context, drugs mean something different to each person. To some, drugs are a necessity for sustaining and prolonging life; to others, drugs provide an escape from the pressures of life; to still others, they are a means of ending it.

Considering the wide application and acceptance of drugs in our society, it was perhaps inevitable that a segment of our population would use them. During the 1960s, successive waves of hallucinogens, amphetamines, and barbiturates found their way out of laboratories, pharmacies, and medicine chests and into the streets. During this decade, marijuana became the most widely used illicit drug in the United States, and alcohol consumption continued to rise—today 90 million Americans drink alcohol regularly, and 10 million of these are addicted or have severe problems in coping with their drinking habits. In the 1970s, heroin addiction emerged as a national problem, and today, the United States is in the midst of an epidemic of cocaine use.

Drug use has grown from a problem generally associated with members of the lower end of the socioeconomic ladder to one that cuts across all social and ethnic classes of society. Today, approximately 23 million people in the United States use illicit drugs, including about a half million users of heroin and nearly six million users of cocaine.

In the United States, more than 75 percent of the evidence evaluated in crime laboratories is drug related. The deluge of drug specimens has forced the expansion of existing crime laboratories and the creation of new ones. For many concerned forensic scientists, the crime laboratory's preoccupation with drug evidence represents a serious distraction from time that could be devoted to evaluating evidence related to homicides and other types of serious crimes. However, the increasing caseloads associated with drug evidence have justified the expansion of forensic laboratory services. This expansion has increased the overall analytical capabilities of crime laboratories.

Drug Dependence

In assessing the potential danger of drugs, society has become particularly conscious of their effects on human behavior. In fact, the first drugs to be regulated by law in the early years of the 20th century were those deemed to have "habit-forming" properties. The early laws were aimed primarily at controlling opium and its derivatives, cocaine, and later marijuana. Today, it is known that the ability of a drug to induce dependence after repeated use is submerged in a complex array of physiological and social factors.

Dependence on drugs exists in numerous patterns and in all degrees of intensity, depending on the nature of the drug, the route of administration, the dose, the frequency of administration, and the individual's rate of metabolism. Furthermore, nondrug factors play an equally crucial role in determining the behavioral patterns associated with drug use. The personal characteristics of the user, the user's expectations about the drug experience, society's attitudes and possible responses, and the setting in which the drug is used are all major determinants of drug dependence.

The question of how to define and measure a drug's influence on the individual and its danger to society is difficult to assess. To this end, the nature and significance of drug dependence must be considered from two overlapping points of view: the interaction of the drug with the individual and the drug's impact on society. It will be useful when discussing the nature of the drug experience to approach the problem from two distinctly different aspects of human—behavior—**psychological dependence** and **physical dependence**.

Psychological Dependence

The common denominator that characterizes all types of repeated drug use is the creation of a psychological dependence for continued use of the drug. Most users present quite a typical appearance and remain both socially and economically integrated in the life of the community.

The reasons why some people abstain from drugs while others become moderately or heavily involved are difficult if not impossible to delineate. Psychological needs arise from numerous personal and social factors that stem from the individual's desire to create a sense of well-being

psychological dependence
Conditioned use of a drug caused by underlying emotional needs.

physical dependence
Need for a drug that has been brought about by its regular use; dependence is characterized by withdrawal sickness when administration of the drug is abruptly stopped.

and to escape from reality. In some cases, the individual may be seeking relief from personal problems or stressful situations, or they may be trying to sustain a physical and emotional state that permits an improved level of performance. Whatever the reasons, the underlying psychological needs and the desire to fulfill them create a conditioned pattern of drug use.

The intensity of the psychological dependence associated with a drug's use is difficult to define and largely depends on the nature of the drug used. For drugs such as alcohol, heroin, amphetamines, barbiturates, and cocaine, continued use is likely to result in a high degree of involvement. Other drugs, such as marijuana and codeine, appear to have a considerably lower potential for the development of psychological dependence. However, this does not imply that repeated use of drugs deemed to have a low potential for psychological dependency is safe or will always produce low psychological dependence. We have no precise way of measuring or predicting the impact of drug use on the individual. Even if a system could be devised for controlling the many possible variables affecting a user's response, the unpredictability of the human personality would still have to be considered.

Our general knowledge of alcohol consumption should warn us of the fallacy of generalizing when attempting to describe the danger of drug use. Obviously, not all alcohol drinkers are psychologically addicted to the drug; most are "social" drinkers who drink in reasonable amounts and on an irregular basis. Many people have progressed beyond this stage and consider alcohol a necessary crutch for dealing with life's stresses and anxieties. However, alcohol users exhibit a wide range of behavioral patterns, and to a large extent, the degree of psychological dependency must be determined individually. Likewise, it would be fallacious to generalize that all users of marijuana can at worst develop a low degree of dependency on the drug. A wide range of factors also influence marijuana's effect, and heavy users of the drug expose themselves to the danger of developing a high degree of psychological dependency.

Physical Dependence

Whereas emotional well-being is the primary motive leading to repeated and intensive use of a drug, certain drugs, when taken in sufficient dose and frequency, are capable of producing physiological changes that encourage their continued use. Once the user abstains from such a drug, severe physical illness follows. The desire to avoid this *withdrawal sickness* or *abstinence syndrome* ultimately causes physical dependence, or addiction. Hence, for individuals with heroin use problems who are accustomed to receiving large doses of heroin, the thought of abstaining and encountering body chills, vomiting, stomach cramps, convulsions, insomnia, pain, and hallucinations is a powerful inducement for continued drug use.

Interestingly, some of the more widely used drugs have little or no potential for creating physical dependence. Drugs such as marijuana, lysergic acid diethylamide (LSD), and cocaine create strong anxieties when their repeated use is discontinued; however, no medical evidence attributes these discomforts to physiological reactions that accompany withdrawal sickness. On the other hand, use of alcohol, heroin, and barbiturates can result in development of physical dependency.

Physical dependency develops only when the drug user adheres to a regular schedule of drug intake; that is, the interval between doses must be short enough so that the effects of the drug never wear off completely. For example, the interval between injections of heroin for individuals with heroin use problems probably does not exceed six to eight hours. Beyond this time, the user begins to experience the uncomfortable symptoms of withdrawal. Many heroin users avoid taking the drug regularly for fear of becoming physically addicted to its use. Similarly, the risk of developing physical dependence on alcohol becomes greatest when the consumption is characterized by a continuing pattern of daily use in large quantities.

Table 12–1 categorizes some of the more commonly used drugs according to their effect on the body and summarizes their tendency to produce psychological dependency and to induce physical dependency with repeated use.

Societal Aspects of Drug Use

The social impact of drug dependence is directly related to the extent to which the user has become preoccupied with the drug. Here, the most important element is the extent to which drug use has become interwoven in the fabric of the user's life. The more frequently the drug satisfies the person's need, the greater the likelihood that they will become preoccupied with

TABLE 12–1

The Potential of Some Commonly Used Drugs to Produce Dependency with Regular Use

Drug	Psychological Dependence	Physical Dependence
Narcotics		
Morphine	High	Yes
Heroin	High	Yes
Methadone	High	Yes
Codeine	Low	Yes
Depressants		
Barbiturates (short-acting)	High	Yes
Barbiturates (long-acting)	Low	Yes
Alcohol	High	Yes
Methaqualone (Quaalude)	High	Yes
Meprobamate (Miltown, Equanil)	Moderate	Yes
Diazepam (Valium)	Moderate	Yes
Chlordiazepoxide (Librium)	Moderate	Yes
Stimulants		
Amphetamines	High	?
Cocaine	High	No
Caffeine	Low	No
Nicotine	High	Yes
Hallucinogens		
Marijuana	Low	No
LSD	Low	No
Phencyclidine (PCP)	High	No

its use, with a consequent neglect of individual and social responsibilities. Personal health, economic relationships, and family obligations may all suffer as the drug-seeking behavior increases in frequency and intensity and dominates the individual's life. The extreme of drug dependence may lead to behavior that has serious implications for the public's safety, health, and welfare.

Drug dependence in its broadest sense involves much of the world's population. As a result, a complex array of individual, social, cultural, legal, and medical factors ultimately influence society's decision to prohibit or to impose strict controls on a drug's distribution and use. Invariably, society must weigh the beneficial aspects of the drug against the ultimate harm its use will do to the individual and to society as a whole. Obviously, many forms of drug dependence do not carry sufficient adverse social consequences to warrant their prohibition, as illustrated by the widespread use of such drug-containing substances as tobacco and coffee. Although heavy and prolonged use of these drugs may eventually damage body organs and injure an individual's health, there is no evidence that they result in antisocial behavior, even with prolonged or excessive use. Hence, society is willing to accept widespread use of these substances.

We are certainly all aware of the disastrous failure in the United States to prohibit the use of alcohol during the 1920s and the current debate on whether marijuana should be legalized. Each of these issues emphasizes the delicate balance between individual desires and needs and society's concern with the consequences of drug use; moreover, this balance is continuously subject to change and reevaluation.

Types of Drugs

Narcotic Drugs

The term **narcotic** is derived from the Greek word *narkotikos*, which implies a state of lethargy or sluggishness. Pharmacologists classify narcotic drugs as substances that bring relief from pain and produce sleep. Unfortunately, "narcotic" has come to be popularly associated with any drug

narcotic
An analgesic or painkilling substance that depresses vital body functions such as blood pressure, pulse rate, and breathing rate; regular administration of narcotics produces physical dependence.

that is socially unacceptable. As a consequence of this incorrect usage, many drugs are improperly called narcotics.

Furthermore, this confusion has produced legal definitions that are at variance with the pharmacological actions of many drugs. For example, until the early 1970s, most drug laws in the United States incorrectly designated marijuana as a narcotic; even now, many drug-control laws in the United States, including the federal law, classify cocaine as a narcotic drug. Pharmacologically, cocaine is actually a powerful central nervous system stimulant, possessing properties opposite to those normally associated with the depressant effects of a narcotic.

OPIATES   Medical professionals apply the term *opiate* to most of the drugs properly classified as narcotics. Narcotic drugs are **analgesics**—that is, they relieve pain by depressing the central nervous system. Regular use of a narcotic drug leads to physical dependence, with all of its dire consequences. The source of most analgesic narcotics is opium, a gummy, milky juice exuded through a cut made in the unripe pod of the poppy (*Papaver somniferium*), a plant grown mostly in parts of Asia. Opium is brownish in color and has a morphine content ranging from 4 to 21 percent.

Although morphine is readily extracted from opium, for reasons that are not totally known, most users prefer to use one of its derivatives, *heroin*. Heroin is made rather simply by reacting morphine with acetic anhydride or acetyl chloride (see Figure 12–1). Heroin's high solubility in water makes its street preparation for intravenous administration rather simple, for only by injection are heroin's effects almost instantaneously felt and with maximum sensitivity. To prepare the drug for injection, the individual frequently dissolves it in a small quantity of water in a spoon. The process can be speeded up by heating the spoon over a candle or several matches. The solution is then drawn into a syringe or eyedropper for injection beneath the skin. Figure 12–2 shows some of the paraphernalia typically associated with street administration of heroin. Besides being a powerful analgesic, heroin produces a "high" that is accompanied by drowsiness and a deep sense of well-being; however, the effect is short, generally lasting only three to four hours. Regular use of heroin—or any other narcotic drug—invariably leads to physical dependence, with all of its dire consequences.

Codeine is also present in opium, but it is usually prepared synthetically from morphine. It is commonly used as a cough suppressant in prescription cough syrup. Codeine, only one-sixth as strong as morphine, is not an attractive street drug for individuals with drug use problems.

SYNTHETIC OPIATES   A number of narcotic drugs are not naturally derived from opium. However, because they have physiological effects on the body that are similar to those of the opium narcotics, they are also commonly referred to as opiates.

analgesic
A drug or substance that lessens or eliminates pain.

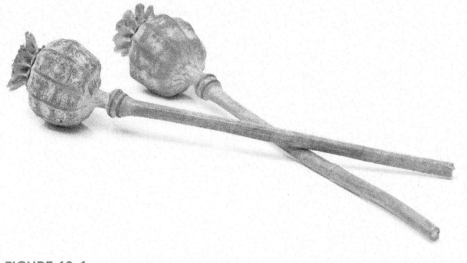

Zcw/Shutterstock

FIGURE 12–1
The opium poppy from which morphine is extracted, which ultimately is used to synthesize heroin.

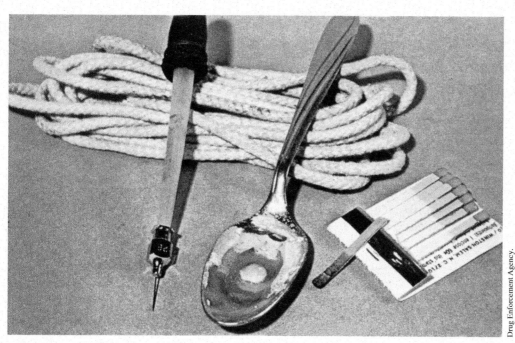

Drug Enforcement Agency.

FIGURE 12–2
Heroin paraphernalia.

In 1995, the U.S. Food and Drug Administration approved for use the painkilling drug *OxyContin*. The active ingredient in OxyContin is oxycodone, a synthetic closely related to morphine and heroin in its chemical structure. OxyContin is an analgesic narcotic that has effects similar to those of heroin. It is prescribed to a million patients for treatment of chronic pain, with doctors writing close to seven million OxyContin prescriptions each year. The drug is compounded with a time-release formulation that the manufacturer initially believed would reduce the risk of use and addiction. This has not turned out to be the case. It is estimated that close to a quarter of a million individuals use the drug.

Because it is a legal drug that is diverted from legitimate sources, OxyContin is obtained differently than illegal drugs. Pharmacy robberies, forged prescriptions, and theft from patients with a legitimate prescription are ways in which users access OxyContin. Some users visit numerous doctors and receive prescriptions even though their medical condition may not warrant it.

Methadone is another well-known synthetic opiate. In the 1960s, scientists discovered that a person receiving methadone periodically in oral doses of 80–120 milligrams a day would not get high if they then took heroin or morphine. Clearly, although methadone is a narcotic pharmacologically related to heroin, its administration appears to eliminate the individual's desire for heroin while producing minimal side effects. Critics of the controversial methadone maintenance programs claim that methadone use is just substituting one narcotic drug for another, and supporters argue that this is the only known treatment for keeping the individuals off heroin and offering some hope for eventual abstention from narcotics.

Physicians are increasingly prescribing methadone for pain relief. Unfortunately, in recent years, the wide availability of the drug for legitimate medical purposes has led to greater quantities of the drug being diverted into the illicit market. Methadone is being used increasingly and is causing an alarming number of overdoses and deaths.

Hallucinogens

Hallucinogens are drugs that can cause marked alterations in mood, attitude, thought processes, and perceptions. Perhaps the most popular and controversial member of this class of drugs is marijuana.

hallucinogen
A substance that induces changes in mood, attitude, thought processes, and perceptions.

Inside the Science

What's in the Bag

The content of a typical bag of heroin is an excellent example of the uncertainty attached to buying illicit drugs. For many years in the 1960s and into early 1970s, the average bag contained 15 to 20 percent heroin. Currently, the average purity of heroin obtained in the illicit U.S. market is approximately 35 percent. The individual with a heroin use problem rarely knows or cares what composes the other 65 percent or so of the material. Traditionally, quinine has been the most common diluent of heroin. Like heroin, it has a bitter taste and was probably originally used to obscure the actual potency of a heroin preparation from those who wished to taste-test the material before buying it. Other diluents commonly added to heroin are starch, lactose, procaine (Novocain), and mannitol.

MARIJUANA   Marijuana is the popular name of the plant *Cannabis sativa*, a weed that will grow wild in most climates. Marijuana easily qualifies as the most widely used illicit drug in the United States today. Marijuana is a preparation derived from the plant *Cannabis*. Most botanists believe there is only one species of the plant, *Cannabis sativa L.* The marijuana preparation normally consists of crushed leaves mixed in varying proportions with the plant's flower, stem, and seed. The plant secretes a sticky resin known as *hashish*. The resinous material can also be extracted from the plant by soaking in a solvent, such as alcohol. On the illicit-drug market, hashish usually appears in the form of compressed vegetation containing a high percentage of resin. A potent form of marijuana is known as *sinsemilla*. This is made from the unfertilized flowering tops of the female *Cannabis* plants, attained by removing all male plants from the growing field at the first sign of their appearance. It follows that the production of sinsemilla requires a great deal of attention and care, and the plant is therefore cultivated on small plots. The *Cannabis* plant contains a chemical known as *tetrahydrocannabinol*, or THC, which produces the psychoactive effects experienced by users. The THC content of *Cannabis* varies in different parts of the plant. The greatest concentration is usually found in hashish. Declining concentrations are typically found in the flowers and leaves, respectively. Little THC is found in the stem, roots, or seeds of the plant. The potency and resulting effect of the drug fluctuate, depending on the relative proportion of these plant parts in the marijuana mixture consumed by the user. The most common method of administration is by smoking either the dried flowers and leaves or various preparations of hashish (see Figure 12–3). Marijuana is also occasionally taken orally, typically baked in sweets, such as brownies or cookies.

Any study that relates to marijuana's effect on humans must consider the potency of the marijuana preparation. An interesting insight into the relationship between dosage level and marijuana's pharmacological effect was presented in the first report of the National Commission of Marijuana and Drug Abuse:

> At low, usual "social" doses the user may experience an increased sense of well-being; initial restlessness and hilarity followed by a dreamy, carefree state of relaxation; alteration of sensory perceptions including expansion of space and time; and a more vivid sense of touch, sight, smell, taste and sound; a feeling of hunger, especially a craving for sweets; and subtle changes in thought formation and expression. To an unknowing observer, an individual in this state of consciousness would not appear noticeably different from his normal state.

> At higher, moderate doses these same reactions are intensified but the changes in the individual would still be scarcely noticeable to an observer. . . . At very high doses, psychotomimetic phenomena may be experienced. These include distortion of body image, loss of personal identity, sensory and mental illusions, fantasies and hallucinations.[1]

[1] *Marijuana—A Signal of Misunderstanding* (Washington, D.C.: U.S. Government Printing Office, 1972), p. 56.

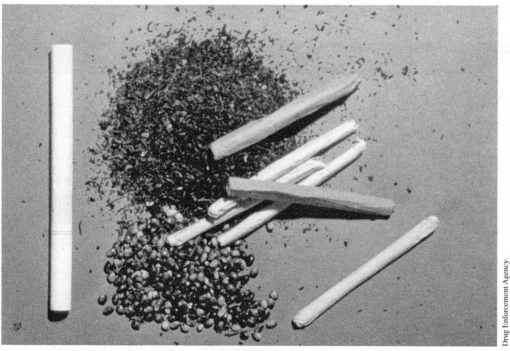

Drug Enforcement Agency.

FIGURE 12–3
Several rolled marijuana cigarettes lie on a pile of crushed dried marijuana leaves next to a tobacco cigarette.

Marijuana easily qualifies as the most widely used illicit drug in the United States. For instance, more than 43 million Americans have tried marijuana, according to the latest surveys, and almost half that number may be regular users. In addition to its widespread illegal use, accumulating evidence suggests that marijuana has potential medical uses. Two promising areas of research are marijuana's reduction of excessive eye pressure in sufferers of glaucoma and the lessening of nausea caused by powerful anticancer drugs. Marijuana may also be useful as a muscle relaxant.

No current evidence suggests that experimental or intermittent use causes physical or psychological harm. Marijuana does not cause physical dependency. However, the risk of harm lies instead in heavy, long-term use of the drug, particularly of the more potent preparations. Heavy users can develop a strong psychological dependence on the drug. Some effects of marijuana use include increased heart rate, dry mouth, reddened eyes, impaired motor skills and concentration, and frequently hunger and an increased desire for sweets.

OTHER HALLUCINOGENS   A substantial number of substances of widely varying chemical compositions have become part of the drug culture because of their hallucinogenic properties. These include LSD, mescaline, phencyclidine (PCP), psilocybin, and methylenedioxymethamphetamine, also known as MDMA or Ecstasy.

LSD is synthesized from lysergic acid, a substance derived from ergot, which is a type of fungus that attacks certain grasses and grains. Its hallucinogenic effects were first described by the Swiss chemist Albert Hofmann after he accidentally ingested some of the material in his laboratory in 1943. The drug is very potent; as little as 25 micrograms is enough to start vivid visual hallucinations that can last for about 12 hours. The drug also produces marked changes in mood, leading to laughing or crying at the slightest provocation. Feelings of anxiety and tension almost always accompany LSD use. Although physical dependence does not develop with continued use, the individual user may be prone to flashbacks and psychotic reactions even after use is discontinued.

In recent years, use of phencyclidine, commonly called PCP, has grown to alarming proportions. Because this drug can be synthesized by rather simple chemical processes, it is

Inside the Science

Marijuana and Hashish

Marijuana grows to a height of 5 to 15 feet and is characterized by an odd number of leaflets on each leaf. Normally each leaf contains five to nine leaflets, all with serrated or sawtooth edges.

The potency of marijuana depends on its form. Marijuana in the form of loose vegetation has an average THC content of about 3 to 4.5 percent.

Hashish preparations average about 2 to 8 percent THC. On the illicit-drug market, hashish (see photo) usually appears in the form of compressed vegetation containing a high percentage of resin. A particularly potent form of hashish is known as *liquid hashish* or *hashish oil*. Hashish in this form is normally a viscous substance, dark green with a tarry consistency. Liquid hashish is produced by efficiently extracting the THC-rich resin from the marijuana plant with an appropriate solvent, such as alcohol. The THC content of liquid hashish typically varies from 8 to 22 percent. Because of its extraordinary potency, one drop of the material can produce a "high."

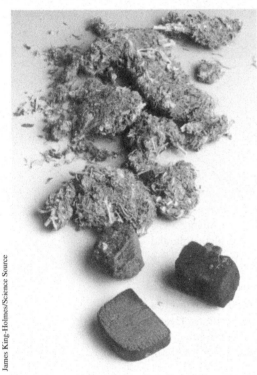

James King-Holmes/Science Source

Blocks of hashish in front of leaves and flowering tops of the marijuana plant.

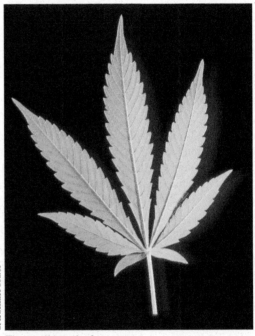

SPL/Science Source

The marijuana leaf.

manufactured surreptitiously for the illicit market in so-called clandestine laboratories (see Figure 12–4). These laboratories range from large, sophisticated operations to small labs located in a bathroom. Small-time operators normally have little or no training in chemistry and employ "cookbook" methods to synthesize the drug. Some of the more knowledgeable and experienced operators have been able to achieve clandestine production levels that approach a commercial level of operation.

PCP is often mixed with other drugs, such as LSD or amphetamine, and is sold as a powder ("angel dust"), capsule, or tablet, or as a liquid sprayed on plant leaves. The drug is smoked,

Inside the Science

Synthetic Cannabis

Synthetic cannabinoids are chemicals designed to mimic the pharmacological effects of naturally occurring cannabinoids. These drugs are generally sold in retail establishments or over the Internet as herbal procedures, potpourri, or incense. Users generally spray the chemicals onto botanical materials and inhale the drug through burning or smoking.

Synthetic cannabinoids derive their pharmacological activity from their affinity toward cannabinoid (CB) receptor sites in the brain. Early in their availability, these synthetics went by the common names "K2" and "spice"; however, currently their chemical composition and names have become quite varied as clandestine laboratories have become adept and innovative in modifying their chemical structures seeking to circumvent control by drug laws. Because the chemical structures of synthetic cannabinoids do not resemble marijuana constituents, they cannot be detected by routine drug screening tests.

The symptomology associated with the use of synthetic cannabinoids can result in anxiety, agitation, and nausea. A federal law, the Food and Drug Administration Safety and Innovation Act, broadly covers any material that contains a synthetic cannabinoid.

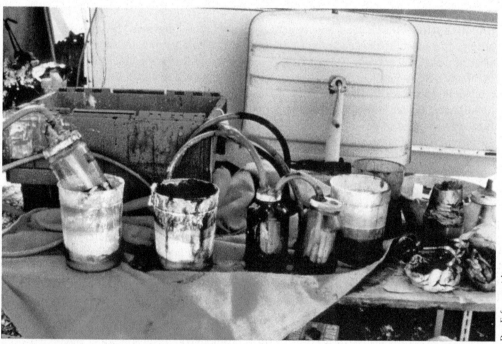

Drug Enforcement Agency.

FIGURE 12–4
Scene from a clandestine drug laboratory.

ingested, or sniffed. Following oral intake of moderate doses (1–6 milligrams), the user first experiences feelings of strength and invulnerability, along with a dreamy sense of detachment. However, the user soon becomes unresponsive, confused, and agitated. Depression, irritability, feelings of isolation, audio and visual hallucinations, and sometimes paranoia accompany PCP use. Severe depression, tendencies toward violence, and suicide accompany long-term daily use of the drug. In some cases, the PCP user experiences sudden schizophrenic behavior days after the drug has been taken.

Depressants

Depressants are drugs that slow down, or depress, the central nervous system. Several types of drugs fall under this category, including the most widely used drug in the United States—alcohol.

ALCOHOL (ETHYL ALCOHOL)   Many people overlook the fact that alcohol is a drug; its major behavioral effects derive from its depressant action on the central nervous system. In the United States, the alcohol industry annually produces more than one billion gallons of spirits, wine, and beer for which 90 million consumers pay nearly $40 billion. Unquestionably, these and other statistics support the fact that alcohol is the most widely used drug.

The behavioral patterns of alcohol intoxication vary and depend in part on such factors as social setting, amount consumed, and the personal expectation of the individual with regard to alcohol. When alcohol enters the body's bloodstream, it quickly travels to the brain, where it suppresses the brain's control of thought processes and muscle coordination.

Low doses of alcohol tend to inhibit the mental processes of judgment, memory, and concentration. The drinker's personality becomes expansive, and they exude confidence. When taken in moderate doses, alcohol reduces coordination substantially, inhibits orderly thought processes and speech patterns, and slows reaction times. Under these conditions, the ability to walk or drive becomes noticeably impaired. In the next chapter, we examine in greater detail the relationship between alcohol blood levels and driving ability. Higher doses of alcohol may cause the user to become highly irritable and emotional; displays of anger and crying are not uncommon. Extremely high doses may cause an individual to lapse into unconsciousness or even a comatose state that may precede a fatal depression of circulatory and respiratory functions.

BARBITURATES   Barbiturates are commonly referred to as "downers" because they relax, create a feeling of well-being, and produce sleep. Like alcohol, barbiturates suppress the vital functions of the central nervous system. Collectively, barbiturates can be described as derivatives of barbituric acid, which was first synthesized by a German chemist, Adolf von Bayer, more than a hundred years ago. Twenty-five barbiturate derivatives are currently used in medical practice in the United States; however, five—amobarbital, secobarbital, phenobarbital, pentobarbital, and butabarbital—tend to be used for most medical applications. Slang terms for "barbs" usually stem from the color of the capsule or tablet (for example, "yellow jackets," "blue devils," and "reds").

Normally, barbiturate users take these drugs orally. The average sedative dose is about 10–70 milligrams. When taken in this fashion, the drug enters the blood through the walls of the small intestine. Some barbiturates, such as phenobarbital, are absorbed more slowly than others and are therefore classified as long-acting barbiturates. Undoubtedly, the slow action of phenobarbital accounts for its low incidence of use. Apparently, barbiturate users prefer the faster-acting ones—secobarbital, pentobarbital, and amobarbital. When taken in prescribed amounts, barbiturates are relatively safe, but in instances of extensive and prolonged use, physical dependence can develop. Since the early 1970s, a nonbarbiturate depressant, methaqualone (Quaalude), has appeared on the illicit-drug scene. Methaqualone is a powerful sedative and muscle relaxant that possesses many of the depressant properties of barbiturates.

ANTIPSYCHOTICS AND ANTIANXIETY DRUGS   Although antipsychotics and antianxiety drugs can be considered depressants, they differ from barbiturates in the extent of their actions on the central nervous system. Generally, these drugs produce a relaxing tranquility without impairing high-thinking faculties or inducing sleep. Antipsychotics, such as reserpine and chlorpromazine, have been used to reduce the anxieties and tensions of people diagnosed with anxiety disorders.

A group of antianxiety drugs is commonly prescribed to deal with the everyday tensions of many healthy people. These drugs include meprobamate (Miltown), chlordiazepoxide (Librium), diazepam (Valium), and Xanax. In the past 45 years, the use of tranquilizers has grown dramatically. Medical evidence shows that these drugs produce psychological and physical dependency with repeated and high levels of usage. For this reason, widespread prescribing of these substances as a means of overcoming the pressures and tensions of life has worried many who fear the creation of a legalized drug culture.

"HUFFING"   Since the early 1960s, "huffing," the practice of sniffing materials containing volatile solvents (airplane glue or model cement, for example) has grown in popularity. Within recent years, another dimension has been added to the problem with the increasing number of incidents involving the sniffing of aerosol gas propellants, such as freon. All materials used in sniffing contain volatile or gaseous substances that are primarily central nervous system depressants. Although toluene seems to be the most popular solvent to sniff, others can produce comparable physiological effects. These chemicals include naphtha, methyl ethyl ketone (antifreeze), gasoline, and trichloroethylene (dry-cleaning solvent).

The usual immediate effects of sniffing are a feeling of exhilaration and euphoria combined with slurred speech, impaired judgment, and double vision. Finally, the user may experience drowsiness and stupor, with these depressant effects slowly wearing off as the user returns to a normal state. Most experts believe that users become physiologically dependent on the effects achieved by sniffing. There is, however, little evidence to suggest that solvent inhalation is addictive. But sniffers expose themselves to the danger of liver, heart, and brain damage from the chemicals they have inhaled. Even worse, sniffing of some solvents, particularly halogenated hydrocarbons, is accompanied by a significant risk of death.

Stimulants

The term **stimulant** refers to a range of drugs that stimulate, or speed up, the central nervous system.

stimulant
A substance taken to increase alertness or activity.

AMPHETAMINES   Amphetamines are a group of synthetic drugs that stimulate the central nervous system. They are commonly referred to in the terminology of the drug culture as "uppers" or "speed." Ordinary therapeutic doses of 5–20 milligrams per day, taken orally, provide a feeling of well-being and increased alertness that is followed by a decrease in fatigue and a loss of appetite. However, these apparent benefits of the drug are accompanied by restlessness and instability or apprehension, and once the stimulant effect wears off, depression may set in.

In the United States, the most serious form of amphetamine use stems from the intravenous injection of amphetamine or its chemical derivative, methamphetamine (see Figure 12–5). The desire for a more intense amphetamine experience is the primary motive for this route of administration. The initial sensation of a "flash" or "rush," followed by an intense feeling of pleasure, constitutes the principal appeal of the intravenous route for the "speed freak." During a "speed binge," the individual may inject 500–1,000 milligrams of amphetamines every two to three hours. Users have reported experiencing a euphoria that produces hyperactivity, with a feeling of clarity of vision as well as hallucinations. As the effect of the amphetamines wears off, the individual lapses into a period of exhaustion and may sleep continuously for one or two days. Following this, the user often experiences a prolonged period of severe depression, lasting from days to weeks.

A new smokable form of methamphetamine known as "ice" is reportedly in heavy demand in some areas of the United States. Ice is prepared by slow evaporation of a methamphetamine solution to produce large, crystal-clear "rocks." Like crack cocaine (discussed next), ice is smoked and produces effects similar to those of crack cocaine, but the effects last for a longer period of time. Once the effects of ice wear off, users often become depressed and may sleep for days. Chronic users exhibit violent destructive behavior and acute psychosis similar to paranoid schizophrenia. Repeated use of amphetamines leads to a strong psychological dependency, which encourages their continued administration.

COCAINE   Between 1884 and 1887, Sigmund Freud created something of a sensation in European medical circles by describing his experiments with a new drug. He reported a substance of seemingly limitless potential as a source of "exhilaration and lasting euphoria" that permitted "intensive mental or physical work [to be] performed without fatigue. . . . It is as though the need for food and sleep was completely banished."

The object of Freud's enthusiasm was cocaine, a drug stimulant extracted from the leaves of *Erythroxylon coca*, a plant grown in tropical Asia and the Andes Mountains of South America (see Figure 12–6). At one time, cocaine

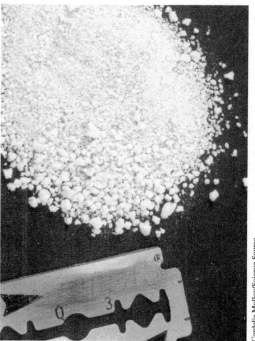

Cordelia Molloy/Science Source

FIGURE 12–5
Granular amphetamine beside a razor blade.

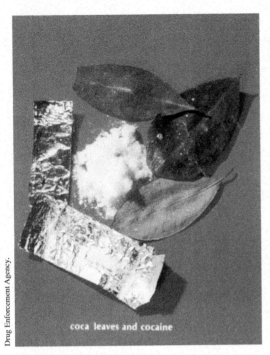

coca leaves and cocaine

FIGURE 12–6
Coca leaves and illicit forms of cocaine.

Drug Enforcement Agency.

had wide medical application as a local painkiller or anesthetic. However, this function has now been largely replaced by other drugs, primarily procaine and lidocaine. Cocaine is also a powerful stimulant to the central nervous system, and its effects resemble those caused by the amphetamines—namely, increased alertness and vigor, accompanied by the suppression of hunger, fatigue, and boredom. Most commonly, cocaine is sniffed or "snorted" and is absorbed into the body through the mucous membranes of the nose.

Crack   A particularly potent form of cocaine known as "crack" can be produced by mixing cocaine with baking soda and water and then heating the resulting solution. This material is then dried and broken into tiny chunks that dealers sell as crack "rocks" that are sufficiently volatile to be smoked. The faster the cocaine level rises in the brain, the greater the euphoria, and the fastest way to obtain a rise in the brain's cocaine level is to smoke crack. Inhaling the cocaine vapor delivers the drug to the brain in less than 15 seconds—about as fast as injecting it and much faster than snorting it. The dark side of crack, however, is that the euphoria fades quickly as the cocaine levels rapidly drop, leaving the user feeling depressed, anxious, and pleasureless. The desire to return to the euphoric feeling is so intense that crack users quickly develop a habit for the drug that is almost impossible to overcome. Only a small percentage of crack users are ever cured of this drug habit. When a person uses large amounts of crack cocaine numerous times, they usually develop a sense of paranoia. Paranoid delusions cause users to lose their sense of reality, leaving them trapped in a world full of voices, whispers, and suspicions. Sufferers come to believe that they are being followed and that their drug use is being watched.

Effects of Use   In the United States, cocaine use is on the rise. Cocaine generates confidence and produces increased alertness, giving a false illusion that one is doing well at an assigned task. However, some regular users of cocaine report accompanying feelings of restlessness, irritability, and anxiety. Cocaine used chronically or at high doses can have toxic effects. Cocaine-related deaths are a result of cardiac arrest or seizures followed by respiratory arrest. Many people are apparently using cocaine to improve their ability to work and to keep going when tired. Although there is no evidence of physical dependency accompanying cocaine's repeated use, abstention from cocaine after prolonged use brings on severe bouts of mental depression, which produce a strong compulsion to resume using the drug. In fact, laboratory experiments with animals have demonstrated that of all the commonly used drugs, cocaine produces the strongest psychological compulsions for continued use.

The United States spends millions of dollars annually in attempting to control cultivation of the coca leaf in various South American countries and to prevent cocaine trafficking into the United States. Three-quarters of the cocaine smuggled into the United States is refined in clandestine laboratories in Colombia. The profits are astronomical. Peruvian farmers may be paid $200 for enough coca leaves to make one pound of cocaine. The refined cocaine is worth $1,000 when it leaves Colombia and sells at retail in the United States for up to $20,000.

Club Drugs

The term *club drugs* refers to synthetic drugs that are used at nightclubs, bars, and raves (all-night dance parties). Substances that are often used as club drugs include, but are not limited to, MDMA (Ecstasy), gamma hydroxybutyrate (GHB), Rohypnol ("roofies"), ketamine, and methamphetamine. These drugs have become popular at the dance scene to stimulate the rave experience. A high incidence of use has been found among teens and young adults.

The rave scene supports this type of drug use. Tablets can be easily hidden in various containers, such as Pez dispensers and other items not usually thought of as drug paraphernalia. The rave scene is often depicted as a room filled with people jumping and bouncing in unison for hours to loud, rhythmic, trancelike music. The stimulatory effects of some of the club drugs allow the users to be active for hours.

GHB and Rohypnol are central nervous system depressants that are often connected with drug-facilitated sexual assault, rape, and robbery. Effects accompanying the use of GHB include dizziness, sedation, headache, and nausea. Recreational users have reported euphoria, relaxation,

Inside the Science

Bath Salts

It has become trendy in the drug culture to use a group of illicit substances known as "bath salts." These drugs are a mix of chemical derivatives derived from cathinone, a naturally occurring substance found in the khat plant. Cathinone is a stimulant having about half the potency of amphetamine. The allure of abusing cathinone and its chemical derivatives is to simulate the high associated with methamphetamine and cocaine use.

Synthetic derivatives of cathinone are commonly sold in powder, crystal, and liquid forms, but they are also available as tablets and capsules. They are sold in packages to be snorted, ingested, smoked, or injected. Like the side effects associated with methamphetamine or cocaine use, bath salts can induce agitation, violent behavior, and paranoia on the part of the user.

A federal law, the Food and Drug Administration Safety and Innovation Act, outlaws two synthetic cathinones, mephidrone and 3,4-methylenedioxypyrovalerone (MDPV), that are common constituents of bath salts.

disinhibition, and increased libido. Rohypnol causes muscle relaxation, loss of consciousness, and an inability to remember what happened during the hours after ingesting the drug. This is particularly a concern in a sexual assault because victims are physically unable to resist the attack. Unsuspecting victims become drowsy or dizzy. Effects are even stronger when the drug is combined with alcohol because the user experiences memory loss, blackouts, and disinhibition. Law enforcement agencies have warned multitudes of partygoers that drugs, such as Rohypnol and GHB, are odorless, colorless, and tasteless and so will remain undetected when slipped into a drink.

Methylenedioxymethamphetamine, also known as MDMA or Ecstasy (see Figure 12–7), is the most popular drug at rave club scenes. Ecstasy is a synthetic, mind-altering drug that exhibits many hallucinogenic and amphetamine-like effects. Ecstasy was originally patented as an appetite suppressant and was later discovered to induce feelings of happiness and relaxation.

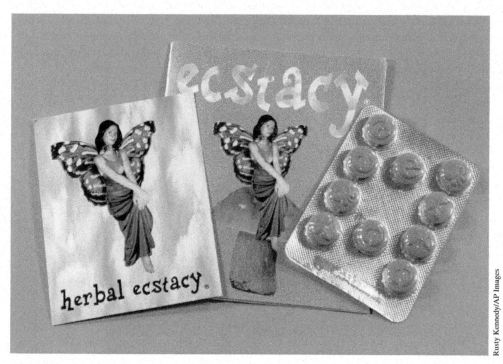

Rusty Kennedy/AP Images

FIGURE 12–7
Ecstasy, a popular club drug.

Recreational drug users find that Ecstasy enhances self-awareness and decreases inhibitions. However, seizures, muscle breakdown, stroke, kidney failure, and cardiovascular system failure often accompany chronic use of Ecstasy. In addition, chronic use of Ecstasy leads to serious damage to the areas of the brain responsible for thought and memory. Ecstasy increases the heart rate and blood pressure; produces muscle tension, teeth grinding, and nausea; and causes psychological difficulties, such as confusion, severe anxiety, and paranoia episodes. The drug can cause significant increases in body temperature from the combination of the drug's stimulant effect with the often hot, crowded atmosphere of a rave club.

Ketamine is primarily used in veterinary medicine as an animal anesthetic. When used by humans, the drug can cause euphoria and feelings of unreality accompanied by visual hallucinations. Ketamine can also cause impaired motor function, high blood pressure, amnesia, and mild respiratory depression.

Anabolic Steroids

anabolic steroids
Steroids that promote muscle growth.

Anabolic steroids are synthetic compounds that are chemically related to the male sex hormone testosterone. Testosterone has two different effects on the body. It promotes the development of secondary male characteristics (androgen effects), and it accelerates muscle growth (anabolic effects). Efforts to promote muscle growth and to minimize the hormone's androgenic effects have led to the synthesis of numerous anabolic steroids. However, a steroid free of the accompanying harmful side effects of an androgen drug has not yet been developed.

Incidence of steroid use first received widespread public attention when both amateur and professional athletes were discovered using these substances to enhance their performance (see Figure 12–8). Interestingly, current research on male athletes given anabolic steroids has generally found little or, at best, marginal evidence of enhanced strength or performance. Although the full extent of anabolic steroid use by the general public is not fully known, the U.S. government is sufficiently concerned to regulate the availability of these drugs to the general population and to severely punish individuals for illegal possession and distribution of anabolic steroids. In 1991, anabolic steroids were classified as controlled dangerous substances, and the Drug Enforcement Administration was given enforcement power to prevent their illegal use and distribution.

Anabolic steroids are usually taken by individuals who are unfamiliar with the harmful medical side effects. Liver cancer and other liver malfunctions have been linked to steroid use. These drugs also cause masculinizing effects in females, infertility, and diminished sex drive in males. For teenagers, anabolic steroids result in premature halting of bone growth. Anabolic steroids can also cause unpredictable effects on mood and personality, leading to unprovoked acts of anger and destructive behavior. Depression is also a frequent side effect of anabolic steroid use.

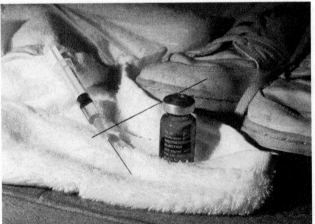

SPL/Science Source

FIGURE 12–8
Anabolic steroids: a vial of testosterone and a syringe. Testosterone, the male sex hormone, is sometimes used by athletes for its protein-building (anabolic) effect.

Drug-Control Laws

Although the previous sections have attempted to classify drugs according to their physiological effects on the body, for practical purposes of law enforcement, the legal community requires a thorough knowledge of drug classification and definitions as they are delineated by drug laws. The medical and legal definitions or classifications of a drug often bear little resemblance. The provisions of drug laws are of particular interest to the criminalist because they may impose specific analytical requirements on drug analysis. For example, the severity of a penalty associated with the manufacture, distribution, possession, and use of a drug may depend on the weight of the drug or its concentration in a mixture. In such cases, the chemist's report must contain all information that is needed to properly charge a suspect under the provisions of the existing law.

The provisions of any drug-control law are an outgrowth of national and local law enforcement requirements and customs, as well as the result of moral and political philosophies. These factors have produced a wide spectrum of national and local drug-control laws. Although their detailed discussion is beyond the intended scope of this book, a brief description of the U.S. federal law known as the Controlled Substances Act will illustrate a legal drug classification system that has been created to prevent and control drug use. Many states have modeled their own drug-control laws after this act, an important step in establishing uniform drug-control laws throughout the United States.

Controlled Substances Act

The federal law establishes five schedules of classification (as outlined next) for controlled dangerous substances on the basis of a drug's potential for use, potential for physical and psychological dependence, and medical value. This classification system is extremely flexible in that the U.S. attorney general has the authority to add, delete, or reschedule a drug as more information becomes available. In addition, controlled dangerous substances listed in schedules I and II are subject to manufacturing quotas set by the attorney general. For example, eight billion doses of amphetamines were manufactured in the United States in 1971. In 1972, production quotas reduced amphetamine production approximately 80 percent below 1971 levels.

CONTROL MECHANISMS AND PENALTIES   The criminal penalties for unauthorized manufacture, sale, or possession of controlled dangerous substances are related to the schedules as well. The most severe penalties are associated with drugs listed in schedules I and II. For example, for drugs included in schedules I and II, a first offense is punishable by up to 20 years in prison and/or a fine of up to $1 million for an individual or up to $5 million for other than individuals. Table 12–2 summarizes the control mechanisms and penalties for each schedule of the Controlled Substances Act.

Schedule I   Schedule I drugs are deemed to have a high potential for use, have no currently accepted medical use in the United States, and/or lack accepted safety for use in treatment under medical supervision. Drugs controlled under this schedule include heroin, marijuana, methaqualone, and LSD.

Schedule II   Schedule II drugs have a high potential for use, a currently accepted medical use or a medical use with severe restrictions, and a potential for severe psychological or physical dependence. Schedule II drugs include opium and its derivatives not listed in schedule I; cocaine; methadone; PCP; most amphetamine preparations; and most barbiturate preparations containing amobarbital, secobarbital, and pentobarbital. Dronabinol, the synthetic equivalent of the active ingredient in marijuana, has been placed in schedule II in recognition of its growing medical uses in treating glaucoma and chemotherapy patients.

Schedule III   Schedule III drugs have less potential for use than those in schedules I and II, a currently accepted medical use in the United States, and a potential for low or moderate physical dependence or high psychological dependence. Schedule III controls, among other substances, all barbiturate preparations (except phenobarbital) not covered under schedule II and certain codeine preparations. Anabolic steroids were added to this schedule in 1991.

TABLE 12–2

Control Mechanisms of the Controlled Substances Act

Schedule	Registration	Record Keeping	Manufacturing Quotas	Distribution Restrictions	Dispensing Limits
I	Required	Separate	Yes	Order forms	Research use only
II	Required	Separate	Yes	Order forms	Rx: written; no refills
III	Required	Readily retrievable	No, but some drugs limited by schedule II quotas	Records required	Rx: written or oral; with medical authorization refills up to five times in six months
IV	Required	Readily retrievable	No, but some drugs limited by schedule II quotas	Records required	Rx: written or oral; with medical authorization refills up to five times in six months
V	Required	Readily retrievable	No, but some drugs limited by schedule II quotas	Records required	Over-the-counter (Rx drugs limited to MD's order; refills up to five times)

Source: Drug Enforcement Administration, Washington, D.C.

Schedule IV   Schedule IV drugs have a low potential for use relative to schedule III drugs and have a current medical use in the United States; their use may lead to limited dependence relative to schedule III drugs. Drugs controlled in this schedule include propoxyphene (Darvon); phenobarbital; and tranquilizers such as meprobamate (Miltown), diazepam (Valium), and chlordiazepoxide (Librium).

Schedule V   Schedule V drugs must show low use potential, have medical use in the United States, and have less potential for producing dependence than schedule IV drugs. Schedule V controls certain opiate drug mixtures that contain nonnarcotic medicinal ingredients.

Other Provisions of the Act

The Controlled Substances Act stipulates that an offense involving a controlled substance analog, a chemical substance substantially similar in chemical structure to a controlled substance, shall trigger penalties as if it were a controlled substance listed in schedule I. This section is designed to combat the proliferation of so-called designer drugs. *Designer drugs* are substances that are chemically related to some controlled drugs and are pharmacologically potent. These substances are manufactured by skilled individuals in clandestine laboratories, with the knowledge that their products will not be covered by the schedules of the Controlled Substances Act. For instance, fentanyl is a powerful narcotic that is commercially marketed for medical use and is also listed as a controlled dangerous substance. This drug is about 100 times as potent as morphine. Currently, a number of substances chemically related to fentanyl have been synthesized by underground chemists and sold on the street. The first such substance encountered was sold under the street name "China White." These drugs have been responsible for more than 100 overdose deaths in California and nearly 20 deaths in western Pennsylvania. As designer drugs, such as China White, are identified and linked to drug use, they are placed in appropriate schedules.

The Controlled Substances Act also reflects an effort to decrease the prevalence of clandestine drug laboratories designed to manufacture controlled substances. The act regulates the manufacture and distribution of *precursors*, the chemical compounds used by clandestine drug laboratories to synthesize drugs used. Targeted precursor chemicals are listed in the definition section of the Controlled Substances Act. Severe penalties are provided for a person who possesses a listed precursor chemical with the intent to manufacture a controlled substance or who possesses or distributes a listed chemical knowing, or having reasonable cause to believe, that the listed chemical will be used to manufacture a controlled substance. In addition, precursors to

	Import–Export		Security	Manufacturer/ Distributor Reports to Drug Enforcement Administration	Criminal Penalties for Individual Trafficking (First Offense)
Narcotic	Nonnarcotic				
Permit	Permit		Vault/safe	Yes	0–20 years/$1 million
Permit	Permit		Vault/safe	Yes	0–20 years/$1 million
Permit	Declaration		Secure storage area	Yes, narcotic No, nonnarcotic	0–5 years/$250,000
Permit	Declaration		Secure storage area	Manufacturer only, narcotic No, nonnarcotic	0–3 years/$250,000
Permit to import; declaration to export	Declaration		Secure storage area	Manufacturer only, narcotic No, nonnarcotic	0–1 year/$100,000

PCP, amphetamines, and methamphetamines are enumerated specifically in schedule II, making them subject to regulation in the same manner as other schedule II substances.

Collection and Preservation of Drug Evidence

Preparation of drug evidence for submission to the crime laboratory is normally a relatively simple task, accomplished with minimal precautions in the field. The field investigator is responsible for ensuring that the evidence is properly packaged and labeled for delivery to the laboratory. Considering the countless forms and varieties of drug evidence seized, it is not practical to prescribe any single packaging procedure for fulfilling these requirements. Generally, common sense is the best guide in such situations, keeping in mind that the package must prevent the loss and/or cross-contamination of the contents. Often, the original container in which the drug was seized will suffice to meet these requirements. Specimens suspected of containing volatile solvents, such as those involved in glue-sniffing cases, must be packaged in an airtight container to prevent evaporation of the solvent.

All packages must be marked with sufficient information to ensure identification by the officer in future legal proceedings and to establish the chain of custody.

To aid the drug analyst, the investigator should supply any background information that may relate to a drug's identity. Analysis time can be markedly reduced when this information is at the disposal of the chemist. For the same reason, the results of drug-screening tests used in the field must also be transmitted to the laboratory. Although these tests may indicate the presence of a drug and may help the officer establish probable cause to search and arrest a suspect, they do *not* offer conclusive evidence of a drug's identity.

Forensic Drug Analysis

One only has to look into the evidence vaults of crime laboratories to appreciate the assortment of drug specimens that confront the criminalist. The presence of a huge array of powders, tablets, capsules, vegetable matter, liquids, pipes, cigarettes, cookers, and syringes is testimony to the vitality and sophistication of the illicit-drug market. If outward appearance is not evidence enough of the difficult analytical chore facing the forensic chemist, consider the complexity of the drug preparations themselves. Usually, these contain active drug ingredients of unknown origin and identity, as well as additives—for example, sugar, starch, and quinine—that dilute their potency and stretch their value on the illicit-drug market. Do not forget that illicit-drug dealers are not hampered by governmental regulations that ensure the quality and consistency of a product.

When a forensic chemist picks up a drug specimen for analysis, they can expect to find just about anything, so all contingencies must be prepared for. The analysis must leave no room for error because its results will have a direct bearing on the process of determining the guilt or innocence of a defendant. There is no middle ground in drug identification—either the specimen is a specific drug or it is not—and once a positive conclusion is drawn, the chemist must be prepared to support and defend the validity of the results in a court of law.

The Analytical Process

The challenge or difficulty of forensic drug identification comes in selecting analytical procedures that will ensure a specific identification of a drug. Presented with a substance of unknown origin and composition, the forensic chemist must develop a plan of action that will ultimately yield the drug's identity. This plan, or scheme of analysis, is divided into two phases.

screening test
A test that is nonspecific and preliminary in nature.

SCREENING   First, faced with the prospect that the unknown substance may be any one of a thousand or more commonly encountered drugs, the analyst must employ **screening tests** to reduce these possibilities to a small and manageable number. This objective is often accomplished by subjecting the material to a series of color tests that produce characteristic colors for the more commonly encountered illicit drugs. Even if these tests produce negative results, their value lies in having excluded certain drugs from further consideration.

CONFIRMATION   Once the number of possibilities has been substantially reduced, the second phase of the analysis is devoted to pinpointing and confirming the drug's identity. In an era in which crime laboratories receive voluminous quantities of drug evidence, it is impractical to subject a drug to all of the chemical and instrumental tests available. Indeed, it is more realistic to view these techniques as a large analytical arsenal. The chemist, aided by training and experience, must choose tests that will most conveniently furnish the identity of a particular drug.

confirmation
A single test that specifically identifies a substance.

Forensic chemists often use a specific test (such as infrared spectrophotometry or mass spectrometry) to identify a drug substance to the exclusion of all other known chemical substances. A single test that identifies a substance is known as a **confirmation**. The analytical scheme sometimes consists of a series of nonspecific or presumptive tests. Each test in itself is insufficient to prove the drug's identity; however, the proper analytical scheme encompasses a combination of test results that characterize one and only one chemical substance—the drug under investigation. Furthermore, experimental evidence must confirm that the probability of any other substance responding in an identical manner to the scheme selected is so small as to be beyond any reasonable scientific certainty.

QUANTITATIVE VS. QUALITATIVE DETERMINATION   Another consideration in selecting an analytical technique is the need for either a *qualitative* or a *quantitative* determination. The former relates just to the identity of the material, whereas the latter refers to the percentage combination of the components of a mixture. Hence, a qualitative identification of a powder may reveal the presence of heroin and quinine, whereas a quantitative analysis may conclude the presence of 10 percent heroin and 90 percent quinine.

Obviously, a qualitative identification must precede any attempt at quantitation, for little value is served by attempting to quantitate a material without first determining its identity. Essentially, a qualitative analysis of a material requires the determination of numerous properties using a variety of analytical techniques. On the other hand, a quantitative measurement is usually accomplished by precise measurement of a single property of the material.

Forensic chemists normally rely on several tests for a routine drug-identification scheme: color tests, microcrystalline tests, chromatography, spectrophotometry, and mass spectrometry.

Color Tests

Many drugs yield characteristic colors when brought into contact with specific chemical reagents. Not only do these tests provide a useful indicator of a drug's presence, but they are also used by

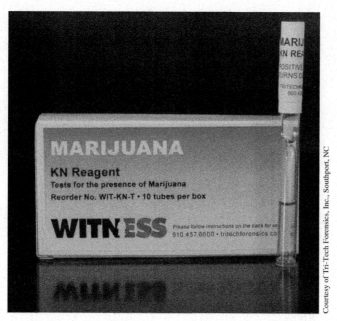

FIGURE 12–9
A field color test kit for marijuana.

investigators in the field to examine materials suspected of containing a drug (see Figure 12–9).[2] However, color tests are useful for screening purposes only and are never taken as conclusive identification of unknown drugs.

Five primary color test reagents are as follows:

1. *Marquis* (2 percent formaldehyde in sulfuric acid). The reagent turns purple in the presence of heroin and morphine and most opium derivatives. Marquis also becomes orange-brown when mixed with amphetamines and methamphetamines.
2. *Dillie–Koppanyi* (1 percent cobalt acetate in methanol is first added to the suspect material, followed by 5 percent isopropylamine in methanol). This is a valuable screening test for barbiturates, in whose presence the reagent turns violet-blue in color.
3. *Duquenois–Levine* (solution A is a mixture of 2 percent vanillin and 1 percent acetaldehyde in ethyl alcohol; solution B is concentrated hydrochloric acid; solution C is chloroform). This is a valuable color test for marijuana, performed by adding solutions A, B, and C, respectively, to the suspect vegetation. A positive result is shown by a purple color in the chloroform layer.
4. *Van Urk* (1 percent solution of *p*-dimethylaminobenzaldehyde in 10 percent concentrated hydrochloric acid and ethyl alcohol). The reagent turns blue-purple in the presence of LSD. However, owing to the extremely small quantities of LSD in illicit preparations, this test is difficult to conduct under field conditions.
5. *Scott Test* (solution A is 2 percent cobalt thiocyanate dissolved in water and glycerine [1:1]; solution B is concentrated hydrochloric acid; solution C is chloroform). This is a color test for cocaine. A powder containing cocaine turns solution A blue. Upon addition of B, the blue color is transformed to a clear pink color. Upon addition of C, if cocaine is present, the blue color reappears in the chloroform layer.

Microcrystalline Tests

A technique considerably more specific than color tests is the **microcrystalline test**. A drop of a chemical reagent is added to a small quantity of the drug on a microscope slide. After a short time, a chemical reaction ensues, producing a crystalline precipitate. The size and shape of the

microcrystalline tests
Tests to identify specific substances by the color and morphology of the crystals formed when the substance is mixed with specific reagents.

---

[2] Field-color test kits for drugs can be purchased from various commercial manufacturers.

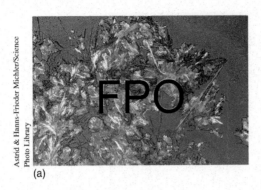
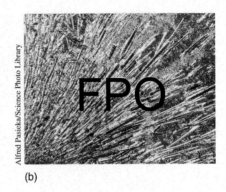

(a)
(b)

FIGURE 12–10

(a) A photomicrograph of a cocaine crystal formed in platinum chloride (400×).
(b) A photomicrograph of a methamphetamine crystal formed in gold chloride (400×).

crystals, under microscope examination, are highly characteristic of the drug. Crystal tests for cocaine and methamphetamine are illustrated in Figure 12–10.

Over the years, analysts have developed hundreds of crystal tests to characterize the most commonly used drugs. These tests are rapid and often do not require the isolation of a drug from its diluents; however, because diluents can sometimes alter or modify the shape of the crystal, the examiner must develop experience in interpreting the results of the test.

Most color and crystal tests are largely empirical—that is, scientists do not fully understand why they produce the results that they do. From the forensic chemist's point of view, this is not important. When the tests are properly chosen and are used in proper combination, their results constitute an analytical scheme that is characteristic for one and only one drug.

Chromatography

chromatography
Any of several analytical techniques for separating organic or carbon-containing mixtures into their components by attraction to a stationary phase while being propelled by a moving phase.

Chromatography as a technique for separating the components of a mixture is particularly useful for analyzing the multicomponent specimens that are frequently received in the crime laboratory. For example, illicit drugs sold on the street are not manufactured to meet government labeling standards; instead, they may be diluted with practically any material at the disposal of the drug dealer to increase the quantity of product available to prospective customers. Hence, the task of identifying an illicit-drug preparation would be arduous without the aid of chromatographic methods to first separate the mixture into its components.

Gas Chromatography (GC)

Gas chromatography (GC) separates mixtures on the basis of their distribution between a stationary liquid phase and a moving gas phase. This technique is widely used because of its ability to resolve a highly complex mixture into its components, usually within minutes.

BASIC THEORY OF GC   In GC, the moving phase is actually a gas called the *carrier gas*, which flows through a column constructed of stainless steel or glass. The stationary phase is a thin film of liquid within the column. Two types of columns are used: the *packed column* and the *capillary column*. With the packed column, the stationary phase is a thin film of liquid that is fixed onto small granular particles packed into the column. This column is usually constructed of stainless steel or glass and is 2 to 6 meters long and about 3 millimeters in diameter. Capillary columns are composed of glass and are much longer than packed columns—15 to 60 meters long. These types of columns are very narrow, ranging from 0.25 to 0.75 millimeter in diameter. Capillary columns can be made narrower than packed columns because their stationary liquid phase is actually coated as a very thin film directly onto the column's inner wall. In any case, as the carrier gas flows through the packed or capillary column, it carries with it the components of a mixture that have been injected into the column. Components with a greater affinity for the moving gas phase travel through the column more quickly than those with a greater affinity for the stationary liquid phase. Eventually, after the mixture has traversed the length of the column, it emerges separated into its components.

Inside the Science

The Chromatographic Process

The theory of chromatography is based on the observation that chemical substances tend to partially escape into the surrounding environment when dissolved in a liquid or when absorbed on a solid surface. This is best illustrated by a gas dissolved in a beaker of water kept at a constant temperature. It will be convenient for us to characterize the water in the beaker as the liquid phase and the air above it as the gas phase. If the beaker is covered with a bell jar, as shown in the figure, some of the gas molecules (represented by the green balls) escape from the water into the surrounding enclosed air. The molecules that remain are said to be in the liquid phase; the molecules that have escaped into the air are said to be in the gas phase. As the gas molecules escape into the surrounding air, they accumulate above the water; here, random motion carries some of them back into the water. Eventually, a point is reached at which the number of molecules leaving the water is equal to the number returning. At this time, the liquid and gas phases are in *equilibrium*. If the temperature of the water is increased, the equilibrium state readjusts itself to a point at which more gas molecules move into the gas phase.

This behavior was first observed in 1803 by a British chemist, William Henry. His explanation of this phenomenon, known appropriately as Henry's law, may be stated as follows: *When a volatile chemical compound is dissolved in a liquid and is brought to equilibrium with air, there is a fixed ratio between the concentration of the volatile compound in air and its concentration in the liquid, and this ratio remains constant for a given temperature.*

The distribution or partitioning of a gas between the liquid and gas phases is determined by the solubility of the gas in the liquid. The higher its solubility, the greater the tendency of the gas molecules to remain in the liquid phase. If two different gases are simultaneously dissolved in the same liquid, each will reach a state of equilibrium with the surrounding air independently of the other. For example, as shown in the figure, gas A (green balls) and gas B (blue balls) are both dissolved in water. At equilibrium, gas A has a greater number of molecules dissolved in the water than does gas B. This is so because gas A is more soluble in water than gas B.

Now return to the concept of chromatography. In the preceding figures, both phases—liquid and gas—were kept stationary; that is, they were not moving. During a chromatographic process, this is not the case; instead, one phase is always made to move continuously in one direction over a stationary or fixed phase. For example, in the figure, which shows the two gases represented by blue and green balls dissolved in water, chromatography will occur only when the air is forced to move continuously in one direction over the water. Because gas B has a greater percentage of its molecules in the moving gas phase than does gas A, its molecules will travel over the liquid at a faster pace than those of gas A. Eventually, when the moving phase has advanced a reasonable distance, gas B will become entirely separated from gas A and the chromatographic process will be complete. This process is illustrated in the figure.

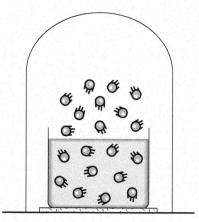

Evaporation of a liquid.

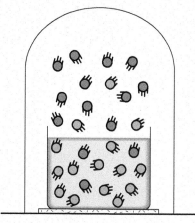

At equilibrium, there are more gas A molecules (green balls) than gas B molecules (blue balls) in the liquid phase.

(continued)

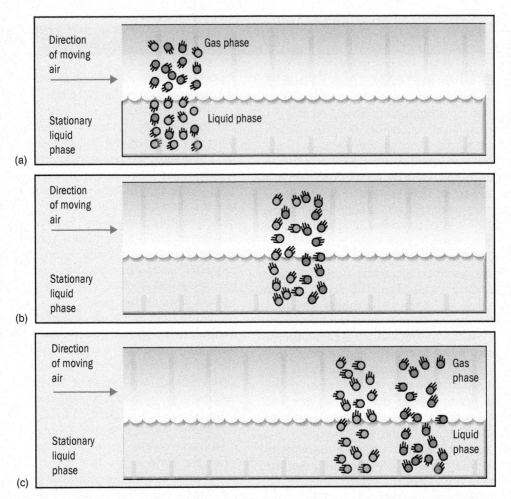

In this illustration of chromatography, the molecules represented by the blue balls have a greater affinity for the upper phase and hence will be pushed along at a faster rate by the moving air. Eventually, the two sets of molecules will separate from each other, completing the chromatographic process.

Simply, we can think of chromatography as being analogous to a race between chemical compounds. At the starting line, all the participating substances are mixed together; however, as the race progresses, materials that prefer the moving phase slowly pull ahead of those that prefer to remain in the stationary phase. Finally, at the end of the race, all the participants are separated, each crossing the finish line at different times.

The different types of chromatographic systems are as varied as the number of stationary and moving-phase combinations that can be devised. However, three chromatographic processes—gas chromatography, high-performance liquid chromatography, and thin-layer chromatography—are most applicable for solving many analytical problems in the crime laboratory.

The time required for a component to emerge from the column from the time of its injection into the column is known as the *retention time*, which is a useful identifying characteristic of a material. Figure 12–11(a) shows the chromatogram of two barbiturates; each barbiturate has tentatively been identified by comparing its retention time to those of known barbiturates, shown in Figure 12–11(b). However, because other substances may have comparable retention times under similar chromatographic conditions, GC cannot be considered an absolute means of identification. Conclusions derived from this technique must be confirmed by other testing procedures.

An added advantage of GC is that it is extremely sensitive and can yield quantitative results. The amount of substance passing through the GC detector is proportional to the peak area recorded;

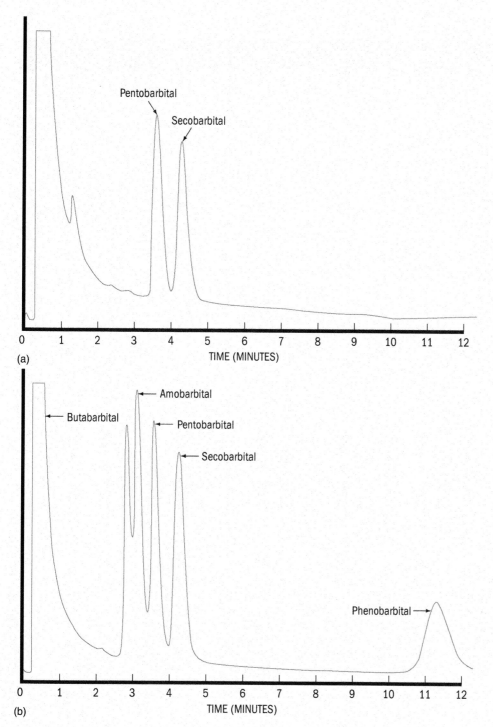

FIGURE 12–11

(a) An unknown mixture of barbiturates is identified by comparing its retention times to (b), a known mixture of barbiturates.

therefore, by chromatographing a known concentration of a material and comparing it to the unknown, the amount of the sample may be determined by proportion. GC has sufficient sensitivity to detect and quantitate materials at the nanogram (0.000000001 gram or 1×10^{-9} gram) level.

Thin-Layer Chromatography (TLC)

The technique of thin-layer chromatography (TLC) uses a solid stationary phase and a moving liquid phase to separate the constituents of a mixture.

Inside the Science

The Gas Chromatograph

A simplified scheme of the gas chromatograph is shown in the figure. The operation of the instrument can be summed up briefly as follows: A gas stream, the so-called carrier gas, is fed into the column at a constant rate. The carrier gas is chemically inert and is generally nitrogen or helium. The sample under investigation is injected as a liquid into a heated injection port with a syringe, where it is immediately vaporized and swept into the column by the carrier gas. The column itself is heated in an oven in order to keep the sample in a vapor state as it travels through the column. In the column, the components of the sample travel in the direction of the carrier gas flow at speeds that are determined by their distribution between the stationary and moving phases. If the analyst has selected the proper liquid phase and has made the column long enough, the components of the sample will be completely separated as they emerge from the column.

As each component emerges from the column, it enters a detector. One type of detector uses a flame to ionize the emerging chemical substance, thus generating an electrical signal. The signal is recorded onto a strip-chart recorder as a function of time. This written record of the separation is called a *chromatogram*. A gas chromatogram is a plot of the recorder response (vertical axis) versus time (horizontal axis). A typical chromatogram shows a series of peaks, each peak corresponding to one component of the mixture.

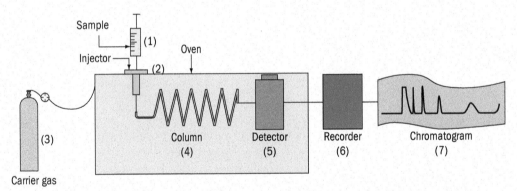

Basic gas chromatography. Gas chromatography permits rapid separation of complex mixtures into individual compounds and allows identification and quantitative determination of each compound. As shown, a sample is introduced by a syringe (1) into a heated injection chamber (2). A constant stream of nitrogen gas (3) flows through the injector, carrying the sample into the column (4), which contains a thin film of liquid. The sample is separated in the column, and the carrier gas and separated components emerge from the column and enter the detector (5). Signals developed by the detector activate the recorder (6), which makes a permanent record of the separation by tracing a series of peaks on the chromatograph (7). The time of elution identifies the component present, and the peak area identifies the concentration.

THE TLC PROCESS   A thin-layer plate is prepared by coating a glass plate with a thin film of a granular material, usually silica gel or aluminum oxide. This granular material serves as the solid stationary phase and is usually held in place on the plate with a binding agent, such as plaster of paris. If the sample to be analyzed is a solid, it must first be dissolved in a suitable solvent and a few microliters of the solution spotted with a capillary tube onto the granular surface near the lower edge of the plate. A liquid sample may be applied directly to the plate in the same manner. The plate is then placed upright into a closed chamber that contains a selected liquid, with care that the liquid does not touch the sample spot.

The liquid slowly rises up the plate by capillary action. This rising liquid is the moving phase in TLC. As the liquid moves past the sample spot, the components of the sample become distributed between the stationary solid phase and the moving liquid phase. The components with the greatest affinity for the moving phase travel up the plate faster than those that have greater affinity for the stationary phase. When the liquid front has moved a sufficient distance (usually 10 centimeters), the development is complete, and the plate is removed from the chamber and dried (see Figure 12–12). An example of the chromatographic separation of ink is shown in Figure 12–13.

VISUALIZING SUBSTANCES   Because most compounds are colorless, no separation will be noticed after development unless the materials are *visualized*. To accomplish this, the plates are

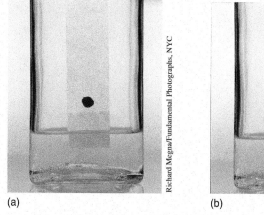
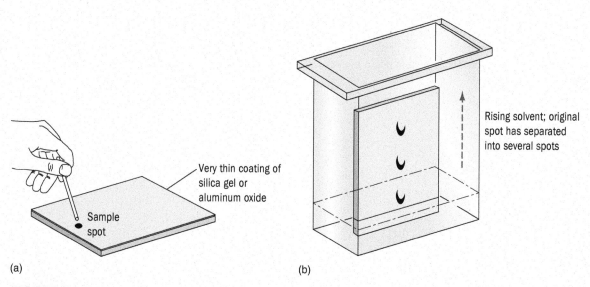

Very thin coating of silica gel or aluminum oxide

Sample spot

Rising solvent; original spot has separated into several spots

(a)   (b)

FIGURE 12–12

(a) In thin-layer chromatography, a liquid sample is spotted onto the granular surface of a gel-coated plate. (b) The plate is placed into a closed chamber that contains a liquid. As the liquid rises up the plate, the components of the sample distribute themselves between the coating and the moving liquid. The mixture is separated, with substances with a greater affinity for the moving liquid traveling up the plate at a faster speed.

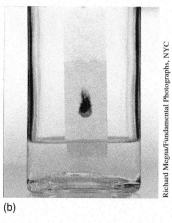
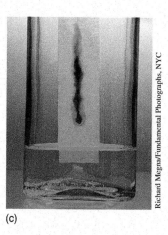

Richard Megna/Fundamental Photographs, NYC

(a)   (b)   (c)

FIGURE 12–13

(a) The liquid phase begins to move up the stationary phase. (b) Liquid moves past the ink spot carrying the ink components up the stationary phase. (c) The moving liquid has separated the ink into its several components.

placed under ultraviolet light, revealing select materials that **fluoresce** as bright spots on a dark background. When a fluorescent dye has been incorporated into the solid phase, nonfluorescent substances appear as dark spots against a fluorescent background when exposed to the ultraviolet light. In a second method of visualization, the plate is sprayed with a chemical reagent that reacts with the separated substances and causes them to form colored spots. Figure 12–14 shows the chromatogram of a marijuana extract that has been separated into its components by TLC and visualized by having been sprayed with a chemical reagent.

Once the components of a sample have been separated, their identification must follow. For this, the questioned sample must be developed alongside an authentic or standard sample on the same TLC plate. If both the standard and the unknown travel the same distance up the plate from their origins, they can tentatively be identified as being the same. For example, suppose a sample suspected of containing heroin and quinine is analyzed alongside known heroin and quinine standards, as shown in Figure 12–15. The identity of the suspect material is confirmed by comparing the migration distances of the heroin and quinine standards against those of the components of the unknown material. If the distances are the same, a tentative identification can be made.

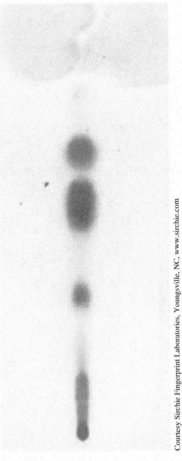

Courtesy Sirchie Fingerprint Laboratories, Youngsville, NC, www.sirchie.com

FIGURE 12–14
Thin-layer chromatogram of a marijuana extract.

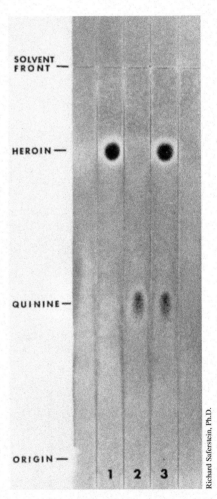

Richard Saferstein, Ph.D.

FIGURE 12–15
Chromatograms of known heroin (1) and quinine (2) standards alongside suspect sample (3).

Inside the Science

Identifying Drugs by TLC

Drug identifications by TLC are only tentative. Such an identification cannot be considered definitive because numerous other substances can migrate the same distance up the plate when chromatographed under similar conditions. Thus, thin-layer chromatography alone cannot provide an absolute identification; it must be used in conjunction with other testing procedures to prove absolute identity.

The distance a spot has traveled up a thin-layer plate can be assigned a numerical value known as the *Rf* value. This value is defined as the distance traveled by the component divided by the distance traveled by the moving liquid phase. For example, in Figure 12–15, the moving phase traveled 10 centimeters up the plate before the plate was removed from the tank. After visualization, the heroin spot moved 8 centimeters, which has an *Rf* value of 0.8; the quinine migrated 4 centimeters, for an *Rf* value of 0.4.

Thousands of possible combinations of liquid and solid phases can be chosen in thin-layer chromatography. Fortunately, years of research have produced much published data relating to the proper selection of TLC conditions for separating and identifying specific classes of substances—for example, drugs, dyes, and petroleum products. These references, along with the experience of the analyst, will aid in the proper selection of TLC conditions for specific problems.

Thin-layer chromatography is a powerful tool for solving many of the analytical problems presented to the forensic scientist. The method is both rapid and sensitive; moreover, less than 100 micrograms of suspect material are required for the analysis. In addition, the equipment necessary for TLC work has minimal cost and space requirements. Importantly, numerous samples can be analyzed simultaneously on one thin-layer plate. The principal application of this technique is in the detection and identification of components in complex mixtures.

Inside the Science

High-Performance Liquid Chromatography (HPLC)

Recall that a chromatographic system requires a moving phase and a stationary phase in contact with each other. The previous section described gas chromatography, in which the stationary phase is a thin film and the moving phase is a gas. However, by changing the nature of these phases, one can create different forms of chromatography. One form finding increasing utility in crime laboratories is high-performance liquid chromatography (HPLC). Its moving phase is a liquid that is pumped through a column filled with fine solid particles. In one form of HPLC, the surfaces of these solid particles are chemically treated and act as the stationary phase. As the liquid moving phase is

pumped through the column, a sample is injected into the column. As the liquid carries the sample through the column, different components are retarded to different degrees, depending on their interaction with the stationary phase. This leads to a separation of the different components making up the sample mixture.

The major advantage of HPLC is that the entire process takes place at room temperature. With GC, the sample must first be vaporized and made to travel through a heated column. Hence, any materials sensitive to high temperatures may not survive their passage through the column. In such situations, the analyst may turn to HPLC as the method of choice. Organic explosives are generally heat sensitive and therefore more readily separated by HPLC. Likewise, heat-sensitive drugs, such as LSD, lend themselves to analysis by HPLC.

Spectrophotometry

Absorption of Electromagnetic Radiation

spectrophotometry
An analytical method for identifying a substance by its selective absorption of different wavelengths of light.

Just as a substance can absorb visible light to produce color, many of the invisible radiations of the electromagnetic spectrum are likewise absorbed. This absorption phenomenon is the basis for **spectrophotometry**, an important analytical technique in chemical identification. Spectrophotometry measures the quantity of radiation that a particular material absorbs as a function of wavelength or frequency.

We have already observed in the description of color in Chapter 10 that an object does not absorb all the visible light it is exposed to; instead, it selectively absorbs some frequencies and reflects or transmits others. Similarly, the absorption of other types of electromagnetic radiation by chemical substances is also selective. These key questions must be asked: Why does a particular substance absorb only at certain frequencies and not at others? And are these frequencies predictable? The answers are not simple. Scientists find it difficult to predict with certainty all the frequencies at which any one substance will absorb in a particular region of the electromagnetic spectrum. What is known, however, is that a chemical substance absorbs photons of radiation with a frequency that corresponds to an energy requirement of the substance, as defined by Equation (10–4). Different materials have different energy requirements and therefore absorb at different frequencies. Most important to the analyst is that these absorbed frequencies are measurable and can be used to characterize a material.

The selective absorption of a substance is measured by an instrument called a *spectrophotometer*, which produces a graph or *absorption spectrum* that depicts the absorption of light as a function of wavelength or frequency. The absorption of UV, visible, and IR radiation is particularly applicable for obtaining qualitative data pertaining to the identification of organic or carbon-containing substances.

Absorption at a single wavelength or frequency of light is not 100 percent complete—some radiation is transmitted or reflected by the material. Just how much radiation a substance absorbs is defined by a fundamental relationship known as Beer's law, shown in Equation (12–1):

$$A = kc \tag{12–1}$$

WEBEXTRA 12.2
See How a Spectrophotometer Works

Here, A symbolizes the absorption or the quantity of light taken up at a single frequency, c is the concentration of the absorbing material, and k is a proportionality constant. This relationship shows that the quantity of light absorbed at any frequency is directly proportional to the concentration of the absorbing species; the more material you have, the more radiation it will absorb. By defining the relationship between absorbance and concentration, Beer's law permits spectrophotometry to be used as a technique for quantification.

Ultraviolet, Visible, and Infrared Spectrophotometry

ultraviolet
Invisible high frequencies of light beyond violet in the visible spectrum.

Ultraviolet and visible spectrophotometry measure the absorbance of UV and visible light as a function of wavelength or frequency. For example, the UV absorption spectrum of heroin shows a maximum absorption band at a wavelength of 278 nanometers (see Figure 12–16). This shows that the simplicity of a UV spectrum facilitates its use as a tool for determining a material's probable identity. For instance, a white powder may have a UV spectrum comparable to heroin and therefore may be tentatively identified as such. (Fortunately, sugar and starch, common diluents of heroin, do not absorb UV light.)

infrared
Invisible short frequencies of light before red in the visible spectrum.

This technique, however, will not provide a definitive result; other drugs or materials may have a UV absorption spectrum similar to that of heroin. Nevertheless, UV spectrophotometry is often used in establishing the probable identity of a drug. For example, if an unknown substance yields a UV spectrum that resembles amphetamine (see Figure 12–17), thousands of substances are immediately eliminated from consideration, and the analyst can begin to identify the material from a relatively small number of possibilities. A comprehensive collection of UV drug spectra provides an index that can rapidly be searched in order to tentatively identify a drug or, failing that, at least to exclude certain drugs from consideration.

monochromator
A device for isolating individual wavelengths or frequencies of light.

monochromatic light
Light having a single wavelength or frequency.

In contrast to the simplicity of a UV spectrum, absorption in the **infrared** region provides a far more complex pattern. Figure 12–18 depicts the IR spectra of heroin and secobarbital. Here, the absorption bands are so numerous that each spectrum can provide enough characteristics

Inside the Science

The Spectrophotometer

The spectrophotometer measures and records the absorption spectrum of a chemical substance. The basic components of a simple spectrophotometer are the same regardless of whether it is designed to measure the absorption of UV, visible, or IR radiation. These components are illustrated in the figure. They include (1) a radiation source, (2) a monochromator or frequency selector, (3) a sample holder, (4) a detector to convert electromagnetic radiation into an electrical signal, and (5) a recorder to produce a record of the signal.

The choice of source will vary with the type of radiation desired. For visible radiation, an ordinary tungsten bulb provides a convenient source of radiation. In the UV region, a hydrogen or deuterium discharge lamp is normally used, and a heated molded rod containing a mixture of rare-earth oxides is a good source of IR light.

The function of the **monochromator** is to select a single wavelength or frequency of light from the source—**monochromatic light**. Some inexpensive spectrophotometers pass the light through colored glass filters to remove all radiation from the beam except for a desired range of wavelengths. More precise spectrophotometers use a prism or diffraction grating to disperse radiation into its component wavelengths or frequencies.[3] The desired wavelength is obtained when the dispersed radiation is focused onto a narrow slit that permits only selected wavelengths to pass through.

Most laboratory infrared spectrophotometers use Fourier transform analysis to measure the wavelengths of light at which a material will absorb in the infrared spectrum. This approach does not use any dispersive elements that select single wavelengths or frequencies of light emitted from a source; instead, the heart of a *Fourier transform infrared* (FT-IR) *spectrometer* is the Michelson interferometer. The interferometer uses a beam-splitting prism and two mirrors, one movable and one stationary, to direct light toward a sample. As the wavelengths pass through the sample and reach a detector, they are all measured simultaneously. A mathematical operation, the Fourier transform method, is used to decode the measured signals and record the wavelength data. These Fourier calculations are rapidly carried out by a computer. In a matter of seconds, a computer-operated FT-IR instrument can produce an infrared absorption pattern compatible to one generated by a prism instrument.

Sample preparation varies with the type of radiation being studied. Absorption spectra in the UV and

[3] A diffraction grating is made by scratching thousands of parallel lines on a transparent surface such as glass. As light passes through the narrow spacings between the lines, it spreads out and produces a spectrum similar to that formed by a prism.

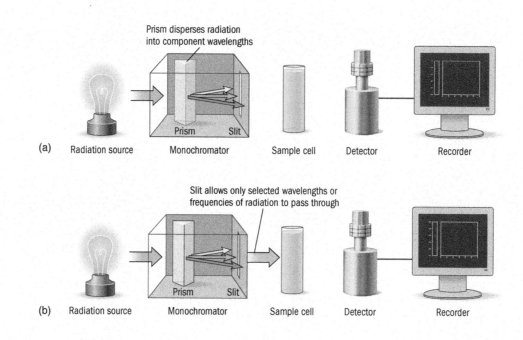

(a)   Radiation source   Monochromator   Sample cell   Detector   Recorder

Prism disperses radiation into component wavelengths

Prism   Slit

Slit allows only selected wavelengths or frequencies of radiation to pass through

(b)   Radiation source   Monochromator   Sample cell   Detector   Recorder

Prism   Slit

(continued)

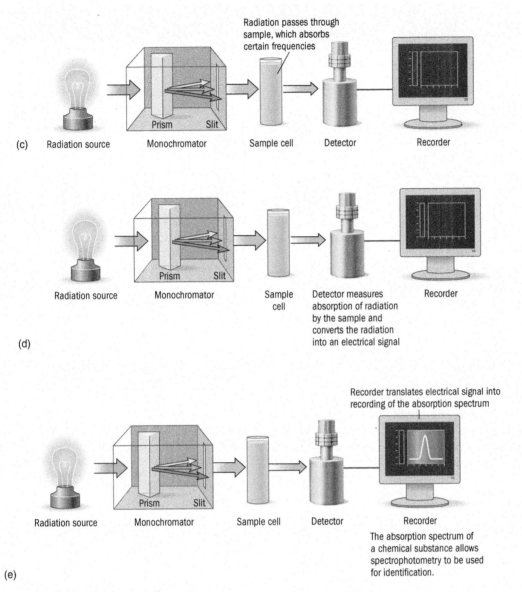

(c)   Radiation source   Monochromator   Sample cell   Detector   Recorder

Radiation passes through
sample, which absorbs
certain frequencies

Prism   Slit

(d)   Radiation source   Monochromator   Sample
cell   Detector measures
absorption of radiation
by the sample and
converts the radiation
into an electrical signal   Recorder

Prism   Slit

Recorder translates electrical signal into
recording of the absorption spectrum

(e)   Radiation source   Monochromator   Sample cell   Detector   Recorder

The absorption spectrum of
a chemical substance allows
spectrophotometry to be used
for identification.

Prism   Slit

The parts of a simple spectrophotometer.

visible regions are usually obtained from samples that have been dissolved in an appropriate solvent. Because the cells holding the solution must be transparent to the light being measured, glass cells are used in the visible region and quartz cells in the ultraviolet region. Practically, all substances absorb in some region of the IR spectrum, so sampling techniques must be modified to measure absorption in this spectral region; special cells made out of sodium chloride or potassium bromide are commonly used because they will not absorb light over a wide range of the IR portion of the electromagnetic spectrum.

The detector measures the quantity of radiation that passes through the sample by converting it to an electrical signal. UV and visible spectrophotometers employ photoelectric tube detectors. A signal is generated when the photons strike the tube surface to produce a current that is directly proportional to the intensity of the light transmitted through the sample. When this signal is compared to the intensity of light that is transmitted to the detector in the absence of an absorbing material, the absorbance of a substance can be determined at each wavelength or frequency of light selected. The signal from the detection system is then fed into a recorder, which plots absorbance as a function of wavelength or frequency. Modern spectrophotometers are designed to trace an entire absorption spectrum automatically.

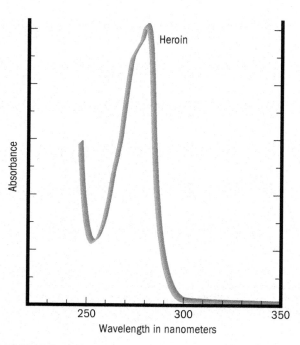

FIGURE 12–16

The ultraviolet spectrum of heroin.

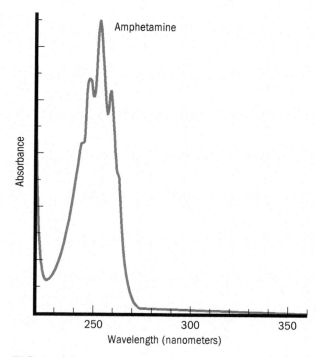

FIGURE 12–17

The ultraviolet spectrum of amphetamine.

to identify a substance specifically. **Different materials always have distinctively different infrared spectra; each IR spectrum is therefore equivalent to a "fingerprint" of that substance and no other.** This technique is one of the few tests available to the forensic scientist that can be considered specific in itself for identification. The IR spectra of thousands of compounds have been collected, indexed, and cataloged to serve as invaluable references for identifying substances.

Mass Spectrometry

A previous section discussed the operation of the gas chromatograph. This instrument is one of the most important tools in a crime laboratory. Its ability to separate the components of a complex mixture is unsurpassed. However, GC does have one important drawback—its inability to produce specific identification. A forensic chemist cannot unequivocally state the identification of a substance based solely on a retention time as determined by the gas chromatograph. Fortunately, coupling the gas chromatograph to a mass spectrometer has largely overcome this problem.

The separation of a mixture's components is first accomplished on the gas chromatograph. A direct connection between the GC column and the mass spectrometer then allows each component to flow into the spectrometer as it emerges from the gas chromatograph. In the mass spectrometer, the material enters a high-vacuum chamber where a beam of high-energy electrons is aimed at the sample molecules. The electrons collide with the molecules, causing them to lose electrons and to acquire a positive charge (commonly called **ions**). These positively charged molecules or ions are unstable or are formed with excess energy and almost instantaneously decompose into numerous smaller fragments. The fragments then pass through an electric or magnetic field, where they are separated according to their masses. The unique feature of mass spectrometry is that under carefully controlled conditions, no two substances produce the same fragmentation pattern. In essence, one can think of this pattern as a "fingerprint" of the substance being examined (see Figure 12–19).

ion

An atom or molecule bearing a positive or negative charge.

FIGURE 12–18
(a) Infrared spectrum of
heroin. (b) Infrared spectrum
of secobarbital.

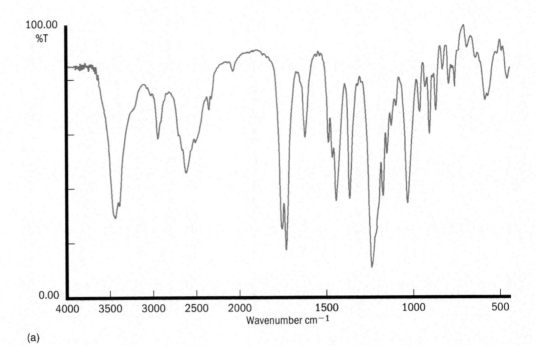

(a)

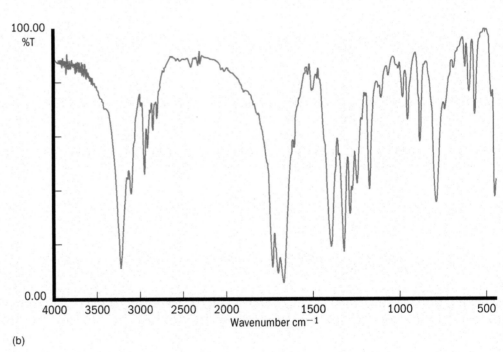

(b)

The technique thus provides a specific means for identifying a chemical structure. It is also sensitive to minute concentrations. At present, mass spectrometry finds its widest application in the identification of drugs; however, further research is expected to yield significant applications for identifying other types of physical evidence. Figure 12–20 illustrates the mass spectra of heroin and cocaine; each line represents a fragment of a different mass (actually the ratio of mass to charge), and the line height reflects the relative abundance of each fragment. Note how different the fragmentation patterns of heroin and cocaine are. Each mass spectrum is unique to each drug and therefore serves as a specific test for identifying it.

The combination of the gas chromatograph and mass spectrometer is further enhanced when a computer is added to the system. The integrated gas chromatograph/mass spectrometer/computer system provides the ultimate in speed, accuracy, and sensitivity. With the ability to record

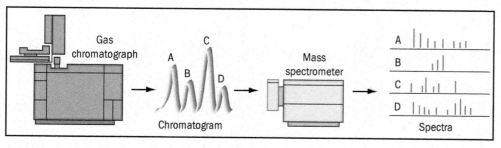

FIGURE 12–19

How GC/MS works. Left to right, the sample is separated into its components by the gas chromatograph, and then the components are ionized and identified by characteristic fragmentation patterns of the spectra produced by the mass spectrometer.

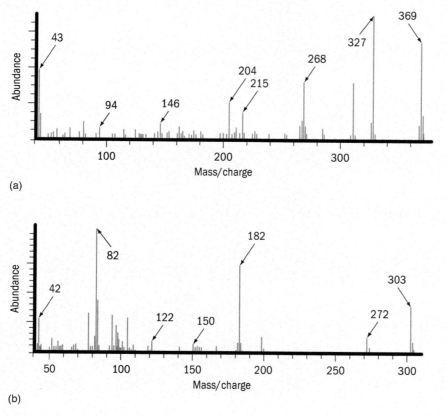

(a)

(b)

FIGURE 12–20

(a) Mass spectrum of heroin. (b) Mass spectrum of cocaine.

and store in its memory several hundred mass spectra, such a system can detect and identify substances present in only one-millionth-of-a-gram quantities. Furthermore, the computer can be programmed to compare an unknown spectrum against a comprehensive library of mass spectra stored in its memory. The advent of personal computers and microcircuitry has made it possible to design mass spectrometer systems that can fit on a small table. Such a unit is pictured in Figure 12–21. Research-grade mass spectrometers are found in laboratories as larger floor-model units (see Figure 12–22).

FIGURE 12–21

A tabletop mass spectrometer.
(1) The sample is injected into a heated inlet port, and a carrier gas sweeps it into the column.
(2) The GC column separates the mixture into its components.
(3) In the ion source, a filament wire emits electrons that strike the sample molecules, causing them to fragment as they leave the GC column. (4) The quadrupole, consisting of four rods, separates the fragments according to their mass. (5) The detector counts the fragments passing through the quadrupole. The signal is small and must be amplified. (6) The data system is responsible for total control of the entire GC/MS system. It detects and measures the abundance of each fragment and displays the mass spectrum.

Source: Agilent Technologies, Inc. 2013 Reproduced with permission, courtesy of Agilent Technologies, Inc.

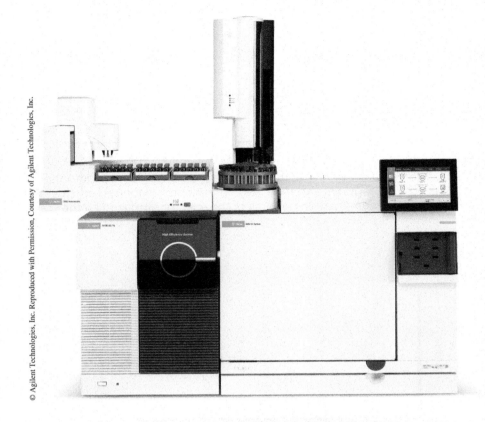

© Agilent Technologies, Inc. Reproduced with Permission, Courtesy of Agilent Technologies, Inc.

FIGURE 12–22

A scientist injecting a sample into a research-grade mass spectrometer.

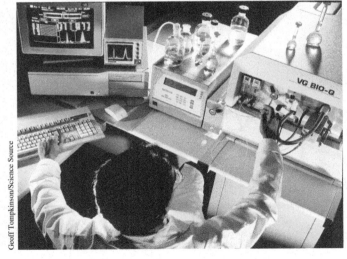

Geoff Tompkinson/Science Source

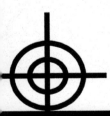

Chapter Summary > > > > > > > > > > > > >

A drug can be defined as a natural or synthetic substance that is used to produce physiological or psychological effects in humans or other higher-order animals.

Narcotic drugs are analgesics, meaning they relieve pain by depressing the central nervous system. Regular use of a narcotic drug leads to physical dependence. The most common source of narcotic drugs is opium. Morphine is readily extracted from opium and is used to synthesize heroin. Opiates, which include methadone and OxyContin (oxycodone),

are not derived from opium or morphine, but they have the same physiological effects on the body as do opium narcotics. Another class of drugs is hallucinogens; marijuana is the most well-known member of this class. Hallucinogens cause marked changes in mood, attitude, thought processes, and perceptions. Marijuana is the most controversial drug in this class because its long-term effects on health are still largely unknown. Other hallucinogens include LSD, mescaline, PCP, psilocybin, and MDMA (Ecstasy).

Depressants are another class of drugs. These include alcohol (ethanol), barbiturates, tranquilizers, and various substances that can be sniffed, such as airplane glue and model cement. Stimulants include amphetamines, sometimes known as "uppers" or "speed," and cocaine, which in its freebase form is known as *crack*. The term *club drugs* refers to synthetic drugs that are used at nightclubs, bars, and raves (all-night dance parties). Substances that are often used as club drugs include, but are not limited to, MDMA (Ecstasy), GHB (gamma hydroxybutyrate), Rohypnol ("roofies"), ketamine, and methamphetamine. Yet another category of drugs is anabolic steroids, which are synthetic compounds chemically related to the male sex hormone testosterone. Anabolic steroids are often used by individuals who want to accelerate muscle growth. Federal law establishes five schedules of classification for controlled dangerous substances on the basis of a drug's potential for use, potential for physical and psychological dependence, and medical value.

The package in which a drug is collected must prevent the loss and/or cross-contamination of the contents. Often, the original container in which the drug was seized will suffice to meet these requirements. Specimens suspected of containing volatile solvents, such as those involved in glue-sniffing cases, must be packaged in an airtight container to prevent evaporation of the solvent.

Faced with the prospect that the unknown substance may be any one of a thousand or more commonly encountered drugs, the analyst must employ screening tests to reduce these possibilities to a small and manageable number. Another consideration in selecting an analytical technique is the need for either a qualitative or a quantitative determination. The former relates just to the identity of the material, whereas the latter requires the determination of the percentage composition of the components of a mixture.

Chromatography, spectrophotometry, and mass spectrometry are all readily used by a forensic scientist to identify or compare organic or carbon-containing materials. Chromatography is a means of separating and tentatively identifying the components of a mixture. Spectrophotometry is the study of the absorption of light by chemical substances. Mass spectrometry characterizes molecules by observing their fragmentation pattern after their collision with a beam of high-energy electrons. GC separates mixtures on the basis of their distribution between a stationary liquid phase and a mobile gas phase. In GC, the moving phase is actually a gas called the carrier gas, which flows through a column. The stationary phase is a thin film of liquid contained within the column. After a mixture has traversed the length of the column, it emerges separated into its components. The written record of this separation is called a chromatogram. A direct connection between the GC column and the mass spectrometer allows each component to flow into the mass spectrometer as it emerges from the GC. Fragmentation of each component by high-energy electrons produces a "fingerprint" pattern of the substance being examined.

Other forms of chromatography applicable to forensic science are high-performance liquid chromatography (HPLC) and TLC. HPLC separates compounds using a stationary phase and a mobile liquid phase and is used with temperature-sensitive compounds. TLC uses a solid stationary phase, usually coated onto a glass plate, and a mobile liquid phase to separate the components of the mixture. Most forensic laboratories use ultraviolet (UV) and infrared (IR) spectrophotometers to characterize chemical compounds. In contrast to the simplicity of a UV spectrum, absorption in the IR region provides a far more complex pattern. Different materials always have distinctively different IR spectra; each IR spectrum is therefore equivalent to a "fingerprint" of that substance. This objective is often accomplished by subjecting the material to a series of color tests that produce characteristic colors for the more commonly encountered illicit drugs. Once this preliminary analysis is completed, a confirmation is pursued. Forensic chemists use a specific test to identify a drug substance to the exclusion of all other known chemical substances. Typically, IR spectrophotometry or mass spectrometry is used to specifically identify a drug substance.

Review Questions

1. True or False: Underlying emotional factors are the primary motives leading to the repeated use of a drug. _____

2. Drugs such as alcohol, heroin, amphetamines, barbiturates, and cocaine can lead to a (high, low) degree of psychological dependence with repeated use.

3. The development of (psychological, physical) dependence on a drug is shown by withdrawal symptoms such as convulsions when the user stops taking the drug.

4. True or False: Use of barbiturates can lead to physical dependency. _____

5. True or False: Repeated use of LSD leads to physical dependency. _____

6. Physical dependency develops only when the drug user adheres to a(n) _____ schedule of drug intake.

7. Narcotic drugs are _____ that _____ the central nervous system.

8. _____ is a gummy, milky juice exuded through a cut made in the unripe pod of the opium poppy.

9. The primary constituent of opium is _____.

10. _____ is a chemical derivative of morphine made by reacting morphine with acetic anhydride.

11. A legally manufactured drug that is chemically related to heroin and heavily used is _____.

12. True or False: Methadone is classified as a narcotic drug, even though it is not derived from opium or morphine. _____

13. Drugs that cause marked alterations in mood, attitude, thought processes, and perceptions are called _____.

14. _____ is the sticky resin extracted from the marijuana plant.

15. The active ingredient of marijuana largely responsible for its hallucinogenic properties is _____.

16. True or False: The potency of a marijuana preparation depends on the proportion of the various plant parts in the mixture. _____

17. The marijuana preparation with the highest THC content is _____.

18. LSD is a chemical derivative of _____, a chemical obtained from the ergot fungus that grows on certain grasses and grains.

19. The drug phencyclidine is often manufactured for the illicit-drug market in _____ laboratories.

20. Alcohol (stimulates, depresses) the central nervous system.

21. _____ are called "downers" because they depress the central nervous system.

22. Phenobarbital is an example of a (short-, long-) acting barbiturate.

23. _____ is a powerful sedative and muscle relaxant that possesses many of the depressant properties of barbiturates.

24. _____ and _____ drugs are used to relieve anxiety and tension without inducing sleep.

25. True or False: Glue sniffing stimulates the central nervous system. _____

26. _____ are a group of synthetic drugs that stimulate the central nervous system.

27. The most severe form of amphetamine use stems from its (oral, intravenous) administration.

28. An increasing percentage of amphetamines available on the illicit-drug market originate from _____ drug laboratories.

29. _____ is extracted from the leaf of the coca plant.

30. Traditionally, cocaine is _____ into the nostrils.

31. True or False: Cocaine is a powerful central nervous system depressant. _____

32. The two drugs usually associated with drug-facilitated sexual assaults are _____ and _____.

33. _____ steroids are designed to promote muscle growth but have harmful side effects.

34. The federal drug-control law is known as _____.

35. Federal law establishes _____ schedules of classification for the control of dangerous drugs.

36. Drugs that have no accepted medical use are placed in schedule _____.

37. Librium and Valium are listed in schedule _____.

38. A(n) _____ analysis describes the identity of a material, and a(n) _____ analysis relates to a determination of the quantity of a substance.

39. True or False: Color tests are used to identify drugs conclusively. _____

40. The _____ color test reagent turns purple in the presence of heroin.

41. The _____ color test reagent turns orange-brown in the presence of amphetamines.

42. The Duquenois–Levine test is a valuable color test for _____.

43. The _____ test is a widely used color test for cocaine.

44. _____ tests tentatively identify drugs by the size and shape of crystals formed when the drug is mixed with specific reagents.

45. A mixture's components can be separated by the technique of _____.

46. The time required for a substance to travel through the gas chromatographic column is a useful identifying characteristic known as _____.

47. A technique that uses a moving liquid phase and a stationary solid phase to separate mixtures is _____.

48. True or False: Thin-layer chromatography yields the positive identification of a material. _____

49. Because most chemical compounds are colorless, the final step of the thin-layer development usually requires that they be _____ by spraying with a chemical reagent.

50. True or False: Color is a usual indication that substances selectively absorb light. _____

51. The study of the absorption of light by chemical substances is known as _____.

52. An (ultraviolet, infrared) absorption spectrum provides a unique "fingerprint" of a chemical substance.

53. The gas chromatograph, in combination with the _____, can separate the components of a drug mixture and then unequivocally identify each substance present in the mixture.

54. The selective absorption of electromagnetic radiation by materials (can, cannot) be used as an aid for identification.

55. The pattern of a(n) _____ absorption spectrum is unique for each drug and thus is a specific test for identification.

56. The technique of _____ exposes molecules to a beam of high-energy electrons in order to fragment them.

57. True or False: A mass spectrum is normally considered a specific means for identifying a chemical substance. _____

58. All packages containing drugs must be marked for identification by the police officer before being sent to the laboratory in order to maintain the _____.

Review Questions for Inside the Science

1. True or False: Henry's law describes the distribution of a volatile chemical compound between its liquid and gas phases. _____

2. The (higher, lower) the solubility of a gas in a liquid, the greater its tendency to remain dissolved in that liquid.

3. True or False: In order for chromatography to occur, one phase must move continuously in one direction over a stationary phase. _____

4. A technique that separates mixtures on the basis of their distribution between a stationary liquid phase and a moving gas phase is _____.

5. The distance a spot has traveled up a thin-layer plate can be assigned a numerical value known as the _____ value.

6. A major advantage of high-performance liquid chromatography is that the entire process takes place at _____ temperature.

7. The amount of radiation a substance will absorb is directly proportional to its concentration as defined by _____ law.

8. The _____ is the instrument used to measure and record the absorption spectrum of a chemical substance.

9. The function of the _____ is to select a single frequency of light emanating from the spectrophotometer's source.

Application and Critical Thinking

1. An individual who has been using a drug for an extended period of time suddenly finds himself unable to secure more of the drug. He acts nervous and irritable and is hyperactive. He seems almost desperate to find more of the drug, but experiences no sickness, pain, or other outward physical discomfort. Based on his behavior, what drugs might he possibly have been using? Explain your answer.

2. Following are descriptions of behavior that are characteristic among users of certain classes of drugs. For each description, indicate the class of drug (narcotics, stimulants, and so on) for which the behavior is most characteristic. For each description, also name at least one drug that produces the described effects.

   a. Slurred speech, slow reaction time, impaired judgment, reduced coordination

   b. Intense emotional responses, anxiety, altered sensory perceptions

   c. Alertness, feelings of strength and confidence, rapid speech and movement, decreased appetite

   d. Drowsiness, intense feeling of well-being, relief from pain

3. Following are descriptions of four hypothetical drugs. According to the Controlled Substances Act, under which drug schedule would each substance be classified?

   a. This drug has a high potential for psychological dependence, it currently has accepted medical uses in the United States, and the distributor is not required to report to the U.S. Drug Enforcement Administration.

   b. This drug has medical use in the United States, is not limited by manufacturing quotas, and may be exported without a permit.

   c. This drug must be stored in a vault or safe, requires separate record keeping, and may be distributed with a prescription.

   d. This drug may not be imported or exported without a permit, is subject to manufacturing quotas, and currently has no medical use in the United States.

4. A police officer stops a motorist who is driving erratically and notices a bag of white powder on the front seat of the car that he suspects contains heroin. The officer brings the bag to you, a forensic scientist in the local crime lab. Name one screening test that you might perform to determine the presence of heroin. Assuming the powder tests positive for heroin, what should you do next?

5. The following figure shows a chromatogram of a known mixture of barbiturates. Based on this figure, answer the following questions:

   a. What barbiturate detected by the chromatogram had the longest retention time?

   b. Which barbiturate had the shortest retention time?

   c. What is the approximate retention time of amobarbital?

6. When investigating a potential warehouse for storing illegal drugs, the police collected a variety of drugs. The drugs were tested with presumptive color tests for determining their possible identity. The test tubes shown in the following figure display the positive color tests. Match the drugs on the right with the color tests on the left and name the test.

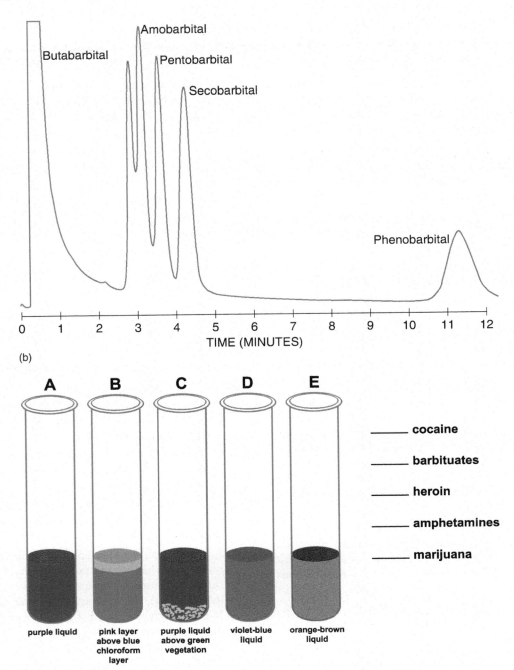

(b)

TIME (MINUTES)

Butabarbital
Amobarbital
Pentobarbital
Secobarbital
Phenobarbital

A   B   C   D   E

_____ cocaine

_____ barbituates

_____ heroin

_____ amphetamines

_____ marijuana

purple liquid | pink layer above blue chloroform layer | purple liquid above green vegetation | violet-blue liquid | orange-brown liquid

Further References

Bono, J. P., "Criminalistics—Introduction to Controlled Substances," in S. B. Karch, ed., *Drug Abuse Handbook*, 2nd ed. Boca Raton, FL: CRC Press, 2007.

Brinsko, K. M., et al., *A Modern Compendium of Microcrystal Tests for Illicit Drugs and Diverted Pharmaceuticals, Compendium*, http://mcri.org/uploads/A_Modern_Compendium_of_Microcrystal_Tests.pdf

Christian, D. R., and S. Bell, "Seized Drug Analysis," in S. H. James, J. J. Nordby, and S. Bell, eds.,

Forensic Science: An Introduction to Scientific and Investigative Techniques, 4th ed. Boca Raton, FL: CRC Press, 2014.

Siegel, J. A., "Forensic Identification of Controlled Substances," in R. Saferstein, ed., *Forensic Science Handbook*, vol. 2, 2nd ed. Upper Saddle River, NJ: Prentice Hall, 2005.

Smith, F., and J. A. Siegel, eds., *Handbook of Forensic Drug Analysis*. Boca Raton, FL: CRC Press, 2005.

Chapter 13

Forensic Toxicology

KEY TERMS

absorption
acid
alveoli
anticoagulant
artery
base
capillary
excretion
fuel cell detector
metabolism
oxidation
pH scale
preservative
toxicologist
vein

Learning Objectives

After studying this chapter, you should be able to:

13.1 Explain how alcohol is absorbed into the bloodstream, transported throughout the body, and eliminated by oxidation and excretion

13.2 Describe the process by which alcohol is excreted in the breath via the lungs

13.3 Discuss the methods used to determine alcohol intoxication

13.4 Discuss the process involved in the analysis of blood for alcohol

13.5 Explain how the "implied consent" law recommended by the NHTSA addressed the constitutional issues raised against blood-alcohol laws

13.6 Describe the role of the forensic toxicologist and the techniques they use to identify substances

13.7 Explain how to coordinate the drug recognition expert program with a forensic toxicology result

Go to www.pearsonhighered.com/careersresources to access Webextras for this chapter.

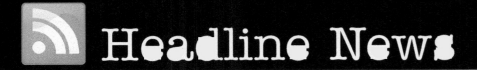

Headline News

Motherisk Drug Testing Laboratory Scandal

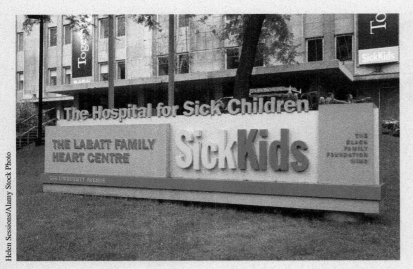

Helen Sessions/Alamy Stock Photo

The Hospital for Sick Children in Ontario, Canada, had been engaged in drug testing hair for child protective services from 2005 to 2015. The laboratory in the hospital responsible for the testing was Motherisk Drug Testing Laboratory, or MDTL. MDTL was one facet of the Hospital's Motherisk Program, which provided information and guidance to members of the public and to physicians about the potential risks to a developing fetus or infant from exposure to drugs, chemicals, diseases, radiation, and environmental agents. MDTL began as a research laboratory, carrying out cutting-edge research on neonatal hair analysis. By the late 1990s, MDTL was receiving an increasing number of requests from child protection agencies to test hair samples for drug use. In 2001, the Laboratory began to promote its hair-testing services to child protection agencies through a variety of presentations and seminars.

In 2005, MDTL tested more than 1,500 samples at the request of child protection agencies, and that number continued to increase over the ensuing years. From time to time, MDTL tests were also used in criminal cases, one of which led directly to this Independent Review. On October 14, 2014, the Court of Appeal for Ontario allowed the appeal of two criminal convictions on charges that a woman had administered cocaine to her 2½-year-old child over a 14-month period. The defendant was convicted, in part, on the results of MDTL hair tests performed on her child. The defense called the deputy chief toxicologist in the Office of the Chief Medical Examiner of Alberta, who criticized MDTL's hair-testing methodology and its interpretation of the hair test results.

Based on this new evidence, the cabinet of the Government of Ontario established an independent review of the lab and its practices. The independent reviewer found, "that the hair-strand drug and alcohol testing used by the Motherisk Drug Testing Laboratory between 2005 and 2015 was inadequate and unreliable for use in child protection and criminal proceedings and that the Laboratory did not meet internationally recognized forensic standards. The use of the Laboratory's hair-testing evidence in child protection and criminal proceedings has serious implications for the fairness of those proceedings and warrants an additional review[1]." Following this criticism, the lab was permanently closed in 2015.

---

[1] "Report of the Motherisk Hair Analysis Independent Review." *Report of the Motherisk Hair Analysis Independent Review*, 2015. www.attorneygeneral.jus.gov. on.ca/english/about/pubs/lang/.

It is no secret that in spite of the concerted efforts of law enforcement agencies to prevent distribution and sale of illicit drugs, thousands die every year from intentional or unintentional administration of drugs, and many more innocent lives are lost as a result of the erratic and frequently uncontrollable behavior of individuals under the influence of drugs. But one should not automatically attribute these occurrences to the wide proliferation of illicit-drug markets. For example, in the United States alone, drug manufacturers produce enough sedatives and antidepressants each year to provide every adult and child with about 40 pills. All of the statistical and medical evidence shows ethyl alcohol, a legal over-the-counter drug, to be the most heavily used drug in Western countries.

Because the uncontrolled use of drugs has become a worldwide problem affecting all segments of society, the role of the toxicologist has taken on new and added significance. Toxicologists detect and identify drugs and poisons in body fluids, tissues, and organs. Their services are required not only in such legal institutions as crime laboratories and medical examiners' offices, they also reach into hospital laboratories—where the possibility of identifying a drug overdose may represent the difference between life and death—and into various health facilities responsible for monitoring the intake of drugs and other toxic substances. Primary examples include performing blood tests on children exposed to leaded paints or analyzing the urine of individuals enrolled in methadone maintenance programs.

The role of the forensic toxicologist is limited to matters that pertain to violations of criminal law. However, the responsibility for performing toxicological services in a criminal justice system varies considerably throughout the United States. In systems, with a crime laboratory independent of the medical examiner, this responsibility may reside with one or the other or may be shared by both. Some systems, however, take advantage of the expertise residing in governmental health department laboratories and assign this role to them. Nevertheless, whatever facility handles this work, its caseload will reflect the prevailing popularity of the drugs that are used in the community. In most cases, this means that the forensic toxicologist handles numerous requests relating to the determination of the presence of alcohol in the body.

All of the statistical and medical evidence shows that ethyl alcohol—a legal, over-the-counter substance—is the most heavily used drug in Western countries. Twenty-nine percent of all traffic deaths in the United States, nearly 10,900 fatalities per year, are alcohol related, along with more than 2 million injuries each year requiring hospital treatment. This highway death toll, as well as the untold damage to life, limb, and property, shows the dangerous consequences of alcohol use. Because of the prevalence of alcohol in the toxicologist's work, we will begin by taking a closer look at how the body processes and responds to alcohol.

Toxicology of Alcohol

The subject of alcohol analysis immediately confronts us with the primary objective of forensic toxicology: to detect and isolate drugs in the body so that their influence on human behavior can be determined. Knowing how the body metabolizes alcohol provides the key to understanding its effects on human behavior. This knowledge has also made possible the development of instruments that measure the presence and concentration of alcohol in individuals suspected of driving while under its influence.

Metabolism of Alcohol

All chemicals that enter the body are eventually broken down by enzymes within the body and transformed into other chemicals that are easier to eliminate. This process of transformation, called **metabolism**, consists of three basic steps: absorption, distribution, and elimination.

ABSORPTION AND DISTRIBUTION   Alcohol, or ethyl alcohol, is a colorless liquid normally diluted with water and consumed as a beverage. Alcohol appears in the blood within minutes after it has been consumed and slowly increases in concentration while it is being absorbed from

metabolism
The transformation of a chemical in the body to another chemical to facilitate its elimination from the body.

absorption
Passage of alcohol across the wall of the stomach and small intestine into the bloodstream.

the stomach and the small intestine into the bloodstream. During the **absorption** phase, alcohol slowly enters the body's bloodstream and is carried to all parts of the body. When the absorption period is completed, the alcohol becomes distributed uniformly throughout the watery portions of the body—that is, throughout about two-thirds of the body volume. Fat, bones, and hair are low in water content and therefore contain little alcohol, whereas alcohol concentration in the rest of the body is fairly uniform. After absorption is completed, a maximum alcohol level is reached in the blood, and the postabsorption period begins. Then the alcohol concentration slowly decreases until it reaches zero again.

Many factors determine the rate at which alcohol is absorbed into the bloodstream, including the total time taken to consume the drink, the alcohol content of the beverage, the amount consumed, and the quantity and type of food present in the stomach at the time of drinking. With so many variables, it is difficult to predict just how long the absorption process will require. For example, beer is absorbed more slowly than an equivalent concentration of alcohol in water, apparently because of the carbohydrates in beer. Also, alcohol consumed on an empty stomach is absorbed faster than an equivalent amount of alcohol taken when there is food in the stomach (see Figure 13–1).

The longer the total time required for complete absorption to occur, the lower the peak alcohol concentration in the blood. Depending on a combination of factors, maximum blood-alcohol concentration may not be reached until two or three hours have elapsed from the time of consumption. However, under normal social drinking conditions, it takes anywhere from 30 to 90 minutes from the time of the final drink until the absorption process is completed.

oxidation
The combination of oxygen with other substances to produce new products.

excretion
Elimination of alcohol from the body in an unchanged state; alcohol is normally excreted in breath and urine.

ELIMINATION   As the alcohol is circulated by the bloodstream, the body begins to eliminate it. Alcohol is eliminated through two mechanisms: **oxidation** and **excretion**. Nearly all of the alcohol consumed (95–98 percent) is eventually oxidized to carbon dioxide and water. Oxidation takes place almost entirely in the liver. There, in the presence of the enzyme *alcohol dehydrogenase*, the alcohol is converted into acetaldehyde and then to acetic acid. The acetic acid is subsequently oxidized in practically all parts of the body, becoming carbon dioxide and water.

The remaining alcohol is excreted, unchanged, in the breath, urine, and perspiration. Most significant, the amount of alcohol exhaled in the breath is in direct proportion to the concentration of alcohol in the blood. This observation has had a tremendous impact on the technology

FIGURE 13–1

Blood-alcohol concentrations after ingestion of 2 ounces of pure alcohol mixed in 8 ounces of water (equivalent to about 5 ounces of 80-proof vodka). *Source:* Courtesy U.S. Department of Transportation, Washington, D.C.

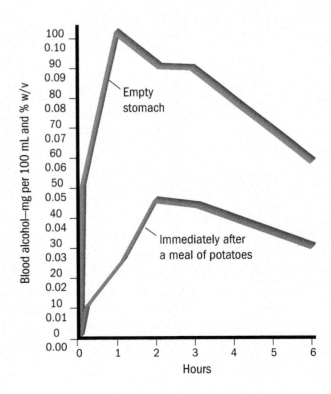

Inside the Science

Alcohol in the Circulatory System

The extent to which an individual may be under the influence of alcohol is usually determined by measuring the quantity of alcohol present in the blood system. Normally, this is accomplished in one of two ways: (1) by direct chemical analysis of the blood for its alcohol content or (2) by measurement of the alcohol content of the breath. In either case, the significance and meaning of the results can better be understood when the movement of alcohol through the circulatory system is studied.

Humans, like all vertebrates, have a closed circulatory system, which consists basically of a heart and numerous arteries, capillaries, and veins. An **artery** is a blood vessel carrying blood away from the heart, and a **vein** is a vessel carrying blood back toward the heart. **Capillaries** are tiny blood vessels that interconnect the arteries with the veins. The exchange of materials between the blood and the other tissues takes place across the thin walls of the capillaries. A schematic diagram of the circulatory system is shown in the figure.

Ingestion and Absorption

Let us now trace the movement of alcohol through the human circulatory system. After alcohol is ingested, it

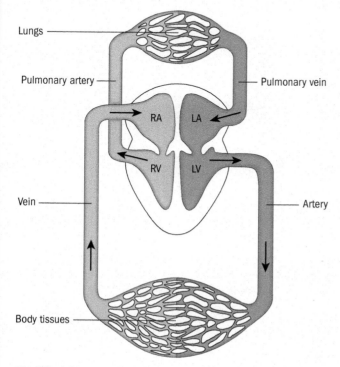

Simplified diagram of the human circulatory system. Dark vessels contain oxygenated blood; light vessels contain deoxygenated blood.

moves down the esophagus into the stomach. About 20 percent of the alcohol is absorbed through the stomach walls into the portal vein of the blood system. The remaining alcohol passes into the blood through the walls of the small intestine. Once in the blood, the alcohol is carried to the liver, where its destruction starts as the blood (carrying the alcohol) moves up to the heart.

The blood enters the upper right chamber of the heart, called the right atrium (or auricle), and is forced into the lower right chamber of the heart, known as the right ventricle. Having returned to the heart from its circulation through the tissues, the blood at this time contains very little oxygen and much carbon dioxide. Consequently, the blood must be pumped up to the lungs, through the pulmonary artery, to be replenished with oxygen.

Aeration

The respiratory system bridges with the circulatory system in the lungs, so that oxygen can enter the blood and carbon dioxide can leave it. As shown in the figure, the pulmonary artery branches into capillaries lying close to tiny pear-shaped sacs called **alveoli**. The lungs contain about 250 million alveoli, all located at the ends of the bronchial tubes. The bronchial tubes connect to the windpipe (trachea), which leads up to the mouth and nose (see the figure). At the surface of the alveolar sacs, blood flowing through the capillaries comes in contact with fresh oxygenated air in the sacs. A rapid exchange now proceeds to take place between the fresh air in the sacs and the spent air in the blood. Oxygen passes through the walls of the alveoli into the blood while carbon dioxide is discharged from the blood into the air (see the figure). If, during this exchange, alcohol or any other volatile substance is in the blood, it too will pass into the alveoli. During breathing, the carbon dioxide and alcohol are expelled through the nose and mouth, and the alveoli sacs are replenished with fresh oxygenated air breathed into the lungs, allowing the process to begin all over again.

The distribution of alcohol between the blood and alveolar air is similar to the example of a gas dissolved in an enclosed beaker of water, as described on page 300. Here again, one can use Henry's law to explain how the alcohol divides itself between the air and blood. Henry's law may now be restated as follows: **When a volatile chemical (alcohol) is dissolved in a liquid (blood) and is brought to equilibrium with air (alveolar breath), there is a fixed ratio between the concentration of the volatile compound (alcohol) in air (alveolar breath) and its concentration in the liquid (blood), and this ratio is constant for a given temperature.**

(continued)

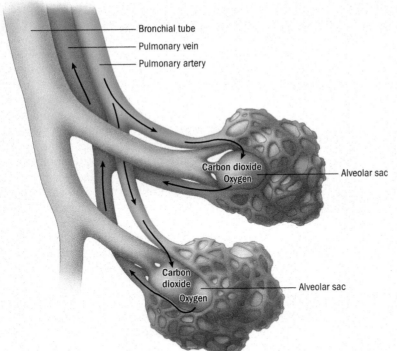

Gas exchange in the lungs. Blood flows from the pulmonary artery into vessels that lie close to the walls of the alveoli sacs. Here, the blood gives up its carbon dioxide and absorbs oxygen. The oxygenated blood leaves the lungs via the pulmonary vein and returns to the heart.

The temperature at which the breath leaves the mouth is normally 34°C. **At this temperature, experimental evidence has shown that the ratio of alcohol in the blood to alcohol in alveoli air is approximately 2,100 to 1. In other words, 1 milliliter of blood will contain nearly the same amount of alcohol as 2,100 milliliters of alveolar breath. Henry's law thus becomes a basis for relating breath to blood-alcohol concentration.**

Recirculation and Distribution

Now let's return to the circulating blood. After emerging from the lungs, the oxygenated blood is rushed back to the upper left chamber of the heart (left atrium) by the pulmonary vein. When the left atrium contracts, it forces the blood through a valve into the left ventricle, which is the lower left chamber of the heart. The left ventricle then pumps the freshly oxygenated blood into the arteries, which carry the blood to all parts of the body. Each of these arteries, in turn, branches into smaller arteries, which eventually connect with the numerous tiny capillaries embedded in the tissues. Here the alcohol moves out of the blood and into the tissues. The blood then runs from the capillaries into tiny veins that fuse to form

larger veins. These veins eventually lead back to the heart to complete the circuit.

During absorption, the concentration of alcohol in the arterial blood is considerably higher than the concentration of alcohol in the venous blood. One typical study revealed a subject's arterial blood-alcohol level to be 41 percent higher than the venous level 30 minutes after the last drink.[2] This difference is thought to exist because of the rapid diffusion of alcohol into the body tissues from venous blood during the early phases of absorption. Because the administration of a blood test requires drawing venous blood from the arm, this test is clearly to the advantage of a subject who may still be in the absorption stage. However, once absorption is complete, the alcohol becomes equally distributed throughout the blood system.

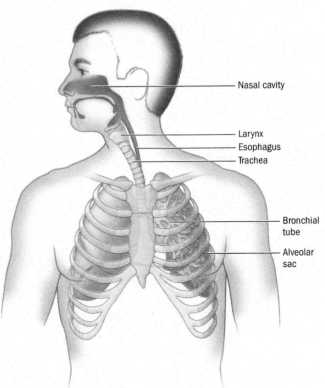

The respiratory system. The trachea connects the nose and mouth to the bronchial tubes. The bronchial tubes divide into numerous branches that terminate in the alveoli sacs in the lungs.

[2]R. B. Forney et al., "Alcohol Distribution in the Vascular System: Concentrations of Orally Administered Alcohol in Blood from Various Points in the Vascular System and in Rebreathed Air during Absorption," *Quarterly Journal of Studies on Alcohol* 25 (1964): 205.

and procedures used for blood-alcohol testing. The development of instruments to reliably measure breath for its alcohol content has made possible the testing of millions of people in a quick, safe, and convenient manner.

The fate of alcohol in the body is therefore relatively simple—namely, absorption into the bloodstream, distribution throughout the body's water, and finally, elimination by oxidation and excretion. The elimination, or "burn-off," rate of alcohol varies in different individuals; 0.015 percent w/v (weight per volume) per hour is the average rate after the absorption process is complete.[3] However, this figure is an average that varies by as much as 30 percent among individuals.

BLOOD-ALCOHOL CONCENTRATION   Logically, the most obvious measure of intoxication would be the amount of liquor a person has consumed. Unfortunately, most arrests are made after the fact, when such information is not available to legal authorities; furthermore, even if these data could be collected, numerous related factors, such as body weight and the rate of alcohol's absorption into the body, are so variable that it would be impossible to prescribe uniform standards that would yield reliable alcohol intoxication levels for all individuals.

Theoretically, for a true determination of the quantity of alcohol impairing an individual's normal body functions, it would be best to remove a portion of brain tissue and analyze it for alcohol content. For obvious reasons, this cannot be done on living subjects. Consequently, toxicologists concentrate on the blood, which provides the medium for circulating alcohol throughout the body, carrying it to all tissues including the brain. Fortunately, experimental evidence supports this approach and shows blood-alcohol concentration to be directly proportional to the concentration of alcohol in the brain. From the medicolegal point of view, blood-alcohol levels have become the accepted standard for relating alcohol intake to its effect on the body.

As noted earlier, alcohol becomes concentrated evenly throughout the watery portions of the body. This knowledge can be useful for the toxicologist analyzing a body for the presence of alcohol. If blood is not available, as in some postmortem situations, a medical examiner can select a water-rich organ or fluid—for example, the brain, cerebrospinal fluid, or vitreous humor—to estimate the body's equivalent alcohol level.

artery
A blood vessel that carries blood away from the heart.

vein
A blood vessel that transports blood toward the heart.

capillary
A tiny blood vessel across whose walls exchange of materials between the blood and the tissues takes place; it receives blood from arteries and carries it to veins.

alveoli
Small sacs in the lungs through whose walls air and other vapors are exchanged between the breath and the blood.

Testing for Intoxication

From a practical point of view, drawing blood from veins of motorists suspected of being under the influence of alcohol is simply not convenient. The need to transport each suspect to a location where a medically qualified person can draw blood would be costly and time consuming, considering the hundreds of suspects that the average police department must test every year. The methods used must be designed to test hundreds of thousands of motorists annually, without causing them undue physical harm or unreasonable inconvenience, and provide a reliable diagnosis that can be supported and defended within the framework of the legal system. This means that toxicologists have had to devise rapid and specific procedures for measuring a driver's degree of alcohol intoxication that can be easily administered in the field.

Breath Testing for Alcohol

The most widespread method for rapidly determining alcohol intoxication is breath testing. A breath tester is simply a device for collecting and measuring the alcohol content of alveolar breath. Alcohol is expelled, unchanged, in the breath of a person who has been drinking. A breath test measures the alcohol concentration in the pulmonary artery by measuring its concentration in alveolar breath. Thus, breath analysis provides an easily obtainable specimen along with a rapid and accurate result.

---

[3]In the United States, laws that define blood-alcohol levels almost exclusively use the unit *percent weight per volume*—% w/v. Hence, 0.015 percent w/v is equivalent to 0.015 gram of alcohol per 100 milliliters of blood, or 15 milligrams of alcohol per 100 milliliters.

Breath-test results obtained during the absorption phase may be higher than results obtained from a simultaneous analysis of venous blood. However, the former are more reflective of the concentration of alcohol reaching the brain and therefore more accurately reflect the effects of alcohol on the subject. Again, once absorption is complete, the difference between a blood test and a breath test should be minimal.

BREATH-TEST INSTRUMENTS   The first widely used instrument for measuring the alcohol content of alveolar breath was the *Breathalyzer*, developed in 1954 by R. F. Borkenstein, who was a captain in the Indiana State Police. Starting in the 1970s, the Breathalyzer was phased out and replaced by other instruments. Like the Breathalyzer, they assume that the ratio of alcohol in the blood to alcohol in alveolar breath is 2,100 to 1 at a mouth temperature of 34°C. In other words, 1 milliliter of blood contains nearly the same amount of alcohol as 2,100 milliliters of alveolar breath. Unlike the Breathalyzer, modern breath testers are free of chemicals. These devices include infrared light–absorption devices and **fuel cell detectors** (described in the following "Inside the Science" box).

fuel cell detector
A detector in which chemical reactions produce electricity.

Infrared and fuel-cell-based breath testers are microprocessor controlled, so all an operator has to do is to press a start button; the instrument automatically moves through a sequence of steps and produces a readout of the subject's test results. These instruments also perform self-diagnostic tests to ascertain whether they are in proper operating condition.

CONSIDERATIONS IN BREATH TESTING   An important feature of these instruments is that they can be connected to an external alcohol standard or simulator in the form of either a liquid or a gas. The liquid simulator contains a known concentration of alcohol in water. It is heated to a controlled temperature and the vapor formed above the liquid is pumped into the instrument. Dry-gas standards typically consist of a known concentration of alcohol mixed with an inert gas and compressed in cylinders. The external standard is automatically sampled by the breath-test instrument before and/or after the subject's breath sample is taken and recorded. Thus, the operator can check the accuracy of the instrument against the known alcohol standard.

The key to the accuracy of a breath-testing device is to ensure that the unit captures the alcohol in the alveolar (i.e., deep-lung) breath of the subject. This is typically accomplished by programming the unit to accept no less than 1.1 to 1.5 liters of breath from the subject. Also, the subject must blow for a minimum time (such as 6 seconds) with a minimum breath flow rate (such as 3 liters per minute).

The breath-test instruments just described feature a *slope detector*, which ensures that the breath sample is alveolar, or deep-lung, breath. As the subject blows into the instrument, the breath-alcohol concentration is continuously monitored. The instrument accepts a breath sample only when consecutive measurements fall within a predetermined rate of change. This approach ensures that the sample measurement is deep-lung breath and closely relates to the true blood-alcohol concentration of the subject being tested.

A breath-test operator must take other steps to ensure that the breath-test result truly reflects the actual blood-alcohol concentration within the subject. A major consideration is to avoid measuring "mouth alcohol" resulting from regurgitation, belching, or recent intake of an alcoholic beverage. Also, recent gargling with an alcohol-containing mouthwash can lead to the presence of mouth alcohol. As a result, the alcohol concentration detected in the exhaled breath is higher than the concentration in the alveolar breath. To avoid this possibility, the operator must not allow the subject to take any foreign material into their mouth for at least 15 minutes before the breath test. Likewise, the subject should be observed not to have belched or regurgitated during this period. Mouth alcohol has been shown to dissipate after 15 to 20 minutes from its inception.

Measurement of independent breath samples taken within a few minutes of each other is another extremely important check of the integrity of the breath test. Acceptable agreement between the two tests taken minutes apart significantly reduces the possibility of errors caused by the operator, mouth alcohol, instrument component failures, and spurious electric signals.

Inside the Science

Infrared Light Absorption

In principle, infrared instruments operate no differently than the spectrophotometers described in Chapter 12. An evidential testing instrument that incorporates the principle of infrared light absorption is shown in Figure (a). Any alcohol present in the subject's breath flows into the instrument's breath chamber. As shown in Figure (b), a beam of infrared light is aimed through the chamber. A filter is used to select a wavelength of infrared light at which alcohol will absorb. As the infrared light passes through the chamber, it interacts with the alcohol and causes the light to decrease in intensity. The decrease in light intensity is measured by a photoelectric detector that gives a signal proportional to the concentration of alcohol present in the breath sample. This information is processed by an electronic microprocessor, and the percent blood-alcohol concentration is displayed on a digital readout. Most infrared breath testers aim a second infrared beam into the same chamber to check for acetone or other chemical interferences on the breath. If the instrument detects differences in the relative response of the two infrared beams that does not conform to ethyl alcohol, the operator is immediately informed of the presence of an "interferant."

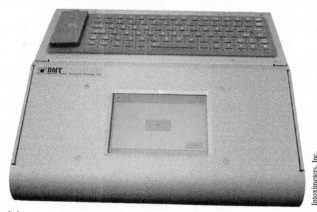

(a)

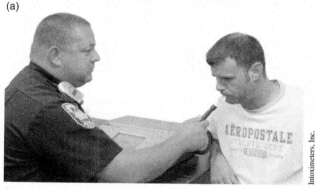

(b)

(a) An infrared breath-testing instrument—the Data Master DMT.
(b) A subject blowing into the DMT breath tester.

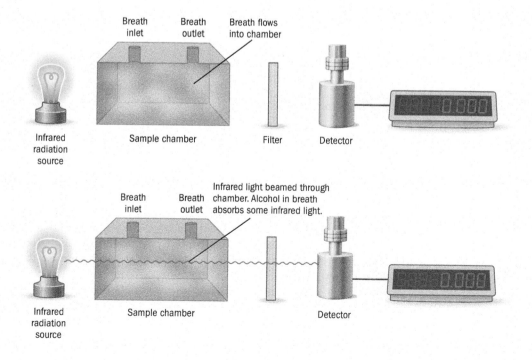

(*continued*)

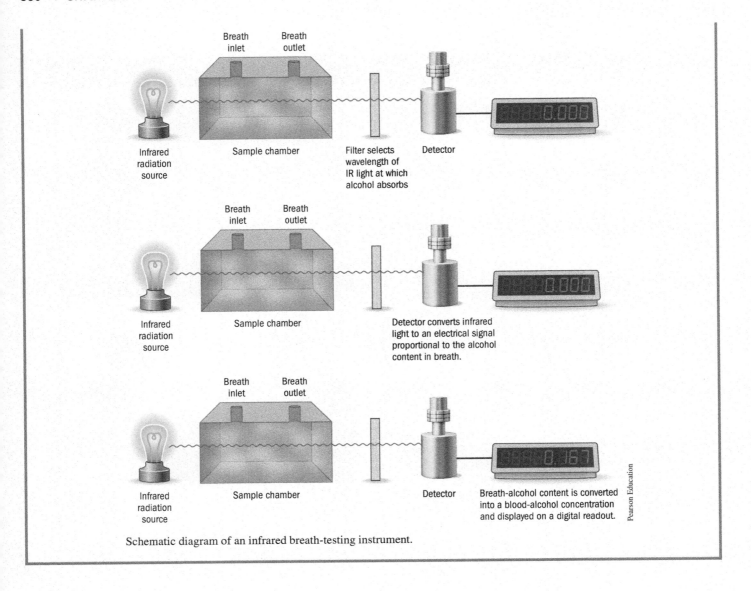

Breath inlet   Breath outlet

Infrared radiation source

Sample chamber

Filter selects wavelength of IR light at which alcohol absorbs

Detector

Breath inlet   Breath outlet

Infrared radiation source

Sample chamber

Detector converts infrared light to an electrical signal proportional to the alcohol content in breath.

Breath inlet   Breath outlet

Infrared radiation source

Sample chamber

Detector

Breath-alcohol content is converted into a blood-alcohol concentration and displayed on a digital readout.

Pearson Education

Schematic diagram of an infrared breath-testing instrument.

Field Sobriety Testing

A police officer who suspects that an individual is under the influence of alcohol usually conducts a series of preliminary tests before ordering the suspect to submit to an evidential breath or blood test. **These preliminary, or field sobriety, tests are normally performed to ascertain the degree of the suspect's physical impairment and whether an evidential test is justified.**

Field sobriety tests usually consist of a series of psychophysical tests and a preliminary breath test (if such devices are authorized and available for use). A portable handheld roadside breath tester is shown in Figure 13–2. This pocket-sized device weighs 5 ounces and uses a fuel cell to measure the alcohol content of a breath sample. The fuel cell absorbs the alcohol from the breath sample, oxidizes it, and produces an electrical current proportional to the breath-alcohol content. This instrument Figure 13–2 can typically perform for years before the fuel cell needs to be replaced. Its been approved for use as an evidential breath tester by the National Highway Traffic Safety Administration.

Horizontal-gaze nystagmus, walk and turn, and the one-leg stand constitute a series of reliable and effective psychophysical tests. Horizontal-gaze nystagmus is an involuntary jerking of the eye as it moves to the side. A person experiencing nystagmus is usually unaware that

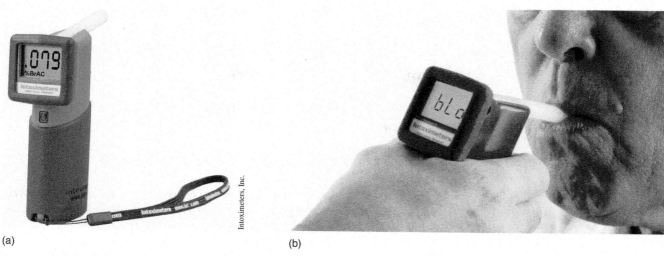

(a)   (b)

FIGURE 13–2
(a) The Alco-Sensor FST. (b) A subject blowing into the roadside tester device.

Inside the Science

The Fuel Cell

A fuel cell converts energy arising from a chemical re-action into electrochemical energy. A typical fuel cell consists of two platinum electrodes separated by an acid- or base-containing porous membrane. A platinum wire connects the electrodes and allows a current to flow between them. In the alcohol fuel cell, one of the electrodes is positioned to come into contact with a subject's breath sample. If alcohol is present in the breath, a reaction at the electrode's surface converts the alcohol to acetic acid. One by-product of this conversion is free electrons, which flow through the connecting wire to the opposite electrode, where they interact with atmospheric oxygen to form water (see the figure). The fuel cell also requires the migration of hydrogen ions across the acidic porous membrane to complete the circuit. The strength of the current flow between the two electrodes is proportional to the concentration of alcohol in the breath.

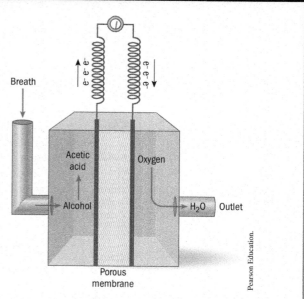

A fuel cell detector in which chemical reactions are used to produce electricity.

the jerking is happening and is unable to stop or control it. The subject being tested is asked to follow a penlight or some other object with their eye as far to the side as the eye can go. The more intoxicated the person is, the less the eye has to move toward the side before jerking or nystagmus begins. Usually, when a person's blood-alcohol concentration is in the range of 0.10 percent, the jerking begins before the eyeball has moved 45 degrees to the side (see Figure 13–3).

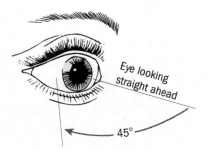

FIGURE 13–3

When a person's blood-alcohol level is in the range of 0.10 percent, jerking of the eye during the horizontal-gaze nystagmus test begins before the eyeball has moved 45 degrees to the side.

Higher blood-alcohol concentration causes jerking at smaller angles. Also, if the suspect has taken a drug that also causes nystagmus (such as phencyclidine, barbiturates, and other depressants), the nystagmus onset angle may occur much earlier than would be expected from alcohol alone.

Walk and turn and the one-leg stand are divided-attention tasks, testing the subject's ability to comprehend and execute two or more simple instructions at one time. The ability to understand and simultaneously carry out more than two instructions is significantly affected by increasing blood-alcohol levels. Walk and turn requires the suspect to maintain balance while standing heel-to-toe and at the same time listening to and comprehending the test instructions. During the walking stage, the suspect must walk a straight line, touching heel-to-toe for nine steps, then turn around on the line and repeat the process. The one-leg stand requires the suspect to maintain balance while standing with heels together listening to the instructions. During the balancing stage, the suspect must stand on one foot while holding the other foot several inches off the ground for 30 seconds; simultaneously, the suspect must count out loud during the 30-second time period.

Analysis of Blood for Alcohol

Gas chromatography is the approach most widely used by forensic toxicologists for determining alcohol levels in blood. Under proper gas chromatographic conditions, ethanol can be separated from other volatile substances in the blood. By comparing the resultant ethanol peak area to ones obtained from known blood-ethanol standards, the investigator can calculate the ethanol level with a high degree of accuracy (see Figure 13–4).

Another procedure for alcohol analysis involves the oxidation of ethanol to acetaldehyde. This reaction is carried out in the presence of the enzyme alcohol dehydrogenase and the coenzyme nicotin-amide-adenine dinucleotide (NAD). As the oxidation proceeds, NAD is converted into another chemical species, NADH. The extent of this conversion is measured by a spectrophotometer and is related to ethanol concentration. This approach to blood-alcohol

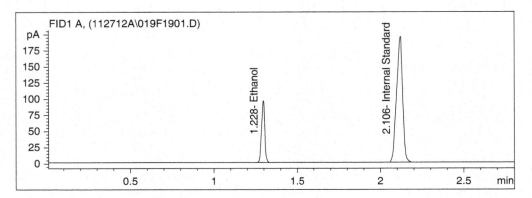

FIGURE 13–4

A gas chromatogram showing ethyl alcohol (ethanol) in whole blood.

testing is normally associated with instruments used in clinical or hospital settings. Instead, forensic laboratories normally use gas chromatography for determining blood-ethanol content.

Collection and Preservation of Blood

Blood must always be drawn under medically acceptable conditions by a qualified individual. A nonalcoholic disinfectant should be applied before the suspect's skin is penetrated with a sterile needle or lancet. It is important to eliminate any possibility that an alcoholic disinfectant could inadvertently contribute to a falsely high blood-alcohol result. Nonalcoholic disinfectants such as aqueous benzalkonium chloride (Zepiran), aqueous mercuric chloride, or povidone-iodine (Betadine) are recommended for this purpose.

Once blood is removed from an individual, it is best preserved sealed in an airtight container after adding an anticoagulant and a preservative. The blood should be stored in a refrigerator until delivery to the toxicology laboratory. The addition of an **anticoagulant**, such as potassium oxalate, prevents clotting; a **preservative**, such as sodium fluoride, inhibits the growth of microorganisms capable of destroying alcohol.

One study performed to determine the stability of alcohol in blood removed from living individuals found that the most significant factors affecting alcohol's stability in blood are storage temperature, the presence of a preservative, and the length of storage.[4] Not a single blood specimen examined showed an increase in alcohol level with time. Failure to keep the blood refrigerated or to add sodium fluoride resulted in a substantial decline in alcohol concentration. Longer storage times also reduced blood-alcohol levels.[5] Hence, failure to adhere to any of the proper preservation requirements for blood works to the benefit of the suspect and to the detriment of society.

The collection of postmortem blood samples for alcohol-level determinations requires added precautions. Ethyl alcohol may be generated in the body of a deceased individual as a result of bacterial action. Therefore, it is best to collect a number of blood samples from different body sites. For example, blood may be removed from the heart and from the femoral vein (in the leg) and cubital vein (in the arm). Each sample should be placed in a clean, airtight container containing an anticoagulant and sodium fluoride preservative and should be refrigerated. Blood-alcohol levels can be attributed solely to alcohol consumption if they are nearly similar in all blood samples collected from the same person. As an alternative to blood collection, the collection of vitreous humor and urine is recommended. Vitreous humor and urine usually do not experience any significant postmortem ethyl alcohol production.

anticoagulant
A substance that prevents coagulation or clotting of blood.

preservative
A substance that stops the growth of microorganisms in blood.

Alcohol and the Law

Constitutionally, every state in the United States is charged with establishing and administering statutes regulating the operation of motor vehicles. Although such an arrangement might encourage diverse laws defining permissible blood-alcohol levels, this has not been the case. Both the American Medical Association and the National Safety Council have exerted considerable influence in persuading the states to establish uniform and reasonable blood-alcohol standards.

Blood-Alcohol Laws

Between 1939 and 1964, 39 states and the District of Columbia enacted legislation that followed the recommendations of the American Medical Association and the National Safety Council in specifying that a person with a blood-alcohol concentration in excess of 0.15 percent w/v was to be considered under the influence of alcohol.[6] However, continued experimental studies have since shown a clear correlation between drinking and driving impairment for blood-alcohol levels much below 0.15 percent w/v. As a result of these studies, in 1960 the American Medical Association and in 1965 the National Safety Council recommended lowering the presumptive

[4] G. A. Brown et al., "The Stability of Ethanol in Stored Blood," *Analytica Chemica Acta* 66 (1973): 271.

[5] N. B. Tisclone, et al., "Long-term Blood Stability in Forensic Antemortem Whole Blood Samples," *Journal of Analytical Toxicology* 39 (2015): 119.

[6] 0.15 percent w/v is equivalent to 0.15 grams of alcohol per 100 milliliters of blood, or 150 milligrams per 100 milliliters.

level at which an individual was considered to be under the influence of alcohol to 0.10 percent w/v. In 2000, U.S. federal law established 0.08 percent as the *per se* blood-alcohol level, meaning that any individual meeting or exceeding this blood-alcohol level shall be deemed intoxicated. No other proof of alcohol impairment is necessary. The 0.08 percent level applies only to noncommercial drivers, as the federal government has set the maximum allowable blood-alcohol concentration for commercial truck and bus drivers at 0.04 percent. The state of Utah has a 0.05 percent *per se* law.

Several Western countries have also set 0.08 percent w/v as the blood-alcohol level above which it is an offense to drive a motor vehicle. Those countries include Canada, Italy, Switzerland, and the United Kingdom. Finland, France, Germany, Ireland, Japan, the Netherlands, and Norway have a 0.05 percent limit. Australian states have adopted a 0.05 percent blood-alcohol concentration level. Sweden has lowered its blood-alcohol concentration limit to 0.02 percent.

As shown in Figure 13–5, one is about four times as likely to become involved in an automobile accident at the 0.08 percent level as a sober individual. At the 0.15 percent level, the chances are 25 times as much for involvement in an automobile accident compared to a sober driver. The reader can *estimate* the relationship of blood-alcohol levels to body weight and the quantity of 80-proof liquor consumed by referring to Figure 13–6.

Constitutional Issues

The Fifth Amendment to the U.S. Constitution guarantees all citizens protection against *self-incrimination*—that is, against being forced to make an admission that would prove one's own guilt in a legal matter. To prevent a person's refusal to take a test for alcohol intoxication on the constitutional grounds of self-incrimination, the National Highway Traffic Safety Administration (NHTSA) recommended an "implied consent" law. By 1973, all the states had complied with this recommendation. In accordance with this statute, operating a motor vehicle on a public highway automatically carries with it the stipulation that the driver must either submit to a test for alcohol intoxication if requested or lose their license for some designated period—usually six months to one year.

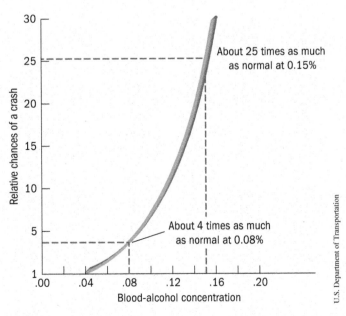

FIGURE 13–5

Diagram of increased driving risk in relation to blood-alcohol concentration.

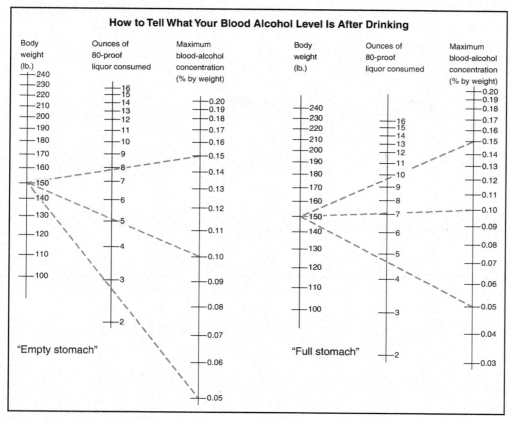

How to Tell What Your Blood Alcohol Level Is After Drinking

FIGURE 13–6

To use this diagram, lay a straightedge across your weight and the number of ounces of liquor you've consumed on an empty or full stomach. The point where the edge hits the right-hand column is your maximum blood-alcohol level. The rate of elimination of alcohol from the bloodstream is approximately 0.015 percent per hour. Therefore, to calculate your actual blood-alcohol level, subtract 0.015 from the number in the right-hand column for each hour from the start of drinking.

Source: U.S. Department of Transportation.

In 1966, the Supreme Court, in *Schmerber* v. *California*,[7] addressed the constitutionality of collecting a blood specimen for alcohol testing, as well as for obtaining other types of physical evidence from a suspect without consent. While being treated at a Los Angeles hospital for injuries sustained in an automobile collision, Schmerber was arrested for driving under the influence of alcohol. A physician took a blood sample from Schmerber at the direction of the police, over the objection of the defendant. On appeal to the U.S. Supreme Court, the defendant argued that his privilege against self-incrimination had been violated by the introduction of the results of the blood test at his trial. The Court ruled against the defendant, reasoning that the Fifth Amendment only prohibits compelling a suspect to give "testimonial" evidence that may be self-incriminating; being compelled to furnish "physical" evidence, such as fingerprints, photographs, measurements, and blood samples, the Court ruled, was not protected by the Fifth Amendment.

The Court also addressed the question of whether Schmerber was subjected to an unreasonable search and seizure by the taking of a blood specimen without a search warrant. In the 1966 decision, the Court upheld the blood removal, reasoning that the natural body elimination of alcohol created an emergency situation allowing for a warrantless search. The Court revisited this issue once again 47 years after Schmerber in the case of *Missouri* v. *McNeely*.[8]

[7] 384 U.S. 757 (1966).
[8] 133 S. Ct. 932 (2013).

Here, the Court addressed the issue as to whether the natural elimination of alcohol in blood categorically justifies a warrantless intrusion. The Court noted that advances in communication technology now allow police to obtain warrant quickly by phone, e-mail, or teleconferencing.

In those drunk-driving investigations where police officers can reasonably obtain a warrant before a blood sample can be drawn without significantly undermining the efficacy of the search, the Fourth Amendment mandates that they do so... . In short, while the natural dissipation of alcohol in the blood may support a finding of exigency in a specific case, as it did in *Schmerber*, it does not do so categorically. Whether a warrantless blood test of a drunk-driving suspect is reasonable must be determined case by case based on the totality of the circumstances.

WEBEXTRA 13.1
Calculate Your Blood-Alcohol Level

WEBEXTRA 13.2
See How Alcohol Affects Your Behavior

toxicologist
An individual charged with the responsibility of detecting and identifying the presence of drugs and poisons in body fluids, tissues, and organs.

The Role of the Toxicologist

Once the forensic **toxicologist** ventures beyond the analysis of alcohol, the toxicologist encounters an encyclopedic maze of drugs and poisons. Even a cursory discussion of the problems and handicaps imposed on toxicologists is enough to develop a sense of appreciation for their accomplishments and ingenuity.

Challenges Facing the Toxicologist

The toxicologist is presented with body fluids and/or organs and asked to examine them for the presence of drugs and poisons. If the toxicologist is fortunate, which is not often, some clue to the type of toxic substance present may develop from the victim's symptoms, a postmortem pathological examination, an examination of the victim's personal effects, or the nearby presence of empty drug containers or household chemicals. Without such supportive information, the toxicologist must use general screening procedures with the hope of narrowing thousands of possibilities to one.

If this task does not seem monumental, consider that the toxicologist is not dealing with drugs at the concentration levels found in powders and pills. By the time a drug specimen reaches the toxicology laboratory, it has been dissipated and distributed throughout the body. Whereas the drug analyst may have gram or milligram quantities of material to work with, the toxicologist must be satisfied with nanogram or at best microgram amounts, acquired only after careful extraction from body fluids and organs.

Furthermore, the body is an active chemistry laboratory, and no one can appreciate this observation more than a toxicologist. Few substances enter and completely leave the body in the same chemical state. The drug that is injected is not always the substance extracted from the body tissues. Therefore, a thorough understanding of how the body alters or metabolizes the chemical structure of a drug is essential in detecting its presence.

It would, for example, be futile and frustrating to search exhaustively for heroin in the human body. This drug is almost immediately metabolized to 6-acetylmorphine which metabolizes to morphine on entering the bloodstream. Even with this information, the search may still prove impossible unless the examiner also knows that only a small percentage of morphine is excreted unchanged in urine. For the most part, morphine becomes chemically bonded to body carbohydrates before elimination in urine. Thus, successful detection of morphine requires that its extraction be planned in accordance with a knowledge of its chemical fate in the body.

Another example of how one needs to know how a drug metabolizes itself in the body is exemplified by the investigation of the death of Anna Nicole Smith. In her case, the sedative chloral hydrate was a major contributor to her death, and its presence was detected by its active metabolite, trichloroethanol (see the following case files box).

Last, when and if the toxicologist has surmounted all of these obstacles and has finally detected, identified, and quantitated a drug or poison, the toxicologist must assess the substance's toxicity. Fortunately, there is published information relating to the toxic levels of most drugs; however, when such data are available, their interpretation must assume that the victim's physiological behavior agrees with that of the subjects of previous studies. In some cases,

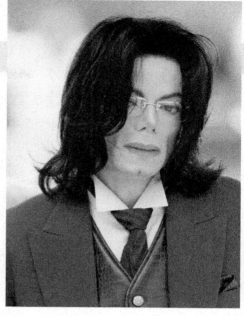

Michael Jackson.

Case Files

> > > > > > > > > >

Michael Jackson: The Demise of a Superstar

A call to 911 had the desperate tone of urgency. The voice of a young man implored an ambulance to hurry to the home of pop star Michael Jackson. The unconscious performer was in cardiac arrest and was not responding to CPR. The 50-year-old Jackson was pronounced dead upon arrival at a regional medical center. When the initial autopsy results revealed no signs of foul play, rumors immediately began to swirl around a drug-related death. News media coverage showed investigators carrying bags full of drugs and syringes out of the Jackson residence. So, it came as no surprise that the forensic toxicology report accompanying Jackson's autopsy showed that the entertainer had died of a drug overdose.

Apparently Jackson had become accustomed to receiving sedatives to help him sleep. Early on the morning of his death, his physician gave Jackson a tab of Valium. At 2 a.m., he administered the sedative lorazepam, and at 3 a.m. the physician administered another sedative, midazolam. Those drugs were administered again at 5 a.m. and 7:30 a.m., but Jackson still was unable to sleep. Finally, at about 10:40 a.m., Jackson's doctor gave him 25 milligrams of propofol, at which point

Jackson went to sleep. Propofol is a powerful sedative used primarily in the maintenance of surgical anesthesia. All of the drugs administered to Jackson were sedatives, which can act in concert to depress the activities of the central nervous system. Therefore, it comes as no surprise that this drug cocktail resulted in cardiac arrest and death.

such an assumption may not be entirely valid without knowing the subject's case history. No experienced toxicologist would be surprised to find an individual tolerating a toxic level of a drug that would have killed most other people.

Collection and Preservation of Toxicological Evidence

Toxicology is made infinitely easier once it is recognized that the toxicologist's capabilities are directly dependent on the input received from the attending physician, medical examiner, and police investigator. It is a tribute to forensic toxicologists, who must often labor under conditions that do not afford such cooperation, that they can achieve such a high level of proficiency.

Generally, with a deceased person, the medical examiner decides what biological specimens must be shipped to the toxicology laboratory for analysis. However, a living person suspected of being under the influence of a drug presents a completely different problem, and few options are available. When possible, both blood and urine are taken from any suspected drug user. The entire urine void is collected and submitted for toxicological analysis. Preferably, two consecutive voids should be collected in separate specimen containers.

When a licensed physician or registered nurse is available, a sample of blood should also be collected. The amount of blood taken depends on the type of examination to be conducted. Comprehensive toxicological tests for drugs and poisons can conveniently be carried out on a minimum of 10 cc of blood. A determination solely for the presence of alcohol will require much less—depending on how analyzed can be less than 1 mL for just alcohol analysis. However, many therapeutic drugs, such as tranquilizers and barbiturates, when taken in combination with a small, nonintoxicating amount of alcohol, produce behavioral patterns resembling alcohol intoxication. For this reason, the toxicologist must be given an adequate amount of blood so he

Case Files

Accidental Overdose: The Tragedy of Anna Nicole Smith

Rumors exploded in the media when former model, Playboy playmate, reality television star, and favorite tabloid subject Anna Nicole Smith was found unconscious in her hotel room at the Seminole Hard Rock Hotel and Casino in Hollywood, Florida. She was taken to Memorial Legal Hospital, where she was declared dead at age 39. Analysis of Smith's blood postmortem revealed an array of prescribed medications. Most pronounced was a toxic level of the sedative chloral hydrate. A part of the contents of the toxicology report from Smith's autopsy are shown here.

Although many of the drugs present were detected at levels consistent with typical doses of the prescribed medications, it was their presence in combination with chloral hydrate that exacerbated the toxic level of chloral hydrate. The lethal combination of these prescription drugs caused failure of both her circulatory and respiratory systems and resulted in her death. The investigators determined that the overdose of chloral hydrate and other drugs was accidental and not a suicide. This was due to the nonexcessive levels of most of the prescription medications and the discovery of a significant amount of chloral hydrate still remaining in its original container; had she intended to kill herself, she would have likely downed it all. Anna Nicole Smith was a victim of accidental overmedication.

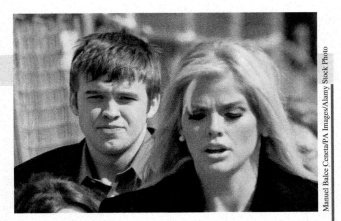

Anna Nicole Smith.

Final Pathological Diagnoses

I. Acute Combined Drug Intoxication
  A. Toxic/legal drug:
     Chloral Hydrate (Noctec)
     1. Trichloroethanol (TCE) 75 mg/L (active metabolite)
     2. Trichloroacetic acid (TCA) 85 mg/L (inactive metabolite)
  B. Therapeutic drugs:

Drug	Level
1. Diphenhydramine (Benadryl)	0.11 mg/L
2. Clonazepam (Klonopin)	0.04 mg/L
3. Diazepam (Valium)	0.21 mg/L
4. Nordiazepam (metabolite)	0.38 mg/L
5. Temazepam (metabolite)	0.09 mg/L
6. Oxazepam	0.09 mg/L
7. Lorazepam	0.022 mg/L

  C. Other noncontributory drugs present (atropine, topiramate, ciprofloxacin, acetaminophen)

or she will have the option of performing a comprehensive analysis for drugs in cases of low alcohol concentrations.

Techniques Used in Toxicology

For the toxicologist, the upsurge in drug use has meant that the overwhelming majority of fatal and nonfatal toxic agents are drugs. Not surprisingly, a relatively small number of drugs—namely, those discussed in Chapter 12—comprise nearly all the toxic agents encountered. Of these, alcohol, marijuana, and cocaine normally account for 90 percent or more of the drugs encountered in a typical toxicology laboratory.

ACIDS AND BASES   Like the drug analyst, the toxicologist must devise an analytical scheme to detect, isolate, and identify a toxic substance. The first chore is to selectively remove and isolate drugs and other toxic agents from the biological materials submitted as evidence. Because drugs constitute a large portion of the toxic materials found, a good deal of effort must be devoted to their extraction and detection. The procedures are numerous, and a useful description of them would be too detailed for this text. We can best understand the underlying principle of drug extraction by observing that many drugs fall into the categories of **acids** and **bases**.

Although several definitions exist for these two classes, a simple one states that an acid is a compound that sheds a hydrogen ion (or a hydrogen atom minus its electron) with reasonable ease. Conversely, a base is a compound that can pick up a hydrogen ion shed by an acid. The idea of acidity and basicity can be expressed in terms of a simple numerical value that relates to the

acid
A compound capable of donating a hydrogen ion (H⁺) to another compound.

base
A compound capable of accepting a hydrogen ion (H⁺).

concentration of the hydrogen ion (H^+) in a liquid medium such as water. Chemists use the **pH scale** to do this. This scale runs from 0 to 14:

$$pH = \frac{0 \quad 1 \quad 2 \quad 3 \quad 4 \quad 5 \quad 6 \quad 7 \quad 8 \quad 9 \quad 10 \quad 11 \quad 12 \quad 13 \quad 14}{\leftarrow \text{Increasing acidity—Neutral—Increasing basicity} \rightarrow}$$

pH scale

A scale used to express the basicity or acidity of a substance; a pH of 7 is neutral, whereas lower values are acidic and higher values are basic.

Normally, water is neither acidic nor basic—in other words, it is neutral, with a pH of 7. However, when an acidic substance—for example, sulfuric acid or hydrochloric acid—is added to the water, it adds excess hydrogen ions, and the pH value becomes less than 7. The lower the number, the more acidic the water. Similarly, when a basic substance—for example, sodium hydroxide or ammonium hydroxide—is added to water, it removes hydrogen ions, thus making water basic. The more basic the water, the higher its pH value.

By controlling the pH of a water solution into which blood, urine, or tissues are dissolved, the toxicologist can conveniently control the type of drug that is recovered. For example, acidic drugs are easily extracted from an acidified water solution (pH less than 7) with organic solvents such as n-butyl chloride or ethyl acetate. Similarly, basic drugs are readily removed from a basic water solution (pH greater than 7) with organic solvents. This simple approach gives the toxicologist a general technique for extracting and categorizing drugs. Some of the more commonly encountered drugs may be classified as follows:

Acid Drugs	Basic Drugs
Barbiturates	Phencyclidine
Acetylsalicylic acid (aspirin)	Methadone
	Amphetamines
	Cocaine

SCREENING AND CONFIRMATION   Once the specimen has been extracted and divided into acidic and basic fractions, the toxicologist can identify the drugs present. The strategy for identifying used drugs entails a two-step approach: *screening* and *confirmation* (see Figure 13–7). A screening test is normally employed to give the analyst quick insight into the likelihood that a specimen contains a drug substance. Many labs will screen using GC/MS or LC-TOF. This test allows a toxicologist to examine a large number of specimens within a short period of time for a wide range of drugs. Any positive results from a screening test are tentative at best and must be verified with a confirmation test. Quantification and confirmation can be done on Gas Chromatography—Nitrogen Phosphorous Detector (GC/NPD) or GC/MS.

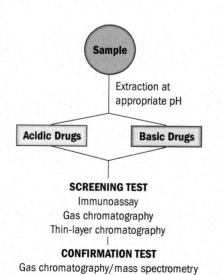

FIGURE 13–7

Biological fluids and tissues are extracted for acidic and basic drugs by controlling the pH of a water solution in which they are dissolved. Once this is accomplished, the toxicologist analyzes for drugs by using screening and confirmation test procedures.

The most widely used screening tests are gas chromatography (GC), and immunoassay. The techniques of GC have already been described on pages 300–302. An immunoassay has proven to be a useful screening tool in toxicology laboratories. Its principles are very different from any of the analytical techniques we have discussed so far. Basically, immunoassay is based on specific drug antibody reactions. We will learn about this concept in Chapter 15. The primary advantage of immunoassay is its ability to detect small concentrations of drugs in body fluids and organs. In fact, this technique provides the best approach for detecting the low drug levels normally associated with the consumption of marijuana.

The necessity of eliminating the possibility that a positive screening test may be due to a substance having a close chemical structure to a drug requires the toxicologist to follow up a positive screening test with a confirmation test. Because of the potential impact of the results of a drug finding on an individual, only the most conclusive confirmation procedures should be used. **Gas chromatography/mass spectrometry is generally accepted as the confirmation test of choice.** The combination of gas chromatography and mass spectrometry provides the toxicologist with a one-step confirmation test of unequaled sensitivity and specificity (see pages 310–313). As shown in Figure 13–8, the sample is separated into its components by the gas chromatograph. When the separated sample component leaves the column of the gas chromatograph, it enters the mass spectrometer, where it is bombarded with high-energy electrons. This bombardment causes the sample to break up into fragments, producing a fragmentation pattern or mass spectrum for each sample. For most compounds, the mass spectrum represents a unique "fingerprint" pattern that can be used for identification.

There is tremendous interest in drug-testing programs conducted not only in criminal matters but for industry and government as well. Urine testing for drugs is becoming common for job applicants and employees in the workplace. Likewise, the U.S. military has an extensive drug urine-testing program for its members. Many urine-testing programs rely on private laboratories to perform the analyses. In any case, when the test results form the basis for taking action against an individual, both a screening and confirmation test must be incorporated into the testing protocol to ensure the integrity of the laboratory's conclusions.

DETECTING DRUGS IN HAIR   When a forensic toxicological examination on a living person is required, practicality limits available specimens to blood and urine. Most drugs remain in the bloodstream for about 24 hours; in urine, they normally are present up to 72 hours. However, it may be necessary to go further back in time to ascertain whether a subject has been abusing a drug. If so, the only viable alternative to blood and urine is head hair.

Hair is nourished by blood flowing through capillaries located close to the hair root. Drugs present in blood diffuse through the capillary walls into the base of the hair and become permanently entrapped in the hair's hardening protein structure. As the hair continues to grow, the drug's location on the hair shaft becomes a historical marker for

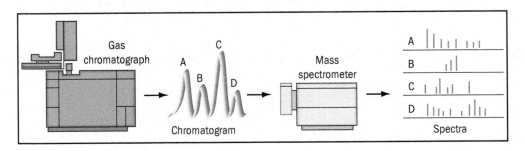

FIGURE 13–8

The combination of the gas chromatograph and the mass spectrometer enables forensic toxicologists to separate the components of a drug mixture and provides specific identification of a drug substance.

delineating drug intake. Given that the average human head hair grows at the rate of 1 centimeter per month, analyzing segments of hair for drug content may define the timeline for drug use, dating it back over a period of weeks, months, or even years, depending on the hair's length.

However, caution is required in interpreting the timeline. The chronology of drug intake may be distorted by drugs penetrating the hair's surface as a result of environmental exposure, or drugs may enter the hair's surface through sweat. Nevertheless, drug hair analysis is the only viable approach for measuring long-term use of a drug.

Detecting Nondrug Poisons

Although forensic toxicologists devote most of their efforts to detecting drugs, they also test for a wide variety of other toxic substances. Some of these are rare elements, not widely or commercially available. Others are so common that virtually everyone is exposed to nontoxic amounts of them every day.

HEAVY METALS   The forensic toxicologist only occasionally encounters a group of poisons known as *heavy metals*. These include arsenic, bismuth, antimony, mercury, and thallium. To screen for many of these metals, the investigator may dissolve the suspect's body fluid or tissue in a hydrochloric acid solution and insert a copper strip into the solution (the Reinsch test). The appearance of a silvery or dark coating on the copper indicates the presence of a heavy metal. Such a finding must be confirmed by the use of analytical techniques suitable for inorganic analysis—namely, inductively coupled plasma or inductively coupled plasma mass spectrometry (ICP-MS).

CARBON MONOXIDE   Unlike heavy metals, *carbon monoxide* still represents one of the most common poisons encountered in a forensic laboratory. When carbon monoxide enters the human body, it combines with hemoglobin found in red blood cells to form carboxyhemoglobin. An average red blood cell contains about 280 million molecules of hemoglobin. Oxygen normally combines with hemoglobin, which transports the oxygen throughout the body. However, if a high percentage of the hemoglobin combines with carbon monoxide, not enough is left to carry sufficient oxygen to the tissues, and death by asphyxiation quickly follows.

There are two basic methods for measuring the concentration of carbon monoxide in the blood. Spectrophotometric methods examine the visible spectrum of blood to determine the amount of carboxyhemoglobin relative to oxyhemoglobin or total hemoglobin; also, a volume of blood can be treated with a reagent to liberate the carbon monoxide, which is then measured by gas chromatography or microdiffusion.

The amount of carbon monoxide in blood is generally expressed as *percent saturation*. This represents the extent to which the available hemoglobin has been converted to carboxyhemoglobin. The transition from normal or occupational levels of carbon monoxide to toxic levels is not sharply defined. It depends, among other things, on the age, health, and general fitness of each individual. In a healthy middle-aged individual, a carbon monoxide blood saturation greater than 50 to 60 percent is considered fatal. However, in combination with alcohol or other depressants, fatal levels may be significantly lower. For instance, a carbon monoxide saturation of 35 to 40 percent may prove fatal in the presence of a blood-alcohol concentration of 0.20 percent w/v. Interestingly, chain smokers may have a constant carbon monoxide level of 8 to 10 percent from the carbon monoxide in cigarette smoke.

Inhaling automobile fumes is a relatively common way to commit suicide. A garden or vacuum cleaner hose is often used to connect the tailpipe with the vehicle's interior, or the engine is allowed to run in a closed garage. A level of carbon monoxide sufficient to cause death accumulates in 5 to 10 minutes in a closed single-car garage. Newer versions of vehicles that have a catalytic converter reduce the amount of carbon monoxide produced; so many newer automobiles may not produce enough carbon monoxide for a suicide.

The level of carbon monoxide in the blood of a victim found dead at the scene of a fire is significant in ascertaining whether foul play has occurred. High levels of carbon monoxide in the blood prove that the victim breathed the combustion products of the fire and was alive when the fire began. Many attempts at covering up a murder by setting fire to a victim's house or car have been uncovered in this manner.

Significance of Toxicological Findings

Once a drug is found and identified, the toxicologist assesses its influence on the behavior of the individual. Interpreting the results of a toxicology find is one of the toxicologist's more difficult chores. Recall that many of the world's countries have designated a specific blood-alcohol level at which an individual is deemed under the influence of alcohol. These levels were established as a result of numerous studies conducted over several years to measure the effects of alcohol levels on driving performance. However, no such legal guidelines are available to the toxicologist who must judge how a drug other than alcohol affects an individual's performance or physical state.

For many drugs, blood concentration levels are readily determined and can be used to *estimate* the pharmacological effects of the drug on the individual. Often, when dealing with a living person, the toxicologist has the added benefit of knowing what a police officer may have observed about an individual's behavior and motor skills, as well as the outcome of a drug influence evaluation conducted by a police officer trained to be a drug recognition expert (discussed shortly). For a deceased person, drug levels in various body organs and tissues provide additional information about the individual's state at the time of death. However, before conclusions can be drawn about a drug-induced death, other factors must also be considered, including the age, physical condition, and tolerance of the drug user.

> > > > > > > > > > >

Case Files

Joann Curley: Caught by a Hair

A vibrant young woman named Joann Curley rushed to the Wilkes-Barre (Pennsylvania) General Hospital—her husband, Bobby, was having an attack and required immediate medical attention. Bobby was experiencing a burning sensation in his feet, numbness in his hands, a flushed face, and intense sweating. He was diagnosed with Guillain-Barré syndrome, an acute inflammation of the nervous system that accounted for all of Bobby's symptoms. After being discharged, Bobby experienced another bout of debilitating pain and numbness. He was admitted to another hospital, the larger and more capable Hershey Medical Center in Hershey, Pennsylvania. There doctors observed extreme alopecia, or hair loss.

Test results of Bobby's urine showed high levels of the heavy metal thallium in his body. Thallium, a rare and highly toxic metal that was used decades ago in substances such as rat poison and to treat ringworm and gout, was found in sufficient quantities to cause Bobby's sickness. The use of thallium was banned in the United States in 1984. Now, at least, Bobby could be treated. However, before Bobby's doctors could treat him for thallium poisoning, he experienced cardiac arrest and slipped into a coma. Joann Curley made the difficult decision to remove her husband of 13 months from life support equipment. He died shortly thereafter.

Bobby Curley was an electrician and, for five months before his death, he worked in the chemistry department at nearby Wilkes University. Authorities suspected that Bobby had been accidentally exposed to thallium there among old chemicals and laboratory equipment. The laboratory was searched and several old bottles of powdered thallium salts were discovered in a storage closet. After testing of the air and surfaces, these were eliminated as possible sources for exposure. This finding was supported by the discovery that none of Bobby's co-workers had any thallium in their systems. The next most logical route of exposure was in the home; thus, the Curley kitchen was sampled. Of the hundreds of items tested, three thermoses were found to contain traces of thallium.

Investigators also learned that Bobby had changed his life insurance to list his wife, Joann, as the beneficiary of his $300,000 policy. Based on this information, police consulted a forensic toxicologist in an effort to glean as much from the physical evidence in Bobby Curley's body as possible. The toxicologist conducted segmental analysis of Bobby's hair, an analytical method based on the predictable rate of hair growth on the human scalp: an average of 1 centimeter per month. Bobby had approximately 5 inches (12.5 centimeters) of hair, which represents almost 12 months of hair growth. Each section tested represented a specific period of time in Bobby's final year of life.

The hair analysis proved that Bobby Curley was poisoned with thallium long before he began working at Wilkes University. The first few doses were small, which probably barely made him sick at the time. Gradually, over a year or more, Bobby was receiving more doses of thallium until he finally succumbed to a massive dose three or four days before his death. After careful scrutiny of the timeline, investigators concluded that only Joann Curley had access to Bobby during each of these intervals. She also had motive, in the amount of $300,000.

Presented with the timeline and the solid toxicological evidence against her, Joann Curley pleaded guilty to murder. As part of her plea agreement, she provided a 40-page written confession of how she haphazardly dosed Bobby with some rat poison she found in her basement. She admitted that she murdered him for the money she would receive from Bobby's life insurance policy.

With prolonged use of a drug, an individual may become less responsive to a drug's effects and tolerate blood-drug concentrations that would kill a casual drug user. Therefore, knowledge of an individual's history of drug use is important in evaluating drug concentrations. Another consideration is additive or synergistic effects of the interaction of two or more drugs, which may produce a highly intoxicated or comatose state even though none of the drugs alone is present at high or toxic levels. The combination of alcohol with tranquilizers or narcotics is a common example of a potentially lethal drug combination.

The presence of a drug present in urine is a poor indicator of how extensively an individual's behavior or state is influenced by the drug. Urine is formed outside the body's circulatory system, and consequently drug levels can build up in it over a long period. Some drugs are found in the urine one to three days after they have been taken and long after their effects on the user have disappeared. Nevertheless, the value of this information should not be discounted. Urine drug levels, like blood levels, are best used by law enforcement authorities and the courts to corroborate other investigative and medical findings regarding an individual's condition. Hence, for an individual who is arrested for suspicion of being under the influence of a drug, a toxicologist's determinations supplement the observations of the arresting officer, including the results of a drug influence evaluation (discussed next).

For a deceased person, the responsibility for establishing a cause of death rests with the medical examiner or coroner. However, before a conclusive determination is made, the examining physician depends on the forensic toxicologist to demonstrate the presence or absence of a drug or poison in the tissues or body fluids of the deceased. Only through the combined efforts of the toxicologist and the medical examiner (or coroner) can society be assured that death investigations achieve high professional and legal standards.

The Drug Recognition Expert

Whereas recognizing alcohol-impaired performance is an expertise generally accorded to police officers by the courts, recognizing drug-induced intoxication is much more difficult and generally not part of police training. During the 1970s, the Los Angeles Police Department developed and tested a series of clinical and psychophysical examinations that a trained police officer could use to identify and differentiate between types of drug impairment. This program has evolved into a national program to train police as *drug recognition experts*. Normally, a three- to five-month training program is required to certify an officer as a drug recognition expert (DRE).

The DRE program incorporates standardized methods for examining suspects to determine whether they have taken one or more drugs. The process is systematic and standard; to ensure that each subject has been tested in a routine fashion, each DRE must complete a standard Drug Influence Evaluation form (see Figure 13–9). The entire drug evaluation takes approximately 30 to 40 minutes. The components of the 12-step process are summarized in Table 13–1.

The DRE evaluation process can suggest the presence of the following seven broad categories of drugs:

1. Central nervous system depressants
2. Central nervous system stimulants
3. Hallucinogens
4. Dissociative anesthetics (includes phencyclidine and its analogs)
5. Inhalants
6. Narcotic analgesics
7. Cannabis

The DRE program is not designed to be a substitute for toxicological testing. The toxicologist can often determine that a suspect has a particular drug in their body. But the toxicologist often cannot infer with reasonable certainty that the suspect was impaired at a specific time. On the other hand, the DRE can supply credible evidence that the suspect was impaired at a specific time and that the nature of the impairment was consistent with a particular family of drugs. But the DRE program usually cannot determine which specific drug was ingested. Proving drug intoxication requires a coordinated effort and the production of competent data from both the DRE and the forensic toxicologist.

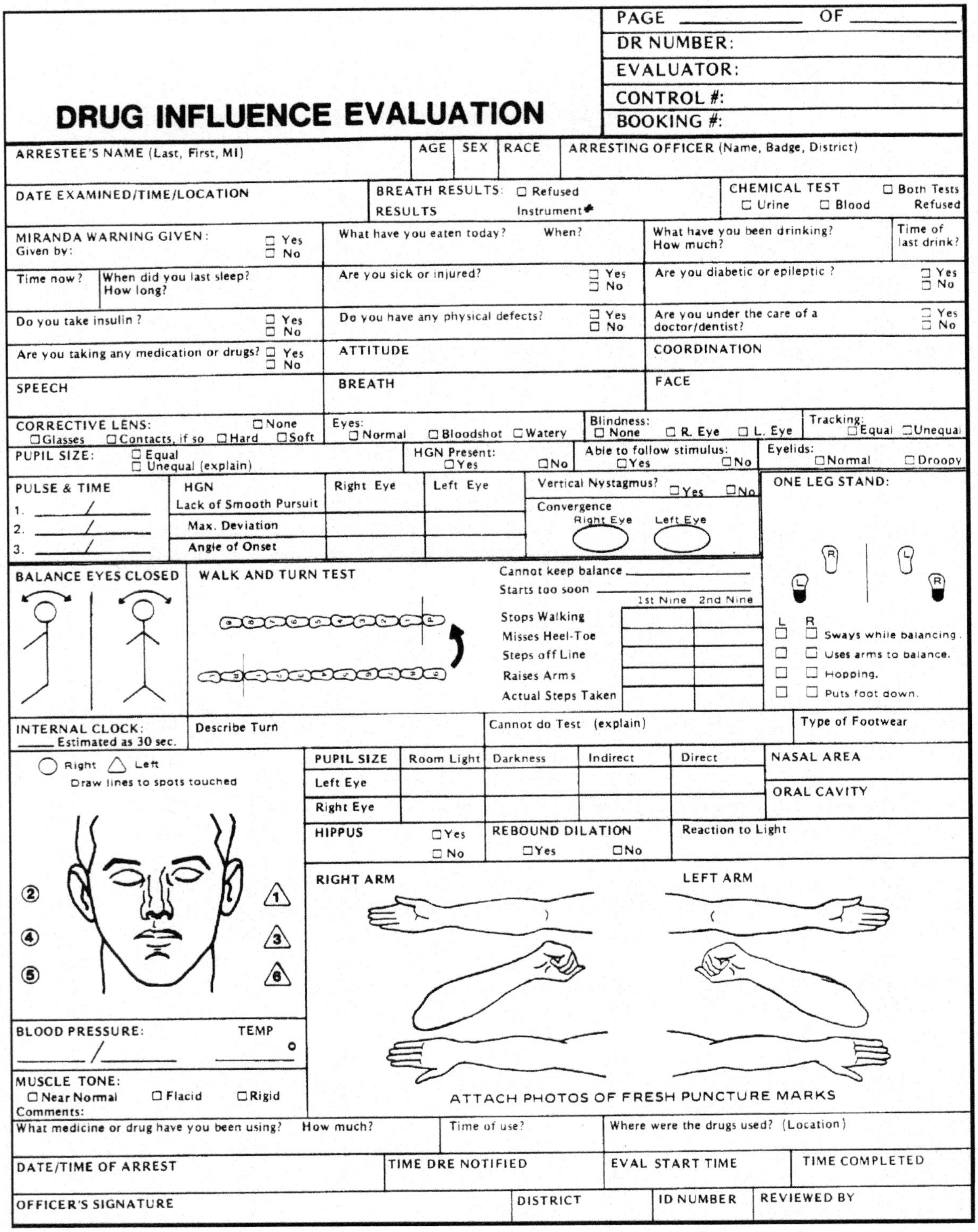

DRUG INFLUENCE EVALUATION

PAGE _____ OF _____
DR NUMBER:
EVALUATOR:
CONTROL #:
BOOKING #:

ARRESTEE'S NAME (Last, First, MI) | AGE | SEX | RACE | ARRESTING OFFICER (Name, Badge, District)

DATE EXAMINED/TIME/LOCATION

BREATH RESULTS: ☐ Refused
RESULTS   Instrument ✦

CHEMICAL TEST ☐ Both Tests
☐ Urine   ☐ Blood   Refused

MIRANDA WARNING GIVEN: ☐ Yes ☐ No
Given by:

What have you eaten today?   When?

What have you been drinking? How much?

Time of last drink?

Time now? When did you last sleep? How long?

Are you sick or injured? ☐ Yes ☐ No

Are you diabetic or epileptic ? ☐ Yes ☐ No

Do you take insulin ? ☐ Yes ☐ No

Do you have any physical defects? ☐ Yes ☐ No

Are you under the care of a doctor/dentist? ☐ Yes ☐ No

Are you taking any medication or drugs? ☐ Yes ☐ No

ATTITUDE

COORDINATION

SPEECH

BREATH

FACE

CORRECTIVE LENS: ☐ None
☐ Glasses ☐ Contacts, if so ☐ Hard ☐ Soft

Eyes: ☐ Normal ☐ Bloodshot ☐ Watery

Blindness: ☐ None ☐ R. Eye ☐ L. Eye

Tracking: ☐ Equal ☐ Unequal

PUPIL SIZE: ☐ Equal ☐ Unequal (explain)

HGN Present: ☐ Yes ☐ No

Able to follow stimulus: ☐ Yes ☐ No

Eyelids: ☐ Normal ☐ Droopy

PULSE & TIME	HGN	Right Eye	Left Eye	Vertical Nystagmus? ☐ Yes ☐ No	ONE LEG STAND:
1. ___/___	Lack of Smooth Pursuit			Convergence	
2. ___/___	Max. Deviation			Right Eye Left Eye	
3. ___/___	Angle of Onset				

BALANCE EYES CLOSED

WALK AND TURN TEST

Cannot keep balance _____
Starts too soon _____

	1st Nine	2nd Nine
Stops Walking		
Misses Heel-Toe		
Steps off Line		
Raises Arms		
Actual Steps Taken		

L R
☐ ☐ Sways while balancing.
☐ ☐ Uses arms to balance.
☐ ☐ Hopping.
☐ ☐ Puts foot down.

INTERNAL CLOCK: _____ Estimated as 30 sec.

Describe Turn

Cannot do Test (explain)

Type of Footwear

○ Right △ Left
Draw lines to spots touched

PUPIL SIZE	Room Light	Darkness	Indirect	Direct	NASAL AREA
Left Eye					
Right Eye					ORAL CAVITY

HIPPUS ☐ Yes ☐ No

REBOUND DILATION ☐ Yes ☐ No

Reaction to Light

RIGHT ARM

LEFT ARM

BLOOD PRESSURE: _____/_____   TEMP _____°

MUSCLE TONE: ☐ Near Normal ☐ Flacid ☐ Rigid
Comments:

ATTACH PHOTOS OF FRESH PUNCTURE MARKS

What medicine or drug have you been using? How much? Time of use? Where were the drugs used? (Location)

DATE/TIME OF ARREST | TIME DRE NOTIFIED | EVAL START TIME | TIME COMPLETED

OFFICER'S SIGNATURE | DISTRICT | ID NUMBER | REVIEWED BY

National Highway Traffic Safety Administration

FIGURE 13–9

Drug Influence Evaluation form.

TABLE 13–1

Components of the Drug Recognition Process

1. *The Breath-Alcohol Test.* By obtaining an accurate and immediate measurement of the suspect's blood-alcohol concentration, the drug recognition expert (DRE) can determine whether alcohol may be contributing to the suspect's observable impairment and whether the concentration of alcohol is sufficient to be the sole cause of that impairment.

2. *Interview with the Arresting Officer.* Spending a few minutes with the arresting officer often enables the DRE to determine the most promising areas of investigation.

3. *The Preliminary Examination.* This structured series of questions, specific observations, and simple tests provide the first opportunity to examine the suspect closely. It is designed to determine whether the suspect is suffering from an injury or from another condition unrelated to drug consumption. It also affords an opportunity to begin assessing the suspect's appearance and behavior for signs of possible drug influence.

4. *The Eye Examination.* Certain categories of drugs induce nystagmus, an involuntary, spasmodic motion of the eyeball. Nystagmus is an indicator of drug-induced impairment. The inability of the eyes to converge toward the bridge of the nose also indicates the possible presence of certain types of drugs.

5. *Divided-Attention Psychophysical Tests.* These tests check balance and physical orientation and include the walk and turn, the one-leg stand, the Romberg balance, and the finger-to-nose.

6. *Vital Signs Examinations.* Precise measurements of blood pressure, pulse rate, and body temperature are taken. Certain drugs elevate these signs; others depress them.

7. *Dark Room Examinations.* The size of the suspect's pupils in room light, near-total darkness, indirect light, and direct light is checked. Some drugs cause the pupils to either dilate or constrict.

8. *Examination for Muscle Rigidity.* Certain categories of drugs cause the muscles to become hypertense and quite rigid. Others may cause the muscles to relax and become flaccid.

9. *Examination for Injection Sites.* Users of certain categories of drugs routinely or occasionally inject their drugs. Evidence of needle use may be found on veins along the neck, arms, and hands.

10. *Suspect's Statements and Other Observations.* The next step is to attempt to interview the suspect concerning the drug or drugs the suspect has ingested. Of course, the interview must be conducted in full compliance with the suspect's constitutional rights.

11. *Opinions of the Evaluator.* Using the information obtained in the previous 10 steps, the DRE can make an informed decision about whether the suspect is impaired by drugs and, if so, what category or combination of categories is the probable cause of the impairment.

12. *The Toxicological Examination.* The DRE should obtain a blood or urine sample from the suspect for laboratory analysis in order to secure scientific, admissible evidence to substantiate their conclusions.

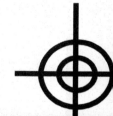

Chapter Summary > > > > > > > > > >

Toxicologists detect and identify the presence of drugs and poisons in body fluids, tissues, and organs. A major branch of forensic toxicology deals with the measurement of alcohol in the body for matters that pertain to violations of criminal law. Alcohol appears in the blood within minutes after it has been taken by mouth and slowly increases in concentration while it is being absorbed from the stomach and the small intestine into the bloodstream. When all the alcohol has been absorbed, a maximum alcohol level is reached in the blood and the postabsorption period begins. Then the alcohol concentration slowly decreases until a zero level is again reached. Alcohol is eliminated from the body through oxidation and excretion. Oxidation takes place almost entirely in the liver, whereas alcohol is excreted unchanged in the breath, urine, and perspiration. The extent to which an individual is under the influence of alcohol is usually determined by measuring the quantity of alcohol in the blood or the breath. Breath testers that operate on the principle of infrared light absorption are becoming increasingly popular within the law enforcement community.

Many types of breath testers analyze a set volume of breath. The sampled breath is exposed to infrared light. The degree of interaction of the light with alcohol in the breath sample allows the instrument to measure a blood-alcohol concentration in breath. These breath-testing devices operate on the principle that the ratio between the concentration of alcohol in deep-lung or alveolar breath and its concentration in blood is fixed. Most breath-test devices have set the ratio of alcohol in the blood to alcohol in alveolar air at 2,100 to 1.

Law enforcement officers typically use field sobriety tests to estimate a motorist's degree of physical impairment by alcohol and whether an evidential test for alcohol is justified. The horizontal-gaze nystagmus test, walk and turn, and the one-leg stand are all reliable and effective psychophysical tests.

Gas chromatography is the most widely used approach for determining alcohol levels in blood. Blood must always be drawn under medically accepted conditions by a qualified individual. A nonalcoholic disinfectant must be applied before the suspect's skin is penetrated with a sterile needle or lancet. Once blood is removed from an individual, it is best preserved sealed in an airtight container after adding an anticoagulant and a preservative.

The Fifth Amendment to the U.S. Constitution guarantees all citizens protection against *self-incrimination*—that is, against being forced to make an admission that would prove one's own guilt in a legal matter. To prevent a person's refusal to take a test for alcohol intoxication on the constitutional grounds of self-incrimination, "implied consent"

laws were implemented in every state by 1973. In accordance with this statute, operating a motor vehicle on a public highway automatically carries with it the stipulation that the driver must either submit to a test for alcohol intoxication if requested or lose their license for some designated period— usually six months to one year.

The forensic toxicologist must devise an analytical scheme to detect, isolate, and identify toxic drug substances. Once the drug has been extracted from appropriate biological fluids, tissues, and organs, the forensic toxicologist can identify the drug substance. The strategy for identifying drugs entails a two-step approach: screening and confirmation. A screening test gives the analyst quick insight into the likelihood that a specimen contains a drug substance. Positive results from a screening test are tentative at best and must be verified with a confirmation test. The most widely used screening tests are thin-layer chromatography, gas chromatography, and immunoassay. Gas chromatography/mass spectrometry is generally accepted as the confirmation test of choice. Once the drug is extracted and identified, the toxicologist may be required to judge the drug's effect on an individual's natural performance or physical state. The Drug Recognition Expert program incorporates standardized methods for examining automobile drivers suspected of being under the influence of drugs. But the DRE program usually cannot determine which specific drug was ingested. Hence, reliable data from both the DRE and the forensic toxicologist are required to prove drug intoxication.

Review Questions

1. The most heavily used drug in the Western world is _____.

2. True or False: Toxicologists are employed only by crime laboratories. _____

3. The amount of alcohol in the blood (is, is not) directly proportional to the concentration of alcohol in the brain.

4. True or False: Blood levels have become the accepted standard for relating alcohol intake to its effect on the body. _____

5. Alcohol consumed on an empty stomach is absorbed (faster, slower) than an equivalent amount of alcohol taken when there is food in the stomach.

6. Under normal drinking conditions, alcohol concentration in the blood peaks in _____ to _____ minutes.

7. In the postabsorption period, alcohol is distributed uniformly among the _____ portions of the body.

8. Alcohol is eliminated from the body by _____ and _____.

9. Ninety-five to 98 percent of the alcohol consumed is _____ to carbon dioxide and water.

10. Oxidation of alcohol takes place almost entirely in the _____.

11. The amount of alcohol exhaled in the _____ is directly proportional to the concentration of alcohol in the blood.

12. Alcohol is eliminated from the blood at an average rate of _____ percent w/v.

13. Alcohol is absorbed into the blood from the _____ and _____.

14. Most modern breath testers use _____ radiation to detect and measure alcohol in the breath.

15. To avoid the possibility of "mouth alcohol," the operator of a breath tester must not allow the subject to take any foreign materials into the mouth for _____ minutes before the test.

16. Alcohol can be separated from other volatiles in blood and quantitated by the technique of _____.

17. Roadside breath testers that use a(n) _____ detector are becoming increasingly popular with the law enforcement community.

18. True or False: Portable handheld roadside breath testers for alcohol provide evidential test results. _____

19. Usually, when a person's blood-alcohol concentration is in the range of 0.10 percent, horizontal-gaze nystagmus begins before the eyeball has moved _____ degrees to the side.

20. When drawing blood for alcohol testing, the suspect's skin must first be wiped with a(n) _____ disinfectant.

21. Failure to add a preservative, such as sodium fluoride, to blood removed from a living person may lead to a(n) (decline, increase) in alcohol concentration.

22. Most states have established _____ percent w/v as the impairment limit for blood-alcohol concentration.

23. In the case of _____, the Supreme Court ruled that taking nontestimonial evidence, such as a blood sample, did not violate a suspect's Fifth Amendment rights.

24. Heroin is changed upon entering the body into _____.

25. The body fluids _____ and _____ are both desirable for the toxicological examination of a living person suspected of being under the influence of a drug.

26. A large number of drugs can be classified chemically as _____ and _____.

27. Water with a pH value (less, greater) than 7 is basic.

28. Barbiturates are classified as _____ drugs.

29. Drugs are extracted from body fluids and tissues by carefully controlling the _____ of the medium in which the sample has been dissolved.

30. The technique of _____ is based on specific drug antibody reactions.

31. Both _____ and _____ tests must be incorporated into the drug-testing protocol of a toxicology laboratory to ensure the correctness of the laboratory's conclusions.

32. The gas _____ combines with hemoglobin in the blood to form carboxyhemoglobin, thus interfering with the transportation of oxygen in the blood.

33. The amount of carbon monoxide in blood is usually expressed as _____.

34. True or False: Blood levels of drugs can alone be used to draw definitive conclusions about the effects of a drug on an individual. _____

35. Interaction of alcohol and barbiturates in the body can produce a(n) _____ effect.

36. The level of a drug present in the urine is by itself a (good, poor) indicator of how extensively an individual is affected by a drug.

37. Urine and blood drug levels are best used by law enforcement authorities and the courts to _____ other investigative and medical findings pertaining to an individual's condition.

38. The _____ program incorporates standardized methods for examining suspects to determine whether they have taken one or more drugs.

Review Questions for Inside the Science

1. A(n) _____ carries blood away from the heart; a(n) _____ carries blood back to the heart.

2. The _____ artery carries deoxygenated blood from the heart to the lungs.

3. Alcohol passes from the blood capillaries into the _____ sacs in the lungs.

4. One milliliter of blood contains the same amount of alcohol as approximately _____ milliliters of alveolar breath.

5. When alcohol is being absorbed into the blood, the alcohol concentration in venous blood is (higher, lower) than that in arterial blood.

Application and Critical Thinking

1. Answer the following questions about driving risk associated with drinking and blood-alcohol concentration:

   a. Randy is just barely legally intoxicated. How much more likely is he to have an accident than someone who is sober?

   b. Marissa, who has been drinking, is 15 times as likely to have an accident as her sober friend, Christine. What is Marissa's approximate blood-alcohol concentration?

   c. After several drinks, Charles is 10 times as likely to have an accident as a sober person. Is he more or less intoxicated than James, whose blood-alcohol level is 0.10?

   d. Under the original blood-alcohol standards recommended by NHTSA, a person considered just barely legally intoxicated was how much more likely to have an accident than a sober individual?

2. Following is a description of four individuals who have been drinking. Rank them from highest to lowest blood-alcohol concentration:

   a. John, who weighs 200 pounds and has consumed eight 8-ounce drinks on a full stomach

   b. Frank, who weighs 170 pounds and has consumed four 8-ounce drinks on an empty stomach

   c. Gary, who weighs 240 pounds and has consumed six 8-ounce drinks on an empty stomach

   d. Stephen, who weighs 180 pounds and has consumed six 8-ounce drinks on a full stomach

3. Following is a description of four individuals who have been drinking. In which (if any) of the following countries would each be considered legally drunk: the United States, Australia, Sweden?

   a. Bill, who weighs 150 pounds and has consumed three 8-ounce drinks on an empty stomach

   b. Sally, who weighs 110 pounds and has consumed three 8-ounce drinks on a full stomach

   c. Rich, who weighs 200 pounds and has consumed six 8-ounce drinks on an empty stomach

   d. Carrie, who weighs 140 pounds and has consumed four 8-ounce drinks on a full stomach

4. You are a forensic scientist who has been asked to test two blood samples. You know that one sample is suspected of containing barbiturates and the other contains no drugs; however, you cannot tell the two samples apart. Describe how you would use the concept of pH to determine which sample contains barbiturates. Explain your reasoning.

5. You are investigating an arson scene and you find a corpse in the rubble, but you suspect that the victim did not die as a result of the fire. Instead, you suspect that the victim was murdered earlier, and that the blaze was started to cover up the murder. How would you go about determining whether the victim died before the fire?

Further References

Benjamin, David M., "Forensic Pharmacology," in R. Saferstein, ed., *Forensic Science Handbook*, vol. 3, 2nd ed. Upper Saddle River, NJ: Prentice Hall, 2010.

Caplan, Y. H., and B. A. Goldberger, eds., *Garriott's Medicolegal Aspects of Alcohol,* 6th ed. Tucson, AZ: Lawyers and Judges, 2015.

Caplan, Y. H., and J. R. Zettl, "The Determination of Alcohol in Blood and Breath," in R. Saferstein, ed., *Forensic Science Handbook*, vol. 1, 2nd ed. Upper Saddle River, NJ: Prentice Hall, 2002.

Couper, F. J., and B. K. Logan, *Drugs and Human Performance* Washington, D.C.: National Highway Traffic Safety Administration, 2004, http://www.nhtsa.dot.gov/people/injury/research/job185drugs/technical-page.htm

Levine, B., ed., *Principles of Forensic Toxicology*, 4th ed. Washington, D.C.: AACC Press, 2013.

Ropero-Miller, J. D., and B. A. Goldberger, eds., *Handbook of Workplace Drug Testing*, 2013 ed. Washington, D.C.: AACC Press, 2013.

Metals, Paint, and Soil

Learning Objectives

After studying this chapter, you should be able to:

14.1 Describe the utility of trace elements for forensic comparison of various types of physical evidence

14.2 Describe the Emission Spectrum of Elements as it relates to the analysis of trace evidence

14.3 Explain how paint is examined, collected, and preserved in the laboratory

14.4 Discuss the processes in the forensic analysis of soil

14.5 Describe the proper collection of soil evidence

The Green River Killer

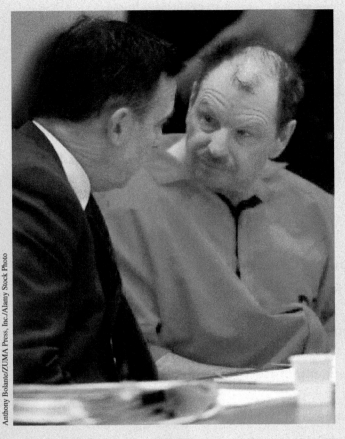

This case takes its name from the Green River, which flows through Washington state and empties into Puget Sound in Seattle. In 1982, within six months the bodies of five females were discovered in or near the river. Most of the victims were known prostitutes who were strangled and apparently raped. As police focused their attention on an area known as Sea-Tac Strip, a haven for prostitutes, girls mysteriously disappeared with increasing frequency. By the end of 1986, the body count in the Seattle region rose to 40, all of whom were believed to have been murdered by the Green River Killer. As the investigation pressed on into 1987, the police renewed their interest in one suspect, Gary Ridgway, a local truck painter. Interestingly, in 1984 Ridgway had passed a lie detector test. Now with a search warrant in hand, police searched the Ridgway residence and also obtained hair and saliva samples from Ridgway. Again, insufficient evidence caused Ridgway to be released from custody. However, as the investigation proceeded, a DNA link between Ridgway and his victims eluded investigators. Ultimately, a careful microscopic search of Ridgway's clothing revealed the presence of paint spheres of various colors, which compared to spheres on the clothing of six of the victims. The paint was microscopically and chemically identified as Imron, a high-end specialty paint that was manufactured before 1984. This product had been used at the truck plant where Ridgway worked and was identified as dried paint spheres emanating from a spray paint. Two of the victims were further linked to Ridgway through DNA, further solidifying the case against Ridgway. Ridgway avoided the death penalty by confessing to the murders of 48 women.

Forensic Analysis of Trace Elements

Considering that most of our raw materials originate from the earth's crust, it is not surprising that they are rarely obtained in pure form; instead, they include numerous elemental impurities that usually have to be eliminated through industrial processing. However, in most cases it is not economically feasible to completely exclude all such minor impurities, especially when their presence will have no effect on the appearance or performance of the final product. For this reason, many manufactured products, and even most natural materials, contain small quantities of elements present in concentrations of less than 1 percent.

For the criminalist, the presence of *trace elements* is particularly useful because they provide "invisible" markers that may establish the source of a material or at least provide additional points for comparison. Glass fragments represent a valuable type of trace evidence; however, generally because of their minute size they present the criminalist with two distinct issues. First is classifying the type of glass being examined. Three types of glass are normally encountered as forensic evidence: float glass (windows, windshields), container glass (bottles, jars), and borosilicates (kitchenware). Figure 14–1 depicts an elemental analysis comparing three different glasses and clearly shows how they are distinguished by the intensity of the peaks associated with Boron (B) and Magnesium (Mg).

Similarly, the comparison of trace elements present in glass may provide particularly meaningful data with respect to source or origin. Technological advances in the manufacture of glass have led to more uniformity in the final product. Unfortunately, this has the consequence of diminishing the value of the most important comparative physical property—refractive index. Fortunately, minor variations in the chemical composition of glass remain between and within batches because of the presence of natural contaminants in raw materials. Up to 25 different elements have been identified in glass. The forensic discrimination associated with glass comparisons can now be enhanced by combining elemental analysis with refractive index (see Figure 14–2). Forensic investigators have also examined the evidential value of trace elements present in soil,

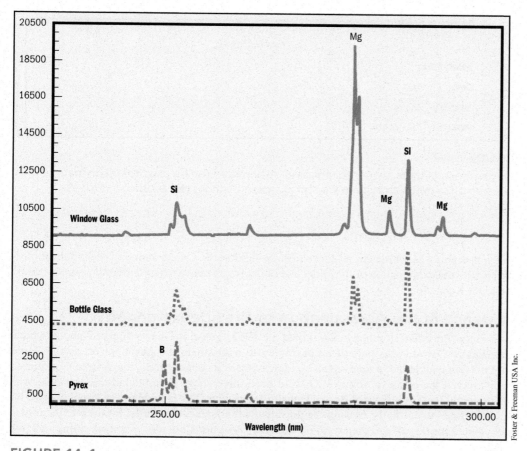

Foster & Freeman USA Inc.

FIGURE 14–1

The presence of trace elements in glass as shown above can be used to identify glass types.

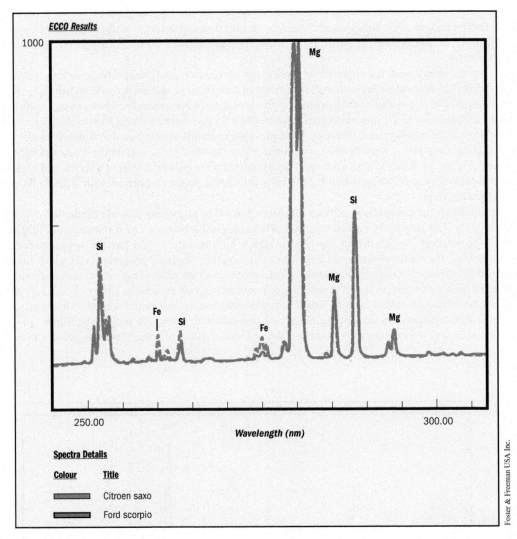

FIGURE 14–2

The presence of trace elements in glass as shown here can be used to discriminate between glass particles that are indistinguishable by other test protocols, such as refractive index.

fibers, and paint, as well as in all types of metallic objects. One example of this application occurred with the examination of the bullet and bullet fragments recovered after the assassination of President Kennedy.

Evidence in the Assassination of President Kennedy

Ever since President Kennedy was killed in 1963, questions have lingered about whether Lee Harvey Oswald was part of a conspiracy to assassinate the president or, as the Warren Commission concluded, a lone assassin. In arriving at its conclusions, the Warren Commission reconstructed the crime as follows: Oswald fired three shots from behind the president while positioned in the Texas School Book Depository building. The president was struck by two bullets, with one bullet totally missing the president's limousine. One bullet hit the president in the back, exited his throat, and then went on to strike Governor Connally, who was sitting in a jump seat in front of the president. The bullet hit Connally first in his back, then exited his chest, struck his right wrist, and temporarily lodged in his left thigh. This bullet was later found on the governor's stretcher at the hospital. A second bullet in the skull fatally wounded the president (see Figure 14–3).

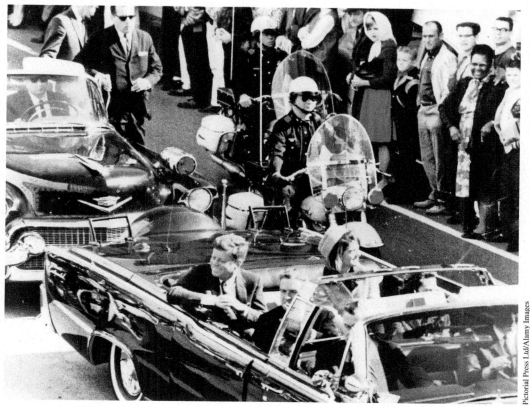

Pictorial Press Ltd/Alamy Images

FIGURE 14–3

President John F. Kennedy, Governor John Connally of Texas, and Mrs. Jacqueline Kennedy ride through Dallas moments before the assassination.

In a room at the Texas School Book Depository, a 6.5-mm Mannlicher-Carcano military rifle was found with Oswald's palm print on it. Also found were three spent 6.5-mm Western Cartridge Co./Mannlicher-Carcano (WCC/MC) cartridge cases. Oswald, an employee of the depository, had been seen there that morning and also a few minutes after the assassination, disappearing soon thereafter. He was apprehended a few miles from the depository nearly two hours after the shooting.

Critics of the Warren Commission have long argued that evidence exists that would prove Oswald did not act alone. Eyewitness accounts and acoustical data interpreted by some experts have been used to advocate the contention that someone else fired at the president from a region in front of the limousine (the so-called grassy knoll). Furthermore, it is argued that the Warren Commission's reconstruction of the crime relied on the assumption that only one bullet caused both the president's throat wound and Connally's back wound. Critics contend that such damage would have deformed and mutilated a bullet. Instead, the recovered bullet showed some flattening, no deformity, and only about 1 percent weight loss.

In 1977, at the request of the U.S. House of Representatives Select Committee on Assassinations, the bullet taken from Connally's stretcher along with bullet fragments recovered from the car and various wound areas were examined for trace element levels.

Lead alloys used for the manufacture of bullets contain an assortment of trace elements. For example, antimony is often added to lead as a hardening agent; copper, bismuth, and silver are other trace elements commonly found in bullet lead. In this case, the bullet and bullet fragments were compared for their antimony and silver content. Previous studies had amply demonstrated that the levels of these two elements are particularly important for characterizing WCC/MC bullets. Bullet lead from this type of ammunition ranges in antimony concentration from 20 to 1,200 parts per million (ppm) and 5 to 15 ppm in silver content.

As can be seen in Table 14–1, the samples designated Q1 and Q9 (the Connally stretcher bullet and fragments from Connally's wrist, respectively) are indistinguishable from one another in antimony and silver content. The samples Q2, Q4, Q5, and Q14 (Q4 and Q5 being fragments from

TABLE 14-1

Bullet and Bullet Fragments Examined in the Kennedy Assassination Investigation

Sample	Description
Q1	Connally stretcher bullet
Q9	Fragments from Connally's wrist
Q2	Large fragment from car
Q4, Q5	Fragments from Kennedy's brain
Q14	Small fragment found in car

Elemental analysis classified the bullets and fragments into two distinctly different groups. Q1 and Q9 were of similar composition containing 815 ppm[1] of antimony and 9.3 ppm of silver, respectively. Q2, Q4, Q5, and Q14 fell into a second group comprised of 622 ppm of antimony and 8.1 ppm of silver, respectively. All the samples examined were consistent with WCC/MC bullet lead, although other sources could not be entirely ruled out.

[1] One part per million equals 0.0001 percent.

Kennedy's brain, and Q2 and Q14 being fragments recovered from two different areas in the car) also are indistinguishable in antimony and silver content but are different from Q1 and Q9.

The conclusions derived from studying these results are as follows:

1. There is evidence of only two bullets—one composed of 815 ppm antimony and 9.3 ppm silver, the other composed of 622 ppm antimony and 8.1 ppm silver.
2. Both bullets have a composition highly consistent with WCC/MC bullet lead, although other sources cannot entirely be ruled out.
3. The bullet found on the Connally stretcher also damaged Connally's wrist. The absence of bullet fragments from the back wounds of Kennedy and Connally prevented any effort at linking these wounds to the stretcher bullet.

None of these conclusions can totally verify the Warren Commission's reconstruction of the assassination, but the results are at least consistent with the commission's findings that two WCC/MC bullets struck the occupants of the President's limousine. Further, in 2003, an ABC television broadcast showed the results of a 10-year 3-D computer animation study of the events of November 22, 1963. The animation graphically showed that the bullet wounds were completely consistent with Kennedy's and Connally's positions at the time of shooting, and that by following the bullet's trajectory backward they could be found to have originated from a narrow cone including only a few windows of the sixth floor of the Texas School Book Depository.

Principles and Technology of Trace Analysis

The Emission Spectrum of Elements

We have already observed that molecules can readily be characterized by their selective absorption of ultraviolet, visible, or infrared radiation. Equally significant to the analytical chemist is the knowledge that elements also selectively absorb and emit light. These observations form the basis of an important analytical technique designed to determine the elemental composition of materials—*emission spectroscopy*.

TYPES OF SPECTRA   The statement that elements emit light should not come as a total surprise, for one need only observe the common tungsten incandescent lightbulb or the glow of a neon light to confirm this observation. When the light emitted from a bulb or from any other light source is passed through a prism, it is separated into its component colors or frequencies. The resulting display of colors is called an **emission spectrum**. When sunlight or the light from an incandescent bulb is passed through a prism, a range of rainbow colors is produced. This emission spectrum is called a **continuous spectrum** because all the colors merge or blend into one another to form a continuous band. However, not all light sources produce such a spectrum. For example, if the light from a sodium lamp, a mercury arc lamp, or a neon light were passed

emission spectrum
Light emitted from a source and separated into its component colors or frequencies.

continuous spectrum
A type of emission spectrum showing a continuous band of colors all blending into one another.

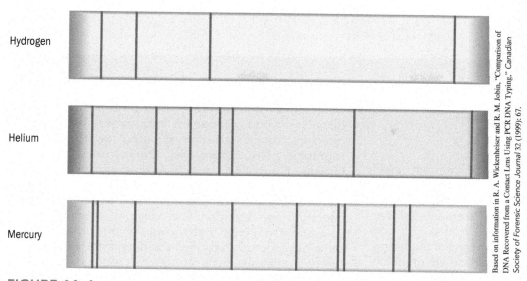

Hydrogen

Helium

Mercury

Based on information in R. A. Wickenheiser and R. M. Jobin, "Comparison of DNA Recovered from a Contact Lens Using PCR DNA Typing," *Canadian Society of Forensic Science Journal* 32 (1999): 67.

FIGURE 14–4

Some characteristic emission spectra.

through a prism, the resultant spectrum would consist not of a continuous band but of several individual colored lines separated by dark spaces. Here, each line represents a definite wavelength or frequency of light that is separate and distinct from all others present in the spectrum. This type of spectrum is called a **line spectrum**. Figure 14–4 shows the line spectra of three elements.

If a solid or liquid is vaporized and "excited" by exposure to a high temperature, each element present emits light composed of select frequencies that are characteristic of the element. This spectrum is in essence a "fingerprint" of an element and offers a practical method of identification. Sodium vapor, for example, always shows the same line spectrum, which differs from the spectrum of all other elements.

Atomic Structure

Any proposed theory that attempts to explain the origin of emission spectra must relate to the fundamental structure of the element—the atom. Scientists now know that the atom is composed of even more elementary particles that are collectively known as *subatomic particles*. The most important subatomic particles are the **proton**, **electron**, and **neutron**. The masses of the proton and neutron are each about 1,837 times the mass of an electron. The proton has a positive electrical charge, the electron has a negative charge equal in magnitude to that of the proton, and the neutron is a neutral particle having neither a positive nor a negative charge. The properties of the proton, neutron, and electron are summarized in the following table:

Particle	Symbol	Relative Mass	Electrical Charge
Proton	P	1	+1
Neutron	n	1	0
Electron	e	1/1,837	−1

A popular descriptive model of the atom, and the one that will be adopted for the purpose of this discussion, pictures an atom as consisting of electrons orbiting around a central nucleus—an image that is analogous to our solar system, in which the planets revolve around the sun.[1] The **nucleus** of the atom is composed of positively charged protons and neutrons, which have no charge. Because the atom has no net electrical charge, the number of protons must always be equal to the number of negatively charged electrons in orbit around the nucleus.

With this knowledge, we can now begin to describe the atomic structure of the elements; for example, hydrogen has a nucleus consisting of one proton and no neutrons, and it has one orbiting electron. Helium has a nucleus comprising two protons and two neutrons, with two electrons in orbit around the nucleus (see Figure 14–5).

line spectrum
A type of emission spectrum showing a series of lines separated by black areas; each line represents a definite wavelength or frequency.

proton
A positively charged particle that is one of the basic structures in the nucleus of an atom.

electron
A negatively charged particle that is one of the fundamental structural units of the atom.

neutron
A particle with no electrical charge that is one of the basic structures in the nucleus of an atom.

nucleus
The core of an atom, containing the protons and neutrons.

[1] Actually, the electrons are moving so rapidly around the nucleus as to best be visualized as being in the form of an electron cloud spread out over the surface of the atom.

Inside the Science

Carbon Arc Emission Spectrometry

An *emission spectrograph* is an instrument used to obtain and record the line spectra of elements. Essentially, this instrument requires a means for vaporizing and exciting the atoms of elements so that they emit light, a means for separating this light into its component frequencies, and a means of recording the resultant spectrum. A simple carbon arc emission spectrograph is depicted in the figure.

The specimen under investigation is excited when it is inserted between two carbon electrodes through which a direct current arc is passed. The arc produces enough heat to vaporize and excite the specimen's atoms. The resultant emitted light is collected by a lens and focused onto a prism that disperses it into component frequencies. The separated frequencies are then directed toward a photographic plate, where they are recorded as line images. Normally, a specimen consists of numerous elements; hence, the typical emission spectrum contains many lines. Each element present in the spectrum can be identified when it is compared to a standard chart that shows the position of the principal spectral lines of all the elements. However, forensic analysis more commonly requires simply a rapid comparison of the elemental composition of two or more specimens. This can readily be accomplished when the emission spectra are matched line for line, an approach illustrated in the figure, in which the emission spectra of two paint chips are shown to be comparable.

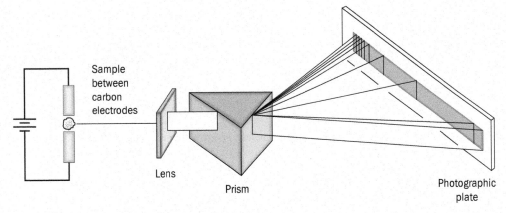

Parts of a simple carbon arc emission spectrograph.

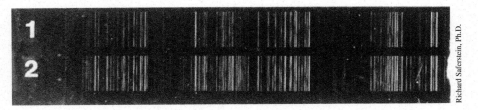

A comparison of paint chips 1 and 2 by emission spectrographic analysis. A line-for-line comparison shows that the paints have the same elemental composition.

FIGURE 14–5

The atomic structures of hydrogen and helium.

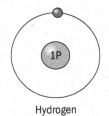

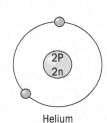

The behavior and properties that distinguish one element from another must be related to the differences in the atomic structure of each element. One such distinction is that each element possesses a different number of protons. This number is called the **atomic number** of the element. As we look back at the periodic table illustrated in Figure 10–1, we see that the elements are numbered consecutively. Those numbers represent the atomic number or number of protons associated with each element. **An element is therefore a collection of atoms that all have the same number of protons.** Thus, each atom of hydrogen has one and only one proton, each atom of helium has two protons, each atom of silver has 47 protons, and each atom of lead has 82 protons in its nucleus.

Inductively Coupled Plasma Emission Spectrometry (ICP)

Carbon arc emission spectrometry has been supplanted by *inductively coupled plasma (ICP) emission spectrometry*. Like the former, ICP identifies and measures elements through light energy emitted by excited atoms. However, instead of using an electrical arc, the atoms are excited by placing the sample in a hot plasma torch. The torch is designed as three concentric quartz tubes through which argon gas flows. A radio frequency (RF) coil that carries a current is wrapped around the tubes. The RF current creates an intense magnetic field.

THE ICP PROCESS   The process begins when a high-voltage spark is applied to the argon gas flowing through the torch. This strips some electrons from the argon atoms. These electrons are then caught and accelerated in the magnetic field such that they collide with other argon atoms, stripping off still more electrons. The collision of electrons and argon atoms continues in a chain reaction, breaking down the gas into argon atoms, argon ions, and electrons and forming an *inductively coupled plasma discharge*. The discharge is sustained by RF energy that is

atomic number
The number of protons in the nucleus of an atom; each element has its own unique atomic number.

electron orbital
The path of electrons as they move around the nuclei of atoms; each orbital is associated with a particular electronic energy level.

excited state
The state in which an atom absorbs energy and an electron moves from a lower to a higher energy level.

Inside the Science

The Origin of Emission Spectra

To explain the origin of atomic spectra, our attention must now focus on the **electron orbitals** of the atom. As electrons move around the nucleus, they are confined to a path from which they cannot stray. This orbital path is associated with a definite amount of energy and is therefore called an *energy level*. Each element has its own set of characteristic energy levels at varying distances from the nucleus. Some levels are occupied by electrons; others are empty.

An atom is in its most stable state when all of its electrons are positioned in their lowest possible energy orbitals in the atom. When an atom absorbs energy, such as heat or light, its electrons are pushed into higher-energy orbitals. In this condition, the atom is in an **excited state**. However, because energy levels have fixed values, only a definite amount of energy can be absorbed in moving an electron from one level to another. This is a most important observation, for it means that atoms absorb only a definite value of energy, and all other energy values will be excluded. In the same manner, if atoms are exposed to intense heat, enough energy is generated to push electrons into unoccupied higher-energy orbitals. Normally, the electron does not remain in this excited state for long, and it quickly falls back to its original energy level. As

the electron falls back, it releases energy. An emission spectrum testifies to the fact that this energy loss comes about in the form of light emission, as shown in the figure. The frequency of light emitted is again determined by the relationship $E = hf$, where E is the energy difference between the upper and lower energy levels, h is a constant known as Planck's constant and f is the frequency of emitted light. Because each element has its own characteristic set of energy levels, each emits a unique set of frequency values. The emission spectrum thus provides a "picture" of the energy levels that surround the nucleus of each element.

Thus, we see that as far as atoms are concerned, energy can be put into the atom at the same time energy is given off; what goes in must come out. The chemist can study the atom using either approach.

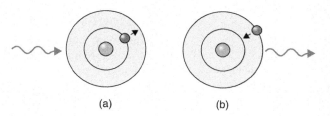

(a)   (b)

(a) The absorption of light by an atom, causing an electron to jump into a higher orbital. (b) The emission of light by an atom, caused by an electron falling back to a lower orbital.

Inside the Science

ICP Analysis of Bullets

Mutilated bullets often are not suitable for traditional microscopic comparisons against an exemplar test-fired bullet. In such situations, ICP has been used to obtain an elemental profile of the questioned bullet fragment for comparison against an unfired bullet, generally found in the possession of the suspect. For a number of years, forensic scientists have taken advantage of significant compositional differences among lead sources for the manufacture of lead-based bullets. Compositional differences in the trace elements that constitute lead bullets are typically reflected in the copper, arsenic, silver, antimony, bismuth, cadmium, and tin profiles of lead bullets. When two or more bullets have comparable elemental compositions, evidence of their similarity may be offered in a court of law.

In this respect, the comparison of lead bullets faces the same quandary as most common types of class physical evidence—how can a forensic analyst explain to a jury that such a finding has meaningful consequences to a criminal inquiry without being able to provide statistical or probability data to support such a contention? Furthermore, the creation of meaningful databases to statistically define the significance of bullets compared by their elemental profiles is currently an unrealistic undertaking. Nevertheless, the significant diversity of bullet lead compositions in our population, like other class evidence such as fibers, hairs, paint, plastics, and glass, makes their chance occurrence at a crime scene and subsequent link to a defendant a highly unlikely event. However, care must be taken to avoid giving the trier of fact the impression that elemental profiles constitute a definitive match. Given the millions of bullets produced each year, one cannot conclusively rule out the possibility of a coincidental match with a non-case-related bullet.

FIGURE 14–6

The creation of charged particles in the torch of an ICP discharge.

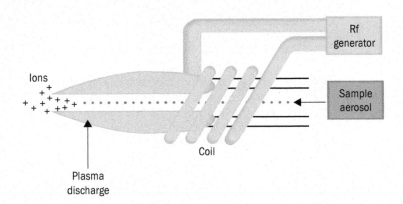

continuously transferred to it from the coil. The plasma discharge acts like an intense continuous flame, generating extremely high temperatures in the range of 7,000–10,000°C. The sample, in the form of an aerosol, is then introduced into the hot plasma, where it collides with the energetic argon electrons, generating charged particles (ions) that emit light of characteristic wavelengths corresponding to the identity of the elements present (see Figure 14–6).

Isotopes and Radioactivity

Until now, our discussion of subatomic particles has been limited to protons and electrons. However, to understand the principles of nuclear chemistry, we must look at the other important subatomic particle, the neutron. Although the atoms of a single element must have the same number of protons, nothing prevents them from having different numbers of neutrons. The total number of protons and neutrons in a nucleus is known as the **atomic mass** number.

Atoms with the same number of protons but differing solely in the number of neutrons are called **isotopes**. For example, hydrogen consists of three isotopes; besides ordinary hydrogen, which has one proton and no neutrons, two other isotopes exist, deuterium and tritium. Deuterium (or heavy hydrogen) also has one proton but contains one neutron as well. Tritium has one proton

atomic mass

The sum of the number of protons and neutrons in the nucleus of an atom.

isotope

An atom differing from another atom of the same element in the number of neutrons in its nucleus.

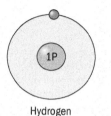
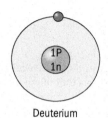
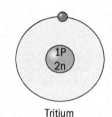

Hydrogen   Deuterium   Tritium

FIGURE 14–7
Isotopes of hydrogen.

and two neutrons in its nucleus. The atomic structures of these isotopes are shown in Figure 14–7. Therefore, all the isotopes of hydrogen have an atomic number of 1 but differ in their atomic mass numbers. Hydrogen has an atomic mass number of 1, deuterium a mass of 2, and tritium a mass of 3. Ordinary hydrogen makes up 99.98 percent of all the hydrogen atoms found in nature.

Like hydrogen, most elements are known to have two or more isotopes. Tin, for example, has 10 isotopes. Many of these isotopes are quite stable, and for all intents and purposes, the isotopes of any one element have indistinguishable properties. Others, however, are not as stable and decompose with time by a process known as *radioactive decay*. **Radioactivity** is the emission of radiation that accompanies the spontaneous disintegration of unstable nuclei. Radioactivity is actually composed of three types of radiation: **alpha particles**, **beta particles**, and **gamma rays**.

Alpha particles are positively charged particles, each with a mass approximately four times that of a hydrogen atom. These particles are helium atoms stripped of their orbiting electrons. Beta particles are actually electrons, and gamma rays are electromagnetic radiations similar to X-rays but of a higher frequency and energy (refer to the electromagnetic spectrum in Figure 10–7). Fortunately, most naturally occurring isotopes are not radioactive, and those that are—radium, uranium, and thorium—are found in such small quantities in the earth's crust that their radioactivity presents no hazard to human survival.

Because of their large mass, alpha particles do not tend to travel far and are not very penetrating; a sheet of paper or your skin easily stops them. However, isotopes that emit alpha particles are dangerous when ingested. The radioisotope polonium-210, an emitter of alpha particles, was implicated in the murder of an ex-KGB agent, as discussed in the following case file.

The existence of isotopes would be of little importance to the forensic chemist were it not for the fact that scientists have mastered the techniques for synthesizing radioactive isotopes. If the only distinction between isotopes of an element is the number of neutrons each possesses, is it not reasonable to assume that when atoms are bombarded with neutrons, some neutrons will be captured to make new isotopes? This is exactly what happens in a nuclear reactor. A nuclear reactor is simply a source of neutrons that can be used to bombard the atoms of a specimen, thereby creating radioactive isotopes. When the nucleus of an atom captures a neutron, a new isotope with one additional neutron is formed. In this state, the nuclei are said to be activated, and many immediately begin to decompose by emitting radioactivity.

Neutron Activation Analysis

Forensic chemists can characterize the trace elements in a specimen by bombarding it with neutrons and measuring the energy of the gamma rays emitted by the activated isotopes. The gamma rays of each element can be associated with a characteristic energy value. Furthermore, once the element has been identified, its concentration can be measured by the intensity of its gamma-ray radiation; intensity is directly proportional to the concentration of the element in a specimen. The technique of bombarding specimens with neutrons and measuring the resultant gamma-ray radioactivity is known as *neutron activation analysis*. The process is depicted in Figure 14–8.

The major advantage of neutron activation analysis is that it provides a nondestructive method for identifying and quantitating trace elements. A median detection sensitivity of one-billionth of a gram (one nanogram) makes neutron activation analysis one of the most sensitive methods available for the quantitative detection of many elements. Further, neutron activation can simultaneously analyze 20 to 30 elements. A major drawback to the technique is its expense and regulatory requirements. Only a handful of crime laboratories worldwide have access to a nuclear reactor; in addition, sophisticated analyzers are needed to detect and discriminate gamma-ray emissions.

As far as forensic analysis is concerned, neutron activation has been used to characterize trace elements present in metals, drugs, paint, soil, gunpowder residues, and hair. A typical illustration

radioactivity
The particle and/or gamma-ray radiation emitted by the unstable nucleus of some isotopes.

alpha particle
A type of radiation emitted by a radioactive element; the radiation is composed of helium atoms minus their orbiting electrons.

beta particle
A type of radiation emitted by a radioactive element; the radiation consists of electrons.

gamma ray
A high-energy form of electromagnetic radiation emitted by a radioactive element.

Death by Radiation Poisoning

In November 2006, Alexander V. Litvinenko lay at death's door in a London hospital. He was in excruciating pain and had symptoms that included hair loss, the inability to make blood cells, and gastrointestinal distress. His organs slowly failed as he lingered for three weeks and then died. British investigators soon confirmed that Litvinenko died from the intake of polonium-210, a radioactive element, in what appeared to be its first use as a murder weapon (see the figure).

Litvinenko's death almost immediately set off an international uproar. Litvinenko, a former KGB operative, had become a vocal critic of the Russian spy agency FSB, the domestic successor to the KGB. In 2000, he fled to London, where he was granted asylum. Litvinenko continued to voice his criticisms of the Russian spy agency and also became highly critical of Russia's president, Vladimir Putin. Just before his death, he was believed to have compiled, on behalf of a British company looking to invest millions in a project in Russia, an incriminating report regarding the activities of senior Kremlin officials.

Suspicions immediately fell onto Andrei Lugovoi and Dmitri Kovtun, business associates of Litvinenko. Lugovoi was himself a former KGB officer. On the day he fell ill, Litvinenko met Lugovoi and Kovtun at the Pine Bar of the Millennium Hotel in London. At the meeting, Litvinenko drank tea out of a teapot.

The forensic evidence shows that the Pine Bar was heavily contaminated with polonium-210. The highest readings were taken from the table where Mr. Litvinenko was sitting and from the inside of one of the teapots. No comparable levels of contamination were found in any of the other places that Mr. Litvinenko visited that day. British officials have accused Lugovoi of poisoning Litvinenko. Investigators have linked him and Kovtun to a trail of polonium-210 radioactivity stretching from hotel rooms, restaurants, bars, and offices in London to Hamburg, Germany. Each man has denied killing Litvinenko.

Polonium-210 is highly radioactive and very toxic. By weight, it is about 250 million times as toxic as cyanide, so a particle the size of a dust particle could be fatal. It emits a radioactive ray known as an alpha particle. This form of radiation cannot penetrate the skin, so polonium-210 is effective as a poison only if it is swallowed, breathed in, or injected. The particles disperse through the body and first destroy fast-growing cells, like those in bone marrow, blood, hair, and the digestive tract. That would be consistent with Litvinenko's symptoms. There is no antidote for polonium poisoning.

Polonium does have industrial uses and is produced by commercial or institutional nuclear reactors. Polonium-210 has been found to be ideal for making antistatic devices that remove dust from film and lenses as well as paper and textile plants. Its non-body-penetrating rays produce an electric charge on nearby air. Bits of dust with static attract the charged air, which neutralizes them. Once free of static, the dust is easy to blow or brush away. Manufacturers of such antistatic devices take great pains to make the polonium hard to remove from their products.

In 2016, a public inquiry into the death of Alexander Litvinenko was completed and published (https://www. litvinenkoinquiry.org/). The inquiry was headed by Robert Owen, a retired High Court judge in Britain. It chronicled the poisoning of Litvenenko by Lugovoi and Kovtun. The report concluded the Russian Federal Security Service plotted the poisoning of Litvinenko, an operation that was probably approved by President Putin.

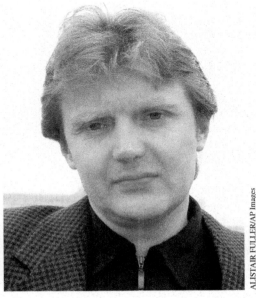

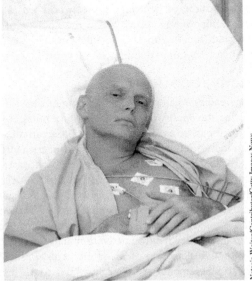

Alexander Litvinenko, former KGB agent, before (right) and after he became sick (left).

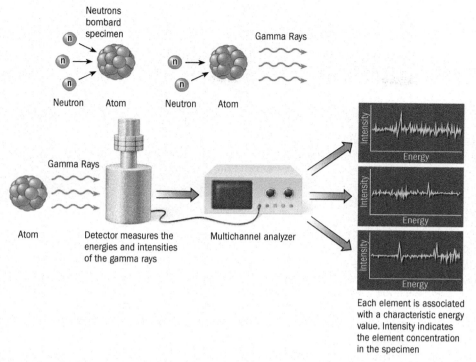

Each element is associated with a characteristic energy value. Intensity indicates the element concentration in the specimen

FIGURE 14–8

The neutron activation process requires the capture of a neutron by the nucleus of an atom. The new atom is now radioactive and emits gamma rays. A detector permits identification of the radioactive atoms present by measuring the energies and intensities of the gamma rays emitted.

TABLE 14–2

Concentration of Trace Elements in Copper Wire

	Selenium	Gold	Antimony	Silver
Control Wire				
A1	2.4	0.047	0.16	12.7
A2	3.5	0.064	0.27	17.2
A3	2.6	0.050	0.20	13.3
A4	1.9	0.034	0.21	12.6
Suspect Wire				
B	2.3	0.042	0.15	13.0

Note: Average concentration measured in parts per million.

Source: R. K. H. Chan, "Identification of Single-Stranded Copper Wires by Nondestructive Neutron Activation Analysis," *Journal of Forensic Sciences* 17 (1972): 93. Reprinted by permission of the American Society for Testing and Materials, copyright 1972.

of its application occurred during the investigation of a theft of copper telegraphic wires in Canada. Four lengths of copper wire (A1, A2, A3, A4) found at the scene of the theft were compared by neutron activation with a length of copper wire (B) seized at a scrap yard and suspected of being stolen. All were bare, single-strand wires with the same general physical appearance and a diameter of 0.28 centimeter. Prior experiments had revealed that significant variations could be expected in the concentration levels of the trace elements selenium, gold, antimony, and silver for wires originating from different sources. A comparison of these elements present in the wires involved in the theft was undertaken. After exposing the wires to neutrons in a nuclear reactor, neutron activation analysis revealed a match between A1 and B that was well within experimental error (see Table 14–2). The findings suggested a common origin of the control and suspect wires.

Inside the Science

Nuclear Forensics

Nuclear forensics has emerged as a critical profession on the forefront in the war on terrorism. Nuclear forensic scientists are responsible for developing ways to analyze nuclear materials recovered from either intercepted intact nuclear materials or postexplosion debris created as a result of a nuclear explosion. Nuclear forensics can trace its origin to the cold war era, when U.S. planes surreptitiously flew over Soviet airspace sampling airborne particles from the country's nuclear bomb tests. Nuclear forensics matured as a science when the Soviet empire disintegrated and concerns arose over the security of nuclear materials located in states of the former Soviet Union. Fears that these materials might fall into the hands of terrorist organizations engendered scenarios of dirty nuclear bomb attacks on the United States and other Western nations.

Nuclear forensics is becoming an increasingly important tool in the fight against illegal smuggling and trafficking of radiological and nuclear materials. These include materials intended for industrial and medical use, nuclear materials such as those produced in the nuclear fuel cycle of a nuclear power plant (see the figure), and much more dangerous nuclear materials that can be used in weapons, such as plutonium and highly enriched uranium. Since the early 1990s, more than 200 cases of illicitly trafficked nuclear materials have been reported.

In the United States, Lawrence Livermore National Laboratory along with seven other Department of Energy (DOE) national laboratories has been tasked by the FBI and the Department of Homeland Security with developing the nation's technical forensics capability for nuclear and radiological materials. Organizations such as the European Commission's Institute for Transuranium Elements, located in Karlsruhe, Germany, have extended nuclear forensic capabilities onto an international scale.

A major focus of nuclear forensics is identifying signatures, which are the physical, chemical, and isotopic characteristics that distinguish one nuclear or radiological material from another. Signatures enable researchers to identify the processes used to initially create a material, which ultimately may yield clues as to the origin of the seized material.

Attribution is the integration of all information, including forensic data, law enforcement and intelligence data, to corroborate or exclude the origin of nuclear materials and devices, routes of transit, and responsible groups or individuals.

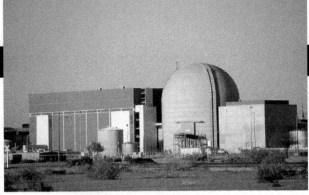

View of a nuclear power plant.

Nuclear forensics can be performed on a broad spectrum of substances. An example is stolen containers of uranium diverted during one of the mining, milling, conversion, enrichment, or fuel fabrication steps used to convert uranium ore to enriched fuel for nuclear power plants; uranium varies in isotopic composition and impurities according to where the uranium was mined and how it was processed. Another example is commercial radioactive materials used in applications such as medical diagnostics and food sterilization.

Researchers analyze the material's chemical and isotopic composition, which includes measuring the amounts of trace elements as well as the ratio of parent isotopes to daughter isotopes. These measurements help determine the source location and sample's age. They also examine the material's morphological characteristics such as shape, size, and texture. Analytical methods include electron microscopy, X-ray diffraction, and mass spectrometry. In addition, as a sample is moved from place to place, it picks up trace evidence such as pollen, hairs, fibers, plant DNA, and fingerprints. These so-called route materials may provide information about who has handled a sample and the path it has traveled.

When comparing a sample's signature against known signatures from uranium mines and fabrication plants, researchers can benefit by assembling a library of nuclear materials of known origin from around the world. Nuclear scientists have developed relationships with domestic suppliers of nuclear materials to assemble such a library. Contracts with major U.S. uranium fuel suppliers have provided researchers with samples and manufacturing data. Forensic scientists are also seeking to obtain samples of uranium products worldwide to analyze the products' isotopic and trace-element content, grain size, and microstructure. Nations with nuclear capabilities are beginning to share information about their nuclear fuel processes and materials. The development of databases is essential to the nuclear forensic scientist's mission of identifying the origin of nuclear materials intercepted in the black market or associated with a terrorist event.

Forensic Examination of Paint

Our environment contains millions of objects whose surfaces are painted. Thus, it is not surprising to observe that paint, in one form or another, is one of the most prevalent types of physical evidence received by the crime laboratory. Paint as physical evidence is perhaps most frequently encountered in hit-and-run and burglary cases. For example, a chip of dried paint or a paint smear may be transferred to the clothing of a hit-and-run victim on impact with an automobile, or paint smears could be transferred onto a tool during the commission of a burglary. Obviously, in many situations a transfer of paint from one surface to another could impart an object with an identifiable forensic characteristic.

In most circumstances, the criminalist must compare two or more paints to establish their common origin. For example, such a comparison may associate an individual or a vehicle with the crime site. However, the criminalist need not be confined to comparisons alone. Crime laboratories often help identify the color, make, and model of an automobile by examining small quantities of paint recovered at an accident scene. Such requests, normally made in connection with hit-and-run cases, can lead to the apprehension of the responsible vehicle.

Composition of Paint

Paint spread onto a surface dries into a hard film consisting of pigments and additives suspended in a binder. Pigments impart color and hiding (or opacity) to paint and are usually mixtures of different inorganic and organic compounds added to the paint by the manufacturer to produce specific colors and properties. The binder provides the support medium for the pigments and additives and is a polymeric substance. Paint is thus composed of a binder and pigments, as well as other additives, all dissolved or dispersed in a suitable solvent. After the paint has been applied to a surface, the solvent evaporates, leaving behind a hard polymeric binder and any pigments that were suspended in it.

One of the most common types of paint examined in the crime laboratory is finishes from automobiles. One interesting fact that is helpful in forensic characterization of automotive paint is that manufacturers apply a variety of coatings to the body of an automobile. This adds significant diversity to automobile paint and contributes to the forensic significance of automobile paint comparisons. The automotive finishing system for steel usually consists of at least four organic coatings:

Electrocoat Primer   The first layer applied to the steel body of a car is the electrocoat primer. The primer, consisting of epoxy-based resins, is electroplated onto the steel body of the automobile to provide corrosion resistance. The resulting coating is uniform in appearance and thickness. The color of these electrodeposition primers ranges from black to gray.

Primer Surfacer   Originally responsible for corrosion control, the surfacer usually follows the electrocoat layer and is applied before the basecoat. Primer surfacers are epoxy-modified polyesters or urethanes. The function of this layer is to completely smooth out and hide any seams or imperfections because the colorcoat will be applied on this surface. This layer is highly pigmented. Color pigments are used to minimize color contrast between primer and topcoats. For example, a light-gray primer may be used under pastel shades of a colored topcoat; a red oxide may be used under a dark-colored topcoat.

Basecoat   The next layer of paint on a car is the basecoat or colorcoat. This layer provides the color and aesthetics of the finish and represents the "eye appeal" of the finished automobile. The integrity of this layer depends on its ability to resist weather, UV radiation, and acid rain. Most commonly, an acrylic-based polymer comprises the binder system of basecoats. Interestingly, the choice of automotive pigments is dictated by toxic and environmental concerns. Thus, the use of lead, chrome, and other heavy-metal pigments has been abandoned in favor of organic-based pigments. There is also a growing trend toward pearl luster or mica pigments. Mica pigments are coated with layers of metal oxide to generate interference colors. Also, the addition of aluminum flakes to automotive paint imparts a metallic look to the paint's finish.

Clearcoat   An unpigmented clearcoat is applied to improve gloss, durability, and appearance. Most clearcoats are acrylic based, but polyurethane clearcoats are increasing in popularity. These topcoats provide outstanding etch resistance and appearance.

Microscopic Examination of Paint

The microscope has traditionally been and remains the most important instrument for locating and comparing paint specimens. Considering the thousands of paint colors and shades, it is quite understandable why color, more than any other property, imparts paint with its most distinctive forensic characteristics. Questioned and known specimens are best compared side by side under a stereoscopic microscope for color, surface texture, and color layer sequence (see Figures 14–9 and 14–10).

The importance of layer structure for evaluating the evidential significance of paint evidence cannot be overemphasized. When paint specimens possess colored layers that match in number and sequence of colors, the examiner can begin to relate the paints to a common origin. How many layers must be matched before the criminalist can conclude that the paints come from the same source? There is no one accepted criterion. Much depends on the uniqueness of each layer's color and texture, as well as the frequency with which the particular combination of colors under investigation is observed to occur. Because no books or journals have compiled this type of information, the criminalist is left to their own experience and knowledge when making this decision.

Unfortunately, most paint specimens presented to the criminalist do not have a layer structure of sufficient complexity to allow them to be individualized to a single source (see Figure 14–11). However, the diverse chemical composition of modern paints provides additional points of comparison between specimens. Specifically, a thorough comparison of paint must include a chemical analysis of the paint's pigments, its binder composition, or both.

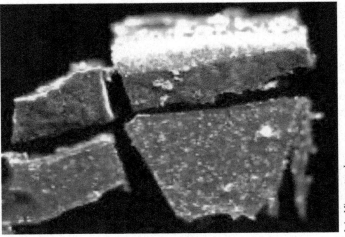

FIGURE 14–9

A stereoscopic microscope comparison of two automotive paints. The questioned paint on the left has a layer structure consistent with P the control paint on the right.

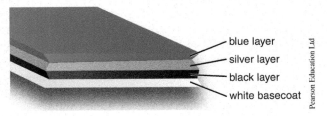

FIGURE 14–10

Diagram of paint taken from crime scene.

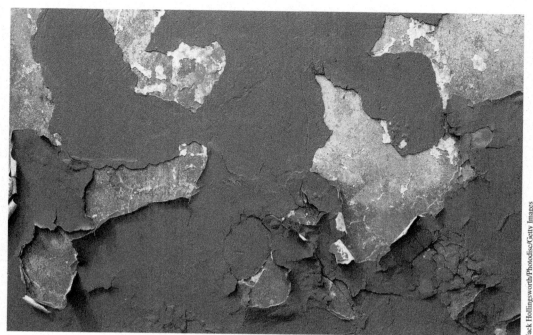

FIGURE 14–11
Red paint chips peeling off a wall revealing underlying layers.

Jack Hollingsworth/Photodisc/Getty Images

Analytical Techniques Used in Paint Comparison

The wide variation in binder formulations in automobile finishes provides particularly significant information. More important, paint manufacturers make automobile finishes in hundreds of varieties; this knowledge is most helpful to the criminalist who is trying to associate a paint chip with one car as distinguished from the thousands of similar models that have been produced in any one year. For instance, there are more than a hundred automobile production plants in the United States and Canada. Each can use one paint supplier for a particular color or vary suppliers during a model year. Although a paint supplier must maintain strict quality control over a paint's color, the batch formulation of any paint binder can vary, depending on the availability and cost of basic ingredients.

CHARACTERIZATION OF PAINT BINDERS **Pyrolysis** gas chromatography has proven to be a particularly invaluable technique for distinguishing most paint formulations. In this process, paint chips as small as 20 micrograms are decomposed by heat into numerous gaseous products and are sent through a gas chromatograph. As shown in Figure 14–12, the polymer chain is decomposed by a heated filament, and the resultant products are swept into and through a gas chromatograph column. The separated decomposition products of the polymer emerge and are recorded. The pattern of this chromatogram or "pyrogram" distinguishes one polymer from another. The result is a pyrogram that is sufficiently detailed to reflect the chemical makeup of the binder. Figure 14–13 illustrates how the patterns produced by paint pyrograms can differentiate acrylic enamel paints removed from two different automobiles. Infrared spectrophotometry is still another analytical technique that provides information about the binder composition of paint.[2] Binders selectively absorb infrared radiation to yield a spectrum that is highly characteristic of a paint specimen.

pyrolysis
The decomposition of organic matter by heat.

CHARACTERIZATION OF PIGMENTS The elements that constitute the inorganic pigments of paints can be identified by a variety of techniques—emission spectroscopy, inductively coupled plasma (ICP), and X-ray spectroscopy (page 182). The emission spectrograph, for instance, can simultaneously detect 15 to 20 elements in most automobile paints. Some of these elements are relatively common to all paints and have little forensic value; others are less frequently encountered and provide excellent points of comparison between paint specimens.

[2] P. G. Rodgers et al., "The Classification of Automobile Paint by Diamond Window Infrared Spectrophotometry, Part I: Binders and Pigments," *Canadian Society of Forensic Science Journal* 9 (1976): 1; T. J. Allen, "Paint Sample Presentation for Fourier Transform Infrared Microscopy," *Vibration Spectroscopy* 3 (1992): 217.

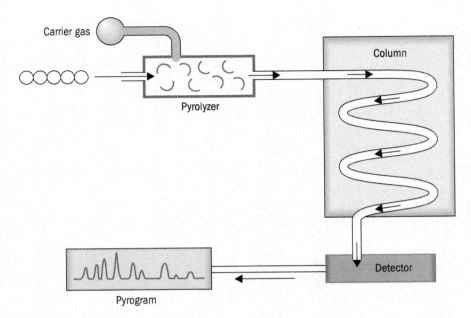

FIGURE 14-12
Schematic diagram of pyrolysis gas chromatography.

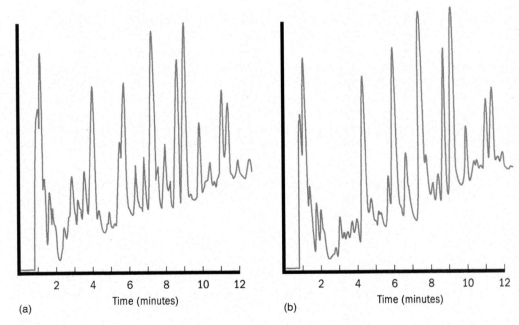

FIGURE 14-13
Paint pyrograms of acrylic enamel paints. (a) Paint from a Ford model and
(b) paint from a Chrysler model.

Significance of Paint Evidence

Once a paint comparison is completed, the task of assessing the significance of the finding begins. How certain can one be that two similar paints came from the same surface? For instance, a casual observer sees countless identically colored automobiles on our roads and streets. If this is the case, what value is a comparison of a paint chip from a hit-and-run scene to paint removed from a suspect car? From previous discussions it should be apparent that far more is involved in paint comparison than matching surface paint colors. Paint layers present beneath a surface layer offer valuable points of comparison. Furthermore, forensic analysts can detect subtle differences in paint binder formulations, as well as major or minor differences in the elemental composition of paint. Obviously, these properties cannot be discerned by the naked eye.

The significance of a paint comparison was convincingly demonstrated from data gathered at the Centre of Forensic Sciences, Toronto, Canada.[3] Paint chips randomly taken from 260 vehicles located in a local wreck yard were compared by color, layer structure, and, when required, by infrared spectroscopy. All were distinguishable except for one pair. In statistical terms, these results signify that if a crime-scene paint sample and a paint standard/reference sample removed from a suspect car compare by the previously discussed tests, the odds against the crime-scene paint originating from another randomly chosen vehicle are approximately 33,000 to 1. Obviously, this type of evidence is bound to forge a strong link between the suspect car and the crime scene.

Crime laboratories are often asked to identify the make and model of a car from a very small amount of paint left behind at a crime scene. Such information is frequently of use in a search for an unknown car involved in a hit-and-run incident. Often, the questioned paint can be identified when its color is compared to color chips representing the various makes and models of manufactured cars. However, in many cases it is not possible to state the exact make or model of the car in question because any one paint color can be found on more than one car model. For example, General Motors may use the same paint color for several production years on cars in its Cadillac, Buick, and Chevrolet lines.

Color charts for automobile finishes are available from various paint manufacturers and refinishers (see Figure 14–14). Starting with the 1974 model year, the Law Enforcement Standards Laboratory at the National Institute of Standards and Technology collected and disseminated to crime laboratories auto paint color samples from U.S. domestic passenger cars. This collection was distributed by Collaborative Testing Services, McLean, Virginia, through 1991. Since 1975, the Royal Canadian Mounted Police Forensic Laboratories have been systematically gathering color and chemical information on automotive paints. This computerized database, known as PDQ (Paint Data Query), allows an analyst to obtain information on paints related to automobile make, model, and year. The database contains such parameters as automotive paint layer colors, primer colors, and binder composition. A number of U.S. laboratories have access to PDQ.[4] Also, some laboratories maintain an in-house collection of automobile paints associated with various makes and models.

After automotive paints, architectural paint comparisons are the most common paint analyses required of forensic laboratories. A large-scale population study of architectural paints collected throughout North America has been conducted for their forensic value.[5] Intercomparisons of nearly 960 randomly collected paints by visual, microscopic, and infrared technology resulted in a 99.99 percent differentiation of the paints, thus demonstrating the high diversity of architectural paints in our environment and their meaningful forensic value as class evidence. A follow-up study on 50 single-layer white architectural paints, selected because of their limited features,

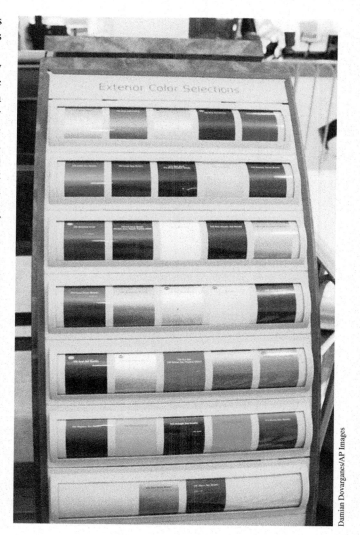

Damian Dovarganes/AP Images

FIGURE 14–14

Automotive color chart of various car models.

---

[3] G. Edmondstone, J. Hellman, K. Legate, G. L. Vardy, and E. Lindsay, "An Assessment of the Evidential Value of Automotive Paint Comparisons," *Canadian Society of Forensic Science Journal* 37 (2004): 147.

[4] J. L. Buckle et al., "PDQ—Paint Data Queries: The History and Technology Behind the Development of the Royal Canadian Mounted Police Laboratory Services Automotive Paint Database," *Canadian Society of Forensic Science Journal* 30 (1997): 199. An excellent discussion of the PDQ database is also available in A. Beveridge, T. Fung, and D. MacDougall, "Use of Infrared Spectroscopy for the Characterisation of Paint Fragments," in B. Caddy, ed., *Forensic Examination of Glass and Paint* (New York: CRC Press, 2001), pp. 222–233.

[5] D. W. Wright et al., "Analysis and Documentation of Architectural Paint Samples via a Population Study," *Forensic Science International* 209 (2011): 86.

> > > > > > > > >

The Predator

September in Arizona is usually hot and dry, much like the rest of the year—but September 1984 was a little different. Unusually heavy rains fell for two days, which must have seemed unfitting to the friends and family of 8-year-old Vicki Lynn Hoskinson. Vicki went missing on September 17 of that year, and her disappearance was investigated as a kidnapping. A schoolteacher who knew Vicki remembered seeing a suspicious vehicle loitering near the school that day, and he happened to jot down the license plate number. This crucial tip led police to 28-year-old Frank Atwood, recently paroled from a California prison. Police soon learned that Atwood had been convicted for committing sex offenses and for kidnapping a boy. This galvanized the investigators, who realized Vicki could be at the mercy of a dangerous and perverse man.

The only evidence the police had to work with was Vicki's bike, which was found abandoned in the middle of the street a few blocks from her home. Police found scrapes from her bike pedal on the underside of the gravel pan on Atwood's car, as well as pink paint on Atwood's front bumper, apparently transferred from Vicki's bike. The police believed that Atwood deliberately struck Vicki while she was riding her bicycle, knocking her to the ground.

The pink paint on Atwood's bumper was first looked at microscopically and then examined by pyrolysis gas chromatography. This technique provides investigators with a "fingerprint" pattern of the paint sample, enabling them to compare this paint to any other paint evidence. In this case, the pink paint on Atwood's bumper matched the paint from Vicki's bicycle.

Vicki's skeletal remains were discovered in the desert, several miles from her home, in the spring of 1985. Positive identification was made using dental records, but investigators wanted to see if the remains could help them determine how long she had been dead. Atwood had been jailed on an unrelated charge three days after Vicki disappeared, so the approximate date of death was very important to proving his guilt.

Investigators found adipocere, a white, fatty residue produced during decomposition, inside Vicki's skull. This provided evidence that moisture was present around Vicki's body after her death, which did not seem to make sense, considering her body was found in the Arizona desert! A check of weather records revealed that there had been an unusual amount of rainfall during only one period of time since Vicki was last seen alive: a mere 48 hours after her disappearance. This put Vicki's death squarely within Frank Atwood's three-day window of opportunity between her disappearance and his arrest. Frank Atwood was sentenced to death in 1987 for the murder of Vicki Lynn Hoskinson. He remains on death row awaiting execution.

demonstrated a high degree of discrimination (99.35 percent) using a series of common forensic testing methods, further providing evidence that architectural paint comparisons can provide strong class evidence.[6]

Collection and Preservation of Paint Evidence

As has already been noted, paint chips are most likely to be found on or near people or objects involved in hit-and-run incidents. The recovery of loose paint chips from a garment or from the road surface must be done with the utmost care to keep the paint chip intact. Paint chips may be picked up with a tweezers or scooped up with a piece of paper. Paper druggist folds and glass or plastic vials make excellent containers for paint. If the paint is smeared on or embedded in garments or objects, the investigator should not attempt to remove it; instead, it is best to package the whole item carefully and send it to the laboratory for examination.

When a transfer of paint occurs in hit-and-run situations, such as to the clothing of a pedestrian victim, uncontaminated standard/reference paint must always be collected from an undamaged area of the vehicle for comparison in the laboratory. It is particularly important that the collected paint be close to the area of the car that was suspected of being in contact with the victim. This is necessary because other portions of the car may have faded or been repainted. Standard/reference samples are always removed so as to include all the paint layers down to the bare metal. This is best accomplished by removing a painted section with a clean scalpel or knife blade. Samples ¼ inch square are sufficient for laboratory examination. Each paint sample should be separately packaged and marked with the exact location of its recovery. When a cross-transfer of paint occurs between two vehicles, again all of the layers, including the foreign as well as the underlying original paints, must be removed from each vehicle. A standard/reference sample from an adjacent undamaged area of each vehicle must also be taken in such cases.

[6] D. W. Wright, et al., "Analysis and Discrimination of Single-Layer White Architectural Paint Samples," *Journal of Forensic Science* 58 (2013): 358.

Carefully wipe the blade of any knife or scraping tool with distilled water before collecting each sample, to avoid cross-contamination of paints.

Tools used to enter buildings or safes often contain traces of paints as well as other substances such as wood and safe insulation. Care must be taken not to lose this type of trace evidence. The scene investigator should not try to remove the paint; instead, the investigator should package the tool for laboratory examination. Standard/reference paint should be collected from all surfaces suspected of having been in contact with the tool. Again, all layers of paint must be included in the sample.

When the tool has left its impression on a surface, standard/reference paint is collected from an uncontaminated area adjacent to the impression. No attempt should be made to collect the paint from the impression itself. If this is done, the impression may be permanently altered and its evidential value lost.

Forensic Analysis of Soil

There are many definitions for the term *soil*; however, for forensic purposes, soil may be thought of as any disintegrated material, natural and/or artificial, that lies on or near the earth's surface. Therefore, forensic examination of soil is not only concerned with the analysis of naturally occurring rocks, minerals, vegetation, and animal matter; it also encompasses the detection of such manufactured objects as glass, paint chips, asphalt, brick fragments, and cinders, whose presence may impart soil with characteristics that make it unique to a particular location. When this material is collected accidentally or deliberately in a manner that associates it with a crime under investigation, it becomes valuable physical evidence.[7]

Significance of Soil Evidence

The value of soil as evidence rests on its prevalence at crime scenes and its transferability between the scene and the person who committed the crime. Thus, soil or dried mud found adhering to a suspect's clothing or shoes or to an automobile, when compared to soil samples collected at the crime site, may link a suspect or object to the crime scene. As with most types of physical evidence, forensic soil analysis is comparative in nature; soil found in the possession of the suspect must be carefully collected and then compared to soil samplings from the crime scene and its vicinity.

However, one should not rule out the value of soil even if the site of the crime has not been ascertained. For instance, small amounts of soil may be found on a person or object far from the actual site of a crime. A geologist who knows the local geology may be able to use geological maps to direct police to the general vicinity where the soil was originally picked up and the crime committed.

Forensic Examination of Soil

Most soils can be differentiated by their gross appearance. A side-by-side visual comparison of the color and texture of soil specimens is easy to perform and provides a sensitive property for distinguishing soils that originate from different locations. Soil is darker when it is wet; therefore, color comparisons must always be made when all the samples are dried under identical laboratory conditions. It is estimated that there are nearly 1,100 distinguishable soil colors; hence, color offers a logical first step in a forensic soil comparison (see Figure 14–15).

Low-power microscopic examination of soil reveals the presence of plant and animal materials as well as artificial debris. Further high-power microscopic examination helps characterize minerals and rocks in earth materials. Although this approach to forensic soil identification requires the expertise of an investigator trained in geology, it can provide the most varied and significant points of comparison between soil samples. Only by carefully examining and comparing the minerals and rocks naturally present in soil can one take advantage of the large number of variations between soils and thus add to the evidential value of a positive comparison.[8]

[7] E. P. Junger, "Assessing the Unique Characteristics of Close-Proximity Soil Samples: Just How Useful Is Soil Evidence?" *Journal of Forensic Sciences* 41 (1996): 27.

[8] W. J. Graves, "A Mineralogical Soil Classification Technique for the Forensic Scientist," *Journal of Forensic Sciences* 24 (1979): 323; M. J. McVicar and W. J. Graves, "The Forensic Comparison of Soil by Automated Scanning Electron Microscopy," *Canadian Society of Forensic Science Journal* 30 (1997): 241.

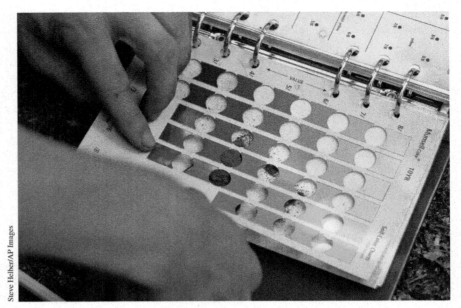

Steve Helber/AP Images

FIGURE 14–15
A technician classifies a soil sample based on a soil color chart.

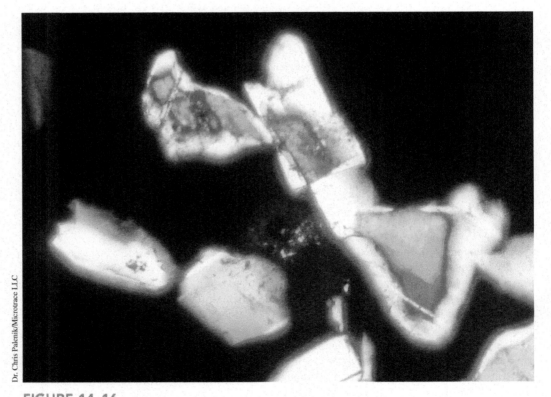

Dr. Chris Palenik/Microtrace LLC

FIGURE 14–16
A mineral viewed under a microscope.

mineral
A naturally occurring crystalline solid.

A **mineral** is a naturally occurring crystal, and like any other crystal, its physical properties—for example, its color, geometric shape, density, and refractive index—are useful for identification. More than 3,800 minerals exist; however, most are so rare that forensic geologists usually encounter only about 20 of them. Rocks are composed of a combination of minerals and therefore exist in thousands of varieties on the earth's surface. They are usually identified by characterizing their mineral content and grain size (see Figure 14–16).

Considering the vast variety of minerals and rocks and the possible presence of artificial debris in soil, the forensic geologist is presented with many points of comparison between two or more specimens. The number of comparative points and their frequency of occurrence must be considered before concluding that specimens are similar and judging the probability of their common origin.

Rocks and minerals not only are present in earth materials but also are used to manufacture a wide variety of industrial and commercial products. For example, the tools and garments of an individual suspected of breaking into a safe often contain traces of safe insulation. Safe insulation may be made from a wide combination of mineral mixtures that provide significant points of identification. Similarly, building materials such as brick, plaster, and concrete blocks are combinations of minerals and rocks that can easily be recognized and compared microscopically to similar minerals found on the breaking-and-entering suspect.

Variations in Soil

The ultimate forensic value of soil evidence depends on its uniqueness at the crime scene. If, for example, soil composition is indistinguishable for miles surrounding the location of a crime, associating soil found on the suspect with that particular site will have limited value. Significant conclusions that link a suspect with a particular location through a soil comparison may be made when variations in soil composition occur every 10 to 100 yards from the crime site. However, even when such variations do exist, the forensic geologist usually cannot individualize soil to any one location unless it contains an unusual combination of rare minerals, rocks, or artificial debris.

No statistically valid forensic studies have examined the variability of soil evidence. A study conducted in southern Ontario, Canada, seems to indicate that soil in that part of Canada shows extensive diversity. It estimates a probability of less than 1 in 50 of finding two soils that are indistinguishable in both color and mineral properties but originate in two different locations separated by a distance of at least 1,000 feet. Based on these preliminary results, similar diversity may be expected in the northern United States, Canada, northern Europe, and eastern Europe. However, such probability values can only generally indicate the variation of soil within these geographical areas. Each crime scene must be evaluated separately to establish its own soil variation probabilities.

> > > > > > > > >

Case Files

Soil: The Silent Witness

Alice Redmond was reported missing by her husband on a Monday night in 1983. Police learned that she had been seen with a co-worker, Mark Miller, after work that evening. When police questioned Miller, he stated that the two just "drove around" after work and then she dropped him off at home. Despite his statement, Miller was the prime suspect because he had a criminal record for burglary and theft.

Alice's car was recovered in town the following morning. The wheel wells were thickly coated in mud, which investigators hoped might provide a good lead. These hopes were dampened when police learned that Alice and her husband had attended a motorcycle race on Sunday, where her car was driven through deep mud.

After careful scrutiny, analysts found two colors of soil on the undercarriage of Alice's car. The thickest soil was brown; on top of the brown layer was a reddish soil that looked unlike anything in the county. Investigators hoped the reddish soil, which had to have been deposited sometime after the Sunday night motorcycle event and before the vehicle was discovered on Tuesday morning, could link the vehicle to the location of Alice Redmond.

An interview with Mark Miller's sister provided a break in the case. She told police that Mark had visited her on Monday evening. During that visit, he confessed that he had driven Alice in her car across the Alabama state line into Georgia, killed her, and buried her in a remote location. Now that investigators had a better idea where to look for Alice, forensic analysts took soil samples that would prove or disprove Miller's sister's story.

Each field sample was dried and compared for color and texture by eye and stereomicroscopy to the reddish-colored soil gathered from the car. Next, soils that compared to the car were passed through a series of mesh filters, each of a finer gauge than the last. In this way, the components of the soil samples were physically separated by size. Finally, each fraction was analyzed and compared for mineral composition with the aid of a polarizing light microscope.

Only samples collected from areas across the Alabama state line near the suspected dump site were consistent with the topmost reddish soil recovered from Alice's car. This finding supported Miller's sister's story and was instrumental in Mark Miller's being charged with murder and kidnapping. After pleading guilty, the defendant led the authorities to where he had buried the body. The burial site was within a half mile of the location where forensic analysts had collected a soil sample consistent with the soil removed from Alice's vehicle.

Collection and Preservation of Soil Evidence

When gathering soil specimens, the evidence collector must give primary consideration to establishing the variation of soil at the crime-scene area. For this reason, standard/reference soils should be collected at various intervals within a 100 foot radius of the crime scene, as well as at the site of the crime, for comparison to the questioned soil. Soil specimens also should be collected at all possible alibi locations that the suspect may have claimed.

All specimens gathered should be representative of the soil that was removed by the suspect. In most cases, only the top layer of soil is picked up during the commission of a crime. Thus, standard/reference specimens must be removed from the surface, without digging into the unrepresentative subsurface layers. Approximately a tablespoon or two of soil in each sample is all the laboratory needs for a thorough comparative analysis. All specimens collected should be packaged in individual containers, such as plastic vials. Each vial should be marked to indicate the location at which the sampling was made.

Soil found on a suspect must be carefully preserved for analysis. If it is found adhering to an object, as in the case of soil on a shoe, the investigator must not remove it. Instead, each object should be individually wrapped in paper, with the soil intact, and transmitted to the laboratory. Similarly, loose soil adhering to garments should not be removed; these items should be carefully and individually wrapped in paper bags and sent to the laboratory for analysis. Care must be taken that particles that may fall off the garment during transportation will remain in the paper bag.

When a lump of soil is found, it should be collected and preserved intact. For example, an automobile tends to collect and build up layers of soil under the fenders, body, and so on. The impact of an automobile with another object may jar some of this soil loose. Once the suspect car has been apprehended, a comparison of the soil left at the scene with soil remaining on the automobile may help establish that the car was present at the accident scene. In these situations, separate samples are collected from under all the fender and frame areas of the vehicle; care is taken to remove the soil in clump form to preserve the order in which the particles of soil adhered to the car and to the other soil on the car. Undoubtedly, during the normal use of an automobile, soil will be picked up from numerous locations over a period of months and years. This layering effect may impart soil with greater variation, and hence greater evidential value, than that normally associated with loose soil.

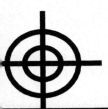

Chapter Summary > > > > > > > > > >

Many manufactured products and even most natural materials contain small quantities of elements in concentrations of less than 1 percent. For the criminalist, the presence of these trace elements is particularly useful because they provide "invisible" markers that may establish the source of a material or at least provide additional points for comparison.

Emission spectroscopy and inductively coupled plasma are techniques available to forensic scientists for determining the elemental composition of materials. An emission spectrograph vaporizes and heats samples to a high temperature so that the atoms present in the material achieve an "excited" state. Under these circumstances, the excited atoms emit light. If the light is separated into its components, one observes a line spectrum. Each element present in the spectrum can be identified by its characteristic line frequencies. In inductively coupled plasma, the sample, in the form of an aerosol, is introduced into a hot plasma, creating charged particles that emit light of characteristic wavelengths corresponding to the identity of the elements present.

Neutron activation analysis measures the gamma-ray frequencies of specimens that have been bombarded with neutrons. This method provides a highly sensitive and nondestructive analysis for simultaneously identifying and quantitating 20 to 30 trace elements. Because this technique requires access to a nuclear reactor, however, it has limited value to forensic analysis.

Paint spread onto a surface dries into a hard film consisting of pigments and additives suspended in the binder. One of the most common types of paint examined in the crime laboratory is finishes from automobiles. Automobile manufacturers normally apply a variety of coatings to the body of an automobile. Hence, the wide diversity of automotive paint contributes to the forensic significance of an automobile paint comparison. Questioned and known specimens are best compared side by side under a stereoscopic microscope for color, surface texture, and color layer sequence. Pyrolysis gas chromatography and infrared spectrophotometry are invaluable techniques for distinguishing most paint binder formulations, adding further significance to a forensic paint comparison.

The value of soil as evidence rests with its prevalence at crime scenes and its transferability between the scene and the criminal. Most soils can be differentiated by their gross appearance. A side-by-side visual comparison of the color and texture of soil specimens is easy to perform and provides a sensitive property for distinguishing soils that originate from different locations. In many forensic laboratories, forensic geologists characterize and compare the mineral content of soils.

Soils should be collected at various intervals within a 100 foot radius of the crime scene, as well as at the site of the crime, for comparison to the questioned soil. Soil specimens also should be collected at all possible alibi locations that the suspect may have claimed. All specimens gathered should be representative of the soil that was removed by the suspect. In most cases, only the top layer of soil is picked up during the commission of a crime. Soil found on a suspect must be carefully preserved for analysis. Items bearing soil should be carefully and individually wrapped in paper bags and sent to the laboratory for analysis. When a lump of soil is found, it should be collected and preserved intact as the composition of the layers in the sample might yield important information.

Review Questions

1. The presence of _____ elements in materials provides useful "invisible" markers when comparing physical evidence.

2. The proton and electron (are, are not) of approximately equal mass.

3. A proton imparts the nucleus of an atom with a _____ charge.

4. The number of protons (is, is not) always equal to the number of electrons in orbit around the nucleus of an atom.

5. Each atom of the same element always has the same number of _____ in its nucleus.

6. The number of protons in the nucleus of an atom is called the _____.

7. The knowledge that elements selectively _____ and _____ light provides the basis for important analytical techniques designed to detect the presence of elements in materials.

8. A(n) _____ is a display of colors or frequencies emitted from a light source.

9. True or False: A continuous spectrum consists of a blending of colors. _____

10. A(n) _____ spectrum shows distinct frequencies or wavelengths of light.

11. A line spectrum of an element (is, is not) characteristic of the element.

12. Three important subatomic particles of the atom are the _____, _____, and _____.

13. The total number of protons and neutrons present in a nucleus is known as the _____.

14. Atoms differing only in the number of neutrons present in their nuclei are called _____.

15. True or False: Deuterium has the greatest number of protons of all the isotopes of hydrogen. _____

16. Radioactivity is composed of the following emissions: _____, _____, and _____.

17. Beta particles are identical to _____.

18. Electromagnetic waves similar to X-rays but of a higher energy are _____.

19. A nuclear reactor is a source of _____.

20. The technique of bombarding specimens with neutrons and measuring the resultant gamma ray emissions is known as _____.

21. The two most important components of dried paint from the criminalist's point of view are the _____ and the _____.

22. The most important physical property of paint in a forensic comparison is _____.

23. Paints can be individualized to a single source only when they have a sufficiently detailed _____.

24. The _____ layer provides corrosion resistance for the automobile.

25. "Eye appeal" of the automobile comes from the _____ layer.

26. Pyrolysis gas chromatography is a particularly valuable technique for characterizing paint's (binder, pigments).

27. True or False: Emission spectroscopy can be used to identify the components of paint's pigments.

28. True or False: Paint samples removed for examination must always include all of the paint layers. _____

29. True or False: Most soils have indistinguishable color and texture. _____

30. Naturally occurring crystals commonly found in soils are _____.

31. True or False: The ultimate value of soil as evidence depends on its variation at the crime scene. _____

32. To develop an idea of the soil variation within the crime-scene area, standard/reference soils should be collected at various intervals within a(n) _____ foot radius of the crime scene.

33. True or False: Each object collected at the crime scene that contains soil evidence must be individually wrapped in plastic, with the soil intact, and transmitted to the laboratory.

Review Questions for Inside the Science

1. True or False: Matter in a solid or liquid state produces an emission spectrum that is characteristic of its composition. _____

2. The _____ is an instrument used to obtain and record the line spectrum of elements.

3. Excitation of a specimen can be accomplished when it is inserted between two _____ electrodes.

4. True or False: Each element has its own characteristic set of energy levels. _____

5. True or False: To move an electron from one energy level to the next requires a definite amount of energy. _____

6. As an electron falls from a higher to a lower energy level, it emits _____.

Application and Critical Thinking

1. You are investigating a hit-and-run accident and have identified a suspect vehicle. Describe how you would collect paint to determine whether the suspect vehicle was involved in the accident. Be sure to indicate the tools you would use and the steps you would take to prevent cross-contamination.

2. A forensic analyst at the local crime lab receives pieces of a disfigured bullet from a crime scene. She then obtains an exemplar bullet fired by the firearms analyst from the suspect's firearm. What is the next step in analysis?

3. Only a handful of crime laboratories worldwide have access to a nuclear reactor to carry out neutron activation analysis. What are some possible reasons why this is so?

4. Criminalist Jared Heath responds to the scene of an assault, on an unpaved lane in a rural neighborhood. Rain had fallen steadily the night before, making the area quite muddy. A suspect with very muddy shoes was apprehended nearby but claims to have picked up the mud either from his garden or from the unpaved parking lot of a local restaurant. Jared uses a spade to remove several samples of soil, each about 2 inches deep, from the immediate crime scene and places each in a separate plastic vial. He collects the muddy shoes and wraps them in plastic as well. At the laboratory, he unpackages the soil samples and examines them carefully, one at a time. He then analyzes the soil on the shoes to see whether it matches the soil from the crime scene. What mistakes, if any, did Jared make in his investigation?

Further References

Caddy, B., ed., *Forensic Examination of Glass and Paint.* Boca Raton, FL: CRC Press, 2001.

Forensic Analysis: Weighing Bullet Lead Evidence. Washington, D.C.: National Academies Press, 2004.

Houck, Max M., ed., *Mute Witnesses: Trace Evidence Analysis.* Burlington, MA: Elsevier Academic Press, 2001.

Houck, Max M., ed., *Trace Evidence Analysis—More Cases in Mute Witnesses.* Burlington, MA: Elsevier Academic Press, 2004.

Murray, R. C., *Evidence from the Earth: Forensic Geology and Criminal Investigation*, 2nd ed. Missoula, MT: Mountain Press, 2014.

Murray, R. C., and L. P. Solebello, "Forensic Examination of Soil," in R. Saferstein, ed. *Forensic Science Handbook*, vol. 1, 2nd ed. Upper Saddle River, NJ: Prentice Hall, 2002.

Pye, K., *Geological and Soil Evidence: Forensic Applications.* Boca Raton, FL: CRC Press, 2007.

Thornton, J. L., "Forensic Paint Examination," in R. Saferstein, ed., *Forensic Science Handbook*, vol. 1, 2nd ed. Upper Saddle River, NJ: Prentice Hall, 2002.

Forensic Serology

After studying this chapter, you should be able to:

15.1 Explain the nature of blood and the concept of antigen–antibody interactions

15.2 Explain the application of serology in typing whole blood

15.3 Describe forensic tests used to characterize a stain as blood

15.4 Discuss the principles of heredity

15.5 Summarize the laboratory tests necessary to characterize seminal stains

15.6 Describe the collection and analysis of physical evidence in a rape investigation

Go to www.pearsonhighered.com/careersresources to access Webextras for this chapter.

KEY TERMS

acid phosphatase
agglutination
allele
antibody
antigen
antiserum
aspermia
chromosome
deoxyribonucleic acid
  (DNA)
egg
erythrocyte
gene
genotype
hemoglobin
heterozygous
homozygous
hybridoma cells
locus
luminol
monoclonal antibodies
oligospermia
phenotype
plasma
polyclonal antibodies
precipitin
serology
serum
sperm
X chromosome
Y chromosome
Zygote

O. J. Simpson—A Mountain of Evidence

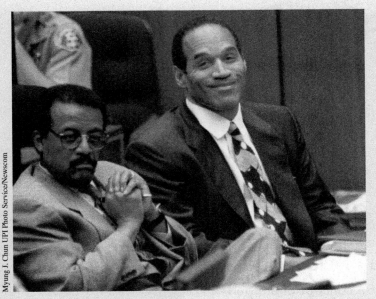

Myung J. Chun UPI Photo Service/Newscom

On June 12, 1994, police arrived at the home of Nicole Simpson only to view a horrific scene. The bodies of O. J. Simpson's estranged wife and her friend Ron Goldman were found on the path leading to the front door of Nicole's home. Both bodies were covered in blood and had suffered deep knife wounds. Nicole's head was nearly severed from her body. This was not a well-planned murder. A trail of blood led away from the murder scene. Blood was found in O. J. Simpson's Bronco. Blood drops were on O. J.'s driveway and in the foyer of his home. A blood-soaked sock was located in O. J. Simpson's bedroom, and a bloodstained glove rested outside his residence.

As DNA was extracted and profiled from each bloodstained article, a picture emerged that seemed to irrefutably link Simpson to the murders. A trail of DNA leaving the crime scene was consistent with O. J.'s profile, as was the DNA found entering Simpson's home. Simpson's DNA profile was found in the Bronco along with that of both victims. The glove contained the DNA profiles of Nicole and Ron, and the sock had Nicole's DNA profile. At trial, the defense team valiantly fought back. Miscues in evidence collection were craftily exploited. The defense strategy was to paint a picture of not only an incompetent investigation, but one that was tinged with dishonest police planting evidence. The strategy worked. O. J. Simpson was acquitted of murder.

In 1901, Karl Landsteiner announced one of the most significant discoveries of the 20th century—the typing of blood—a finding that 29 years later earned him a Nobel Prize. For years, physicians had attempted to transfuse blood from one individual to another. Their efforts often ended in failure because the transfused blood tended to coagulate in the body of the recipient, causing instantaneous death. Landsteiner was the first to recognize that all human blood was not the same; instead, he found that blood is distinguishable by its group or type. Out of Landsteiner's work came the classification system that we call the A-B-O system. Now physicians had the key for properly matching the blood of a donor to a recipient. One blood type cannot be mixed with a different blood type without disastrous consequences. This discovery, of course, had important implications for blood transfusion and the millions of lives it has since saved. Meanwhile, Landsteiner's findings had opened up a completely new field of research in the biological sciences. Others began to pursue the identification of additional characteristics that could further differentiate blood. By 1937, the Rh factor in blood was demonstrated, and shortly thereafter, numerous blood factors or groups were discovered. More than a hundred different blood factors have been shown to exist. However, the ones in the A-B-O system are still the most important for properly matching a donor and recipient for a transfusion.

Until the early 1990s, forensic scientists focused on blood factors, such as A-B-O, as offering the best means for linking blood to an individual. What made these factors so attractive to the forensic scientist was that in theory no two individuals, except for identical twins, could be expected to have the same combination of blood factors. In other words, blood factors are controlled genetically and have the potential of being a highly distinctive feature for personal identification. What makes this observation so relevant is the high frequency of occurrence of bloodstains at crime scenes, especially crimes of the most serious nature—that is, homicides, assaults, and rapes. Consider, for example, a transfer of blood between the victim and assailant during a struggle; that is, the victim's blood is transferred to the suspect's garment, or vice versa. If the criminalist could individualize human blood by identifying all of its known factors, the result would be evidence of the strongest kind for linking the suspect to the crime scene.

The advent of DNA technology has dramatically altered the approach of forensic scientists toward individualization of bloodstains and other biological evidence. The search for genetically controlled blood factors in bloodstains has been abandoned in favor of characterizing biological evidence by select regions of our **deoxyribonucleic acid (DNA)**. The individualization of dried blood and other biological evidence, now a reality, has significantly altered the role that crime laboratories play in criminal investigations. As we will learn in the next chapter, the high sensitivity of DNA analysis has even altered the type of materials collected from crime scenes in the search for DNA. The next chapter is devoted to discussing recent breakthroughs in associating blood and semen stains with a single individual through characterization of DNA. This chapter focuses on underlying biological concepts that forensic scientists historically relied on as they sought to characterize and individualize biological evidence before the dawning of the age of DNA.

deoxyribonucleic acid (DNA)
The molecules carrying the body's genetic information; DNA is double stranded in the shape of a double helix.

The Nature of Blood

The word *blood* actually refers to a highly complex mixture of cells, enzymes, proteins, and inorganic substances. The fluid portion of blood is called **plasma**. Plasma is composed principally of water and accounts for 55 percent of blood content. Suspended in the plasma are solid materials consisting chiefly of cells—that is, red blood cells (**erythrocytes**), white blood cells (leukocytes), and platelets. The solid portion of blood accounts for 45 percent of its content. Blood clots when a protein in the plasma known as fibrin traps and enmeshes the red blood cells. If one were to remove the clotted material, a pale yellowish liquid known as serum would be left.

Obviously, considering the complexity of blood, any discussion of its function and chemistry would have to be extensive, extending beyond the scope of this text. It is certainly far more relevant at this point to concentrate our discussion on the blood components that are directly pertinent to the forensic aspects of blood identification—the red blood cells and the blood **serum**.

plasma
The fluid portion of unclotted blood.

erythrocyte
A red blood cell.

serum
The liquid that separates from the blood when a clot is formed.

Antigens and Antibodies

Functionally, red blood cells transport oxygen from the lungs to the body tissues and in turn remove carbon dioxide from tissues by transporting it back to the lungs, where it is exhaled. However, for reasons unrelated to the red blood cell's transporting mission, on the surface of each cell are millions of characteristic chemical structures called **antigens**. Antigens impart blood-type characteristics to the red blood cells. Blood antigens are grouped

antigen
A substance, usually a protein that stimulates the body to produce antibodies against it.

into systems depending on their relationship to one another. More than 15 blood antigen systems have been identified to date; of these, the A-B-O and Rh systems are the most important.

If an individual is type A, this simply indicates that each red blood cell has A antigens on its surface; similarly, all type B individuals have B antigens; and the red blood cells of type AB contain both A and B antigens. Type O individuals have neither A nor B antigens on their cells. Hence, the presence or absence of the A and B antigens on the red blood cells determines a person's blood type in the A-B-O system.

Another important blood antigen has been designated as the Rh factor, or D antigen. People with the D antigen are said to be Rh positive; those without this antigen are Rh negative. In routine blood banking, the presence or absence of the three antigens—A, B, and D—must be determined in testing for the compatibility of the donor and recipient.

Serum is important because it contains certain proteins known as **antibodies**. The fundamental principle of blood typing is that for every antigen, there exists a specific antibody. Each antibody symbol contains the prefix anti-, followed by the name of the antigen for which it is specific. Hence, anti-A is specific only for A antigen, anti-B for B antigen, and anti-D for D antigen. The serum-containing antibody is referred to as the **antiserum**, meaning a serum that reacts against something (antigens).

An antibody reacts only with its specific antigen, and no other. Thus, if serum containing anti-B is added to red blood cells carrying the B antigen, the two immediately combine, causing the antibody to attach itself to the cell. Antibodies are normally bivalent—that is, they have two reactive sites. This means that each antibody can simultaneously be attached to antigens located on two different red blood cells. This creates a vast network of cross-linked cells usually seen as clumping or **agglutination** (see Figure 15–1).

Let's look a little more closely at this phenomenon. In normal blood, shown in Figure 15–2 (a), antigens on red blood cells and antibodies coexist without destroying each other because the antibodies present are not specific toward any of the antigens. However, suppose a foreign serum added to the blood introduces a new antibody. The occurrence of a specific antigen–antibody reaction immediately causes the red blood cells to link together, or agglutinate, as shown in Figure 15–2(b).

antibody
A protein that destroys or inactivates a specific antigen; antibodies are found in the blood serum.

antiserum
Blood serum that contains specific antibodies.

agglutination
The clumping together of red blood cells by the action of an antibody.

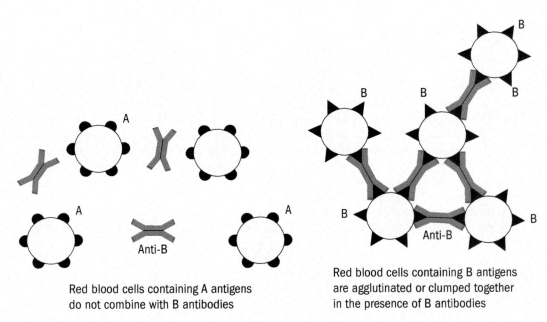

Red blood cells containing A antigens do not combine with B antibodies

Red blood cells containing B antigens are agglutinated or clumped together in the presence of B antibodies

FIGURE 15–1
Agglutination of blood cells.

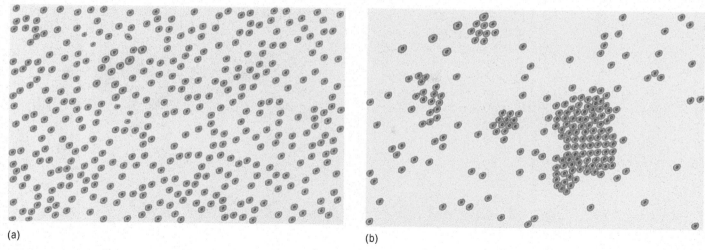

(a)   (b)

FIGURE 15–2

(a) Microscopic view of normal red blood cells (500×). (b) Microscopic view of agglutinated red blood cells (500×).

Evidently, nature has taken this situation into account because when we examine the serum of type A blood, we find anti-B and no anti-A. Similarly, type B blood contains only anti-A, type O blood has both anti-A and anti-B, and type AB blood contains neither anti-A nor anti-B. The antigen and antibody components of normal blood are summarized in the following table:

Blood Type	Antigens on Red Blood Cells	Antibodies in Serum
A	A	Anti-B
B	B	Anti-A
AB	AB	Neither anti-A nor anti-B
O	Neither A nor B	Both anti-A and anti-B

The reasons for the fatal consequences of mixing incompatible blood during a transfusion should now be quite obvious. For example, transfusing type A blood into a type B patient will cause the natural anti-A in the blood of the type B patient to react promptly with the incoming A antigens, resulting in agglutination. In addition, the incoming anti-B of the donor will react with the B antigens of the patient.

Blood Typing

The term **serology** is used to describe a broad scope of laboratory tests that use specific antigen and serum antibody reactions. The most widespread application of serology is the typing of whole blood for its A-B-O identity. In determining the A-B-O blood type, only two antiserums are needed—anti-A and anti-B. For routine blood typing, both of these antiserums are commercially available.

Table 15–1 summarizes how the identity of each of the four blood groups is established when the blood is tested with anti-A and anti-B serum. Type A blood is agglutinated by anti-A serum; type B blood is agglutinated by anti-B serum; type AB blood is agglutinated by both anti-A and anti-B; and type O blood is not agglutinated by either the anti-A or anti-B serum (see Figure 15–3).

serology
The study of antigen–antibody reactions.

FIGURE 15–3

A blood test for types A, B, AB, and O. Commercial antisera are systematically applied to a questioned blood in order to determine blood type.

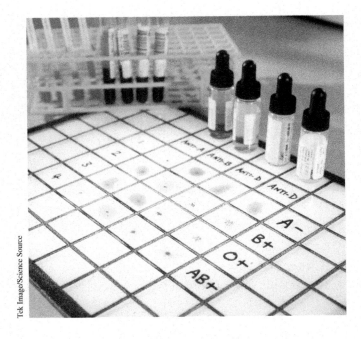

Tek Image/Science Source

The identification of natural antibodies present in blood offers another route to the determination of blood type. Testing blood for the presence of anti-A and anti-B requires using red blood cells that have known antigens. Again, these cells are commercially available. Hence, when A cells are added to a blood specimen, agglutination occurs only in the presence of anti-A. Similarly, B cells agglutinate only in the presence of anti-B. All four A-B-O types can be identified in this manner by testing blood with known A and B cells, as summarized in Table 15–2.

TABLE 15–1

Identification of Blood with Known Antiserum

Anti-A Serum + Whole Blood	Anti-B Serum + Whole Blood	Antigen Present	Blood Type
+	−	A	A
−	+	B	B
+	+	A and B	AB
−	−	Neither A nor B	O

Note: + shows agglutination; − shows absence of agglutination.

TABLE 15–2

Identification of Blood with Known Cells

A Cells + Blood	B Cells + Blood	Antibody Present	Blood Type
+	−	Anti-A	B
−	+	Anti-B	A
+	+	Both anti-A and anti-B	O
−	−	Neither anti-A nor anti-B	AB

Note: + shows agglutination; − shows absence of agglutination.

The population distribution of blood types varies with location and ancestry throughout the world. In the United States, a typical distribution is as follows:

O	A	B	AB
43 %	42 %	12 %	3 %

Immunoassay Techniques

The concept of a specific antigen–antibody reaction is finding application in other areas unrelated to the blood typing of individuals. Most significantly, this approach has been extended to the detection of drugs in blood and urine. Antibodies that react with drugs do not naturally exist; however, they can be produced in animals such as rabbits by first combining the drug with a protein and injecting this combination into the animal. This drug–protein complex acts as an antigen stimulating the animal to produce antibodies (see Figure 15–4). The recovered blood serum of the animal will contain antibodies that are specific or nearly specific to the drug.

Currently, thousands of individuals regularly submit to urinalysis tests for the presence of drugs. These individuals include military personnel, transportation industry employees, police and corrections personnel, and subjects requiring preemployment drug screening. Immunoassay testing for drugs has proven quite suitable for handling the large volume of specimens that must be rapidly analyzed for drug content on a daily basis. Testing laboratories have access to many commercially prepared sera arising from animals being injected with any one of a variety of drugs. A particular serum that has been added to a urine specimen is designed to interact with opiates, cannabinoids, cocaine, amphetamines, phencyclidine, barbiturates, methadone, or other drugs. A word of caution: Immunoassay is only presumptive in nature, and its result must be confirmed by additional testing. Specifically, the confirmation test of choice is gas chromatography-mass spectrometry, which is described in more detail in Chapter 12.

Forensic Characterization of Bloodstains

The criminalist must answer the following questions when examining dried blood: (1) Is it blood? (2) From what species did the blood originate? (3) If the blood is of human origin, how closely can it be associated with a particular individual?

Color Tests

The determination of blood is best made by means of a preliminary color test. For many years, the most commonly used test for this purpose was the benzidine color test; however, because benzidine has been identified as a known carcinogen, its use has generally been discontinued, and the chemical phenolphthalein is usually substituted in its place (this test is also known as the Kastle–Meyer color test).[1] Both the benzidine and Kastle–Meyer color tests are based on the observation that blood **hemoglobin** possesses peroxidase-like activity. Peroxidases are enzymes

hemoglobin
A red blood cell protein that transports oxygen in the bloodstream; it is responsible for the red color of blood.

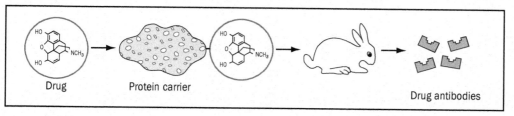

Drug   Protein carrier   Drug antibodies

FIGURE 15–4

Stimulating production of drug antibodies.

[1] S. Tobe et al., "Evaluation of Six Presumptive Tests for Blood, Their Specificity, Sensitivity, and Effect on High Molecular-Weight DNA," *Journal of Forensic Sciences* 52 (2007): 102–109.

Inside the Science

The Enzyme Multiplied Immunoassay Technique

Several immunological assay techniques are commercially available for detecting drugs through an antigen–antibody reaction. One such technique, the *enzyme-multiplied immunoassay technique (EMIT)*, has gained widespread popularity among toxicologists because of its speed and high sensitivity for detecting drugs in urine.

A typical EMIT analysis begins by adding to a subject's urine antibodies that bind to a particular type or class of drug being looked for. This is followed by adding to the urine a chemically labeled version of the drug. As shown in the figure, a competition will ensue between the labeled and unlabeled drug (if it's present in the subject's urine) to bind with the antibody. If this competition does occur in a person's urine, it signifies that the urine screen test was positive for the drug being tested. For example, to check someone's urine for methadone, the analyst would add methadone antibodies and chemically labeled methadone to the urine. Any methadone present in the urine immediately competes with the labeled methadone to bind with the methadone antibodies.

The quantity of chemically labeled methadone left uncombined is then measured, and this value is related to the concentration of methadone originally present in the urine.

One of the most frequent uses of EMIT in forensic laboratories has been for screening the urine of suspected marijuana users. The primary pharmacologically active agent in marijuana is tetrahydrocannabinol, or THC. To facilitate the elimination of THC, the body converts it to a series of substances called *metabolites* that are more readily excreted. The major THC metabolite found in urine is a substance called *THC-9-carboxylic acid*. Antibodies against this metabolite are prepared for EMIT testing. Normally, the urine of marijuana users contains a very small quantity of THC-9-carboxylic acid (less than one-millionth of a gram); however, this level is readily detected by EMIT.

The greatest problem with detecting marijuana in urine is interpretation. Although smoking marijuana will result in the detection of THC metabolite, it is difficult to determine when the individual actually used marijuana. In individuals who smoke marijuana frequently, detection is possible within two to five days after the last use of the drug. However, some individuals may yield positive results up to 30 days after the last use of marijuana.

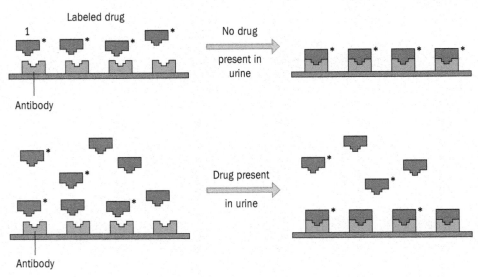

In the EMIT assay, a drug that may be present in a urine specimen will compete with added labeled drugs for a limited number of antibody binding sites. The labeled drugs are indicated by an asterisk. Once the competition for antibody sites is completed, the number of remaining unbound labeled drug is proportional to the drug's concentration in urine.

Inside the Science

Polyclonal and Monoclonal Antibodies

As we have seen in the previous section, when an animal such as a rabbit or mouse is injected with an antigen, the animal responds by producing antibodies designed to bind to the invading antigen. However, the process of producing antibodies designed to respond to foreign antigens is complex. For one, an antigen typically has structurally different sites to which an antibody may bind. So when the animal is actively producing attack antibodies, it produces a series of different antibodies, all of which are designed to attack some particular site on the antigen of interest. These antibodies are known as **polyclonal antibodies**.

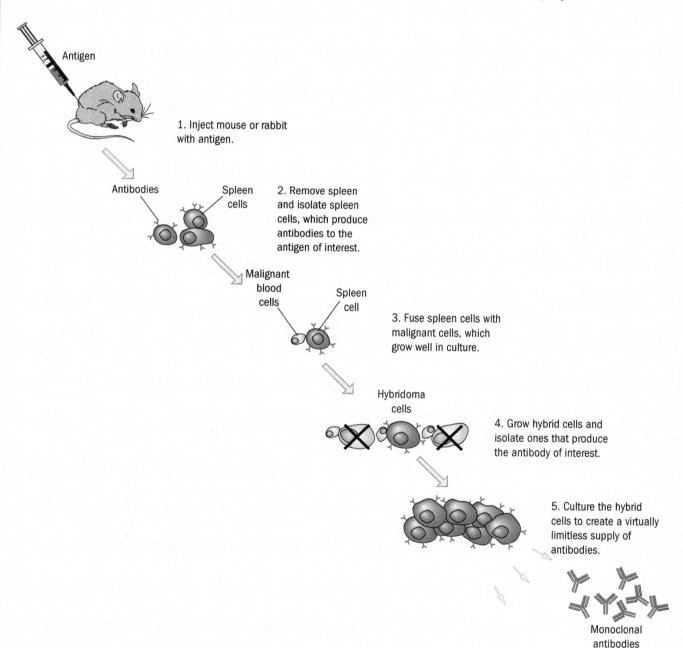

Antigen

1. Inject mouse or rabbit with antigen.

Antibodies   Spleen cells

2. Remove spleen and isolate spleen cells, which produce antibodies to the antigen of interest.

Malignant blood cells   Spleen cell

3. Fuse spleen cells with malignant cells, which grow well in culture.

Hybridoma cells

4. Grow hybrid cells and isolate ones that produce the antibody of interest.

5. Culture the hybrid cells to create a virtually limitless supply of antibodies.

Monoclonal antibodies

Steps required to produce monoclonal antibodies.

(continued)

However, the disadvantage of polyclonal antibodies is that an animal can produce antibodies that vary in composition over time. As a result, different batches of polyclonals may vary in their specificity and their ability to bind to a particular antigen site.

As the technologies associated with forensic science have grown in importance, a need has developed, in some instances, to have access to antibodies that are more uniform in their composition and attack power than the traditional polyclonals. This is best accomplished by adopting a process in which an animal will produce antibodies designed to attack one and only one site on an antigen. Such antibodies are known as **monoclonal antibodies**. How can such monoclonals be produced? The process begins by injecting a mouse with the antigen of interest. In response, the mouse's spleen cells will produce antibodies to fight off the invading antigen. The spleen cells are removed from the animal and are fused to fast-growing blood cancer cells to produce **hybridoma cells**. The hybridoma cells are then allowed to multiply and are screened for their specific antibody activity. The hybridoma cells that bear the antibody activity of interest are then selected and cultured. The rapidly multiplying cancer cells linked to the selected antibody cells produce identical monoclonal antibodies in a limitless supply, as shown in the figure.

Monoclonal antibodies are being incorporated into commercial forensic test kits with increasing frequency. Many immunoassay test kits for drugs of abuse are being formulated with monoclonal antibodies. Also, an immunological test for seminal material that incorporates a monoclonal antibody has found wide popularity in crime laboratories (see pages 392–393).

As a side note, in 1999, the U.S. Food and Drug Administration approved a monoclonal drug treatment for cancer. Rituxin is a nontoxic monoclonal antibody designed to attack and destroy cancerous white blood cells containing an antigen designated as CD20. Other monoclonal drug treatments are in the pipeline. Monoclonals are finally beginning to fulfill their long-held expectation as medicine's version of the "magic bullet."

polyclonal antibodies
Antibodies produced by injecting animals with a specific antigen; a series of antibodies is produced responding to a variety of different sites on the antigen.

monoclonal antibodies
A collection of identical antibodies that interact with a single antigen site.

hybridoma cells
Fused spleen and tumor cells; used to produce identical monoclonal antibodies in a limitless supply.

WEBEXTRA 15.1
See a Color Test for Blood

WEBEXTRA 15.2
See How the Hemastix Test Is Run for Blood

luminol
The most sensitive chemical test that is capable of presumptively detecting bloodstains diluted to as little as 1 in 100,000; its reaction with blood emits light and thus requires the result to be observed in a darkened area.

that accelerate the oxidation of several classes of organic compounds by peroxides. When a bloodstain, phenolphthalein reagent, and hydrogen peroxide are mixed together, the blood's hemoglobin causes the formation of a deep pink color.

The Kastle–Meyer test is not a specific test for blood; some vegetable materials, for instance, may turn Kastle–Meyer pink. These substances include potatoes and horseradish. However, it is unlikely that such materials will be encountered in criminal situations, and thus from a practical point of view, a positive Kastle–Meyer test is highly indicative of blood. Field investigators have found Hemastix strips a useful presumptive field test for blood. Designed as a urine dipstick test for blood, the strip can be moistened with distilled water and placed in contact with a suspect bloodstain. The appearance of a green color is indicative of blood.

Luminol and Bluestar

Another important presumptive identification test for blood is the **luminol** test.[2] Unlike the benzidine and Kastle–Meyer tests, the reaction of luminol with blood produces light rather than color. By spraying luminol reagent onto a suspect item, investigators can quickly screen large areas for bloodstains. The sprayed objects must be located in a darkened area while being viewed for the emission of light (luminescence); any bloodstains produce a faint blue glow. A relatively new product, Bluestar, is now available to be used in place of luminol (http://www.bluestar-forensic.com). Bluestar is easy to mix in the field. Its reaction with blood can be observed readily without having to create complete darkness. The luminol and Bluestar tests are extremely sensitive—capable of detecting bloodstains diluted to as little as 1 in 100,000. For this reason, spraying large areas such as carpets, walls, flooring, or the interior of a vehicle may reveal blood traces or patterns that would have gone unnoticed under normal lighting conditions (see Figure 15–5). It is important to note that luminol and Bluestar do not interfere with any subsequent DNA testing.[3]

[2] The luminol reagent is prepared by mixing 0.1 grams 3-amino-phthalhydrazide and 5.0 grams sodium carbonate in 100 milliliters distilled water. Before use, 0.7 grams sodium perborate is added to the solution.

[3] A. M. Gross et al., "The Effect of Luminol on Presumptive Tests and DNA Analysis Using the Polymerase Chain Reaction," *Journal of Forensic Sciences* 44 (1999): 837.

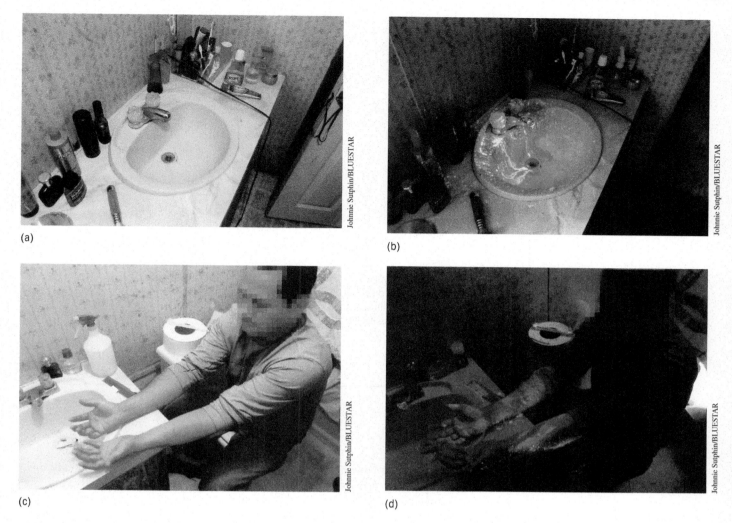

FIGURE 15–5

(a) Sink and arms before applications of Bluestar reagent. (b) Bluestar applications reveals bloodstain patterns.

Microcrystalline Tests

The identification of blood can be made more specific if microcrystalline tests are performed on the material. Several tests are available; the two most popular ones are the Takayama and Teichmann tests. Both of these depend on the addition of specific chemicals to the blood so that characteristic crystals with hemoglobin derivatives will form. Crystal tests are far less sensitive than color tests for blood identification and are more susceptible to interference from contaminants that may be present in the stain.

Precipitin Test

Once the stain has been characterized as blood, the serologist determines whether the stain is of human or animal origin. For this purpose, the standard test used is the **precipitin** test. Precipitin tests are based on the fact that when animals (usually rabbits) are injected with human blood, antibodies form that react with the invading human blood to neutralize its presence. The investigator can recover these antibodies by bleeding the animal and isolating the blood serum. This serum contains antibodies that specifically react with human antigens. For this reason, the serum is known as human antiserum. In the same manner, by injecting rabbits with the blood of other known animals, virtually any kind of animal antiserum can be produced. Currently, antiserums are commercially available for humans and for a variety of commonly encountered animals—for example, dogs, cats, and deer.

precipitin
An antibody that reacts with its corresponding antigen to form a precipitate.

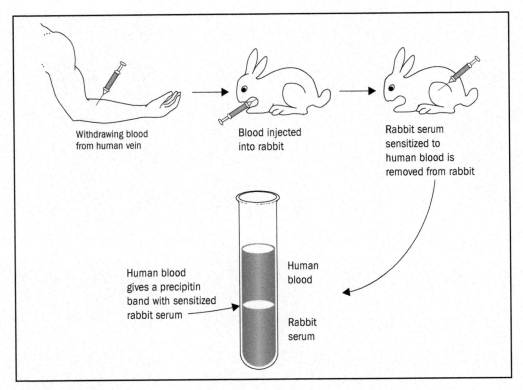

FIGURE 15–6
The precipitin test.

A number of techniques have been devised for performing precipitin tests on bloodstains. The classic method is to layer an extract of the bloodstain on top of the human antiserum in a capillary tube. Human blood, or for that matter, any protein of human origin in the extract, reacts specifically with antibodies present in the antiserum, as indicated by the formation of a cloudy ring or band at the interface of the two liquids (see Figure 15–6).

Gel Diffusion

Another version of the precipitin test, called gel diffusion, takes advantage of the fact that antibodies and antigens diffuse or move toward one another on a plate coated with a gel medium made from a natural polymer called agar. The extracted bloodstain and the human antiserum are placed in separate holes opposite each other on the gel. If the blood is of human origin, a line of precipitation will form where the antigens and antibodies meet.

Similarly, the antigens and antibodies can be induced to move toward one another under the influence of an electrical field. In the electrophoretic method, an electrical potential is applied to the gel medium; a specific antigen–antibody reaction is denoted by a line of precipitation formed between the hole containing the blood extract and the hole containing the human antiserum (see Figure 15–7).

The precipitin test is very sensitive and requires only a small amount of blood for testing. Human bloodstains dried for 10 to 15 years and longer may still give a positive precipitin reaction. Even extracts of tissue from mummies four to five thousand years old have given positive reactions with this test. Furthermore, human bloodstains diluted by washing in water and left with only a faint color may still yield a positive precipitin reaction (see Figure 15–8).

Once it has been determined that the bloodstain is of human origin, an effort must be made to associate or disassociate the stain with a particular individual. Until the mid-1990s, routine characterization of bloodstains included the determination of A-B-O types; however, the widespread use of DNA profiling or typing has relegated this subject to one of historical interest only.

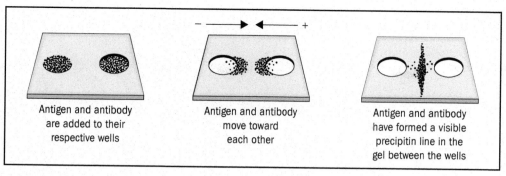

FIGURE 15–7

Antigens and antibodies moving toward one another under the influence of an electrical potential.

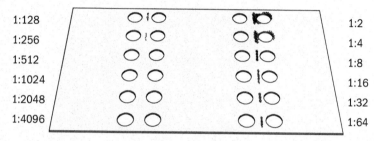

FIGURE 15–8

Results of the precipitin test of dilutions of human serum up to 1 in 4,096 against a human antiserum. A reaction is visible for blood dilutions up to 1 in 256.

Principles of Heredity

All of the antigens that have been described in previous sections are genetically controlled traits. That is, they are inherited from parents and become a permanent feature of a person's biological makeup from the moment the person is conceived. Determining the identity of these traits, then, not only provides us with a picture of how one individual compares to or differs from another, but gives us an insight into the basic biological substances that determine our overall makeup as human beings and the mechanism by which those substances are transmitted from one generation to the next.

Genes and Chromosomes

Hereditary material is transmitted via microscopic units called **genes**. The gene is the basic unit of heredity. Each gene by itself or in concert with other genes controls the development of a specific characteristic in the new individual; the genes determine the nature and growth of virtually every body structure.

The genes are positioned on **chromosomes**, threadlike bodies that appear in the nucleus of every body cell (see Figure 15–9). All nucleated human cells contain 46 chromosomes, mated in 23 pairs. The only exceptions are the nucleated human reproductive cells, the **egg** and **sperm**, which contain only 23 unmated chromosomes. During fertilization, a sperm and egg combine so that each contributes chromosomes to form the new cell (**zygote**). Hence, the new individual begins life properly with 23 mated chromosome pairs. Because the genes are positioned on the chromosomes, the new individual inherits genetic material from each parent.

Actually, two dissimilar chromosomes are involved in the determination of sex. The egg cell always contains a long chromosome known as the **X chromosome**, but the sperm cell may contain either a short chromosome, known as the **Y chromosome**, or a long X chromosome. When an X-carrying sperm fertilizes an egg, the new cell is XX and develops into a female.

WEBEXTRA 15.3
Learn About the Chromosomes
Present in Our Cells

gene
A unit of inheritance consisting of a DNA segment located on a chromosome.

chromosome
A rodlike structure in the cell nucleus, along which the genes are located; it is composed of DNA surrounded by other material, mainly proteins.

egg
The female reproductive cell.

sperm
The male reproductive cell.

zygote
The cell arising from the union of an egg and a sperm cell.

X chromosome
The female sex chromosome.

Y chromosome
The male sex chromosome.

FIGURE 15–9

Computer-enhanced photo-micrograph image of human chromosomes.

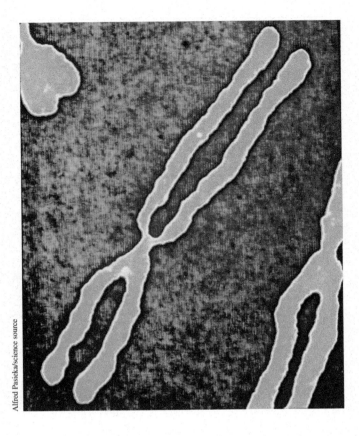

Alfred Pasieka/science source

locus
The physical location of a gene on a chromosome.

allele
Any of several alternative forms of a gene located at the same point on a particular pair of chromosomes; for example, the genes determining the blood types A and B are alleles.

homozygous
Having two identical allelic genes on two corresponding positions of a pair of chromosomes.

heterozygous
Having two different allelic genes on two corresponding positions of a pair of chromosomes.

WEBEXTRA 15.4
Learn About the Structure of Our Genes

WEBEXTRA 15.5
See How Genes Position Themselves on a Chromosome Pair

WEBEXTRA 15.6
See How Genes Define Our Genetic Makeup

A Y-carrying sperm produces an XY fertilized egg and develops into a male. Because the sperm cell ultimately determines the nature of the chromosome pair, we can say that the father biologically determines the sex of the child.

ALLELES   Just as chromosomes come together in pairs, so do the genes they bear. The position a gene occupies on a chromosome is its **locus**. Genes that govern a given characteristic are similarly positioned on the chromosomes inherited from the mother and father. Thus, a gene for eye color on the mother's chromosome will be aligned with a gene for eye color on the corresponding chromosome inherited from the father. Alternative forms of genes that influence a given characteristic and are aligned with one another on a chromosome pair are known as **alleles**.

Another simple example of allele genes in humans is that of blood types belonging to the A-B-O system. Inheritance of the A-B-O type is best described by a theory that uses three genes designated A, B, and O. A gene pair made up of two similar genes—for example, AA and BB—is said to be **homozygous**; a gene pair made up of two different genes—AO, for example—is said to be **heterozygous**. If the chromosome inherited from the father carries the A gene and the chromosome inherited from the mother carries the same gene, the offspring would have an AA combination. Similarly, if one chromosome contains the A gene and the other has the O gene, the genetic makeup of the offspring would be AO.

DOMINANT AND RECESSIVE GENES   When an individual inherits two similar genes from their parents, there is no problem in determining the blood type of that person. Hence, an AA combination will always be type A, a BB type B, and an OO type O. However, when two different genes are inherited, one gene will be dominant. It can be said that the A and B genes are dominant and that the O gene is always recessive—that is, its characteristics remain hidden. For instance, with an AO combination, A is always dominant over O, and the individual will be typed as A. Similarly, a BO combination is typed as B. In the case of AB, the genes are codominant, and the individual's blood type will be AB. The recessive characteristics of O appear only when both recessive genes are present. Hence, the combination OO is typed simply as O.

Inside the Science

Genotypes and Phenotypes

A pair of allele genes together constitutes the **genotype** of the individual. However, no laboratory test can determine an individual's A-B-O genotype. For example, a person's outward characteristic, or **phenotype**, may be type A, but this does not tell us whether their genotype is AA or AO. The genotype can be determined only by studying the family history of the individual. If the genotypes of both parents are known, that of their possible offspring can be forecast.

An easy way to figure this out is to construct a *Punnett square*. To do this, write along a horizontal line the two genes of the male parent, and in the vertical column write the two kinds of female genes present, as shown. In our example, we assume the male parent is type O and therefore has to be an OO genotype; the female parent is type AB and can be only an AB genotype:

Next, write in each box the corresponding gene contributed from the female and then from the male. The squares will contain all the possible genotype combinations that the parents can produce in their offspring:

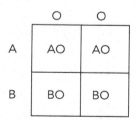

Hence, in this case, 50 percent of the offspring are likely to be AO and the other 50 percent BO. These are the only genotypes possible from this combination. Because O is recessive, 50 percent of the offspring will probably be type A and 50 percent type B. From this example, we can see that no blood group gene can appear in a child unless it is present in at least one of the parents.

Although the genotyping of blood factors has useful applications for studying the transmission of blood characteristics from one generation to the next, it has no direct relevance to criminal investigations. It does, however, have important implications in disputed-paternity cases, which are normally encountered in civil, not criminal, courts.

Many cases of disputed paternity can be resolved when the suspected parents and the offspring are related according to their blood group systems. For instance, in the previous example, had the child been type AB, the suspected father would have been cleared. A type O father and a type AB mother cannot have a type AB child. On the other hand, if the child had been type A or type B, the most that could be said is that the suspect may have been the father; this does not mean that he *is* the father, just that he is not excluded based on blood typing. Obviously, many other males also have type O blood. Of course, the more blood group systems that are tested, the better the chances of excluding an innocent male from involvement. Conversely, if no discrepancies are found between offspring and suspect father, the more certain one can be that the suspect is indeed the father. In fact, routine paternity testing involves characterizing blood factors other than A-B-O. Currently, paternity testing laboratories have implemented tests for DNA alleles that can raise the odds of establishing paternity beyond 99 percent.

Forensic Characterization of Semen

Many cases received in a forensic laboratory involve sexual offenses, making it necessary to examine exhibits for the presence of seminal stains.

The normal male releases 2.5 to 6 milliliters of seminal fluid during an ejaculation. Each milliliter contains 100 million or more spermatozoa, the male reproductive cells. Forensic examination of articles for seminal stains can actually be considered a two-step process. First, before any tests can be conducted, the stain must be located. Considering the number and soiled

genotype
The particular combination of genes present in the cells of an individual.

phenotype
The physical manifestation of a genetic trait such as shape, color, and blood type.

condition of outer garments, undergarments, and possible bedclothing submitted for examination, this may prove to be an arduous task. Once located, the stain will have to be subjected to tests that will prove its identity; it may even be tested for the blood type of the individual from whom it originated.

Testing for Seminal Stains

Often, seminal stains are readily visible on a fabric because they exhibit a stiff, crusty appearance. However, reliance on such appearance for locating the stain is at best unreliable and is useful only when the stain is present in a rather obvious area. Certainly, if the fabric has been washed or contains only minute quantities of semen, visual examination of the article offers little chance of detecting the stain. The best way to locate and characterize a seminal stain is to perform the acid phosphatase color test.

acid phosphatase
An enzyme found in high concentration in semen.

ACID PHOSPHATASE TEST   **Acid phosphatase** is an enzyme that is secreted by the prostate gland into seminal fluid. Its concentrations in seminal fluid are up to 400 times greater than those found in any other body fluid. Its presence can easily be detected when it comes in contact with an acidic solution of sodium alpha naphthylphosphate and Fast Blue B dye. Also, 4-methylumbelliferyl phosphate (MUP) fluoresces under UV light when it comes in contact with acid phosphatase.

The utility of the acid phosphatase test is apparent when it becomes necessary to search numerous garments or large fabric areas for seminal stains. If a filter paper is simply moistened with water and rubbed lightly over the suspect area, acid phosphatase, if present, is transferred to the filter paper. Then, when a drop or two of the sodium alpha naphthylphosphate and Fast Blue B solution are placed on the paper, the appearance of a purple color indicates the acid phosphatase enzyme. In this manner, any fabric or surface can be systematically searched for seminal stains.

WEBEXTRA 15.7
See How the Acid Phosphatase Test for Semen Is Run

If it is necessary to search extremely large areas—for example, a bedsheet or carpet—the article can be tested in sections, narrowing the location of the stain with each successive test. Alternatively, the garment under investigation can be pressed against a suitably sized piece of moistened filter paper. The paper is then sprayed with MUP solution. Semen stains appear as strongly fluorescent areas under UV light. A negative reaction can be interpreted as meaning the absence of semen. Although some vegetable and fruit juices (such as cauliflower and watermelon), fungi, contraceptive creams, and vaginal secretions give a positive response to the acid phosphatase test, none of these substances normally reacts with the speed of seminal fluid. A reaction time of less than 30 seconds is considered a strong indication of the presence of semen.

MICROSCOPIC EXAMINATION OF SEMEN   Semen can be unequivocally identified by the presence of spermatozoa. When spermatozoa are located through a microscope examination, the stain is definitely identified as having been derived from semen. Spermatozoa are slender, elongated structures 50–70 microns long, each with a head and a thin flagellate tail (see Figure 15–10). The criminalist can normally locate them by immersing the stained material in a small volume of water. Rapid stirring of the liquid transfers a small percentage of the spermatozoa present into the water. A drop of the water is dried onto a microscope slide, then stained and examined under a compound microscope at a magnification of approximately 400×.[4] An alternative to the traditional microscopic examination of spermatozoa is searching for spermatozoa with an immunology-fluorescence staining kit which uses a monoclonal antibody to detect an antigen in the sperm head. The kit is designed to have sperm heads fluoresce in green as observed under a properly configured microscope (see Figure 15–11).[5]

Considering the extremely large number of spermatozoa found in seminal fluid, one would think the chance of locating one would be very good; however, this is not always true. One reason is that spermatozoa are bound tightly to cloth materials.[6] Also, spermatozoa are extremely brittle when dry and easily disintegrate if the stain is washed or when the stain is rubbed against another object, as can happen frequently in the handling and packaging of this type of

[4] J. P. Allery et al., "Cytological Detection of Spermatozoa: Comparison of Three Staining Methods," *Journal of Forensic Sciences* 46 (2001): 349.

[5] K. W. P. Miller et al., "Developmental Validation of the SPERM HY-Liter™ for the Identification of Human Spermatozoa in Forensic Samples," *Journal of Forensic Sciences* 56 (2011): 853.

[6] In one study, only a maximum of 4 sperm cells out of 1,000 could be extracted from a cotton patch and observed under the microscope. Edwin Jones (Ventura County Sheriff's Department, Ventura, Calif.), personal communication.

evidence. Furthermore, sexual crimes may involve males who have an abnormally low sperm count, a condition known as **oligospermia**, or they may involve individuals who produce no sperm (**aspermia**). Significantly, aspermatic individuals are increasing in numbers because of the growing popularity of vasectomies.

oligospermia
An abnormally low sperm count.

aspermia
The absence of sperm; sterility in males.

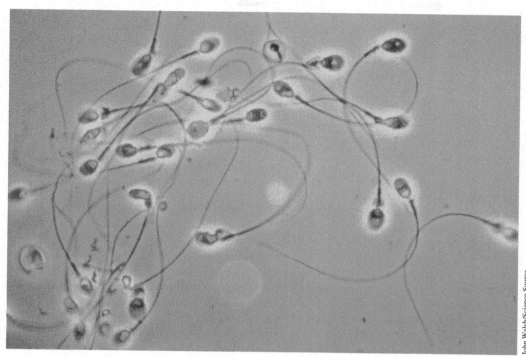

FIGURE 15–10
Photomicrograph of human spermatozoa (300×).

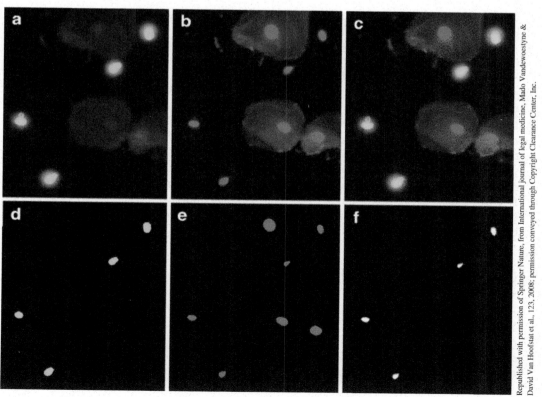

FIGURE 15–11
Fluorescent detection of human sperm heads-sexual assault smear slide.

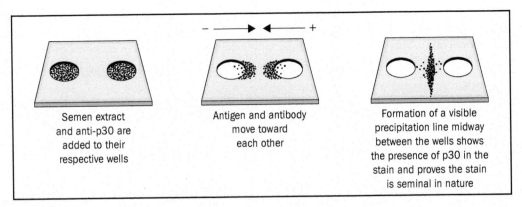

Semen extract
and anti-p30 are
added to their
respective wells

Antigen and antibody
move toward
each other

Formation of a visible
precipitation line midway
between the wells shows
the presence of p30 in the
stain and proves the stain
is seminal in nature

FIGURE 15–12

PSA testing by electrophoresis.

PROSTATE SPECIFIC ANTIGEN (PSA)   Forensic analysts often must examine stains or swabs that they suspect contain semen (because of the presence of acid phosphatase) but that yield no detectable spermatozoa. How, then, can one unequivocally prove the presence of semen? The solution to this problem apparently came with the discovery in the 1970s of a protein called p30 or prostate-specific antigen (PSA). At first, this protein was thought to be prostate specific and hence a unique identifier of semen. However, additional research has shown that low levels of p30 may be detectable in other human tissues. **A more reasonable approach to the unequivocal identification of semen is to use a positive PSA (p30) in combination with an acid phosphatase color test with a reaction time of less than 30 seconds.**[7]

When PSA is isolated and injected into a rabbit, it stimulates the production of polyclonal antibodies (anti-PSA). The sera collected from these immunized rabbits can then be used to test suspected semen stains. As shown in Figure 15–12, the stain extract is placed in one well of an electrophoretic plate and the anti-PSA in an opposite well. When an electric potential is applied, the antigens and antibodies move toward each other. The formation of a visible line midway between the two wells shows the presence of PSA in the stain and proves that the stain was seminal in nature.

A more elegant approach to identifying PSA (p30) involves placing an extract of a questioned sample on a porous membrane in the presence of a monoclonal PSA antibody that is linked to a dye. If PSA is present in the extract, a PSA antigen–monoclonal PSA antibody complex forms. This complex then migrates along the membrane, where it interacts with a polyclonal PSA antibody embedded in the membrane. The antibody–antigen–antibody "sandwich" that forms will be apparent by the presence of a colored line (see Figure 15–13). This monoclonal antibody technique is about a hundred times more sensitive for detecting PSA than the one described in the previous paragraph.

WEBEXTRA 15.8
See How the P30 Test Is Run

Once the material under examination is proven to be semen, the next task is to attempt to associate the semen as closely as possible with a single individual. As we will learn in Chapter 16, forensic scientists can link seminal material to one individual with DNA technology. Just as important is the knowledge that this technology can exonerate many of those wrongfully accused of sexual assault.

Collection and Preservation of Rape Evidence

Seminal constituents on a rape victim are important evidence that sexual intercourse has taken place, but their absence does not necessarily mean that a rape did not occur. Physical injuries such as bruises or bleeding tend to confirm that a violent assault did take place. Furthermore, the forceful physical contact between victim and assailant may result in a transfer of physical

[7] S. Cavness et al., "Hospital Wet Mount Examination for the Presence of Sperm in Sexual Assault Cases Is of Questionable Value," *Journal of forensic Sciences* 59 (2014): 729.

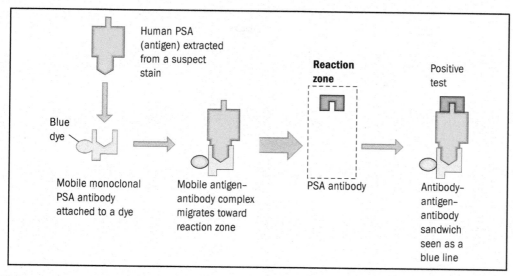

FIGURE 15–13

An antibody–antigen–antibody sandwich or complex is seen as a colored band. This signifies the presence of PSA in the extract of a stain and positively identifies human semen.

evidence—blood, semen, hairs, and fibers. The presence of such physical evidence will help forge a vital link in the chain of circumstances surrounding a sexual crime.

Collection and Handling

To protect this kind of evidence, all the outer garments and undergarments from the involved parties should be carefully removed and packaged separately in paper (not plastic) bags. Place a clean bedsheet on the floor and lay a clean paper sheet over it. The victim must remove their shoes before standing on the paper. Have the person disrobe while standing on the paper in order to collect any loose foreign material falling from the clothing. Collect each piece of clothing as it is removed and place the items in separate paper bags to avoid cross-contamination of physical evidence. Carefully fold the paper sheet so that all foreign materials are contained inside.

If it is deemed appropriate, bedding or the object on which the assault took place should be submitted to the laboratory for processing. Items suspected of containing seminal stains must be handled carefully. Folding an article through the stain may cause it to flake off, as will rubbing the stained area against the surface of the packaging material. If, under unusual circumstances, it is not possible to transport the stained article to the laboratory, the stained area should be cut out and submitted with an unstained piece as a substrate control.

In the laboratory, analysts try to link seminal material to a donor(s) using DNA typing. Because an individual may transfer their DNA types to a stain through perspiration, investigators must handle stained articles with care, minimizing direct personal contact. The evidence collector must wear disposable latex gloves when such evidence must be touched.

The rape victim must undergo a medical examination as soon as possible after the assault. At this time, the appropriate items of physical evidence are collected by trained personnel. Evidence collectors should have an evidence-collection kit from the local crime laboratory (see Figures 15–14, 15–15, and 15–16).

The following items of physical evidence are to be collected:

1. *Pubic combings.* Place a paper towel under the buttocks and comb the pubic area for loose or foreign hairs.
2. *Pubic hair standard/reference samples.* Cut 25 full-length hairs from the pubic area at the skin line.
3. *External genital dry-skin areas.* Swab with at least one dry swab and one moistened swab.
4. *Vaginal swabs and smear.* Using two swabs simultaneously, carefully swab the vaginal area and let the swabs air-dry before packaging. Using two additional swabs, repeat the swabbing procedure and smear the swabs onto separate microscope slides, allowing them to air-dry before packaging.

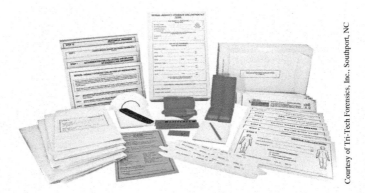

Courtesy of Tri-Tech Forensics, Inc., Southport, NC

FIGURE 15–14

Victim rape collection kit with instructions, and forms for medical history and assault information. Envelope for foreign materials.

Collection bags for outer clothing and underpants. Envelopes for debris, pubic hair combings, and envelope for pulled pubic hair. Envelopes for vaginal swabs and rectal swabs with swap boxes and microscope slides. Envelopes for oral swabs and smear with microscope and a swab box, and envelope for known saliva sample. Known blood sample envelope. Anatomical drawings.

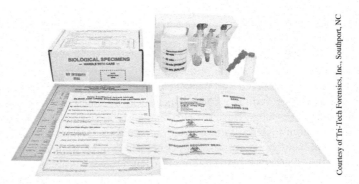

Courtesy of Tri-Tech Forensics, Inc., Southport, NC

FIGURE 15–15

Drug Facilitated Sexual Assault Evidence Toxicology Kit containing a blood tube and urine specimen bottle holder.

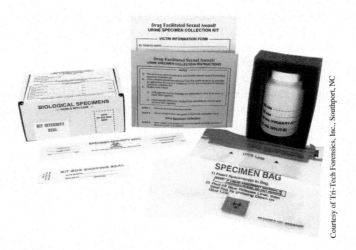

Courtesy of Tri-Tech Forensics, Inc., Southport, NC

FIGURE 15–16

Drug Facilitated Sexual Assault Evidence Toxicology Kit containing a urine specimen bottle.

5. *Cervix swabs.* Using two swabs simultaneously, carefully swab the cervix area and let the swabs air-dry before packaging.

6. *Rectal swabs and smear.* To be taken when warranted by case history. Using two swabs simultaneously, swab the rectal canal, smearing one of the swabs onto a microscope slide. Allow both samples to air-dry before packaging.

7. *Oral swabs and smear.* To be taken if oral–genital contact occurred. Use two swabs simultaneously to swab the buccal area and gum line. Using both swabs, prepare one smear slide. Allow both swabs and the smear to air-dry before packaging.

8. *Swabs of body areas, such as breasts.* To be taken if suspected of being in contact with DNA arising from touching or saliva.

9. *Head hairs.* Cut at skin line a minimum of five full-length hairs from each of the following scalp locations: center, front, back, left side, and right side. It is recommended that a total of at least 25 hairs be cut and submitted to the laboratory.

10. *Blood sample.* Collect at least 20 milliliters in a vacuum tube containing the preservative EDTA. The blood sample can be used for toxicological analysis if required for a drug-facilitated sexual investigation (see pages 294–296).

11. *Collect buccal swab for DNA typing* (see pages 420–421).

12. *Fingernail scrapings.* Scrape the undersurface of the nails with a dull object over a piece of clean paper to collect debris. Use separate paper, one for each hand.

13. *All clothing.* Package as described earlier.

14. *Urine specimen.* Collect 30 milliliters or more of urine from the victim for the purpose of conducting a drug toxicological analysis for Rohypnol, GHB, and other substances associated with drug-facilitated sexual assaults (see pages 294–296).

Often during the investigation of a sexual assault, the victim reports that a perpetrator engaged in biting, sucking, or licking of areas of the victim's body. As we will learn in the next chapter, the tremendous sensitivity associated with DNA technology offers investigators the opportunity to identify a perpetrator's DNA types from saliva residues collected off the skin. The most efficient way to recover saliva residues from the skin is to first swab the suspect area with a rotating motion using a cotton swab moistened with distilled water. A second, dry swab is then rotated over the skin to recover the moist remains on the skin's surface from the wet swab. The swabs are air-dried and packaged together as a single sample.

If a suspect is apprehended, the following items are routinely collected:

1. All clothing and any other items believed to have been worn at the time of assault.
2. Pubic hair combings.
3. Pulled head and pubic hair standard/reference samples.
4. Penile swab within 24 hours of assault when appropriate to case history.
5. Buccal swab (see pages 420–421) for DNA-typing purposes.

The advent of DNA profiling has forced investigators to rethink what items are evidential with respect to a sexual assault. As we will learn in Chapter 16, DNA levels in the range of one-billionth of a gram are now routinely characterized in crime laboratories. In the past, scant

> > > > > > > > > >

Case Files

A DNA Bonus

A common mode of DNA transfer occurs when skin cells from the walls of the victim's vagina are transferred onto the suspect during intercourse. Subsequent penile contact with the inner surface of the suspect's underwear often leads to the recovery of the female victim's DNA from the underwear's inner surface. The power of DNA is aptly illustrated in a case in which the female victim of a rape had consensual sexual intercourse with a male partner prior to being assaulted by a different male. DNA extracted from the inside front area of the suspect's underwear revealed a female DNA profile matching that of the victim. The added bonus in this case was finding male DNA on the same underwear that matched that of the consensual partner.

Based on information contained in Gary G. Verret, "Sexual Assault Cases with No Primary Transfer of Biological Material from Suspect to Victim: Evidence of Secondary and Tertiary Transfer of Biological Material from Victim to Suspect's Undergarments," *Proceedings of the Canadian Society of Forensic Science,* Toronto, ON, November 2001.

attention was paid to the underwear recovered from a male who was suspected of being involved in a sexual assault. From a practical point of view, the presence of seminal constituents on a man's underwear had little or no investigative value. Today, the high sensitivity of DNA analysis has created new areas of investigation. Experience now tells us that it is possible to establish a link between a victim and her assailant by analyzing biological material recovered from the interior front surface of a male suspect's underwear. This is especially important when investigations have failed to yield the presence of a suspect's DNA on exhibits recovered from the victim.

ANALYZING SEMINAL CONSTITUENTS

The persistence of seminal constituents in the vagina may become a factor when trying to ascertain the time of an alleged sexual attack. Although the presence of spermatozoa in the vaginal cavity provides evidence of intercourse, important information regarding the time of sexual activity can be obtained from the knowledge that motile or living sperm generally survive up to four to six hours in the vaginal cavity of a living person. However, a successful search for motile sperm requires a microscopic examination of a vaginal smear immediately after it is taken from the victim. Some investigators question the value of investing time into seeking out motile sperm, noting that such findings may be expected to be found in a relatively small percentage of cases (about 5 percent).[8]

A more extensive examination of vaginal collections is later made at a forensic laboratory. Nonmotile sperm may be found in a living female for up to three days after intercourse and occasionally up to six days later. However, intact sperm (sperm with tails) are not normally found 16 hours after intercourse but have been found as late as 72 hours after intercourse. The likelihood of finding seminal acid phosphatase in the vaginal cavity markedly decreases with time following intercourse, with little chance of identifying this substance 48 hours after intercourse.[7] Hence, with the possibility of the prolonged persistence of both spermatozoa and acid phosphatase in the vaginal cavity after intercourse, investigators should determine when and if voluntary sexual activity last occurred before the sexual assault. This information will be useful for evaluating the significance of finding these seminal constituents in the female victim. Blood or buccal swabs for DNA analysis are to be taken from any consensual partner having sex with the victim within 72 hours prior to the examination.

Another significant indicator of recent sexual activity is PSA. This semen marker normally is not detected in the vaginal cavity beyond 72 hours following intercourse.[7]

WEBEXTRA 15.9
Step into the Role of the First Responding Officer at a Sexual Assault Scene

WEBEXTRA 15.10
Assume the Duties of an Evidence-Collection Technician at a Sexual Assault Scene

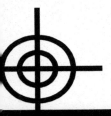

Chapter Summary >>>>>>>>>>>>

There are the three antigens—A, B, and D—which are prevalent in A-B-O blood typing. If an individual is type A, this simply indicates that each red blood cell has A antigens on its surface; similarly, all type B individuals have B antigens; and the red blood cells of type AB contain both A and B antigens. Type O individuals have neither A nor B antigens on their cells. Hence, the presence or absence of the A and B antigens on the red blood cells determines a person's blood type in the A-B-O system.

The term serology describes a broad scope of laboratory tests that use specific antigen and serum antibody reactions. An antibody reacts or agglutinates only with its specific antigen. The identity of each of the four A-B-O blood groups can be established by testing the blood with anti-A and anti-B sera. The concept of specific antigen–antibody reactions has been applied to immunoassay techniques for detecting drugs in blood and urine. When an animal is injected with an antigen, its body produces a series of different antibodies, all of which are designed to attack some particular site on the antigen of interest. This collection of antibodies is known as polyclonal antibodies. Alternately, a more uniform and specific collection of antibodies designed to combine with a single antigen site can be manufactured. Such antibodies are known as monoclonals.

The criminalist must answer the following questions when examining dried blood: (1) Is it blood? (2) From what species did the blood originate? (3) If the blood is of human origin, how closely can it be associated to a particular individual? The determination of blood is best made by means of a preliminary color test. A positive result from

---

[8] R. Dziak et al., "Providing Evidence-Based Opinions on Time Since Intercourse (TSI) Based on Body Fluid Testing Results of Internal Samples," *Canadian Society of Forensic Science Journal* 44 (2011): 59.

the Kastle–Meyer color test is highly indicative of blood. Alternatively, the luminol and Bluestar tests are used to search out trace amounts of blood located at crime scenes. The precipitin test uses antisera normally derived from rabbits that have been injected with the blood of a known animal to determine the species origin of a questioned bloodstain. Before the advent of DNA typing, bloodstains were linked to a source by A-B-O typing. This approach has now been supplanted by the newer DNA technology.

Many cases sent to a forensic laboratory involve sexual offenses, making it necessary to examine exhibits for the presence of seminal stains. The best way to locate and characterize a seminal stain is to perform the acid phosphatase color test. Semen can be uniquely identified by the presence of spermatozoa. Also, the PSA protein in combination with the acid phosphatase color test provides an unequivocal identification of semen. Forensic scientists can link seminal material to an individual by DNA typing. The rape victim must undergo a medical examination as soon as possible after the assault. At that time clothing, hairs, and vaginal and rectal swabs can be collected for subsequent laboratory examination. If a suspect is apprehended within 24 hours of the assault, it may be possible to detect the victim's DNA on the male's underwear or on a penile swab of the suspect.

Review Questions

1. Karl Landsteiner discovered that blood can be classified by its _____.

2. True or False: No two individuals, except for identical twins, can be expected to have the same combination of blood types or antigens. _____

3. _____ is the fluid portion of unclotted blood.

4. The liquid that separates from the blood when a clot is formed is called the _____.

5. _____ transport oxygen from the lungs to the body tissues and carry carbon dioxide back to the lungs.

6. On the surface of red blood cells are chemical substances called _____, which impart blood type characteristics to the cells.

7. Type A individuals have _____ antigens on the surface of their red blood cells.

8. Type O individuals have (both A and B, neither A nor B) antigens on their red blood cells.

9. The presence or absence of the _____ and _____ antigens on the red blood cells determines a person's blood type in the A-B-O system.

10. The D antigen is also known as the _____ antigen.

11. Serum contains proteins known as _____, which destroy or inactivate antigens.

12. An antibody reacts with (any, only a specific) antigen.

13. True or False: Agglutination describes the clumping together of red blood cells by the action of an antibody. _____

14. Type B blood contains _____ antigens and anti-_____ antibodies.

15. Type AB blood has (both anti-A and anti-B, neither anti-A nor anti-B) antigens.

16. A drug–protein complex can be injected into an animal to form specific _____ for that drug.

17. The term _____ describes the study of antigen–antibody reactions.

18. Type AB blood (is, is not) agglutinated by both anti-A and anti-B serum.

19. Type B red blood cells agglutinate when added to type (A, B) blood.

20. Type A red blood cells agglutinate when added to type (AB, O) blood.

21. The distribution of type A blood in the United States is approximately (42, 15) percent.

22. The distribution of type AB blood in the United States is approximately (12, 3) percent.

23. (All, Most) blood hemoglobin has peroxidase-like activity.

24. For many years, the most commonly used color test for identifying blood was the _____ color test.

25. _____ reagent reacts with blood, causing it to luminesce.

26. Blood can be characterized as being of human origin by the _____ test.

27. Antigens and antibodies (can, cannot) be induced to move toward each other under the influence of an electrical field.

28. The basic unit of heredity is the _____.

29. Genes are positioned on threadlike bodies called _____.

30. All nucleated cells in the human body, except the reproductive cells, have _____ pairs of chromosomes.

31. The sex of an offspring is always determined by the (mother, father).

32. Genes that influence a given characteristic and are aligned with one another on a chromosome pair are known as _____.

33. When a pair of allelic genes is identical, the genes are said to be (homozygous, heterozygous).

34. The _____ color test is used to locate and characterize seminal stains.

35. Semen is unequivocally identified by the microscopic appearance of _____.

36. Males with a low sperm count have a condition known as (oligospermia, aspermia).

37. The protein _____ is useful for the characterization of semen.

38. True or False: DNA may be transferred to an object through the medium of perspiration. _____

39. True or False: Seminal constituents may remain in the vagina for up to six days after intercourse. _____

Review Questions for Inside the Science

1. An immunological assay technique used to detect the presence of minute quantities of drugs in blood and urine is _____.

2. Antibodies designed to interact with a specific antigen site are (monoclonal, polyclonal).

3. True or False: Hybridoma cells are used to produce antigens designed to attack one and only one site on an antibody. _____

4. A (phenotype, genotype) is an observable characteristic of an individual.

5. The combination of genes present in the cells of an individual is called the _____.

6. A gene (will, will not) appear in a child when it is present in one of the parents.

7. A type B individual may have the genotype _____ or the genotype _____.

8. A type AB mother and type AB father will have offspring of what possible genotypes? _____

9. A type AB mother and type AB father will have offspring of what possible phenotypes? _____

Application and Critical Thinking

1. Police investigating the scene of a sexual assault recover a large blanket that they believe may contain useful physical evidence. They take it to the laboratory of forensic serologist Scott Alden, asking him to test it for the presence of semen. Noticing faint pink stains on the blanket, Scott asks the investigating detective if he is aware of anything that might recently have been spilled on the blanket. The detective reports that an overturned bowl of grapes and watermelon was found at the scene, as well as a broken glass that had contained wine. After the detective departs, Scott chooses and administers what he considers the best test for analyzing the piece of evidence in his possession. Three minutes after completion of the test, the blanket shows a positive reaction. What test did Scott choose and what was his conclusion? Explain your answer.

2. Criminalist Cathy Richards is collecting evidence from the victim of a sexual assault. She places a sheet on the floor, asks the victim to disrobe, and places the clothing in a paper bag. After collecting pubic combings and pubic hair samples, she takes two vaginal swabs, which she allows to air-dry before packaging. Finally, Cathy collects blood, urine, and scalp hair samples from the victim. What mistakes, if any, did she make in collecting this evidence?

Further References

Jones, E. L., Jr., "The Identification and Individualization of Semen Stains," in R. Saferstein, ed., *Forensic Science Handbook*, vol. 2, 2nd ed. Upper Saddle River, NJ: Prentice Hall, 2005.

Li, Richard, *Forensic Biology*, 2nd ed. Boca Raton, FL: CRC Press, 2015.

Shaler, R. C., "Modern Forensic Biology," in R. Saferstein, ed., *Forensic Science Handbook*, vol. 1, 2nd ed. Upper Saddle River, NJ: Prentice Hall, 2002.

Virkler, K., and I. K. Lednev, "Analysis of Body Fluids for Forensic Purposes: From Laboratory Testing to Non-Destructive Rapid Confirmatory Identification at a Crime Scene," *Forensic Science International* 188 (2009): 1.

Chapter 16

DNA: The Indispensable Forensic Science Tool

Learning Objectives

After studying this chapter, you should be able to:

16.1 Explain DNA and its structure

16.2 Explain how the amino acid sequence in a protein chain is determined by the structure of DNA

16.3 Explain the phenomenon of DNA replication and the impact of the PCR technique on duplicating DNA strands

16.4 Discuss STR analysis and the concept of electrophoresis

16.5 Describe the difference between nuclear and mitochondrial DNA

16.6 List the necessary procedures for the proper preservation of bloodstained evidence for laboratory DNA analysis

KEY TERMS

amelogenin gene
amino acids
buccal cells
chromosome
complementary base
    pairing
deoxyribonucleic acid
    (DNA)
electrophoresis
epithelial cells
human genome
hybridization
low copy number
mitochondria
multiplexing
nucleotide
picogram
polymer
polymerase chain
    reaction (PCR)
primer
proteins
replication
restriction fragment
    length polymorphisms
    (RFLPs)
sequencing
short tandem repeat
    (STR)
substrate control
tandem repeat
touch DNA
Y-STRs

Go to www.pearsonhighered.com/careersresources to access Webextras for this chapter.

The Golden State Killer

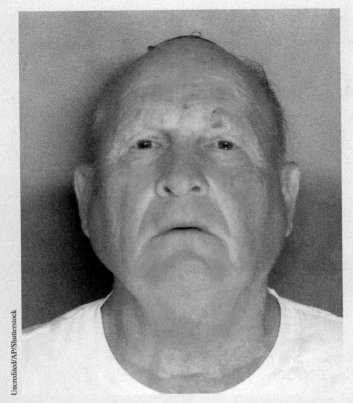

The crime spree began in 1974 in the East Area of Sacramento, California. A serial rapist was at work and over the next 12 years he would be linked to additional attacks in Contra Costa County, Stockton, and Modesto. His modus operandi was unique. He was particularly organized, carefully stalking his victims and becoming familiar with their homes and schedules before executing his attacks. His crimes were so prolific that he garnered several names in the press. Known as the "East Area Rapist" in Northern California and "The Original Night Stalker" in the South, DNA testing revealed three decades later that the crimes were all the work of one man. Over the course of his criminal career, he is suspected of committing at least 13 murders, more than 50 rapes, and over 100 burglaries.

Advancements in DNA testing are credited with linking several rapes and murders in 2001. At that time, authorities had the DNA profile of the killer, but they still didn't know his identity. His DNA wasn't present in the Combined DNA Indexing System (CODIS) database and neither was the DNA of any close relatives. Investigators painstakingly made their way through a list of possible suspects, collecting samples and eventually ruling out each one. In 2016, the Federal Bureau of Investigation and local law enforcement agencies held a news conference to announce a renewed nationwide effort, offering a $50,000 reward for his capture.

In 2017, investigators heard about a new and promising method for identifying individuals based on their DNA. It was being used to help reunite families who had been separated, as in cases of adoption. It was called genetic genealogy, and it involved examining similarities shared by related people for clues about the donor's lineage, as discussed in Chapter 3. By tracing the DNA back to a family tree using parentage and relatedness databases like GEDmatch, investigators could narrow the pool of potential suspects considerably. Investigators, with the help of a genetic genealogist, traced the DNA to a common ancestor and constructed family trees using birth records, newspaper clippings, and social media profiles. It was through this method authorities identified 72-year-old United States Navy veteran and former police officer Joseph James DeAngelo as the Golden State Killer. He is charged with eight counts of first-degree murder and is currently awaiting trial.

The discovery of **deoxyribonucleic acid (DNA)**, the deciphering of its structure, and the decoding of its genetic information were turning points in our understanding of the underlying concepts of inheritance. Now, with incredible speed, as molecular biologists unravel the basic structure of genes, we can create new products through genetic engineering and develop diagnostic tools and treatments for genetic disorders.

For a number of years, these developments were of seemingly peripheral interest to forensic scientists. All that changed when, in 1985, what started out as a more or less routine investigation into the structure of a human gene led to the discovery that portions of the DNA structure of certain genes are as unique to each individual as fingerprints. Alec Jeffreys and his colleagues at Leicester University, England, who were responsible for these revelations, named the process for isolating and reading these DNA markers *DNA fingerprinting*. As researchers uncovered new approaches and variations to the original Jeffreys technique, the terms *DNA profiling* and *DNA typing* came to be applied to describe this relatively new technology.

This discovery caught the imagination of the forensic science community because forensic scientists have long desired to link with certainty biological evidence such as blood, semen, hair, or tissue to a single individual. Although conventional testing procedures had gone a long way toward narrowing the source of biological materials, individualization remained an elusive goal. Now, DNA typing has allowed forensic scientists to accomplish this goal. The technique is still relatively new, but in the few years since its introduction, DNA typing has become routine in public crime laboratories and has been made available to interested parties through the services of a number of skilled private laboratories. In the United States, courts have overwhelmingly admitted DNA evidence and accepted the reliability of its scientific underpinnings.

deoxyribonucleic acid (DNA)
The molecules carrying the body's genetic information; DNA is double stranded in the shape of a double helix.

chromosome
A rod-like structure in the cell nucleus, along which the genes are located; it is composed of DNA surrounded by other material, mainly proteins.

polymer
A substance composed of a large number of atoms; these atoms are usually arranged in repeating units, or monomers.

nucleotide
The unit of DNA consisting of one of four bases—adenine, guanine, cytosine, or thymine—attached to a phosphate–sugar group.

What Is DNA?

Inside each of 60 trillion cells in the human body are strands of genetic material called **chromosomes**. Arranged along the chromosomes, like beads on a thread, are nearly 25,000 genes. The gene is the fundamental unit of heredity. It instructs the body cells to make proteins that determine everything from hair color to our susceptibility to diseases. Each gene is actually composed of DNA specifically designed to carry out a single body function.

Interestingly, although DNA was first discovered in 1868, scientists were slow to understand and appreciate its fundamental role in inheritance. Painstakingly, researchers developed evidence that DNA was probably the substance by which genetic instructions are passed from one generation to the next. But the major breakthrough in comprehending how DNA works did not occur until the early 1950s, when two researchers, James Watson and Francis Crick, deduced the structure of DNA. It turns out that DNA is an extraordinary molecule skillfully designed to carry out the task of controlling the genetic traits of all living cells, plant and animal.

Structure of DNA

Before examining the implications of Watson and Crick's discovery, let's see how DNA is constructed. DNA is a **polymer**. As we will learn in this chapter, a polymer is a very large molecule made by linking a series of repeating units.

NUCLEOTIDES   In the case of DNA, the repeating units are known as **nucleotides**. A nucleotide is composed of a sugar molecule, a phosphorus-containing group, and a nitrogen-containing molecule called a *base*. Figure 16–1 shows how nucleotides can be strung together to form a DNA strand. In this figure, S designates the sugar component, which is joined with a phosphate group to form the backbone of the DNA strand. Projecting from the backbone are the bases.

The key to understanding how DNA works is to appreciate the fact that only four types of bases are associated with DNA: adenine, cytosine, guanine, and thymine. To simplify our discussion of DNA, we will designate each of these bases by the first letter of their names. Hence, *A* will stand for adenine, *C* will stand for cytosine, *G* will stand for guanine, and *T* will represent thymine.

Again, notice in Figure 16–1 how the bases project from the backbone of DNA. Also, although this figure shows a DNA strand of four bases, keep in mind that in theory there is no limit to the length of the DNA strand; in fact, a DNA strand can be composed of a long chain with millions of bases. The information just discussed was well known to Watson and Crick by

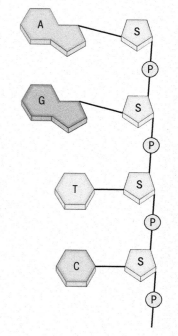

FIGURE 16–1

How nucleotides can be linked to form a DNA strand. S designates the sugar component, which is joined with phosphate groups (P) to form the backbone of DNA. Projecting from the backbone are four bases: A, adenine; G, guanine; T, thymine; and C, cytosine.

the time they set about detailing the structure of DNA. Their efforts led to the discovery that the DNA molecule is actually composed of two DNA strands coiled into a *double helix*. This can be thought of as resembling two wires twisted around each other.

As these researchers manipulated scale models of DNA strands, they realized that the only way the bases on each strand could be properly aligned with each other in a double-helix configuration was to place base *A* opposite *T* and *G* opposite *C*. Watson and Crick had solved the puzzle of the double helix and presented the world with a simple but elegant picture of DNA (see Figure 16–2).

COMPLEMENTARY BASE PAIRING   The only arrangement possible in the double-helix configuration was the pairing of bases *A* to *T* and *G* to *C*, a concept that has become known as **complementary base pairing**. Although *A–T* and *G–C* pairs are always required, there are no restrictions on how the bases are to be sequenced on a DNA strand. Thus, one can observe the sequences *T–A–T–T* or *G–T–A–A* or *G–T–C–A*. When these sequences are joined with their complements in a double-helix configuration, they pair as follows:

T A T T   G T A A   G T C A
| | | | | | | | | | | |
A T A A   C A T T   C A G T

Any base can follow another on a DNA strand, which means that the possible number of different sequence combinations is staggering! Consider that the average human chromosome has DNA containing 100 million base pairs. All of the human chromosomes taken together contain about 3 billion base pairs. From these numbers, we can begin to appreciate the diversity of DNA

complementary base pairing
The specific pairing of base *A* with *T* and base *G* with *C* in double-stranded DNA.

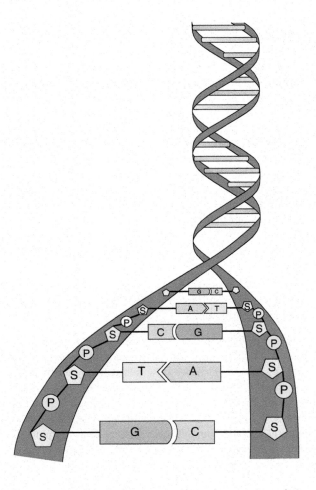

FIGURE 16–2

A representation of a DNA double helix. Notice how bases *G* and *C* pair with each other, as do bases *A* and *T*. This is the only arrangement in which two DNA strands can align with each other in a double-helix configuration.

and hence the diversity of living organisms. DNA is like a book of instructions. The alphabet used to create the book is simple enough: *A*, *T*, *G*, and *C*. The order in which these letters are arranged defines the role and function of a DNA molecule.

WEBEXTRA 16.1
What Is DNA?

DNA at Work

The inheritable traits that are controlled by DNA arise out of its ability to direct the production of complex molecules called **proteins**. Proteins are actually made by linking a combination of **amino acids**. Although thousands of proteins exist, they can all be derived from a combination of up to 20 known amino acids. The sequence of amino acids in a protein chain determines the shape and function of the protein. Let's look at one example: The protein hemoglobin is found in our red blood cells. It carries oxygen to our body cells and removes carbon dioxide from these cells. One of the four amino acid chains of "normal" hemoglobin is shown in Figure 16–3(a). Studies of individuals with sickle-cell anemia show that this inheritable disorder arises from the presence of "abnormal" hemoglobin in their red blood cells. An amino acid chain for "abnormal" hemoglobin is shown in Figure 16–3(b). Note that the sole difference between "normal" and "abnormal" or sickle-cell hemoglobin arises from the substitution of one amino acid for another in the protein chain.

proteins
Polymers of amino acids that play basic roles in the structures and functions of living things.

amino acids
The building blocks of proteins; there are 20 common amino acids; amino acids are linked to form a protein; the types of amino acids and the order in which they're linked determine the character of each protein.

The Combined DNA Index System (CODIS)

Perhaps the most significant investigative tool to arise from a DNA-typing program is CODIS (Combined DNA Index System), a computer software program developed by the FBI that maintains local, state, and national databases of DNA profiles from convicted offenders, unsolved crime-scene evidence, and profiles of missing people. CODIS allows crime laboratories to compare DNA types recovered from crime-scene evidence to those of convicted sex offenders and others who are convicted of crimes.

Thousands of CODIS matches have linked serial crimes to each other and have solved crimes by allowing investigators to match crime-scene evidence to known convicted offenders. This capability is of tremendous value to investigators in cases in which the police have not been able to identify a suspect. The CODIS concept has already had a significant impact on police investigations in various states, as shown in the Case Files feature on page 73.

The genetic information that determines the amino acid sequence for every protein manufactured in the human body is stored in DNA in a genetic code that relies on the sequence of bases along the DNA strand. The alphabet of DNA is simple—*A*, *T*, *G*, and *C*—but the key to deciphering the genetic code is to know that each amino acid is coded by a sequence of three bases. Thus, the amino acid alanine is coded by the combination *C–G–T*; the amino acid aspartate is coded by the combination *C–T–A*; and the amino acid phenylalanine is coded by the combination *A–A–A*. With this code in hand, we can now see how the amino acid sequence in a protein chain is determined by the structure of DNA. Consider the DNA segment

–C–G–T–C–T–A–A–A–A–C–G–T–

The triplet code contained within this segment translates into

[*C–G–T*] – [*C–T–A*] – [*A–A–T*] – [*C–G–T*]
alanine   aspartate   phenylalanine alanine

or the protein chain

| alanine | aspartate | phenylalanine | alanine |

Interestingly, this code is not restricted to humans. Almost all living cells studied to date use the same genetic code as the language of protein synthesis.[1]

If we look at the difference between "normal" and sickle-cell hemoglobin (see Figure 16–3), we see that the latter is formed by substituting one amino acid (valine) for another (glutamate).

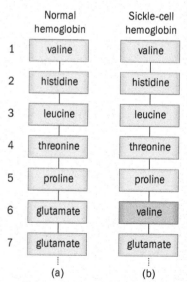

	Normal hemoglobin	Sickle-cell hemoglobin
1	valine	valine
2	histidine	histidine
3	leucine	leucine
4	threonine	threonine
5	proline	proline
6	glutamate	valine
7	glutamate	glutamate
	(a)	(b)

FIGURE 16–3

(a) A string of amino acids composes one of the protein chains of hemoglobin. (b) Substitution of just one amino acid for another in the protein chain results in sickle-cell hemoglobin.

---

[1] Instructions for assembling proteins are actually carried from DNA to another region of the cell by ribonucleic acid (RNA). RNA is directly involved in the assembly of the protein using the genetic code it received from DNA.

Within the DNA segment that codes for the production of normal hemoglobin, the letter sequence is

$$-[C–C–T]–[G–A–G]–[G–A–G]–$$
proline glutamate glutamate

Individuals with sickle-cell disease carry the sequence

$$-[C–C–T]–[G–T–G]–[G–A–G]–$$
proline valine glutamate

Thus, we see that a single base or letter change (*T* has been substituted for *A* in valine) is the underlying cause of sickle-cell anemia, demonstrating the delicate chemical balance between health and disease in the human body.

As scientists unravel the base sequences of DNA, they obtain a greater appreciation for the roles that proteins play in the chemistry of life. Already the genes responsible for hemophilia, Duchenne muscular dystrophy, and Huntington's disease have been located. Once scientists have isolated a disease-causing gene, they can determine the protein that the gene has directed the cell to manufacture. By studying these proteins—or the absence of them—scientists will be able to devise a treatment for genetic disorders.

A 13-year project to determine the order of bases on all 23 pairs of human chromosomes (also called the **human genome**) is now complete. Knowing where on a specific chromosome DNA codes for the production of a particular protein is useful for diagnosing and treating genetic diseases. This information is crucial for understanding the underlying causes of cancer. Also, comparing the human genome with that of other organisms will help us understand the role and implications of evolution.

Replication of DNA

Once the double-helix structure of DNA was discovered, how DNA duplicated itself before cell division became apparent. The concept of base pairing in DNA suggests the analogy of positive and negative photographic film. Each strand of DNA in the double helix has the same information; one can make a positive print from a negative or a negative from a positive.

The Process of Replication

The synthesis of new DNA from existing DNA begins with the unwinding of the DNA strands in the double helix. Each strand is then exposed to a collection of free nucleotides. Letter by letter, the double helix is re-created as the nucleotides are assembled in the proper order, as dictated by the principle of base pairing (*A* with *T* and *G* with *C*). The result is the emergence of two identical copies of DNA where before there was only one (see Figure 16–4). A cell can now pass on its genetic identity when it divides.

Many enzymes and proteins are involved in unwinding the DNA strands, keeping the two DNA strands apart, and assembling the new DNA strands. For example, DNA *polymerases* are enzymes that assemble a new DNA strand in the proper base sequence determined by the original, or parent, DNA strand. DNA polymerases also "proofread" the growing DNA double helices for mismatched base pairs, which are replaced with correct bases.

Until recently, the phenomenon of DNA **replication** appeared to be of only academic interest to forensic scientists interested in DNA for identification. However, this changed when researchers perfected the technology of using DNA polymerases to copy a DNA strand located outside a living cell. This laboratory technique is known as **polymerase chain reaction (PCR)**. Put simply, PCR is a technique designed to copy or multiply DNA strands in a laboratory test tube.

In PCR, small quantities of DNA or broken pieces of DNA found in crime-scene evidence can be copied with the aid of a DNA polymerase. The copying process is highly temperature dependent and can be accomplished in an automated fashion using a DNA thermal cycler

human genome

The total DNA content found within the nucleus of a human cell; it is composed of approximately three billion base pairs of genetic information.

replication

The synthesis of new DNA from existing DNA.

polymerase chain reaction (PCR)

A technique for replicating or copying a portion of a DNA strand outside a living cell; this technique leads to millions of copies of the DNA strand.

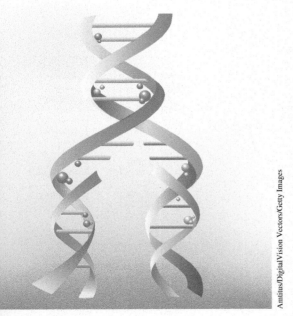

FIGURE 16–4

Replication of DNA. The strands of the original DNA molecule are separated, and two new strands are assembled.

Amitius/DigitalVision Vectors/Getty Images

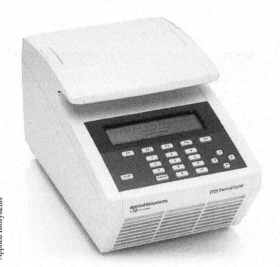

FIGURE 16–5

The DNA thermal cycler, an instrument that automates the rapid and precise temperature changes required to copy a DNA strand. Within a matter of hours, DNA can be multiplied a millionfold.

Applied Biosystems

(see Figure 16–5). Each cycle of the PCR technique results in a doubling of the DNA, as shown in Figure 16–4. Within a few hours, 30 cycles can multiply DNA a billionfold. Once DNA copies are in hand, they can be analyzed by any of the methods of modern molecular biology. The ability to multiply small bits of DNA opens new and exciting avenues for forensic scientists to explore. It means that sample size is no longer a limitation in characterizing DNA recovered from crime-scene evidence.

DNA Typing with Short Tandem Repeats

Tandem Repeats

Geneticists have discovered that portions of the DNA molecule contain sequences of letters that are repeated numerous times. In fact, more than 30 percent of the human genome is composed of repeating segments of DNA. These repeating sequences, or **tandem repeats**, seem to act as filler or spacers between the coding regions of DNA. Although these repeating segments do not seem to affect our outward appearance or control any other basic genetic function, they are nevertheless part of our genetic makeup, inherited from our parents in the manner illustrated by the Punnett square (page 386). The origin and significance of these tandem repeats is a mystery, but to forensic scientists they offer a means of distinguishing one individual from another through DNA typing.

Forensic scientists first began applying DNA technology to human identity in 1985. From the beginning, attention has focused on the tandem repeats of the genome. These repeats can be visualized as a string of connected boxes with each box having the same core sequence of DNA bases (see Figure 16–6). All humans have the same type of repeats, but there is tremendous variation in the number of repeats that each of us has.

tandem repeat
A region of a chromosome that contains multiple copies of a core DNA sequence that are arranged in a repeating fashion.

WEBEXTRA 16.2
Polymerase Chain Reaction

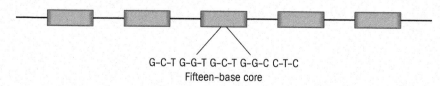

G-C-T G-G-T G-C-T G-G-C C-T-C
Fifteen-base core

FIGURE 16–6

A DNA segment consisting of a series of repeating DNA units. In this illustration, the 15-base core can repeat itself hundreds of times. The entire DNA segment is typically hundreds to thousands of bases long.

Inside the Science

Polymerase Chain Reaction

The most important feature of PCR is the knowledge that an enzyme called *DNA polymerase* can be directed to synthesize a specific region of DNA. In a relatively straightforward manner, PCR can be used to repeatedly duplicate or amplify a strand of DNA millions of times. As an example, let's consider a segment of DNA that we want to duplicate by PCR:

–G–T–C–T–C–A–G–C–T–T–**C–C–A–G**–

–C–A–G–A–G–T–C–G–A–A–A–G–G–T–C–

To perform PCR on this DNA segment, short sequences of DNA on each side of the region of interest must be identified. In the example shown here, the short sequences are designated by boldface letters in the DNA segment. These short DNA segments must be available in a pure form known as a **primer** if the PCR technique is going to work.

The first step in PCR is to heat the DNA strands to about 94°C. At this temperature, the double-stranded DNA molecules separate completely:

–G–T–C–T–C–A–G–C–T–T–C–C–A–G–

–C–A–G–A–G–T–C–G–A–A–A–G–G–T–C–

The second step is to add the primers to the separated strands and allow the primers to combine, or **hybridize**, with the strands by lowering the test-tube temperature to about 60°C.

–G–T–C–T–C–A–G–C–T–T–C–C–A–G–

–C–A–G–A

                    C–C–A–G

–C–A–G–A–G–T–C–G–A–A–A–G–G–T–C–

The third step is to add the DNA polymerase and a mixture of free nucleotides (*A, C, G, T*) to the separated strands. When the test tube is heated to 72°C, the polymerase enzyme directs the rebuilding of a double-stranded DNA molecule, extending the primers by adding the appropriate bases, one at a time, resulting in the production of two complete pairs of double-stranded DNA segments:

–G–T–C–T–C–A–G–C–T–T–C–C–A–G–

C–A–G–A–G–T–C–G–A–A–A–G–G–T–C–

G–T–C–T–C–A–G–C–T–T–C–C–A–G

–C–A–G–A–G–T–C–G–A–A–A–G–G–T–C–

This completes the first cycle of the PCR technique, which results in a doubling of the number of DNA molecules from one to two. The cycle of heating, cooling, and strand rebuilding is then repeated, resulting in a further doubling of the DNA molecules. On completion of the second cycle, four double-stranded DNA molecules have been created from the original double-stranded DNA sample. Typically, 28 to 32 cycles are carried out to yield more than one billion copies of the original DNA molecule. Each cycle takes less than two minutes.

restriction fragment length polymorphisms (RFLPs)
Different fragment lengths of base pairs that result from cutting a DNA molecule with restriction enzymes.

electrophoresis
A technique for separating molecules through their migration on a support medium while under the influence of an electrical potential.

Up until the mid-1990s, the forensic community aimed its efforts at characterizing repeat segments known as **restriction fragment length polymorphisms (RFLPs)**. A number of different RFLPs were selected by the forensic science community for performing DNA typing. Typically a core sequence is 15 to 35 bases long and repeats itself up to one thousand times. These repeats are cut out of the DNA double helix by a restriction enzyme that acts like a pair of scissors. Once the DNA molecules have been cut up by the restriction enzyme, the resulting fragments were sorted out by separating the fragments by a technique known as **electrophoresis**.

RFLP DNA typing has the distinction of being the first scientifically accepted protocol in the United States used for the forensic characterization of DNA. However, its utility has been short lived. New technology incorporating PCR has supplanted RFLP. In its short history, perhaps RFLP's most startling impact related to the impeachment trial of President Bill Clinton. The whole complexion of the investigation regarding the relationship of the president with a White House intern, Monica Lewinsky, changed when it was revealed that Ms. Lewinsky possessed a dress that she claimed was stained with the president's semen. The FBI Laboratory was asked to compare the DNA extracted from the dress stain with that of the president. An RFLP match was obtained between the president's DNA and the stain. The combined frequency of occurrence for the seven DNA types found was nearly one in eight trillion, an undeniable link. The dress and a copy of the FBI DNA report are shown in Figure 16–7.

Why couldn't the PCR technology be applied to RFLP DNA typing? Simply put, the RFLP strands are too long, often containing thousands of bases. PCR is best used with DNA strands that are no longer than a couple of hundred bases. The obvious solution to this problem is to characterize DNA strands that are much shorter than RFLPs. Another advantage in moving to shorter DNA strands is that they would be expected to be more stable and less subject to degradation brought about by adverse environmental conditions. The long RFLP strands tend to break apart under adverse conditions not uncommon at crime scenes.

primer
A short strand of DNA used to target a region of DNA for replication by PCR.

hybridization
The process of joining two complementary strands of DNA to form a double-stranded molecule.

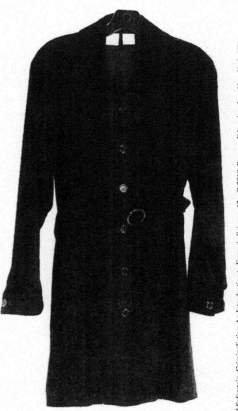

FEDERAL BUREAU OF INVESTIGATION
WASHINGTON, D. C. 20535

Report of Examination

Examiner Name:	~~████████~~	Date:	08/17/98
Unit:	DNA Analysis 1	Phone No.:	202-324-4409
FBI File No.:	29D-OIC-LR-35063	Lab No.:	980730002 S BO
			980803100 S BO

Results of Examinations:

    Deoxyribonucleic acid (DNA) profiles for the genetic loci D2S44, D17S79, D1S7, D4S139, D10S28, D5S110 and D7S467 were developed from HaeIII-digested high molecular weight DNA extracted from specimens K39 and Q3243-1(a semen stain removed from specimen Q3243). Based on the results of these seven genetic loci, specimen K39 (CLINTON) is the source of the DNA obtained from specimen Q3243-1, to a reasonable degree of scientific certainty.

    No DNA-RFLP examinations were conducted on specimen Q3243-2 (a semen stain removed from specimen Q3243).

BLACK — 1,440,000,000,000
CAUC — 7,870,000,000,000
SEH — 3,140,000,000,000
SWH — 943,000,000,000

DNAU1 - Page 1 of 1

This Report Is Furnished For Official Use Only

Q3243

Richard Saferstein, Criminalistics: An Introduction to Forensic Science, 12e, © 2018. Pearson Education, Inc., New York, NY.

FIGURE 16–7

The dress and the FBI Report of Examination for a semen stain located on the dress.

Inside the Science

Gel and Capillary Electrophoresis

Electrophoresis is somewhat related to thin-layer chromatography (discussed in Chapter 12) in that it separates materials according to their migration rates on a stationary solid phase. However, electrophoresis does not use a moving liquid phase to move the material; instead, an electrical potential is placed across the stationary medium (Figure 1). The technique is particularly useful for separating and identifying complex biochemical mixtures. In forensic science, electrophoresis is most useful for characterizing proteins and DNA in dried blood.

Forensic serologists have developed several electrophoretic procedures for characterizing DNA in dried blood. Mixtures of DNA fragments can be separated by gel electrophoresis by taking advantage of the fact that the rate of movement of DNA across a gel-coated plate depends on the molecule's size. Smaller DNA fragments move faster along the plate than larger DNA fragments. After completing the electrophoresis run, the separated DNA is stained with a suitable developing agent for visual observation (see Figure 2).

The separation of STRs can typically be carried out on a flat gel-coated electrophoretic plate, as described earlier. However, the need to reduce analysis time and to automate sampling and data collection has led to the emergence of *capillary electrophoresis* as the preferred technology for characterization of STRs. Capillary electrophoresis is carried out in a thin glass column rather than on the surface of a coated-glass plate.

Capillary electrophoresis technology has evolved from the traditional flat gel electrophoresis approach. The separation of DNA segments is carried out on the interior wall of a glass capillary tube that is kept at a constant voltage. The size of the DNA fragments determines the speed at which they move through the column.

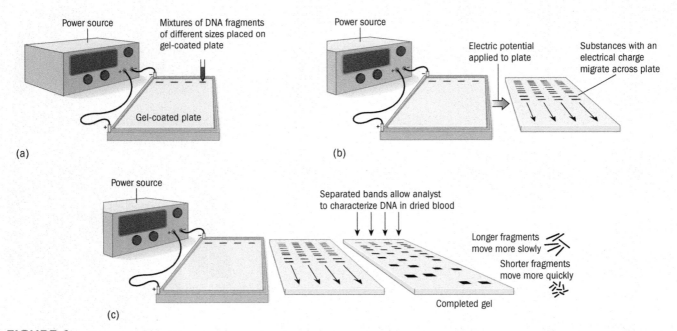

FIGURE 1

The technique of gel electrophoresis. (a) Applying samples to the plate. (b) Applying electric potential to the plate to cause the fragments to migrate. (c) Separation of the fragments on the gel allows for analysis.

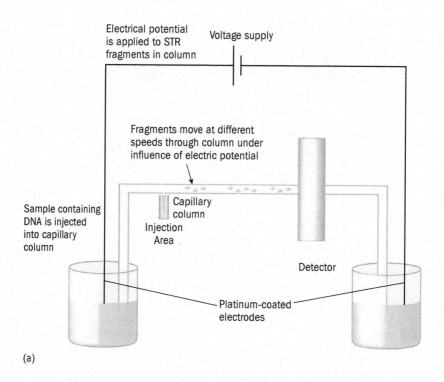

(a)

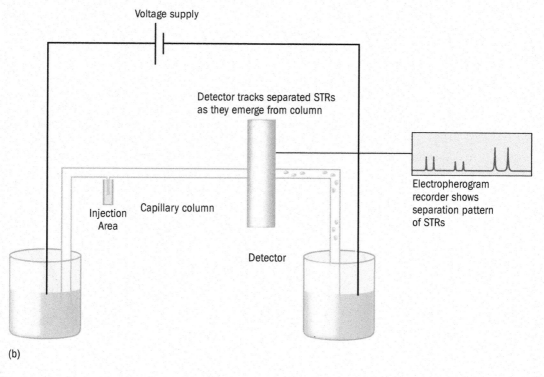

(b)

FIGURE 2

The technique of capillary electrophoresis. (a) Injecting the sample into the capillary by electrokinetic injection. (b) Sample fragments to migrate through the capillary where separation of the fragments in the polymer matrix allows for analysis.

WEBEXTRA 16.3
An Animated Demonstration of Gel
Electrophoresis

short tandem repeat (STR)
A region of a DNA molecule that
contains short segments consisting
of three to seven repeating base
pairs.

Short Tandem Repeats (STRs)

Currently, **short tandem repeat (STR)** analysis has emerged as the most successful and widely used DNA-profiling procedure. STRs are locations (loci) on the chromosome that contain short sequence elements that repeat themselves within the DNA molecule. They serve as helpful markers for identification because they are found in great abundance throughout the human genome.

STRs normally consist of repeating sequences of three to seven bases; the entire strand of an STR is also very short, less than 450 bases long. These strands are significantly shorter than those encountered in other DNA typing procedures. This means that STRs are much less susceptible to degradation and are often recovered from bodies or stains that have been subject to extreme decomposition. Also, because of their shortness, STRs are an ideal candidate for multiplication by PCR, thus overcoming the limited-sample-size problem often associated with crime-scene evidence. Only the equivalent of 18 DNA-containing cells is needed to obtain a DNA profile. For instance, STR profiles have been used to identify the origin of saliva residue on envelopes, stamps, soda cans, and cigarette butts.

To understand the utility of STRs in forensic science, let's look at one commonly used STR known as TH01. This DNA segment contains the repeating sequence *A–A–T–G*. Seven TH01 variants have been identified in the human genome. These variants contain 5 to 11 repeats of *A–A–T–G*. Figure 16–8 illustrates two such TH01 variants, one containing six repeats and the other containing eight repeats of *A–A–T–G*.

During a forensic examination, TH01 is extracted from biological materials and amplified by PCR as described earlier. The ability to copy an STR means that extremely small amounts of the molecule can be detected and analyzed. Once the STRs have been copied or amplified, they are separated by electrophoresis. Here, the STRs are forced to move across a gel-coated plate under the influence of an electrical potential. Smaller DNA fragments move along the plate faster than do larger DNA fragments. By examining the distance the STR has migrated on the electrophoretic plate, one can determine the number of *A–A–T–G* repeats in the STR. Every person has two STR types for TH01, one inherited from each parent. Thus, for example, one may find in a semen stain TH01 with six repeats and eight repeats. This combination of TH01 is found in approximately 3.5 percent of the population. It is important to understand that all humans have the same type of repeats, but there is tremendous variation in the number of repeats each of us has.

When examining an STR DNA pattern, one merely needs to look for a match between peak sets. For example, in Figure 16–9, DNA extracted from a crime-scene stain matches the DNA recovered from one of three suspects. When comparing only one STR, a limited number of people in a population would have the same STR fragment pattern as the suspect. However, by using additional STRs, a high degree of discrimination or complete individualization can be achieved.

FIGURE 16–8

Variants of the short tandem repeat TH01. The upper DNA strand contains six repeats of the sequence *A-A-T-G*; the lower DNA strand contains eight repeats of the sequence *A-A-T-G*. This DNA type is designated as TH01 6,8.

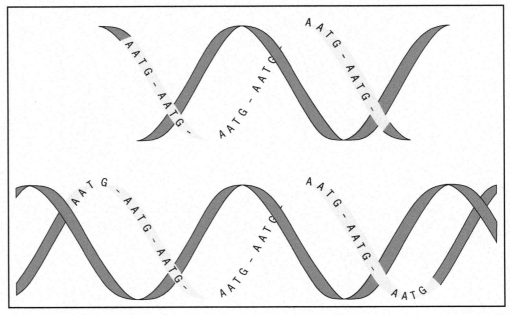

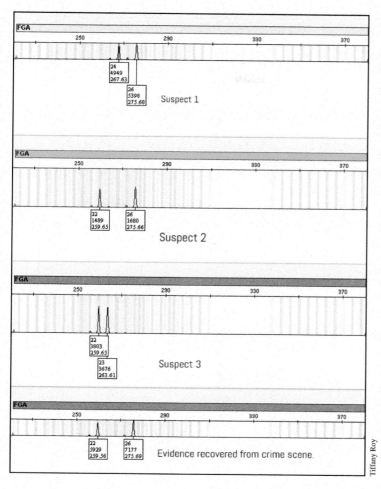

FIGURE 16–9

DNA profile peak pattern analysis of a crime scene stain compared to three suspects at the highly polymorphic FGA locus. Suspect 2 matches the crime scene stain at this locus.

Multiplexing

What makes STRs so attractive to forensic scientists is that hundreds of types of STRs are found in human genes. The more STRs one can characterize, the smaller the percentage of the population from which these STRs can emanate. This gives rise to the concept of **multiplexing**. Using PCR technology, one can simultaneously extract and amplify a combination of different STRs.

    The majority of the STR systems on the commercial market today are multiplex systems. There are kits that can amplify DNA on both the X and Y chromosomes simultaneously, amplifying up to 24 loci at a time. The kits provide the necessary materials for amplifying and detecting the STRs. The design of the system ensures that the size of the STRs does not overlap, thereby allowing each marker to be viewed clearly on an electropherogram, as shown in Figure 16–10. In the United States, the forensic science community had initially standardized 13 STRs for entry into a national database known as the Combined DNA Index System (CODIS). In 2017, seven additional STR loci have been added to the required CODIS database for a total of 20. Since many of these loci are included in global databases, the expanded CODIS loci set will enhance international law enforcement and counter-terrorism investigations to allow for cross comparison of databases in Europe and across the globe.

    When an STR is selected for analysis, not only must the identity and number of core repeats be defined, but the sequence of bases flanking the repeats must also be known. This knowledge allows commercial manufacturers of STR typing kits to prepare the correct primers to delineate the STR segment to be amplified by PCR. Also, a mix of different primers aimed at different STRs will be used to simultaneously amplify a multitude of STRs (i.e., to multiplex). In fact, some STR kits on the commercial market can simultaneously make copies of 24 different STRs (see Figure 16–11).

multiplexing
A technique that simultaneously detects more than one DNA marker in a single analysis.

FIGURE 16-10
A multiplex system containing five loci: D3S1358, vWA, D16S539, CSF1PO and, TPOX indicating a match between the questioned profile and the standard profile.

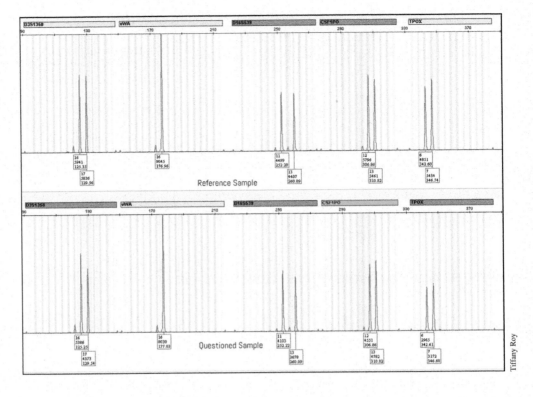

FIGURE 16-11
STR profile for 24 loci.

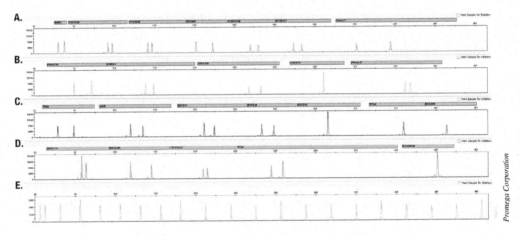

Estimation of Weight Using STRs

DNA matches and inclusions fall on a sliding scale, from weak associations with mixed DNA samples to strong single source DNA matches. It has always been important in forensic DNA to estimate the weight of an association between the DNA profile from an item of evidence and the DNA profile of a known individual. In general, if an analyst reports a match, they have to describe how strong the match is.

In the beginning, the combined probability of inclusion and the random match probability were used to estimate weight. These calculations were first described in 1996 by the National Research Council Report on forensic DNA evidence. They describe the probability that two individuals selected at random will have an identical STR type to that seen in the evidence. The smaller the value of this probability, the more discriminating the match. A high degree of discrimination and even individualization can be attained by analyzing a combination of STRs. Because STRs occur independently of each other, the probability of biological evidence having a particular combination of STR types is determined by the product of their frequency of occurrence in a population. This combination is referred to as the *product rule* (see page 66). Hence,

Inside the Science

Probabilistic Genotyping Software

Probabilistic genotyping is an innovative approach to the statistical analysis of DNA mixtures. It was created in response to the increased difficulty and irregularity in mixture deconvolution procedures in crime labs nationwide. Probabilistic genotyping software can be classified into two categories: semi-continuous or fully continuous. In the semi-continuous method, also known as the drop model or discrete model, profile information like peak heights and peak area are not considered in the analysis. Information is determined solely from the presence or absence of alleles. Fully continuous models attempt to use all of the data, including peak heights and peak area, and incorporates biological parameters to account for stutter, allele drop in and allele drop out.

Probabilistic genotyping software reduces the number of subjective decisions made by an analyst therefore improving consistency. This methodology has allowed laboratories to analyze cases with mixtures previously too complex for traditional methods of interpretation and statistical analysis.

the greater the number of STRs characterized, the smaller the frequency of occurrence of the analyzed sample in the general population.

However, the data produced in the 1990s is different than the data commonly seen today. DNA testing has become increasingly more sensitive. Today, DNA analysts are able to develop DNA profiles from just a few skin cells, where at its inception, analysts required a high quantity and high-quality DNA source, like blood. When testing items that are handled by many different people, like door handles or clothing, the resulting profile can be more complex to interpret. In recognition of this change, the field is moving away from previously established probability methods toward the use of the likelihood ratio.

The likelihood ratio is comparing the probability of observing the mixture data under two (or more) alternative hypotheses. The calculation compares the probability of the evidence if the crime stain originated with the suspect versus the probability of the evidence if the crime stain originated from an unknown, unrelated individual. Likelihood ratios allow the analyst to more completely utilize DNA data in estimating weight. They have been integrated into software programs developed to assist in standardizing DNA interpretation across the nation and around the globe, discussed in more detail in the next section.

WEBEXTRA 16.4
Understand the Operational Principles of Capillary Electrophoresis

Sex Identification Using STRs

Manufacturers of commercial STR kits typically used by crime laboratories provide one additional piece of useful information along with STR types: the sex of the DNA contributor. The focus of attention here is the **amelogenin gene** located on both the X and Y chromosomes. This gene, which is actually the gene for tooth pulp, has an interesting characteristic in that it is shorter by six bases in the X chromosome than in the Y chromosome. Hence, when the amelogenin gene is amplified by PCR and separated by electrophoresis, males, who have an X and a Y chromosome, show two peaks; females, who have two X chromosomes, have just one peak. Typically, these results are obtained in conjunction with STR types.

Another tool in the arsenal of the DNA analyst is the ability to type STRs located on the Y chromosome. The Y chromosome is male specific and is always paired with the X chromosome. Although more than 400 **Y-STRs** have been identified, only a small number of them are being used for forensic applications. One commercial kit allows for the characterization of 17 Y chromosome STRs. When can it be advantageous to seek out Y-STR types? Generally, Y-STRs are useful for analyzing blood, saliva, or a vaginal swab that is a mix originating from more than one male. For example, Y-STRs prove useful when multiple males are involved in a sexual assault. Further simplifying the analysis is that any DNA in the mixture that originates from a female will not show.

Keep in mind that STR types derived from the Y chromosome originate only from this single male chromosome. A female subject, or one with an XX chromosome pattern, does not contribute any DNA information. Also, unlike a conventional STR type that is derived from two chromosomes and typically shows two peaks, a Y-STR has only one peak for each STR type.

amelogenin gene
A genetic locus useful for determining sex.

WEBEXTRA 16.5
The DNA Process: A Review

Y-STRs
Short tandem repeats located on the human Y chromosome.

For example, the traditional STR DNA pattern may prove to be overly complex in the case of a vaginal swab containing the semen of two males. Each STR type would be expected to show four peaks, two from each male. Also complicating the appearance of the DNA profile may be the presence of DNA from skin cells emanating from the walls of the vagina. In this circumstance, homing in on the Y chromosome greatly simplifies the appearance and interpretation of the DNA profile. Thus, when presented with a DNA mixture of two males and one female, Y-STR analysis would show only two peaks (one peak for each male) for each Y-STR type.

When gauging the significance of a Y-STR match between questioned and known specimens, one should take into consideration that all male paternal relatives (e.g., brothers, father, male offspring, and uncles) would be expected to have the same Y-STR profile.

Another advantage of employing STR technology is to extend the success of detecting evidential DNA from vaginal swabs collected from rape victims. Casework experience has demonstrated significant difficulties in obtaining traditional STR DNA profiles for the male donor from vaginal swabs collected after three to four days after intercourse. However, the application of Y-STR technology often extends the routine postcoital detection time to five days for the male donor.

Case Files

Reopening the Boston Strangler Case

Albert DeSalvo's rape and murder of 11 women shocked the country in the early 1960s. Better known as the Boston Strangler, DeSalvo would gain entry to primarily single female's apartments using disguises and tricks. Boston Police finally apprehended DeSalvo through a witness sketch and his confession to the crimes through detailed descriptions. Despite his confession, DeSalvo later recanted, and forensic experts contested his guilt. DeSalvo was sentenced to life in prison for unrelated sexual assaults, but never was charged with the Boston Strangler killings. Albert DeSalvo died in jail in 1973, further complicating the situation.

Through funding by the National Institute of Justice, the Boston Strangler case was reopened and examined with new DNA testing techniques. The Boston Police Department's cold case squad used DNA found on one of the Strangler's victims, Mary Sullivan, to link the crimes back to DeSalvo. Forensic scientists focused their research on the (Y) chromosome, as it relates back to every male in a paternal lineage. DeSalvo's nephew provided the key DNA used to tie Albert to the killings, and a positive match was made. Detectives confirmed these results by exhuming DeSalvo's body; they concluded that the odds of someone else committing these crimes were 1 in 220 billion. The Boston Strangler Case has finally been resolved.

Inside the Science

MiniSTRs

The forensic science community turned to STRs when it became apparent that short segments of DNA would be required to meet the requirements of PCR. Commercial manufacturers of DNA-typing kits prepared a series of 13 STRs for compatibility with the CODIS DNA database that ranged in length from 100 to 450 bases. One obvious benefit in working with short DNA segments was the likelihood that useful information could be extracted even from fragmented DNA. This often proved to be the case, but not always. On occasion, degraded DNA is encountered that is so badly damaged that traditional STR analysis

is not possible. Prolonged exposure of DNA to extreme environmental elements, such as temperature extremes, humidity, or microbial activity, can lead to such degradation. An approach to dealing with this problem is to further shorten the STR strands that emerge from the PCR process.

The approach that has been taken to accomplish this task is to create new primers that can be positioned closer to the STR repeat region (see the figure). The shorter STR products (called *amplicons*) that now emerge from PCR increase the chances of characterizing badly fragmented strands of DNA. These smaller amplicons are called "miniSTRs." One manufacturer of STR kits has produced a miniSTR kit designed to amplify eight miniSTRs, seven of which are totally compatible with the CODIS database. The miniSTRs range in size from 71 to 250 bases. A DNA analyst suspecting a degraded sample now has the option, if sample size permits, of running both traditional STR and miniSTR determinations, or just the latter.

The advent of miniSTRs means that forensic scientists can now analyze samples that were once thought to be of no value. One of the first benefactors of miniSTR technology was the identification of a number of victims from the Waco Branch Davidian fire. Also, a number of World Trade Center victims were identified by miniSTR technology. Another focus of attention has been human hair. In the past, extracting nuclear DNA out of the hair shaft has been enormously difficult; the number of STRs in hair has been found to be very low as well as highly degraded. However, one study has demonstrated that miniSTRs may overcome some of the difficulties in obtaining partial profiles from the degraded DNA present in shed hair.[2]

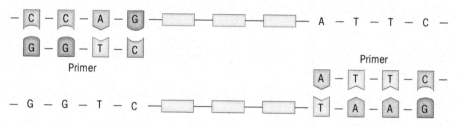

Appropriate primers are positioned close to the repeat units of a DNA segment in order to initiate the PCR process that will create short or mini STRs.

Significance of DNA Typing

STR DNA typing has become an essential and basic investigative tool in the law enforcement community. The technology has progressed at a rapid rate and in only a few years has surmounted numerous legal challenges to become vital evidence for resolving violent crimes and sex offenses. DNA evidence is impartial, implicating the guilty and exonerating the innocent.

In a number of well-publicized cases, DNA evidence has exonerated individuals who have been wrongly convicted and imprisoned. The importance of DNA analyses in criminal investigations has also placed added burdens on crime laboratories to improve their quality-assurance procedures and to ensure the correctness of their results. In several well-publicized instances, the accuracy of DNA tests conducted by government-funded laboratories has been called into question.

WEBEXTRA 16.6
See the 13 CODIS STRs and Their Chromosomal Positions

WEBEXTRA 16.7
See How to Calculate the Frequency of Occurrence of a DNA Profile

WEBEXTRA 16.8
See the Electropherogram Record from One Individual's DNA

WEBEXTRA 16.9
An Animation Depicting Y-STRs

Mitochondrial DNA

Typically, when one describes DNA in the context of a criminal investigation, the subject is assumed to be the DNA in the nucleus of a cell. Actually, a human cell contains two types of DNA—nuclear and mitochondrial. The first constitutes the 23 pairs of chromosomes in the nuclei of our cells. Each parent contributes to the genetic makeup of these chromosomes. Mitochondrial DNA (mtDNA), on the other hand, is found outside the nucleus of the cell and is inherited solely from the mother.

Mitochondria are cell structures found in all human cells. They are the power plants of the body, providing about 90 percent of the energy that the body needs to function. A single mitochondrion contains several loops of DNA, all of which are involved in energy generation. Further, because each cell in our bodies contains hundreds to thousands of mitochondria, there are hundreds to thousands of mtDNA copies in a human cell. This compares to just one set of nuclear DNA located in that same cell. Thus, forensic scientists are offered enhanced sensitivity and the opportunity to characterize mtDNA when nuclear DNA is significantly degraded, such as in charred remains, or when nuclear DNA may be present in a small quantity (such as in a hair shaft). Interestingly, when authorities cannot obtain a reference sample from an individual who may be long deceased or missing, an mtDNA reference sample can be obtained from any maternally related relative. However, all individuals of the same maternal lineage will be indistinguishable by mtDNA analysis.

mitochondria

Small structures located outside the nucleus of a cell; these structures supply energy to the cell; maternally inherited DNA is found in each mitochondrion.

[2] K. E. Opel et al., "Evaluation and Quantification of Nuclear DNA from Human Telogen Hairs," *Journal of Forensic Sciences* 53 (2008): 853.

> > > > > > > > >

Case Files

Cold Case Hit

In 1990, a series of attacks on older victims was committed in Goldsboro, North Carolina, by an unknown individual dubbed the Night Stalker. During one such attack in March, an older woman was brutally sexually assaulted and almost murdered. Her daughter's early arrival home saved the woman's life. The suspect fled, leaving behind materials intended to burn the residence and the victim in an attempt to conceal the crime.

In July 1990, another older woman was sexually assaulted and murdered in her home. Three months later, a third older woman was sexually assaulted and stabbed to death. Her husband was also murdered. Although their house was set alight in an attempt to cover up the crime, fire and rescue personnel pulled the bodies from the house before it was engulfed in flames. DNA analysis of biological evidence collected from vaginal swabs from the three sexual assault victims enabled authorities to conclude that the same perpetrator had committed all three crimes. However, there was no suspect.

More than 10 years after these crimes were committed, law enforcement authorities retested the biological evidence from all three cases using newer DNA technology and entered the DNA profiles into North Carolina's DNA database. The DNA profile developed from the crime-scene evidence was compared to thousands of convicted-offender profiles already in the database.

In April 2001, a "cold hit" was made: The DNA profiles were matched to that of an individual in the convicted-offender DNA database. The perpetrator had been convicted of shooting into an occupied dwelling, an offense that requires inclusion of the convict's DNA in the North Carolina DNA database. The suspect was brought into custody for questioning and was served with a search warrant to obtain a sample of his blood. That sample was analyzed and compared to the crime-scene evidence, confirming the DNA database match. When confronted with the DNA evidence, the suspect confessed to all three crimes.

Source: National Institute of Justice, "Using DNA to Solve Cold Cases" (NIJ Special Report), July 2002.

Inside the Science

Familial DNA—Expanding the DNA Database

In 1984, Deborah Sykes was raped and stabbed to death as she walked to work in Winston-Salem, North Carolina. A month later, Darryl Hunt, then 19 years old, was arrested and eventually convicted of the crime. Hunt insisted that he was innocent, and by 1990, DNA testing of semen found on Sykes proved that he was not its source. Nevertheless, North Carolina prosecutors ignored this new evidence and he remained in jail. Finally, a search against Darryl Hunt's STR profile in the North Carolina DNA database revealed a close but not perfect match to a genetic profile already in the database, that of his brother. Upon further investigation, that man, Willard Brown, confessed to Sykes's murder in 2003, and Hunt was finally freed from prison.

In this case, DNA profiling exonerated an innocent man and helped lead the police to the real culprit. The Sykes case illustrates how the contents of a criminal DNA database can be dramatically expanded to aid the police in identifying people who commit crimes by searching the database for near matches.

Typically, the CODIS database is used to find exact matches with crime-scene DNA. However, taking into account the facts that the 13 STR loci that constitute U.S. offender DNA databases are genetically inherited and

that each individual's DNA profile is genetically determined by one's parents creates opportunities to use the database's raw data to search out close relatives. DNA profiles of related individuals are likely to show a higher proportion of shared STR loci as compared to unrelated individuals. Hence, searching the database for profiles that have a high degree of commonality may lead to the identification of a close relative of the perpetrator. Interestingly, studies have shown that a person's chances of committing a crime increase if a parent or sibling had previously done so. A 1999 U.S. Department of Justice survey found that 46 percent of jail inmates had at least one close relative who had also been incarcerated.

The potential for improving the effectiveness of DNA database searches is considerable. Familial searches of a DNA database would dramatically increase the size of the database by three or more times because every profile that is entered would, in effect, contain genetic information about the STR alleles of the donor's parents, siblings, and children. One study estimates that using familial DNA searches could increase the "cold hit" rates by 40 percent. Considering the fact that there have been about 95,000 cold hits in the United States, familial DNA has the potential for identifying thousands of additional criminal suspects.

The concept of familial DNA searching has been routinely adopted in the United Kingdom. In the United States, the FBI notifies investigators about close matches it finds using its current software, but the agency has no current plans to modify its search algorithms to optimize the database's capacity to ferret out near or close matches. This leaves it up to the states to decide whether to release identifying information about an offender whose DNA closely matches a crime-scene sample from another state. Challengers to familial database searching have cited it as a violation of constitutional protections against unreasonable search and seizure. A number of mixed state court decisions have failed to produce a consensus on the constitutionality of familial DNA database searches.

Although mtDNA analysis is significantly more sensitive than nuclear DNA profiling, forensic analysis of mtDNA is more rigorous, time consuming, and costly than nuclear DNA profiling. For this reason, only a handful of public and private forensic laboratories receive evidence for this type of determination. The FBI Laboratory has imposed strict limitations on the types of cases in which it will apply mtDNA technology.

Inside the Science

Forensic Aspects of Mitochondrial DNA

As was previously discussed, nuclear DNA is composed of a continuous linear strand of nucleotides (*A, T, G,* and *C*). On the other hand, mtDNA is constructed in a circular or loop configuration. Each loop contains enough *A, T, G,* and *C* (approximately 16,569 units) to make up 37 genes involved in mitochondrial energy generation. Two regions of mtDNA have been found to be highly variable in the human population. These two regions have been designated hypervariable region I (HV1) and hypervariable region II (HV2), as

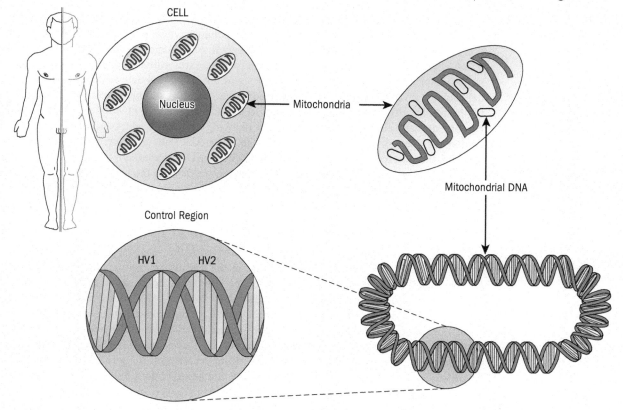

Every cell in the body contains hundreds of mitochondria, which provide energy to the cell. Each mitochondrion contains numerous copies of DNA shaped in the form of a loop. Distinctive differences between individuals in their mitochondrial DNA makeup are found in two specific segments of the control region on the DNA loop known as HV1 and HV2.

(continued)

shown in the figure. As indicated previously, the process for analyzing HV1 and HV2 is tedious. It involves generating many copies of these DNA hypervariable regions by PCR and then determining the order of the A–T–G–C bases constituting the hypervariable regions. This process is known as **sequencing**. The FBI Laboratory, the Armed Forces DNA Identification Laboratory, and other laboratories have collaborated to compile an mtDNA population database containing the base sequences from HV1 and HV2.

Once the sequences of the hypervariable regions from a case sample are obtained, most laboratories simply report the number of times these sequences appear in the mtDNA database maintained by the FBI. The mtDNA database contains about 5,000 sequences. This approach permits an assessment of how common or rare an observed mtDNA sequence is in the database. Interestingly, many of the sequences that have been determined in casework are unique to the existing database, and many types are present at frequencies no greater than 1 percent in the database. Thus it is often possible to demonstrate how uncommon a particular mitochondrial DNA sequence is. However, even under the best circumstances, mtDNA typing does not approach STR analysis in its discrimination power. Thus, mtDNA analysis is best reserved for samples for which nuclear DNA typing is simply not possible.

---

sequencing
A procedure used to determine the order of the base pairs that constitute DNA.

WEBEXTRA 16.10
See How We Inherit Our Mitochondrial DNA

WEBEXTRA 16.11
Look into the Structure of Mitochondrial DNA and See How It Is Used for DNA Typing

picogram
One-trillionth of a gram, or 0.000000000001 gram.

low copy number
Fewer than 18 DNA-bearing cells.

epithelial cells
The outer layer of skin cells; these DNA-bearing cells often fall off or are rubbed off onto objects retrieved from crime scenes.

touch DNA
DNA from skin cells transferred onto the surface of an object by simple contact.

Collection and Preservation of Biological Evidence for DNA Analysis

Since the early 1990s, the advent of DNA profiling has vaulted biological crime-scene evidence to a stature of importance that is eclipsed only by the fingerprint. In fact, the high sensitivity of DNA determinations has even changed the way police investigators define biological evidence.

Just how sensitive is STR profiling? Forensic analysts using currently accepted protocols can reach sensitivity levels as low as 125 **picograms**. Interestingly, a human cell has an estimated 7 picograms of DNA, which means that only 18 DNA-bearing cells are needed to obtain an STR profile. However, modifications in the technology can readily extend the level of detection down to 9 cells. A quantity of DNA that is below the normal level of detection is defined as a **low copy number**. (However, analysts must take extraordinary care in analyzing low-copy-number DNA and often may find that courts will not allow this data to be admissible in a criminal trial.) With this technology in hand, the horizon of the criminal investigator extends beyond the traditional dried blood or semen stain to include stamps and envelopes licked with saliva, a cup or can that has touched a person's lips, chewing gum, the sweat band of a hat, or a bedsheet containing dead skin cells. Likewise, skin or **epithelial cells** transferred onto the surface of a weapon, the interior of a glove, or a pen have yielded DNA results.[3]

The phenomenon of transferring DNA via skin cells onto the surface of an object has come to be called **touch DNA**. Again, keep in mind that, in theory, only 18 skin cells deposited on an object are required to obtain a DNA profile.

Collection and Packaging of Biological Evidence

However, before investigators become enamored with the wonders of DNA, they should first realize that the crime scene must be treated in the traditional manner. Before the collection of evidence begins, biological evidence should be photographed close-up and its location relative to the entire crime scene recorded through notes, sketches, and photographs. If the shape and position of bloodstains may provide information about the circumstances of the crime, an expert must immediately conduct an on-the-spot evaluation of the blood evidence. The significance of the position and shape of bloodstains can best be ascertained when the expert has an on-site overview of the entire crime scene and can better reconstruct the movement of the individuals involved. No attempt should be made to disturb the blood pattern before this phase of the investigation is completed.

---

[3] R. A. Wickenheiser, "Trace DNA: A Review, Discussion of Theory, and Application of the Transfer of Trace Qualities Through Skin Contact," *Journal of Forensic Sciences* 47 (2002): 442.

The evidence collector must handle all body fluids and biologically stained materials with a minimum amount of personal contact. All body fluids must be assumed to be infectious; hence, wearing disposable non-latex powder free gloves (e.g., nitrile) while handling the evidence is required. Double gloving with changes of the top gloves when handling different sample sites or after touching any surface shall be employed. Safety considerations and avoidance of contamination also call for the wearing of face masks, a lab coat, eye protection, shoe covers, and possibly coveralls.

The deposition of DNA onto crime-scene objects via saliva, sweat, skin, blood, and semen has created a vast array of forensic evidence that is quite different from the traditional evidence collected at crime scenes prior to the DNA era (see Table 16–1). Biological evidence should not be packaged in plastic or airtight containers because accumulation of residual moisture could contribute to the growth of DNA-destroying bacteria and fungi. **Each stained article should be packaged separately in a paper bag or a well-ventilated box**. A red biohazard label must be attached to each container. If feasible, the entire stained article should be packaged and submitted for examination. If this is not possible, dried blood is best removed from a surface with a sterile cotton-tipped swab lightly moistened with distilled water from a dropper bottle. A portion of the unstained surface material near the recovered stain must likewise be removed or swabbed and placed in a separate package. This is known as a **substrate control**. The forensic examiner might use the substrate swab to confirm that the results of the tests performed were brought about by the stain and not by the material on which it was deposited. The deposition of biological stains on clothing, bed sheets, and other relevant items involving intrafamilial sexual abuse often requires the examination of a substrate control in the laboratory. The revelation that DNA be transferred between articles during machine laundering is a stark reminder of the ease with which secondary transfer of DNA can occur and the need to ascertain that areas surrounding a stain is free of evidential DNA. This is accomplished by examining cuttings taken in proximity to the stain.[4]

substrate control
An unstained object adjacent to an area on which biological material has been deposited.

One point is critical, and that is that the collected swabs must not be packaged in a wet state. After the collection is made, the swab must be air-dried for approximately 5 to 10 minutes. Then

TABLE 16–1

Location and Sources of DNA at Crime Scenes

Evidence	Possible Location of DNA on the Evidence	Source of DNA
Baseball bat or similar weapon	Handle, end	Sweat, skin, blood, tissue
Hat, bandanna, mask	Inside	Sweat, hair, dandruff
Eyeglasses	Nose or ear pieces, lens	Sweat, skin
Facial tissue, cotton swab	Surface area	Mucus, blood, sweat, semen, ear wax
Dirty laundry	Surface area	Blood, sweat, semen
Toothpick	Tips	Saliva
Used cigarette	Cigarette butt	Saliva
Stamp or envelope	Licked area	Saliva
Tape or ligature	Inside/outside surface	Skin, sweat
Bottle, can, glass	Sides, mouthpiece	Saliva, sweat
Used condom	Inside/outside surface	Semen, vaginal or rectal cells
Blanket, pillow, sheet	Surface area	Sweat, hair, semen, urine, saliva
"Through and through" bullet	Outside surface	Blood, tissue
Bite mark	Person's skin or clothing	Saliva
Fingernail, partial fingernail	Scrapings	Blood, sweat, tissue

Source: From National Institute of Justice, by National Institute of Justice.

[4] S. Noel et al., "DNA Transfer During Laundering May Yield Complete Genetic Profiles," *Forensic Science International: Genetics* 23 (2016): 240.

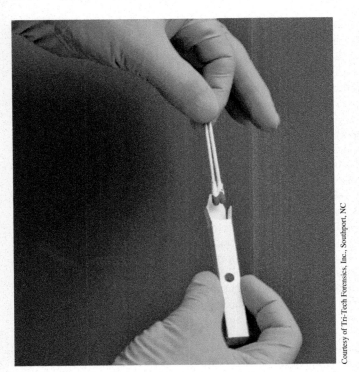

Courtesy of Tri-Tech Forensics, Inc., Southport, NC

FIGURE 16–12
Air-dried swabs are placed in a swab box for delivery to the forensic laboratory.

buccal cells
Cells derived from the inner cheek lining.

WEBEXTRA 16.12
Step into the Role of the First Responding Officer at a Burglary Scene

WEBEXTRA 16.13
Assume the Duties of an Evidence Collection Technician at a Burglary Scene

it is best to place it in a swab box (see Figure 16–12), which has a circular hole to allow air circulation. The swab box can then be placed in a paper or manila envelope.

All packages containing biological evidence should be refrigerated or stored in a cool location out of direct sunlight until delivery to the laboratory.

However, one common exception is blood mixed with soil. Microbes present in soil rapidly degrade DNA. Therefore, blood in soil must be stored in a clean glass or plastic container and immediately frozen.

Obtaining DNA Reference Specimens

Biological evidence attains its full forensic value only when an analyst can compare each of its DNA types to known DNA samples collected from victims and suspects. The least intrusive method for obtaining a DNA standard/reference, one that nonmedical personnel can readily use, is the *buccal swab*. Cotton swabs are placed in the subject's mouth and the inside of the cheek is vigorously swabbed, resulting in the transfer of **buccal cells** onto the swab (see Figure 16–13).

If an individual is not available to give a DNA standard/reference sample, some interesting alternatives are available to evidence collectors, including a toothbrush, combs and hairbrushes, a razor, soiled laundry, used cigarette butts, and earplugs. Any of these items may contain a sufficient quantity of DNA for typing purposes. Interestingly, as investigators worked to identify the remains of victims of the World Trade Center attack on September 11, 2001, the families of the missing were requested to supply the New York City DNA Laboratory with these types of items in an effort to match recovered DNA with human remains.

Contamination of DNA Evidence

One key concern during the collection of a DNA-containing specimen is contamination. Contamination can occur by introducing foreign DNA through coughing or sneezing onto a stain during the collection process, or there can be a transfer of DNA when items of evidence are incorrectly placed in contact with each other during packaging. Fortunately, an examination of DNA peak patterns in the laboratory readily reveals the presence of contamination. For example, with an STR, one will expect to see a two-peak pattern. More than two peaks suggest a mixture of DNA from more than one source.

Crime-scene investigators can take some relatively simple steps to minimize contamination of biological evidence:

1. Use double-layered disposable gloves.
2. Wear a face mask while collecting evidence, a lab coat, eye protection, as well as shoe covers.
3. Change outer glove before handling each new piece of evidence or touching a surface.
4. Collect a substrate control for possible subsequent laboratory examination.
5. Pick up small items of evidence such as cigarette butts and stamps with clean forceps. Disposable forceps are to be used so that they can be discarded after a single evidence collection.
6. Always package each item of evidence in its own well-ventilated container.

A common occurrence at crime scenes is to suspect the presence of blood but not be able to observe any with the naked eye. In these situations, the common test of choice is luminol or Bluestar (see page 381). Interestingly, neither luminol nor Bluestar is expected to inhibit the ability to detect and characterize STRs.[5] Therefore, luminol and Bluestar can be used to locate traces of blood and areas that have been washed nearly free of blood without compromising the potential for DNA typing.

---

[5] A. M. Gross et al., "The Effect of Luminol on Presumptive Tests and DNA Analysis Using the Polymerase Chain Reaction," *Journal of Forensic Sciences* 44 (1999): 837.

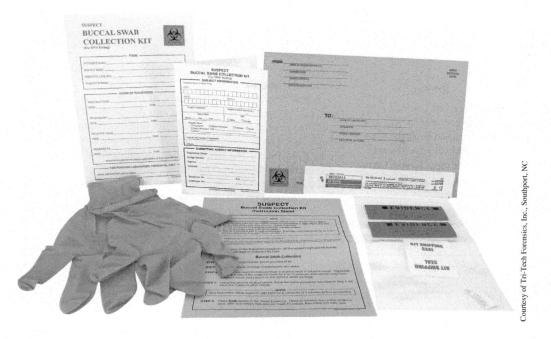

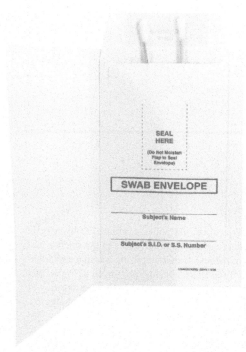

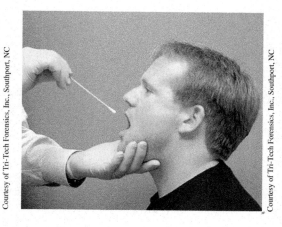

FIGURE 16–13

A buccal swab collection kit is designed for use by nonmedical personnel. The cotton-tipped swabs are placed in the subject's mouth and the inside of the cheek is vigorously swabbed, resulting in the transfer of buccal cells onto the cotton bulb of the swab. The kit is then delivered to the forensic laboratory.

> > > > > > > >

Contact Lens Evidence

A woman alleged that she had been held against her will and sexually assaulted by a male friend in an apartment. During the course of the assault, a contact lens was knocked from the victim's eye. After the assault, she escaped, but because she was afraid of the threats made by her attacker, she did not report the assault to the police for three days. When the police examined the apartment, they noted that it had been thoroughly cleaned. A vacuum cleaner bag was seized for examination, and several pieces of material resembling fragments of a contact lens were discovered within the bag.

In the laboratory, approximately 20 nanograms of human DNA was recovered from the contact lens fragments. Cells from both the eyeball and the interior of the eyelids are naturally replaced every 6 to 24 hours. Therefore, both are potential sources for the DNA found. The DNA profile originating from the fragments matched the victim, thus corroborating the victim's account of the crime. The estimated population frequency of occurrence for the nine matching STRs are approximately 1 in 850 million. The suspect subsequently pleaded guilty to the offense.

STR Locus	Victim's DNA Type	Contact Lens
D3S1358	15, 18	15, 18
FGA	24, 25	24, 25
vWA	17, 17	17, 17
TH01	6, 7	6, 7
F13A1	5, 6	5, 6
fes/fps	11, 12	11, 12
D5S818	11, 12	11, 12
D13S317	11, 12	11, 12
D7S820	10, 12	10, 12

Based on information in R. A. Wickenheiser and R. M. Jobin, "Comparison of DNA Recovered from a Contact Lens Using PCR DNA Typing," *Canadian Society of Forensic Science Journal* 32 (1999): 67.

> > > > > > > >

The JonBenét Ramsey Murder Case

Point–Counterpoint

Point

July 9, 2008

Boulder District Attorney Mary T. Lacy issues the following announcement with regard to the investigation of the murder of JonBenét Ramsey.

On December 25–26, 1996, JonBenét Ramsey was murdered in the home where she lived with her mother, father, and brother. Despite a long and intensive investigation, the death of JonBenét remains unsolved.

The murder has received unprecedented publicity and has been shrouded in controversy. That publicity has led to many theories over the years in which suspicion has focused on one family member or another. However, there has been at least one persistent stumbling block to the possibility of prosecuting any Ramsey family members for the death of JonBenét—DNA.

As part of its investigation of the JonBenét Ramsey homicide, the Boulder Police identified genetic material with apparent evidentiary value. Over time, the police continued to investigate DNA, including taking advantage of advances in the science and methodology. One of the results of their efforts was that they identified genetic material and a DNA profile from drops of JonBenét's blood located in the crotch of the underwear she was wearing at the time her body was discovered. That genetic profile belongs to a male and does not belong to anyone in the Ramsey family.

The police department diligently compared that profile to a very large number of people associated with the victim, with her family, and with the investigation, and has not identified the source, innocent or otherwise, of this DNA. The Boulder Police and prosecutors assigned to this investigation in the past also worked conscientiously with laboratory analysts to obtain better results through new approaches and additional tests as they became available. Those efforts ultimately led to the discovery of sufficient genetic markers from this male profile to enter it into the national DNA data bank.

In December of 2002, the Boulder District Attorney's Office, under Mary T. Lacy, assumed responsibility for the investigation of the JonBenét Ramsey homicide. Since then, this office has worked with the Boulder Police Department to continue the investigation of this crime.

In early August of 2007, District Attorney Lacy attended a Continuing Education Program in West Virginia sponsored by the National Institute of Justice on Forensic Biology and DNA. The presenters discussed successful outcomes from a new methodology described as "touch DNA." One method for sampling for touch DNA is the "scraping method." In this process, forensic scientists scrape a surface where there is no observable stain or other indication of possible DNA in an effort to recover for analysis any genetic material that might nonetheless be present. This methodology was not well known in this country until recently and is still used infrequently.

In October of 2007, we decided to pursue the possibility of submitting additional items from the JonBenét Ramsey homicide to be examined using this methodology. We checked with a number of Colorado sources regarding which private laboratory to use for this work. Based upon multiple recommendations, including that of the Boulder Police Department, we contacted the Bode Technology Group located near Washington, D.C., and initiated discussions with the professionals at that laboratory. First Assistant District Attorney Peter Maguire and Investigator Andy Horita spent a full day with staff members at the Bode facility in early December of 2007.

The Bode Technology laboratory applied the "touch DNA" scraping method to both sides of the waist area of the long johns that JonBenét Ramsey was wearing over her underwear when her body was discovered. These sites were chosen because evidence supports the likelihood that the perpetrator removed and/or replaced the long johns, perhaps by handling them on the sides near the waist.

On March 24, 2008, Bode informed us that they had recovered and identified genetic material from both sides of the waist area of the long johns. The unknown male profile previously identified from the inside crotch area of the underwear matched the DNA recovered from the long johns at Bode.

We consulted with a DNA expert from a different laboratory, who recommended additional investigation into the remote possibility that the DNA might have come from sources at the autopsy when this clothing was removed. Additional samples were obtained and then analyzed by the Colorado Bureau of Investigation to assist us in this effort. We received those results on June 27 of this year and are, as a result, confidant that this DNA did not come from innocent sources at the autopsy. As mentioned above, extensive DNA testing had previously excluded people connected to the family and to the investigation as possible innocent sources.

I want to acknowledge my appreciation for the efforts of the Boulder Police Department, Bode Technology Group, the Colorado Bureau of Investigation, and the Denver Police Department Forensic Laboratory for the great work and assistance they have contributed to this investigation.

The unexplained third party DNA on the clothing of the victim is very significant and powerful evidence. It is very unlikely that there would be an innocent explanation for DNA found at three different locations on two separate items of clothing worn by the victim at the time of her murder. This is particularly true in this case because the matching DNA profiles were found on genetic material from inside the crotch of the victim's underwear and near the waist on both sides of her long johns, and because concerted efforts that might identify a source, and perhaps an innocent explanation, were unsuccessful.

It is therefore the position of the Boulder District Attorney's Office that this profile belongs to the perpetrator of the homicide.

DNA is very often the most reliable forensic evidence we can hope to find during a criminal investigation. We rely on it often to bring to justice those who have committed crimes. It can likewise be reliable evidence upon which to remove people from suspicion in appropriate cases.

The Boulder District Attorney's Office does not consider any member of the Ramsey family, including John, Patsy, or Burke Ramsey, as suspects in this case. We make this announcement now because we have recently obtained this new scientific evidence that adds significantly to the exculpatory value of the previous scientific evidence. We do so with full appreciation for the other evidence in this case.

Local, national, and even international publicity has focused on the murder of JonBenét Ramsey. Many members of the public came to believe that one or more of the Ramseys, including her mother or her father or even her brother, were responsible for this brutal homicide. Those suspicions were not based on evidence that had been tested in court; rather, they were based on evidence reported by the media.

It is the responsibility of every prosecutor to seek justice. That responsibility includes seeking justice for people whose reputations and lives can be damaged irreparably by the lingering specter of suspicion. In a highly publicized case, the detrimental impact of publicity and suspicion on people's lives can be extreme. The suspicions about the Ramseys in this case created an ongoing living hell for the Ramsey family and their friends, which added to their suffering from the unexplained and devastating loss of JonBenét.

For reasons including those discussed above, we believe that justice dictates that the Ramseys be treated only as victims of this very serious crime. We will accord them all the rights guaranteed to the victims of violent crimes under the law in Colorado and all the respect and sympathy due from one human being to another. To the extent that this office has added to the distress suffered by the Ramsey family at any time or to any degree, I offer my deepest apology.

We prefer that any tips related to this ongoing investigation be submitted in writing or via electronic mail to BoulderDA.org, but they can also be submitted to our tip line at (303) 441–1636.

This office will make no further statements.

Counterpoint

Last year, then–Boulder, Colorado, District Attorney Mary Keenan Lacy, who had been "investigating" the Ramsey case for the last few years, wrote a letter to JonBenét's father John, apologizing for having believed he or his wife, the late Patsy, or their son Burke (then nine) had anything to do with their daughter's 1996 death. Lacy indicated that recent tests from the Bode Laboratory of Virginia revealed that their "new methodology" of touch DNA found a match that proves an intruder was culpable of the slaying in which the 6-year-old was molested, strangled, and given a fractured skull.

There has always been unmatched, unknown male DNA—likely from saliva—in the inside crotch of the child's underpants. A minute amount, too degraded to get a proper DNA profile, was mixed with her blood when someone stuck her oh-so-slightly with the pointed end of a broken paintbrush on the night of her death. Because the DNA was so insignificant, it was theorized to have come from someone coughing during the manufacturing process, then the blood drops on top rehydrated

(continued)

it. If the DNA and blood were deposited at the same time, they would have degraded at the same rate—but here the blood sample was robust.

Lacy wrote that the lab discovered that sloughed-off skin cells on the waist area of the long johns JonBenét wore over her underpants can be matched to the underpants' DNA.

That was great news for people who want to believe there was an intruder with no link to the family members. No one imagines a parent could harm a child in such a brutal and horrendous fashion. Only problem is, adults—including parents—kill kids all the time. While this murder is unique in its application and renown, from an investigative point of view it's just another homicide that has to be dissected to be understood. Anyone looking rationally at the evidence here, and assessing it as a whole, cannot be pleased with Lacy's letter to Ramsey or the fact that she cleared the most credible suspects in the case. At the least it sets a terrible precedent where other people "under the umbrella of suspicion" in other cases will demand the same treatment if their investigations take a long time to reach a courtroom. Just because someone isn't on trial, or a case has gone cold, doesn't mean that the right people aren't firmly under the microscope of authorities.

Mary Lacy left office in January 2009, and the new DA, or any in the future, can retract her pronouncement. Frankly, it will take a brave person to go against the sea of public opinion by individuals who want to blame a bogeyman. One note of encouragement is the case has been returned to the Boulder police, who are better equipped to investigate than the DA's office ever was. The case had been moved to Lacy's predecessor when the Ramsey family complained that the police spotlight on them was unfair. As we all know, there's no statute of limitations on homicide.

This doesn't take Lacy off the hook, as I see it. Here are some facts of the case which were ignored by her reckless decision. . . .

Touch DNA is nothing new to law enforcement, although Bode has only tested for it for about three years. For some 10 years, the FBI lab at Quantico and other labs have used it to capture skin cells from inside masks or gloves, and from guns or knives.

Neither Lacy nor Bode will make available their test results so independent experts can critically review the information. If scientific evidence is to be used to make an argument, proof should be offered. Perhaps some media outlet will file a lawsuit to compel the documents.

What Lacy and Bode have said is that the mystery man's DNA is on the waist area, and that the DNA doesn't match any Ramsey family member. Nothing is stated about where and how much Ramsey DNA was discovered. Patsy dressed the child in those long johns before putting her to bed, and the waistband is precisely what John's two hands touched when he carried his daughter's stiff body in a vertical position upstairs from the basement where she was found deceased. And since DNA can survive multiple launderings, we can't pinpoint when that touch DNA was left on the waistband.

Boulder County Coroner Dr. John Meyer's autopsy report is the Rosetta Stone to this case. It explains the type and order of JonBenét's injuries—asphyxiation by a ligature, then a head blow. It does not reveal who killed the girl. Due to the three-page phony ransom note that many analysts believe was penned by Patsy, the working strategy was to consider Mrs. Ramsey as the perpetrator of all the insults inflicted upon the tot. But while there might have been enough evidence for an arrest, there was not enough for a conviction—and among insiders there was debate about who—if anyone in the household—did what. Without a clear through-line that police and prosecutors could agree upon, what chance would a jury have to find its way to a guilty verdict?

What the autopsy report states without equivocation is that the child suffered vaginal injuries that were "chronic," meaning they predated the murder by days or weeks. We're talking repeated digital penetration that eroded—not ruptured—her hymen. Also, the opening of her vagina was twice the size of a similar aged child's. These factors would have been testified to by at least three pediatric gynecological physicians, had the case gone to trial. This unknown pedophile would have needed on-going intimate access to JonBenét before the night she died. Mary Lacy's early prosecutorial career was as a sex crimes expert, so why didn't she recognize the nature of this little girl's injuries?

If some accident led to JonBenét being strangled, then hit violently in the head, a normal reaction would have been for her caretakers to rush her to a hospital. But that didn't happen, I surmise, because her pre-existing genital injuries would have been noticed. And so, a ridiculous—and sadly, effective—cover-up ensued.

Mary Lacy was responsible for the 2006 debacle where she had arrested and brought back from Thailand a false confessor named John Mark Karr. When the underpants' DNA excluded him from being the perpetrator, she let him go and publicly stated: "The DNA could be an artifact. It isn't necessarily the killer's. There's a probability that it's the killer's. But it could be something else."

She added: "No one is really cleared of a homicide until there's a conviction in court, beyond a reasonable doubt. And I don't think you will get any prosecutor, unless they were present with the person at the time of the crime, to clear someone."

What made her change her thinking when she cleared the Ramseys?

More to the point, where are the intruder's skin cells from the rope around the child's neck, the paintbrush, the spoon, and bowl of pineapple she ate from just before she died, the white blanket that covered her, the flashlight believed to have hit her head, and the pen and paper used in the bogus ransom note? And where is the intruder's touch DNA on the waistband of JonBenét's underpants? Did the stranger pull down her long johns, then command her to pull down her own panties? Are we to believe he then put on gloves—or maybe a whole scuba suit, since there were no unidentified footprints, finger- or handprints, hairs or fibers?

Woven inside the rope around the neck, which was wrapped around a piece of a broken paintbrush, were fibers from the distinctive jacket Patsy wore that evening—and, allegedly, inside the underpants were fibers from the wool sweater John had on. Patsy's fibers were also in the tote where the paintbrush came from and on the sticky side of the piece of duct tape that covered JonBenét's mouth—a length of tape so small it could have been easily flicked aside by her tongue if it had been placed on her mouth while she was alive.

Lacy wrote that autopsy personnel were swabbed and tested for a DNA match, and thus excluded. But what about crime-scene workers or lab technicians? And how many markers are in the touch DNA profile? The underpants' DNA was not enough to get a proper match through CODIS, the federal database. That didn't stop Lacy from sending it through on a regular basis—such busy-work has little prospect of ending with a match, but it makes it seem as if something is being done.

Years ago, there was a civil suit in this case wherein a federal judge issued a statement that said, based on her reading of the material submitted to her, there was a higher likelihood of an intruder being the killer than a family member. At that time, Mary Lacy read a statement that suggested the Ramseys were innocent, based on the judicial ruling—though not clearing them. That statement was reportedly dictated to her by a Ramsey associate. What only those close to the case know is that one side of the civil suit completely abandoned its case, never offering paperwork, so the only information the judge had was that which came from the Ramsey camp. Ergo, an easy decision for the judge to make. Since then, Ramsey advisers have pummeled Lacy to clear the family entirely and eventually it happened.

It was widely assumed then that the Boulder Grand Jury, which had spent 13 months hearing testimony and weighing evidence, failed to indict John and Patsy Ramsey for any involvement in their daughter's death. But, in 2013, it was learned that the jurors returned "true bills" against both parents for two felonious criminal counts each: child abuse resulting in death and being accessories to the crime. Despite their strong recommendation, then-District Attorney Alex Hunter refused to proceed to trial, feeling there was not enough evidence to win convictions. Only four pages of the grand jury's 18-page document were released and, to date, reporters and lawyers have been unsuccessful in getting the remaining pages unsealed.

It's egregious when an officer of the court misrepresents scientific evidence to win political favor. Mary Lacy was right to offer up an apology. But it should have been to JonBenét and not her family.

Source: Dawna Kaufmann, investigative journalist. Co-author with Cyril H. Wecht, MD, JD, of A Question of Murder, *Final Exams: True Crime Cases from Cyril Wecht, and From Crime Scene to Courtroom.*

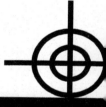

Chapter Summary >>>>>>>>>>>

The key to understanding how DNA works is to appreciate the fact that only four types of bases are associated with DNA: adenine (*A*), cytosine (*C*), guanine (*G*), and thymine (*T*). In general, *A* pairs with *T* and *C* pairs with *G*. The arrangement of these base pairs codes for all the proteins in the body. A DNA strand can be composed of a long chain with millions of bases. The DNA molecule is actually composed of two DNA strands coiled into a *double helix*. This can be thought of as resembling two wires twisted around each other.

The synthesis of new DNA from existing DNA begins with the unwinding of the DNA strands in the double helix. Each strand is then exposed to a collection of free nucleotides. Letter by letter, the double helix is re-created as the nucleotides are assembled in the proper order, as dictated by the principle of base pairing. The result is the emergence of two identical copies of DNA where before there was only one. This laboratory technique is known as **polymerase chain reaction (PCR)**. Put simply, PCR is a technique designed to copy or multiply DNA strands in a laboratory test tube.

Portions of the DNA structure are as unique to each individual as fingerprints. The gene is the fundamental unit of heredity. Each gene is actually composed of DNA specifically designed to control the genetic traits of our cells. DNA

is constructed as a very large molecule made by linking a series of repeating units called nucleotides. Four types of bases are associated with the DNA structure: adenine (*A*), guanine (*G*), cytosine (*C*), and thymine (*T*). The bases on each strand are properly aligned in a double-helix configuration. As a result, adenine pairs with thymine and guanine pairs with cytosine. This concept is known as base pairing. The order of the bases is what distinguishes different DNA strands.

Portions of the DNA molecule contain sequences of bases that are repeated numerous times. To a forensic scientist, these tandem repeats offer a means of distinguishing one individual from another through DNA typing. Length differences associated with relatively short repeating DNA strands are called short tandem repeats (STRs) and form the basis for the current DNA-typing procedure. They serve as useful markers for identification because they are found in great abundance throughout the human genome. STRs normally consist of repeating sequences 3 to 7 bases long, and the entire strand of an STR is also very short, less than 450 bases long. This means that STRs are much less susceptible to degradation and may often be recovered from bodies or stains that have been subjected to decomposition. Also, because of their shortness, STRs are ideal candidates for multiplication by PCR, in which STR strands are multiplied over a billionfold. PCR is responsible for the ability of STR typing to detect the genetic material of as few as 18 DNA-bearing cells. The more STRs one can characterize, the smaller the percentage of the population from which a particular combination of STRs can emanate. This gives rise to the concept of multiplexing. Using the technology of PCR, one can simultaneously extract and amplify a combination of different STRs. Currently, U.S. crime laboratories have standardized on 13 STRs. With STR analysis, as few as 125 picograms of DNA are required.

Another type of DNA used for individual characterization is mitochondrial DNA. Mitochondrial DNA is located outside the cell's nucleus and is inherited from the mother. However, mitochondrial DNA typing does not approach STR analysis in its discrimination power and thus is best reserved for samples, such as hair, for which STR analysis may not be possible.

Bloodstained evidence should not be packaged in plastic or airtight containers because accumulation of residual moisture could contribute to the growth of blood-destroying bacteria and fungi. Each stained article should be packaged separately in a paper bag or in a well-ventilated box.

Review Questions

1. The fundamental unit of heredity is the _____.

2. Each gene is actually composed of _____, specifically designed to carry out a single body function.

3. A(n) _____ is a very large molecule made by linking a series of repeating units.

4. A(n) _____ is composed of a sugar molecule, a phosphorus-containing group, and a nitrogen-containing molecule called a base.

5. DNA is actually a very large molecule made by linking a series of _____ to form a natural polymer.

6. _____ different bases are associated with the makeup of DNA.

7. Watson and Crick demonstrated that DNA is composed of two strands coiled into the shape of a(n) _____.

8. The structure of DNA requires the pairing of base A to _____ and base G to _____.

9. The base sequence T–G–C–A can be paired with the base sequence _____ in a double-helix configuration.

10. The inheritable traits that are controlled by DNA arise out of DNA's ability to direct the production of _____.

11. _____ are derived from a combination of up to 20 known amino acids.

12. The production of an amino acid is controlled by a sequence of _____ bases on the DNA molecule.

13. True or False: Enzymes known as DNA polymerase assemble new DNA strands into a proper base sequence during replication. _____

14. True or False: DNA can be copied outside a living cell. _____

15. True or False: All of the letter sequences in DNA code for the production of proteins. _____

16. In STR DNA typing, a typical DNA pattern shows (two, three) peaks.

17. True or False: Specimens amenable to DNA typing are blood, semen, body tissues, and hair. _____

18. Short DNA segments containing repeating sequences of three to seven bases are called _____.

19. True or False: The longer the DNA strand, the less susceptible it is to degradation. _____

20. The short length of STRs allows them to be replicated by _____.

21. Used as markers for identification purposes, _____ are locations on the chromosome that contain short sequences that repeat themselves within the DNA molecule and in great abundance throughout the human genome.

22. (CODIS, AFIS) maintains local, state, and national databases of DNA profiles from convicted offenders, unsolved crime-scene evidence, and profiles of missing people.

23. Amazingly, the sensitivity of STR profiling requires only _____ DNA-bearing cells to obtain an STR profile.

24. During evidence collection, all body fluids must be assumed to be _____ and handled with latex-gloved hands.

25. The concept of (CODIS, multiplexing) involves simultaneous detection of more than one DNA marker.

26. The amelogenin gene shows two peaks for a (male, female) and one peak for a (male, female).

27. Y-STR typing is useful when one is confronted with a DNA mixture containing more than one (male, female) contributor.

28. Mitochondrial DNA is inherited from the (mother, father).

29. True or False: Mitochondrial DNA is more plentiful in the human cell than is nuclear DNA. _____

30. The national DNA database in the United States has standardized on _____ STRs for entry into the database.

31. True or False: Y-STR data is normally entered into the CODIS database collection. _____.

32. Small amounts of blood are best submitted to a crime laboratory in a (wet, dry) condition.

33. True or False: Airtight packages make the best containers for blood-containing evidence. _____

34. Whole blood collected for DNA-typing purposes must be placed in a vacuum containing the preservative _____.

35. A typical STR DNA type emanating from a single individual shows a (one, two, three)-peak pattern.

Review Questions for Inside the Science

1. True or False: Enzymes known as DNA polymerases assemble new DNA strands into a proper base sequence based off the template strand during replication. _____

2. DNA evidence at a crime scene can be copied by the processes of the _____ with the aid of a DNA polymerase and specific primers.

3. DNA fragments can be separated and identified by (gas chromatography, capillary electrophoresis).

4. (Two, Four) regions of mitochondrial DNA have been found to be highly variable in the human population.

5. True or False: Polymerase chain reaction is a part of the process used in the forensic analysis of RFLP, STRs, and mitochondrial DNA. _____

Application and Critical Thinking

1. The following sequence of bases is located on one strand of a DNA molecule:

   C–G–A–A–T–C–G–C–A–A–T–C–G–A–C–C–T–G

   List the sequence of bases that will form complementary pairs on the other strand of the DNA molecule.

2. Police discover a badly decomposed body buried in an area where a man disappeared some years before. The case was never solved, nor was the victim's body ever recovered. As the lead investigator, you suspect that the newly discovered body is that of the victim. What is your main challenge in using DNA typing to determine whether your suspicion is correct? How would you go about using DNA technology to test your theory?

3. You are a forensic scientist performing DNA typing on a blood sample sent to your laboratory. While performing an STR analysis on the sample, you notice a four-peak pattern. What conclusion should you draw? Why?

4. A woman reports being mugged by a masked assailant, whom she scratched on the arm during a brief struggle. The victim is not sure whether the attacker was male or female. DNA analysts extract and amplify the amelogenin gene from the epithelial cells under the victim's fingernails (allegedly belonging to the attacker) and from a buccal swab of the victim.

The sample is separated by gel electrophoresis with the result shown here. The victim's amelogenin DNA is in lane 2, and the amelogenin DNA from the fingernail scraping is in lane 4. What conclusion can you draw about the attacker from this result? How did you reach this conclusion?

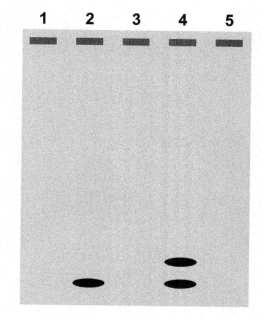

5. At a crime scene, you encounter each of the following items. For each item, indicate the potential sources of DNA. The five possible choices are saliva, skin cells, sweat, blood, and semen.

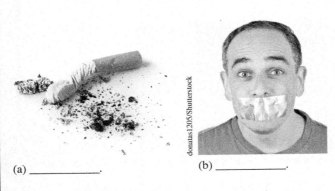

(a) _____.

(b) _____.

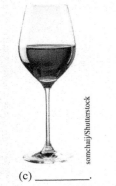

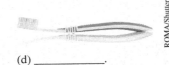

(c) _____.

(d) _____.

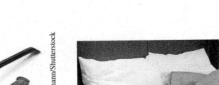

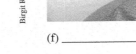

(e) _____.

(f) _____.

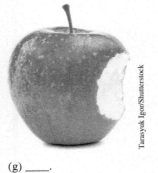

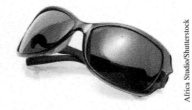

(g) _____.

(h) _____.

6. The 15-STR locus DNA profile of a missing person, James Dittman, is shown in the following table.

STR Loci	Allele
D3S1358	15
THO1	6, 9.3
D21S11	27
D18S51	15, 16
PENTA E	10
D5S818	11
D13S807	10, 13
D7S820	9, 10
D16S539	11, 12
CSF1PO	13
PENTA D	12, 13
AMELOGENIN	XY
VWA	17, 19
D8S1170	10, 13
TPOX	8, 12
FGA	21

Decomposing remains were found deep in the woods near Dittman's house. DNA from these remains was extracted, amplified, and analyzed at 15 STR loci. Compare the STR readout for Dittman in the table with the chart on page 408 to determine whether the remains could belong to James Dittman. If not, at which STR loci do the profiles differ?

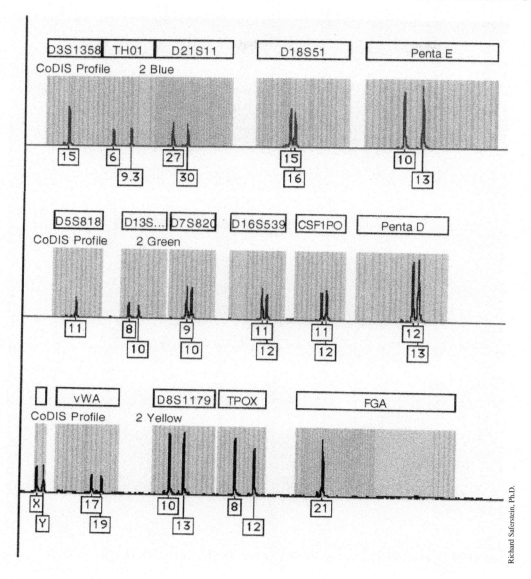

Further References

Butler, M. *Advanced Topics in Forensic DNA Typing: Interpretation.* San Diego, CA: Academic Press, 2015.

Butler, M. *Advanced Topics in Forensic DNA Typing: Methodology.* Burlington, MA: Elsevier Academic Press, 2012.

Butler, M. *Fundamentals of Forensic DNA Typing,* 3rd ed. Burlington, MA: Elsevier Academic Press, 2010.

Isenberg, A. R. "Forensic Mitochondrial DNA Analysis," in R. Saferstein, ed., *Forensic Science Handbook,* vol. 2, 2nd ed. Upper Saddle River, NJ: Prentice Hall, 2005.

Isenberg A. R., and J. M. Moore, "Mitochondrial DNA Analysis at the FBI Laboratory," *Forensic Science Communications* 1, no. 2 (1999), https://www2.fbi.gov/hq/lab/fsc/backissu/july1999/index.htm

Kobilinsky, L. "Deoxyribonucleic Acid Structure and Function—A Review," in R. Saferstein, ed., *Forensic Science Handbook,* vol. 3, 2nd ed. Upper Saddle River, NJ: Prentice Hall, 2010.

The Biological Evidence Preservation Handbook: Best Practices for Evidence Handlers, http://nvlpubs.nist.gov/nistpubs/ir/2013/NIST.IR.7928.pdf

Chapter 17

Forensic Aspects of Fire and Explosion Investigation

Learning Objectives

After studying this chapter, you should be able to:

17.1 Explain the chemical reactions that initiate and sustain fire

17.2 Explain the three mechanisms of heat transfer

17.3 Recognize how to locate the fire's origin along with telltale signs of an accelerant-initiated fire

17.4 Describe how to collect physical evidence at the scene of a suspected arson

17.5 Describe laboratory procedures used to detect and identify hydrocarbon residues

17.6 Explain the chemical reactions that occur during an explosion

17.7 List some common commercial, homemade, and military explosives

17.8 Describe how to collect physical evidence at the scene of an explosion and the procedures for analysis

KEY TERMS

accelerant
black powder
combustion
deflagration
detonating cord
detonation
endothermic reaction
energy
exothermic reaction
explosion
flammable range
flash point
glowing combustion
heat of combustion
high explosive
hydrocarbon
ignition temperature
low explosive
modus operandi
oxidation
oxidizing agent
primary explosive
pyrolysis
safety fuse
secondary explosive
smokeless powder
  (double-base)
smokeless powder
  (single-base)
spontaneous
  combustion

Go to www.pearsonhighered.com/careersresources to access Webextras for this chapter.

The Oklahoma City Bombing

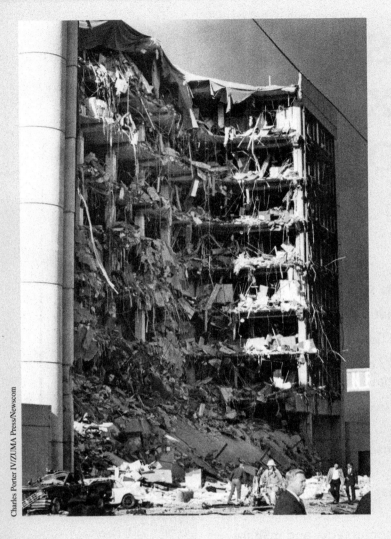

Charles Porter IV/ZUMA Press/Newscom

It was the biggest act of mass murder in U.S. history. On a sunny spring morning in April 1995, a Ryder rental truck pulled into the parking area of the Alfred P. Murrah federal building in Oklahoma City. The driver stepped down from the truck's cab and casually walked away. Minutes later, the truck exploded into a fireball, unleashing enough energy to destroy the building and kill 168 people, including 19 children and infants in the building's day care center.

Later that morning, an Oklahoma Highway Patrol officer pulled over a beat-up 1977 Mercury Marquis being driven without a license plate. On further investigation, the driver, Timothy McVeigh, was found to be in possession of a loaded firearm and charged with transporting a firearm. At the explosion site, remnants of the Ryder truck were located and the truck was quickly traced to a renter—Robert Kling, an alias for Timothy McVeigh. Coincidentally, the rental agreement and McVeigh's driver's license both used the address of McVeigh's friend Terry Nichols.

Investigators later recovered McVeigh's fingerprint on a receipt for two thousand pounds of ammonium nitrate, a basic explosive ingredient. Forensic analysts also located PETN residues on the clothing McVeigh wore on the day of his arrest. PETN is a component of detonating cord. After three days of deliberation, a jury declared McVeigh guilty of the bombing and sentenced him to die by lethal injection.

Arson often presents complex and difficult circumstances to investigate. Normally, these incidents are committed at the convenience of a perpetrator who has thoroughly planned the criminal act and has left the crime scene long before any official investigation is launched. Furthermore, proving commission of the offense is more difficult because of the extensive destruction that frequently dominates the crime scene. The contribution of the criminalist is only one aspect of a comprehensive and difficult investigative process that must establish a motive, the **modus operandi**, and a suspect.

modus operandi
An offender's pattern of operation.

The criminalist's function is limited; usually the criminalist is expected only to detect and identify relevant chemical materials collected at the scene and to reconstruct and identify igniters. Although a chemist can identify trace amounts of gasoline or kerosene in debris, no scientific test can determine whether an arsonist has used a pile of rubbish or paper to start a fire. Furthermore, a fire can have many accidental causes, including faulty wiring, overheated electric motors, improperly cleaned and regulated heating systems, and cigarette smoking—which usually leave no chemical traces. Thus, the final determination of the cause of a fire must consider numerous factors and requires an extensive on-site investigation. The ultimate determination must be made by an investigator whose training and knowledge have been augmented by the practical experiences of fire investigation.

The Chemistry of Fire

Humankind's early search to explain the physical concepts underlying the behavior of matter always bestowed a central and fundamental role on fire. To ancient Greek philosophers, fire was one of the four basic elements from which all matter was derived. The medieval alchemist thought of fire as an instrument of transformation, capable of changing one element into another. One ancient recipe expresses its mystical power as follows: "Now the substance of cinnabar is such that the more it is heated, the more exquisite are its sublimations. Cinnabar will become mercury, and passing through a series of other sublimations, it is again turned into cinnabar, and thus it enables man to enjoy eternal life."

oxidation
The combination of oxygen with other substances to produce new substances.

Today, we know of fire not as an element of matter but as a transformation process during which oxygen is united with some other substance to produce noticeable quantities of heat and light (a flame). Therefore, any insight into why and how a fire is initiated and sustained must begin with the knowledge of the fundamental chemical reaction of fire—**oxidation**.

Oxidation

In a simple description of oxidation, oxygen combines with other substances to produce new products. Thus, we may write the chemical equation for the burning of methane gas, a major component of natural gas, as follows:

$$CH_4 \quad + \quad 2O_2 \quad \rightarrow \quad CO_2 \quad + 2H_2O$$
methane   oxygen   yields   carbon dioxide   water

However, not all oxidation proceeds in the manner that one associates with fire. For example, oxygen combines with many metals to form oxides. Thus, iron forms a red-brown iron oxide, or rust, as follows (see Figure 17–1):

$$4Fe \quad + \quad 3O_2 \quad \rightarrow \quad 2Fe_2O_3$$
iron   oxygen   yields   iron oxide

Yet chemical equations do not give us a complete insight into the oxidation process. We must consider other factors to understand all of the implications of oxidation or, for that matter, any other chemical reaction. Methane burns when it unites with oxygen, but merely mixing methane and oxygen does not produce a fire. Nor, for example, does gasoline burn when it is simply exposed to air. However, lighting a match in the presence of any one of these fuel–air mixtures (assuming proper proportions) produces an instant fire.

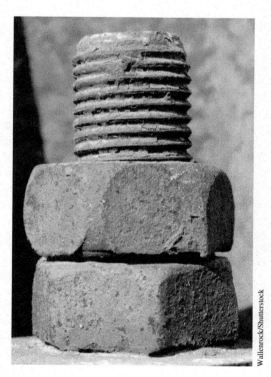

FIGURE 17–1

Rust forming on iron is an example of oxidation.

Wallenrock/Shutterstock

What are the reasons behind these differences? Why do some oxidations proceed with the outward appearances that we associate with a fire, but others do not? Why do we need a match to initiate some oxidations, but others proceed at room temperature? The explanation lies in a fundamental but abstract concept—energy.

Energy

energy
The ability or potential of a system or material to do work.

Energy can be defined as the ability or potential of a system or material to do work. Energy takes many forms, such as heat energy, electrical energy, mechanical energy, nuclear energy, light energy, and chemical energy. For example, when methane is burned, the stored chemical energy in methane is converted to energy in the form of heat and light. This heat may be used to boil water or to provide high-pressure steam to turn a turbine. This is an example of converting chemical energy to heat energy to mechanical energy. The turbine can then be used to generate electricity, transforming mechanical energy to electrical energy. Electrical energy may then be used to turn a motor. In other words, energy can enable work to be done; heat is energy.

The quantity of heat from a chemical reaction comes from the breaking and formation of chemical bonds. Methane is a molecule composed of one carbon atom bonded with four hydrogen atoms:

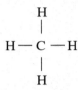

An oxygen molecule forms when two atoms of the element oxygen bond:

$$O=O$$

In chemical changes, atoms are not lost but merely redistributed during the chemical reaction; thus, the products of methane's oxidation will be carbon dioxide:

$$O=C=O$$

and water:

$$H—O—H$$

This rearrangement, however, means that the chemical bonds holding the atoms together must be broken and new bonds formed. We now have arrived at a fundamental observation in our dissection of a chemical reaction—that molecules must absorb energy to break apart their chemical bonds, and that they liberate energy when their bonds are reformed.

The amount of energy needed to break a bond and the amount of energy liberated when a bond is formed are characteristic of the type of chemical bond involved. Hence, a chemical reaction involves a change in energy content; energy is going in and energy is given off. The quantities of energies involved are different for each reaction and are determined by the participants in the chemical reaction.

combustion
Rapid combination of oxygen with another substance, accompanied by production of noticeable heat and light.

exothermic reaction
A chemical transformation in which heat energy is liberated.

heat of combustion
The heat liberated during combustion.

endothermic reaction
A chemical transformation in which heat energy is absorbed from the surroundings.

Combustion

All oxidation reactions, including the **combustion** of methane, are examples of reactions in which more energy is liberated than is required to break the chemical bonds between atoms. Such reactions are said to be **exothermic**. The excess energy is liberated as heat, and often as light, and is known as the **heat of combustion**. Table 17–1 summarizes the heats of combustion of some important fuels in fire investigation.

Although we will not be concerned with them, some reactions require more energy than they eventually liberate. These reactions are known as **endothermic reactions**.

Thus, all reactions require an energy input to start them. We can think of this requirement as an invisible energy barrier between the reactants and the products of a reaction (see Figure 17–2). The higher this barrier, the more energy required to initiate the reaction. Where does this initial energy come from? There are many sources of energy; however, for the purpose of this discussion, we need to look at only one—heat.

TABLE 17–1

Heats of Combustion of Fuels

Fuel	Heat of Combustion[a]
Crude oil	19,650 Btu/gal
Diesel fuel	19,550 Btu/lb
Gasoline	19,250 Btu/lb
Methane	995 Btu/cu ft
Natural gas	128–1,868 Btu/cu ft
Octane	121,300 Btu/gal
Wood	7,500 Btu/lb
Coal, bituminous	11,000–14,000 Btu/lb
Anthracite	13,351 Btu/lb

[a]A BTU (British thermal unit) is defined as the quantity of heat required to raise the temperature of 1 pound of water 1°F at or near its point of maximum density.

Source: John D. DeHaan, *Kirk's Fire Investigation*, 2nd ed. Upper Saddle River, NJ: Prentice Hall, 1983.

HEAT   The energy barrier in the conversion of iron to rust is relatively small, and it can be surmounted with the help of heat energy in the surrounding environment at normal outdoor temperatures. Not so for methane or gasoline; these energy barriers are quite high, and a high temperature must be applied to start the oxidation of these fuels. Hence, before any fire can result, the temperature of these fuels must be raised enough to exceed the energy barrier. Table 17–2 shows that this temperature, known as the **ignition temperature**, is quite high for common fuels.

Once combustion starts, enough heat is liberated to keep the reaction going by itself. In essence, the fire becomes a chain reaction, absorbing a portion of its own liberated heat to generate even more heat. The fire burns until either the oxygen or the fuel is exhausted.

Normally, a lighted match provides a convenient igniter of fuels. However, the fire investigator must also consider other potential sources of ignition—for example, electrical discharges, sparks, and chemicals—while reconstructing the initiation of a fire. All of these sources have temperatures higher than the ignition temperature of most fuels.

ignition temperature
The minimum temperature at which a fuel spontaneously ignites.

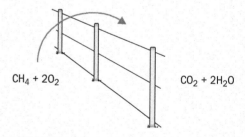

$CH_4 + 2O_2$ $CO_2 + 2H_2O$

FIGURE 17–2

An energy barrier must be hurdled before reactants such as methane and oxygen can combine with one another to form the products of carbon dioxide and water.

SPEED OF REACTION   Although the liberation of energy explains many important features of oxidation, it does not explain all characteristics of the reaction. Obviously, although all oxidations liberate energy, not all are accompanied by a flame; witness the oxidation of iron to rust. Therefore, one other important consideration will make our understanding of oxidation and fire complete: the rate or speed at which the reaction takes place.

A chemical reaction, such as oxidation, takes place when molecules combine or collide with one another. The faster the molecules move, the greater the number of collisions between them and the faster the rate of reaction. Many factors influence the rate of these collisions. In our description of fire and oxidation, we consider only two: the physical state of the fuel and the temperature.

TABLE 17–2

Ignition Temperatures of Some Common Fuels

Fuel	Ignition Temperature, °F
Acetone	869
Benzene	928
Fuel oil #2	495
Gasoline (low octane)	536
Kerosene (fuel oil #1)	410
n-Octane	428
Petroleum ether	550
Turpentine	488

Source: John D. DeHaan, *Kirk's Fire Investigation*, 4th ed. Upper Saddle River, NJ: Prentice Hall, 1997.

Physical State of Fuel   A fuel achieves a reaction rate with oxygen sufficient to produce a flame only when it is in the gaseous state because only in this state can molecules collide frequently enough to support a flaming fire. This remains true whether the fuel is a solid such as wood, paper, cloth, or plastic, or a liquid such as gasoline or kerosene.

For example, the conversion of iron to rust proceeds slowly because the iron atoms cannot achieve a gaseous state. The combination of oxygen with iron is thus restricted to the surface area of the metal exposed to air, a limitation that severely reduces the rate of reaction. On the other hand, the reaction of methane and oxygen proceeds rapidly because all the reactants are in the gaseous state. The speed of the reaction is reflected by the production of noticeable quantities of heat and light (a flame).

Fuel Temperature   How, then, does a liquid or solid maintain a gaseous reaction? In the case of a liquid fuel, the temperature must be high enough to vaporize the fuel. The vapor that forms burns when it mixes with oxygen and combusts as a flame. The **flash point** is the *lowest* temperature at which a liquid gives off sufficient vapor to form a mixture with air that will support combustion. Once the flash point is reached, the fuel can be ignited by some outside source of temperature to start a fire. The ignition temperature of a fuel is always considerably higher than the flash point. For example, gasoline has a flash point of $-50°F$; however, an ignition temperature of $495°F$ is needed to start a gasoline fire.

With a solid fuel such as wood, the process of generating vapor is more complex. A solid fuel burns only when exposed to heat intense enough to decompose the solid into gaseous products. This chemical breakdown of solid material is known as **pyrolysis**. The gaseous products of pyrolysis combine with oxygen to produce a fire (see Figure 17–3). Here again, fire can be described as a chain reaction. A match or other source of heat initiates the pyrolysis of the solid fuel, the gaseous products react with oxygen in the air to produce heat and light, and this heat in turn pyrolyzes more solid fuel into volatile gases.

Typically, the rate of a chemical reaction increases when the temperature is raised. The magnitude of the increase varies from one reaction to another and also from one temperature range to another. For most reactions, a $10°C$ ($18°F$) rise in temperature doubles or triples the reaction rate. This observation explains in part why burning is so rapid. As the fire spreads, it

flash point
The minimum temperature at which a liquid fuel produces enough vapor to burn.

pyrolysis
The decomposition of solid organic matter by heat.

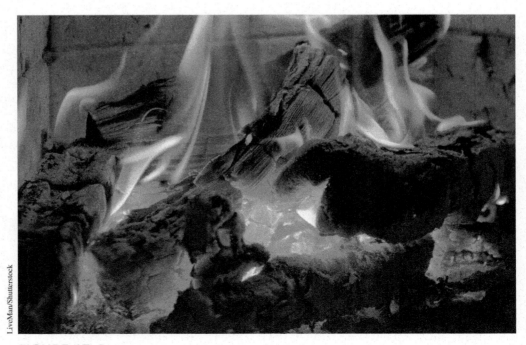

FIGURE 17–3
Intense heat causes solid fuels such as wood to decompose into gaseous products, a process called pyrolysis.

LiveMan/Shutterstock

raises the temperature of the fuel–air mixture, thus increasing the rate of reaction; this in turn generates more heat, again increasing the rate of reaction. Only when the fuel or oxygen is depleted does this vicious cycle come to a halt.

THE FUEL–AIR MIX   As we have seen from our discussion about gaseous fuel, air (oxygen) and sufficient heat are the basic ingredients of a flaming fire. There is also one other consideration—the gas fuel–air mix. A mixture of gaseous fuel and air burns only if its composition lies within certain limits. If the fuel concentration is too low (lean) or too great (rich), combustion does not occur. The concentration range between the upper and lower limits is called the **flammable range**. For example, the flammable range for gasoline is 1.3–6.0 percent. Thus, in order for a gasoline–air mix to burn, gasoline must make up at least 1.3 percent, and no more than 6 percent, of the mixture.

GLOWING COMBUSTION   Although a flaming fire can be supported only by a gaseous fuel, in some instances a fuel can burn without a flame. Witness a burning cigarette or the red glow of hot charcoal (see Figure 17–4). These are examples of **glowing combustion** or *smoldering*. Here, combustion occurs on the surface of a solid fuel in the absence of heat high enough to pyrolyze the fuel. Interestingly, this phenomenon generally ensues long after the flames have gone out. Wood, for example, tends to burn with a flame until all of its pyrolyzable components have been expended; however, wood's carbonaceous residue continues to smolder long after the flame has extinguished itself.

SPONTANEOUS COMBUSTION   One interesting phenomenon often invoked by arson suspects as the cause of a fire is **spontaneous combustion**. Actually, the conditions under which spontaneous combustion can develop are rather limited and rarely account for the cause of a fire. Spontaneous combustion is the result of a natural heat-producing process in poorly ventilated containers or areas. For example, hay stored in barns provides an excellent growing medium for bacteria whose activities generate heat. If the hay is not properly ventilated, the heat builds to a level that supports other types of heat-producing chemical reactions in the hay. Eventually, as the heat rises, the ignition temperature of hay is reached, spontaneously setting off a fire.

Another example of spontaneous combustion involves the ignition of improperly ventilated containers containing rags soaked with certain types of highly unsaturated oils, such as linseed oil. Heat can build up to the point of ignition as a result of a slow heat-producing chemical oxidation

flammable range
The entire range of possible gas or vapor fuel concentrations in air that are capable of burning.

glowing combustion
Combustion on the surface of a solid fuel in the absence of heat high enough to pyrolyze the fuel.

spontaneous combustion
A fire caused by a natural heat-producing process in the presence of sufficient air and fuel.

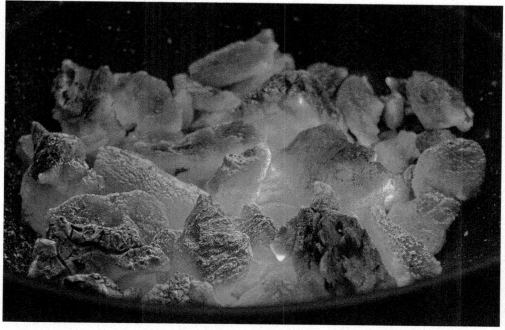

FIGURE 17–4
Glowing red charcoals.

Lev Kropotov/Shutterstock

between the air and the oil. Of course, storage conditions must encourage the accumulation of the heat over a prolonged period of time. However, spontaneous combustion does not occur with hydrocarbon lubricating oils, and it is not expected to occur with most household fats and oils.

In summary, three requirements must be satisfied to initiate and sustain combustion:

1. A fuel must be present.
2. Oxygen must be available in sufficient quantity to combine with the fuel.
3. Heat must be applied to initiate the combustion, and sufficient heat must be generated to sustain the reaction.

Heat Transfer

Consider how a structural fire begins. The typical scenario starts with heat ignition at a single location. It may be an arsonist lighting a gasoline-soaked rag, a malfunctioning electric appliance sparking, or an individual falling asleep while smoking a cigarette in bed. How does a flame initially confined to a single location spread to engulf an entire structure? Understanding the anatomy of a fire begins with comprehending how heat travels through a burning structure.

The previous section stressed the importance of the role of heat in generating sufficient fuel vapors to support combustion, as well as the requirement that the heat source be hot enough to ignite the fuel's vapor. Once the fire begins, the heat generated by the fuel's reaction with air is fed back into the fuel–air mix to keep the chemical reaction going.

As a fire progresses, the heat created by the combustion process tends to move from a high-temperature region to one at a lower temperature. Understanding heat transfer from one location to another is important for reconstructing the origin of a fire, as well as for understanding why and how fire spreads through a structure. The three mechanisms of heat transfer are conduction, radiation, and convection.

Conduction

Movement of heat through a solid object is caused by a process called *conduction*, in which electrons and atoms within the heated object collide with one another. Heat always travels from hot areas of a solid to cold ones by conduction. Solids whose atoms or molecules have loosely

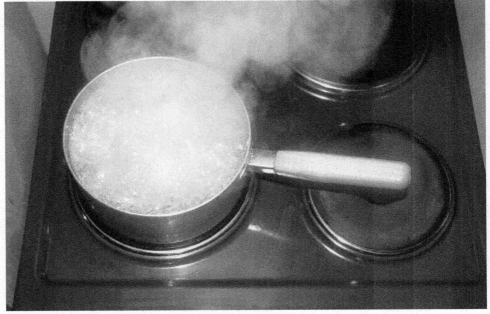

The wooden handle on this saucepan is a poor conductor of heat.

held electrons are good conductors of heat. Metals have the most loosely held electrons and are therefore excellent conductors of heat. Thus, when you insert one end of a metal object into an open flame, the entire object quickly becomes hot to the touch.

Materials that have electrons firmly attached to their molecules are poor conductors of heat. Poor conductors are called *insulators*. Wood is a good insulator; for that reason, metal objects that are subject to intense heat (such as skillets and saucepans) often have wooden handles (see the figure).

In reconstructing a fire scene, it's important to keep in mind that heat may be transported through metals such as beams, nails, fasteners, bolts, and other good conductors to a location far from the initial heat source. Any fuel in contact with the conductor may be ignited, creating a new fire location. On the other hand, the conductivity of wood, plastic, and paper is very low, meaning that heat emanating from these surfaces does not spread well and does not cause ignitions far from the initial heat source.

Radiation

Radiation is the transfer of heat energy from a heated surface to a cooler surface by electromagnetic radiation. A hot surface emits electromagnetic radiation of various wavelengths, and in a fire scene the electromagnetic radiation moves in a straight line from one surface to another. Radiant heat plays a key role in understanding how fire spreads throughout a structure. For example, all surfaces that face the fire are exposed to radiant heat and burst into flames when the surface reaches their ignition temperature. In very large fires, nearby structures and vehicles are often ignited at a distance by radiant heat.

Convection

Convection is the transfer of heat energy by movement of molecules within a liquid or gas. Water being heated on a stove illustrates the concept of convection. As the water molecules on the bottom of the pot move faster, they spread apart and become less dense, causing them to move upward. Denser, cooler water molecules then migrate to the bottom of the pot. In this way convection currents keep the fluid stirred up as warmer fluid moves away from the heat source and cooler fluid moves toward the heat source. Likewise, warm air expands, becoming less dense and causing it to rise and move toward the cooler surrounding air.

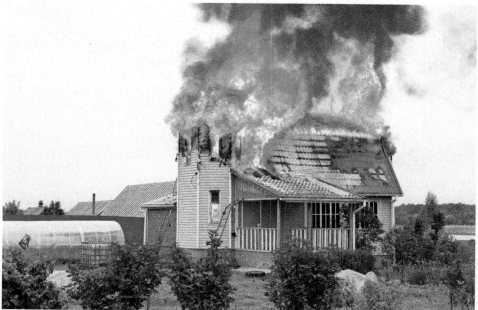

Convection causes flames to rise to the upper floor of a burning structure.

In a structural fire, the gaseous hot products of combustion expand, and convection moves the hot gases to the upper portions of the structure (see the figure). The convected hot gases become a source of heat, radiating heat energy downward onto all the surfaces below them. The hot surfaces of the exposed objects often pyrolyze or break down, releasing gaseous molecules. The phenomenon known as *flashover* occurs when all the combustible fuels simultaneously ignite, engulfing the entire structure in flame.

Searching the Fire Scene

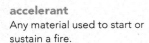

accelerant
Any material used to start or sustain a fire.

The arson investigator should begin examining a fire scene for signs of arson as soon as the fire has been extinguished. Most arsons are started with petroleum-based **accelerants**, such as gasoline or kerosene. Thus, the presence of containers capable of holding an accelerant arouse suspicions of arson. Discovery of an ignition device ranging in sophistication from a candle to a time-delay device is another indication of possible arson. A common telltale sign of arson is an irregularly shaped pattern on a floor or on the ground (see Figure 17–5) resulting from pouring an accelerant onto the surface. Fire investigators are cautioned that irregular patterns are common in post-flashover conditions; hence, if the presence of ignitable liquids is suspected to have caused a fire pattern, supporting evidence from the laboratory for the presence of accelerant residues must confirm its existence. In addition to these visual indicators, investigators should look for signs of breaking and entering and theft, and they should begin interviewing any eyewitnesses to the fire.

Timeliness of Investigation

Time constantly works against the arson investigator. Any accelerant residues that remain after a fire is extinguished may evaporate within a few days or even hours. Furthermore, safety and health conditions may necessitate that cleanup and salvage operations begin as quickly as possible. Once this occurs, a meaningful investigation of the fire scene is impossible. Accelerants in soil and vegetation can be rapidly degraded by bacterial action. Freezing samples containing soil or vegetation is an effective way to prevent this degradation.

The need to begin an *immediate* investigation of the circumstances surrounding a fire even takes precedence over the requirement to obtain a search warrant to enter and search the premises. The Supreme Court, explaining its position on this issue, stated in part:

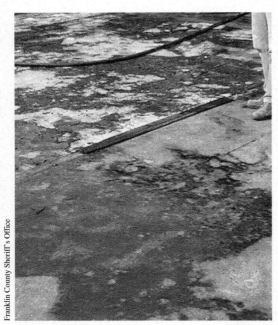

Franklin County Sheriff's Office

> ... Fire officials are charged not only with extinguishing fires, but with finding their causes. Prompt determination of the fire's origin may be necessary to prevent its recurrence, as through the detection of continuing dangers such as faulty wiring or a defective furnace. Immediate investigation may also be necessary to preserve evidence from intentional or accidental destruction. And, of course, the sooner the officials complete their duties, the less will be their subsequent interference with the privacy and the recovery efforts of the victims. For these reasons, officials need no warrant to remain in a building for a reasonable time to investigate the cause of a blaze after it has been extinguished. And if the warrantless entry to put out the fire and determine its cause is constitutional, the warrantless seizure of evidence while inspecting the premises for these purposes also is constitutional....

FIGURE 17–5
Irregularly shaped pattern on the ground resulting from a poured ignitable liquid.

In determining what constitutes a reasonable time to investigate, appropriate recognition must be given to the exigencies that confront officials serving under these conditions, as well as to individuals' reasonable expectations of privacy.[1]

---

[1] *Michigan* v. *Tyler*, 436 U.S. 499 (1978).

Locating the Fire's Origin

A search of the fire scene must focus on finding the fire's origin, which will prove most productive in any search for an accelerant or ignition device. In searching for a fire's specific point of origin, the investigator may uncover telltale signs of arson such as evidence of separate and unconnected fires or the use of "streamers" to spread the fire from one area to another. For example, the arsonist may have spread a trail of gasoline or paper to cause the fire to move rapidly from one room to another.

There are no fast and simple rules for identifying a fire's origin. Normally, a fire tends to move upward, and thus the probable origin is most likely closest to the lowest point that shows the most intense characteristics of burning. Sometimes as the fire burns upward, a V-shaped pattern forms against a vertical wall, as shown in Figure 17–6. Because flammable liquids always flow to the lowest point, more severe burning found on the floor than on the ceiling may indicate the presence of an accelerant. If a flammable liquid was used, charring is expected to be more intense on the bottom of furniture, shelves, and other items rather than the top.

However, many factors can contribute to the deviation of a fire from normal behavior. Using burn patterns, such as depth of char, a V-shaped pattern, or low intense burn area, as indicators of a fire's origin can prove to be misleading, particularly, when a structural fire burns beyond flashover to full-room involvement. Flashover has been defined as the transitional phase in some compartment fires in which temperatures rise to a level sufficient to cause the ignition of all combustible items in the compartment. Studies of this phenomenon show that in some flashovers, the effects of radiation from the layer of hot gases forming at the ceiling level may cause floors, furniture, and baseboards to ignite without direct flame impingement (see Figure 17–7(a)–(c)). As a result, a fire that starts in one area of a structure could, through flashover, ignite fuel in another area of the structure, thus creating the illusion of two or more unrelated fires, a sign mistaken for arson. Further, in these situations, air flow currents through the burning room can become a dominant factor, in creating burn patterns.

Prevailing drafts and winds; secondary fires due to collapsing floors and roofs; the physical arrangement of the burning structure; stairways and elevator shafts; holes in the floor, wall, or

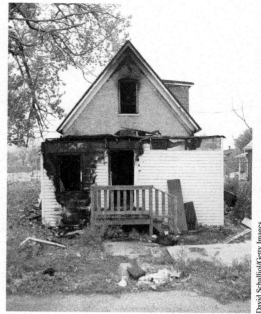

FIGURE 17–6

Typical V pattern illustrating upward movement of the fire.

David Schallio/Getty Images

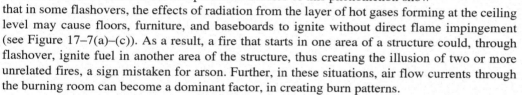

(a)

(b)

Radiant heat

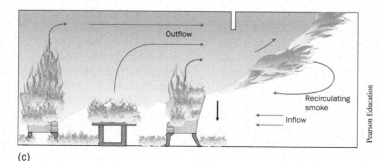

(c)

Outflow

Recirculating smoke

Inflow

Pearson Education

FIGURE 17–7

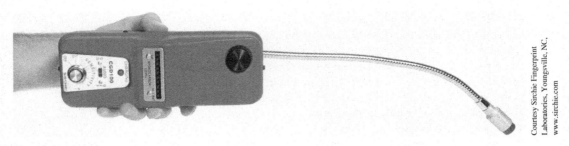

Courtesy Sirchie Fingerprint Laboratories, Youngsville, NC, www.sirchie.com

FIGURE 17–8
Portable hydrocarbon detector.

roof; and the effects of the firefighter in suppressing the fire are other factors that the fire investigator must consider before determining conclusive findings regarding a fire's origin.

Once located, the point of origin should be protected to permit careful investigation. As at any crime scene, nothing should be touched or moved before notes, sketches, and photographs are taken. An examination must also be made for possible accidental causes, as well as for evidence of arson. The most common materials used by an arsonist to ensure the rapid spread and intensity of a fire are gasoline and kerosene or, for that matter, any volatile flammable liquid.

Searching for Accelerants

Fortunately, only under the most ideal conditions will combustible liquids be entirely consumed during a fire. When the liquid is poured over a large area, a portion of it will likely seep into a porous surface, such as cracks in the floor, upholstery, rags, plaster, wallboards, or carpet. Enough of the liquid may remain unchanged to permit its detection in the crime laboratory. In addition, when a fire is extinguished with water, the evaporation rate of volatile fluids may be slowed because water cools and covers materials through which the combustible liquid may have soaked. Fortunately, water does not interfere with laboratory methods used to detect and characterize flammable liquid residues.

The search for traces of flammable liquid residues may be aided by the use of a sensitive portable vapor detector or "sniffer" (see Figure 17–8). This device can rapidly screen suspect materials for volatile residues by sucking in the air surrounding the questioned sample. The air is passed over a heated filament; if a combustible vapor is present, it oxidizes and immediately increases the temperature of the filament. The rise in filament temperature is then registered as a deflection on the detector's meter.

Of course, such a device is not a conclusive test for a flammable vapor, but it is an excellent screening device for checking suspect samples at the fire scene. Another approach is to use dogs that have been trained to recognize the odor of hydrocarbon accelerants.

> > > > > > > > > >

Case Files

The Sackett Street Fire

A two-alarm fire destroyed a townhouse on Sackett Street, Brooklyn, New York, in February 1980. It was a night so cold that the fire hose water froze as fire fighters fought to slow the blaze. Inside the structure, a mother and her five children, ranging in age from 9 months to 9 years, perished. The building's owner had the ear of the fire investigators when she insisted that the cause of the fire was arson, and that she knew the three individuals who had done it. After a trial, those individuals, three men, were convicted of arson and six felony murders. The Fire Marshal determined that the fire had started at two unconnected first floor locations, based on the observations that there was more severe damage in the foyer and the rear bedroom than in the middle of the apartment. The independent origin sites strongly suggested arson, as did a puddle shape left on the on the foyer's tiles, even though laboratory tests failed to detect traces of an accelerant in the puddle area. At trial, the Fire Marshal testified that the foyer showed a "discoloration and a puddle shape configuration which is indicative of a flammable fluid fire."

In 2014, John Lentini, an eminent forensic scientist specializing in fire investigation, was retained. He concluded that the determination that the fire at Sackett Street was intentionally set was not supported by the evidence. "The cause of the fire cannot be proven to an acceptable level of certainty; the proper classification of this fire is undetermined."

The following year, a judge overturned the arson and murder convictions of the three men. Two of the men spent more than 30 years in prison, and the third died. What went wrong? According to Lentini, in 1980, the science of fire dynamics was poorly understood, and much that was believed by well-meaning investigators was false. The problem was a lack of understanding and appreciation for the phenomenon of flashover in fire investigations.

Flashover occurs when a fire gets so hot that the entire room catches fire, and all available fuel, even fuel from places remote from where the fire started—i.e., floors, furniture, baseboards—ignites almost all at once without direct flame impingement. After flashover, a fire might burn more intensely in a few sites where there was better ventilation, thus creating the appearance of a fire originating from multiple locations, which would be a strong sign of arson. Even pour patterns, a traditional sign of arson, are subject to misinterpretation in a flashover environment. In cases of full room involvement, patterns similar in appearance to burn patterns are common and can be produced when no ignitable liquid is present. The Sackett Street fire scene yielded no laboratory evidence for the presence of trace quantities of an accelerant. The intense charring of the baseboards at the Sackett Street's first floor apartment further confirmed the existence of a flashover phenomenon at the fire scene.

According to Lentini, the errors caused by misinterpretations of flashovers were plentiful. They have resulted in numerous wrongful prosecutions and numerous improper denials of insurance proceeds.

Collection and Preservation of Arson Evidence

Two to three quarts of ash and soot debris must be collected at the point of origin of a fire when arson is suspected. The collection should include all porous materials and all other substances thought likely to contain flammable residues. These include such things as wood flooring, rugs, upholstery, and rags.

Packaging and Preservation of Evidence

Specimens should be packaged immediately in airtight containers so possible residues are not lost through evaporation. New, clean paint cans with friction lids are good containers because they are low cost, airtight, unbreakable, and available in a variety of sizes (see Figure 17–9). Wide-mouthed glass jars are also useful for packaging suspect specimens, provided that they have airtight lids. Cans and jars should be filled one-half to two-thirds full, leaving an air space in the container above the debris.

Large bulky samples should be cut to size at the scene as needed so that they will fit into available containers. Plastic polyethylene bags are not suitable for packaging specimens because they react with hydrocarbons and permit volatile hydrocarbon vapors to be depleted. Fluids found in open bottles or cans must be collected and sealed. Even when such containers appear empty, the investigator is wise to seal and preserve them in case they contain trace amounts of liquids or vapors.

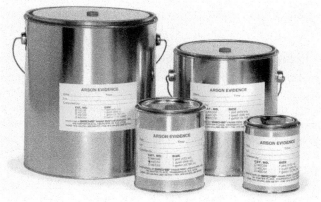

Courtesy Sirchie Fingerprint Laboratories, Youngsville, NC, www.sirchie.com

FIGURE 17–9

Various sizes of paint cans suitable for collecting debris at fire scenes.

Substrate Control

The collection of all materials suspected of containing volatile liquids must be accompanied by a thorough sampling of similar but uncontaminated control specimens from another area of the fire scene. This is known as *substrate control*. For example, if an investigator collects carpeting at the point of origin, the investigator must sample the same carpet from another part of the room, where it can be reasonably assumed that no flammable substance was placed.

In the laboratory, the criminalist checks the substrate control to be sure that it is free of any flammables. This procedure reduces the possibility (and subsequent argument) that the carpet was exposed to a flammable liquid such as a cleaning solution during normal maintenance. In addition, laboratory tests on the unburned control material may help analyze the breakdown products from the material's exposure to intense heat during the fire. Common materials such as plastic floor tiles, carpet, linoleum, and adhesives can produce volatile hydrocarbons when they are burned. These breakdown products can sometimes be mistaken for an accelerant.

Igniters and Other Evidence

The scene should also be thoroughly searched for igniters. The most common igniter is a match. Normally, the match is completely consumed during a fire and is impossible to locate. However, there have been cases in which, by force of habit, matches have been extinguished and tossed aside only to be recovered later by the investigator. This evidence may prove valuable if the criminalist can fit the match to a book found in the possession of a suspect.

Arsonists can construct many other types of devices to start a fire. These include burning cigarettes, firearms, ammunition, a mechanical match striker, electrical sparking devices, and a "Molotov cocktail"—a glass bottle containing flammable liquid with a cloth rag stuffed into it and lit as a fuse. Relatively complex mechanical devices are much more likely to survive the fire for later discovery. The broken glass and wick of the Molotov cocktail, if recovered, must be preserved as well.

One important piece of evidence is the clothing of the suspect perpetrator. If this individual is arrested within a few hours of initiating the fire, residual quantities of the accelerant may still be present in the clothing. As we will see in the next section, the forensic laboratory can detect extremely small quantities of accelerants, making the examination of a suspect's clothing a feasible investigative approach. Each item of clothing should be placed in a separate airtight container, preferably a new, clean paint can.

hydrocarbon
Any compound consisting of only carbon and hydrogen.

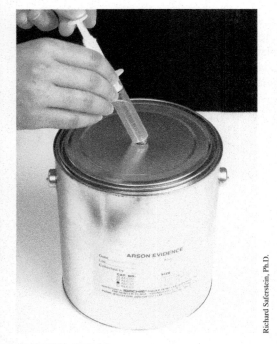

Richard Saferstein, Ph.D.

FIGURE 17–10
Removal of vapor from an enclosed container for gas chromatographic analysis.

Analysis of Flammable Residues

Criminalists are nearly unanimous in judging the gas chromatograph to be the most sensitive and reliable instrument for detecting and characterizing flammable residues. Most arsons are initiated by petroleum distillates, such as gasoline and kerosene, that are composed of a complex mixture of **hydrocarbons**. The gas chromatograph separates the hydrocarbon components of these liquids and produces a chromatographic pattern characteristic of a particular petroleum product.

The Headspace Technique

Before accelerant residues can be analyzed, they first must be recovered from the debris collected at the scene. The easiest way to recover accelerant residues from fire-scene debris is to heat the airtight container in which the sample is sent to the laboratory. When the container is heated, any volatile residue in the debris is driven off and trapped in the container's enclosed airspace. The vapor or *headspace* is then removed with a syringe, as shown in Figure 17–10.

When the vapor is injected into the gas chromatograph, it is separated into its components, and each peak is recorded on the chromatogram. One way of classifying ignitable liquids is by their boiling point range, which is related to the number of carbon molecules that are present in the mixture of hydrocarbons that make up an ignitable fuel. A common classification system characterizes ignitable liquids based on their boiling point ranges and number of carbon

FIGURE 17–11

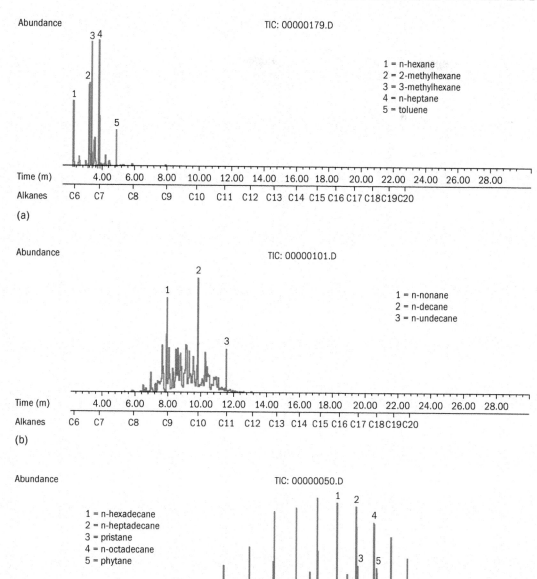

Chromatograms of ignitable liquids. (a) Light petroleum distillate, (b) medium petroleum distillate, and (c) heavy petroleum distillate.

molecules as light, medium, and heavy petroleum distillates. Figure 17–11 illustrates examples of chromatograms for light, medium, and heavy petroleum distillates. The identity of the volatile residue is determined when the pattern of the resultant chromatogram is compared to patterns produced by known petroleum products. For example, in Figure 17–12, a gas chromatographic analysis of debris recovered from a fire site shows a chromatogram similar to a known gasoline standard, thus proving the presence of gasoline.

In the absence of any recognizable pattern, the individual peaks can be identified when the investigator compares their retention times to known hydrocarbon standards (such as hexane, benzene, toluene, and xylenes). The brand name of a gasoline sample cannot currently be determined by gas chromatography or any other technique. Fluctuating gasoline markets and exchange agreements among the various oil companies preclude this possibility.

FIGURE 17–12

(Top) Gas chromatograph of vapor from a genuine gasoline sample. (Bottom) Gas chromatograph of vapor from debris recovered at a fire site. Note the similarity of the known gasoline to vapor removed from the debris.

Source: Richard Saferstein, *Criminalistics: An Introduction to Forensic Science,* 12e, © 2018. Pearson Education, Inc., New York, NY.

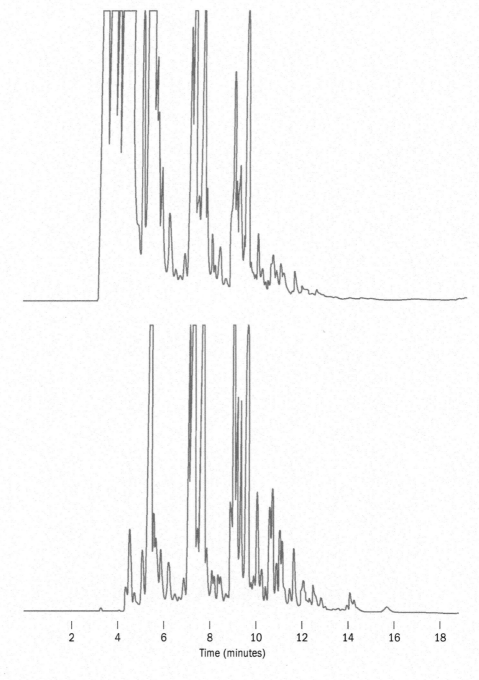

Time (minutes)

Vapor Concentration

One major disadvantage of the headspace technique is that the size of the syringe limits the volume of vapor that can be removed from the container and injected into the gas chromatograph. To overcome this deficiency, many crime laboratories augment the headspace technique with a method called *vapor concentration*. One setup for this analysis is shown in Figure 17–13.

A charcoal-coated strip, similar to that used in environmental monitoring badges, is placed within the container holding the debris that has been collected from the fire scene.[2] The container is then heated to about 60°C for about one hour. At this temperature, a significant quantity of accelerant vaporizes into the container airspace. The charcoal absorbs the accelerant vapor with which it comes into contact. In this manner, over a short period of time a significant quantity of the accelerant will be trapped and concentrated onto the charcoal strip.

[2] R. T. Newman et al., "The Use of Activated Charcoal Strips for Fire Debris Extractions by Passive Diffusion. Part 1: The Effects of Time, Temperature, Strip Size, and Sample Concentration," *Journal of Forensic Sciences* 41 (1996): 361.

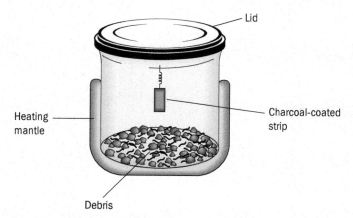

FIGURE 17–13
Apparatus for accelerant recovery by vapor concentration. The vapor in the enclosed container is exposed to charcoal, a chemical absorbent, where it is trapped for later analysis.

Once the heating procedure is complete, the analyst removes the charcoal strip from the container and recovers the accelerant from the strip by washing it with a small volume of solvent (carbon disulfide). The solvent is then injected into the gas chromatograph for analysis. The major advantage of using vapor concentration with gas chromatography is its sensitivity. By absorbing the accelerant into a charcoal strip, the forensic analyst can increase the sensitivity of accelerant detection at least a hundredfold over that of the conventional headspace technique.

An examination of Figure 17–12 shows that identifying an accelerant such as gasoline by gas chromatography is an exercise in pattern recognition. Typically, a forensic analyst compares the pattern generated by the sample to chromatograms from accelerant standards obtained under the same conditions. The pattern of gasoline, as with many other accelerants, can easily be placed in a searchable library. An invaluable reference known as the Ignitable Liquids Reference Collection (ILRC) is found on the Internet at http://ilrc.ucf.edu. The ILRC is a useful collection showing chromatographic patterns for approximately 500 ignitable liquids.

Explosions and Explosives

The ready accessibility of potentially explosive laboratory chemicals, dynamite, and, in some countries, an assortment of military explosives has provided the criminal element of society with a lethal weapon. Unfortunately for society, explosives have become an attractive weapon to criminals bent on revenge, destruction of commercial operations, or just plain mischief.

Inside the Science

Gas Chromatography/Mass Spectrometry

On occasion, discernible patterns are not attainable by gas chromatography. This may be due to a combination of accelerants, or to the mixing of accelerant residue with heat-generated breakdown products of materials burning at the fire scene. Under such conditions, a gas chromatographic pattern can be difficult if not impossible to interpret. In these cases, gas chromatography combined with mass spectrometry (discussed in Chapter 12) has proven valuable for solving difficult problems in the detection of accelerant residues.

Complex chromatographic patterns can be simplified by passing the separated components emerging from the gas chromatographic column through a mass spectrometer. As each component enters the mass spectrometer, it is fragmented into a collection of ions. The analyst can then control which ions will be detected and which will go unnoticed. In essence, the mass spectrometer acts as a filter allowing the analyst to see only the peaks associated with the ions selected for a particular accelerant. In this manner, the chromatographic pattern can be simplified by eliminating extraneous peaks that may obliterate the pattern.[3] The process is illustrated in the figure.

(continued)

[3] M. W. Gilbert, "The Use of Individual Extracted Ion Profiles Versus Summed Extracted Ion Profiles in Fire Debris Analysis," *Journal of Forensic Sciences* 43 (1998): 871.

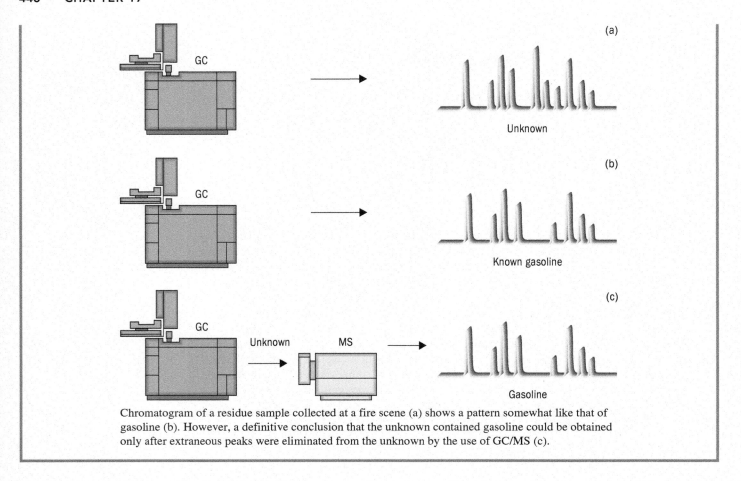

Chromatogram of a residue sample collected at a fire scene (a) shows a pattern somewhat like that of gasoline (b). However, a definitive conclusion that the unknown contained gasoline could be obtained only after extraneous peaks were eliminated from the unknown by the use of GC/MS (c).

Although politically motivated bombings have received considerable publicity worldwide, in the United States, most bombing incidents are perpetrated by isolated individuals rather than by organized terrorists. These incidents typically involve homemade explosives and incendiary devices. The design of such weapons is limited only by the imagination and ingenuity of the bomber.

Like arson investigation, bomb investigation requires close cooperation of a group of highly specialized individuals trained and experienced in bomb disposal, bomb-site investigation, forensic analysis, and criminal investigation. The criminalist must detect and identify explosive chemicals recovered from the crime scene as well as identify the detonating mechanisms. This special responsibility concerns us for the remainder of this chapter.

The Chemistry of Explosions

explosion
A chemical or mechanical action caused by combustion, accompanied by creation of heat and rapid expansion of gases.

Like fire, an **explosion** is the product of combustion accompanied by the creation of gases and heat. However, the distinguishing characteristic of an explosion is the rapid rate of the reaction. The sudden buildup of expanding gas pressure at the origin of the explosion produces the violent physical disruption of the surrounding environment.

Our previous discussion of the chemistry of fire referred only to oxidation reactions that rely on air as the sole source of oxygen. However, we need not restrict ourselves to this type of situation. For example, explosives are substances that undergo a rapid exothermic oxidation reaction, producing large quantities of gases. This sudden buildup of gas pressure constitutes an explosion. Detonation occurs so rapidly that oxygen in the air cannot participate in the reaction; thus, many explosives must have their own source of oxygen.

oxidizing agent
A substance that supplies oxygen to a chemical reaction.
75 percent potassium nitrate (KNO_3)
15 percent charcoal (C)
10 percent sulfur (S)

Chemicals that supply oxygen are known as **oxidizing agents**. One such agent is found in black powder, a *low explosive*, which is composed of a mixture of the following chemical ingredients:

In this combination, oxygen containing potassium nitrate acts as an oxidizing agent for the charcoal and sulfur fuels. As heat is applied to black powder, oxygen is liberated from potassium nitrate and simultaneously combines with charcoal and sulfur to produce heat and gases (symbolized by ↑), as represented in the following chemical equation:

$$3C + S + 2KNO_3 \rightarrow$$
carbon   sulfur   potassium nitrate   yields

$$3CO_2\uparrow + N_2\uparrow + K_2S$$
carbon dioxide   nitrogen   potassium sulfide

Some explosives have their oxygen and fuel components combined within one molecule. For example, the chemical structure of nitroglycerin, the major constituent of dynamite, combines carbon, hydrogen, nitrogen, and oxygen:

$$
\begin{array}{ccccc}
 & H & H & H & \\
 & | & | & | & \\
H - & C & - C & - C & - H \\
 & | & | & | & \\
 & NO_2 & NO_2 & NO_2 &
\end{array}
$$

When nitroglycerin detonates, large quantities of energy are released as the molecule decomposes, and the oxygen recombines to produce large volumes of carbon dioxide, nitrogen, and water.

Consider, for example, the effect of confining an explosive charge to a relatively small, closed container. On detonation, the explosive almost instantaneously produces large volumes of gases that exert enormously high pressures on the interior walls of the container. In addition, the heat energy released by the explosion expands the gases, causing them to push on the walls with an even greater force. If we could observe the effects of an exploding lead pipe in slow motion, we would first see the pipe's walls stretch and balloon under pressures as high as several hundred tons per square inch. Finally, the walls would fragment and fly outward in all directions. This flying debris or shrapnel constitutes a great danger to life and limb in the immediate vicinity.

On release from confinement, the gaseous products of the explosion suddenly expand and compress layers of surrounding air as they move outward from the origin of the explosion. This blast effect, or outward rush of gases, at a rate that may be as high as 7,000 miles per hour creates an artificial gale that can overthrow walls, collapse roofs, and disturb any object in its path. If a bomb is sufficiently powerful, more serious damage will be inflicted by the blast effect than by fragmentation debris (see Figure 17–14).

deflagration
A very rapid oxidation reaction accompanied by the generation of a low-intensity pressure wave that can disrupt the surroundings.

detonation
An extremely rapid oxidation reaction accompanied by a violent disruptive effect and an intense, high-speed shock wave.

low explosive
An explosive with a velocity of detonation less than 1,000 meters per second.

Types of Explosives

The speed at which explosives decompose varies greatly from one to another and permits their classification as *high* and *low explosives*. In a low explosive, this speed is called the speed of **deflagration** (burning). It is characterized by very rapid oxidation that produces heat, light, and a subsonic pressure wave. In a high explosive, it is called the speed of detonation. **Detonation** refers to the creation of a supersonic shock wave within the explosive charge. This shock wave breaks the chemical bonds of the explosive charge, leading to the new instantaneous buildup of heat and gases.

LOW EXPLOSIVES **Low explosives**, such as black and smokeless powders, decompose relatively slowly at rates up to 1,000 meters per second. Because of their slow burning rates, they produce a propelling or throwing action that makes them suitable as propellants for ammunition or skyrockets. However, the danger of this group of explosives

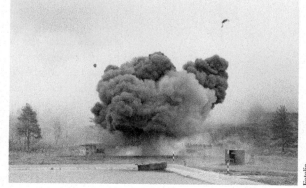

FIGURE 17–14
A violent explosion.

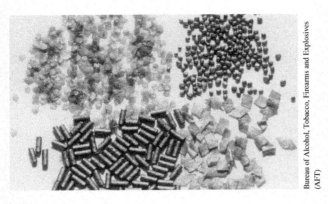

Bureau of Alcohol, Tobacco, Firearms and Explosives (AFT)

FIGURE 17–15
Samples of smokeless powders.

black powder
Normally, a mixture of potassium nitrate, carbon, and sulfur in the ratio 75:15:10.

safety fuse
A cord containing a core of black powder, used to carry a flame at a uniform rate to an explosive charge.

smokeless powder (single-base)
An explosive consisting of nitrated cotton or nitrocellulose.

smokeless powder (double-base)
An explosive consisting of a mixture of nitroglycerin and nitrocellulose.

must not be underestimated because, when any one of them is confined to a relatively small container, it can explode with a force as lethal as that of any known explosive.

Black Powder and Smokeless Powder The most widely used explosives in the low-explosive group are black powder and smokeless powder. The popularity of these two explosives is enhanced by their accessibility to the public. Both are available in any gun store, and black powder can easily be made from ingredients purchased at any chemical supply house as well.

Black powder is a relatively stable mixture of potassium nitrate or sodium nitrate, charcoal, and sulfur. Unconfined, it merely burns; thus, it commonly is used in safety fuses that carry a flame to an explosive charge. A **safety fuse** usually consists of black powder wrapped in a fabric or plastic casing. When ignited, a sufficient length of fuse will burn at a rate slow enough to allow a person adequate time to leave the site of the pending explosion. Black powder, like any other low explosive, becomes explosive and lethal only when it is confined.

The safest and most powerful low explosive is **smokeless powder**. This explosive usually consists of nitrated cotton or nitrocellulose (**single-base powder**) or nitroglycerin mixed with nitrocellulose (**double-base powder**). The powder is manufactured in a variety of grain sizes and shapes, depending on the desired application (see Figure 17–15). The Smokeless Powders Database is a regularly updated reference collection of information and data on single- and double-base smokeless reloading powders obtained from various sources, including law enforcement agencies, vendors, and manufacturers. The database contains a photomicrograph of each powder, physical characteristics, as well as instrumental analytical data. The database is maintained at the University of Central Florida.[4]

Chlorate Mixtures The only ingredients required for a low explosive are fuel and a good oxidizing agent. The oxidizing agent potassium chlorate, for example, when mixed with sugar, produces a popular and accessible explosive mix. When confined to a small container—for example, a pipe—and ignited, this mixture can explode with a force equivalent to a stick of 40 percent dynamite.

Some other commonly encountered ingredients that may be combined with chlorate to produce an explosive are carbon, sulfur, starch, phosphorus, and magnesium filings. Chlorate mixtures may also be ignited by the heat generated from a chemical reaction. For instance, sufficient heat can be generated to initiate combustion when concentrated sulfuric acid comes in contact with a sugar–chlorate mix.

Gas–Air Mixtures Another form of low explosive is created when a considerable quantity of natural gas escapes into a confined area and mixes with a sufficient amount of air. If ignited, this mixture results in simultaneous combustion and sudden production of large volumes of gases and heat. In a building, walls are forced outward by the expanding gases, causing the roof to fall into the interiors, and objects are thrown outward and scattered in erratic directions with no semblance of pattern.

Mixtures of air and a gaseous fuel explode or burn only within a limited concentration range. For example, the concentration limits for methane in air range from 5.3 to 13.9 percent. In the presence of too much air, the fuel becomes too diluted and does not ignite. On the other hand, if the fuel becomes too concentrated, ignition is prevented because there is not enough oxygen to support the combustion.

Mixtures at or near the upper concentration limit ("rich" mixtures) explode; however, some gas remains unconsumed because there is not enough oxygen to complete the combustion. As air rushes back into the origin of the explosion, it combines with the residual hot gas, producing a fire that is characterized by a *whoosh* sound. This fire is often more destructive than the explosion that preceded it. Mixtures near the lower end of the limit ("lean" mixtures) generally cause an explosion without accompanying damage due to fire.

---

[4] The Smokeless Powders Database can be found at http://www.ilrc.ucf.edu/powders/

HIGH EXPLOSIVES **High explosives** include dynamite, TNT, PETN, and RDX. They detonate almost instantaneously at rates of 1,000–8,500 meters per second, producing a smashing or shattering effect on their target. High explosives are classified into two groups—primary and secondary explosives—based on their sensitivity to heat, shock, or friction.

Primary explosives are ultrasensitive to heat, shock, or friction, and under normal conditions they detonate violently instead of burning. For this reason, they are used to detonate other explosives through a chain reaction and are often referred to as *primers*. Primary explosives provide the major ingredients of blasting caps and include lead azide, lead styphnate, and diazodinitrophenol (see Figure 17–16). Because of their extreme sensitivity, these explosives are rarely used as the main charge of a homemade bomb.

Secondary explosives are relatively insensitive to heat, shock, or friction, and they normally burn rather than detonate when ignited in small quantities in open air. This group comprises most high explosives used for commercial and military blasting. Some common examples of secondary explosives are dynamite, TNT (trinitrotoluene), PETN (pentaerythritol tetranitrate), RDX (cyclotrimethylene-trinitramine), and tetryl (2,4,6-trinitrophenylmethylnitramine).

Dynamite   It is an irony of history that the prize most symbolic of humanity's search for peace—the Nobel Peace Prize—should bear the name of the developer of one of our most lethal discoveries—dynamite. In 1867, the Swedish chemist Alfred Nobel, searching for a method to desensitize nitroglycerin, found that when kieselguhr, a variety of diatomaceous earth, absorbed a large portion of nitroglycerin, it became far less sensitive but still retained its explosive force. Nobel later decided to use pulp as an absorbent because kieselguhr was a heat-absorbing material.

This so-called pulp dynamite was the beginning of what is now known as the straight dynamite series. These dynamites are used when a quick shattering action is desired. In addition to nitroglycerine and pulp, present-day straight dynamites also include sodium nitrate (which furnishes oxygen for complete combustion) and a small percentage of a stabilizer, such as calcium carbonate.

All straight dynamite is rated by strength; the strength rating is determined by the weight percentage of nitroglycerin in the formula. Thus, a 40 percent straight dynamite contains 40 percent nitroglycerin, a 60 percent grade contains 60 percent nitroglycerin, and so forth. However, the relative blasting power of different strengths of dynamite is not directly proportional to their strength ratings. A 60 percent straight dynamite, rather than being three times as strong as a 20 percent, is only one and one-half times as strong (see Figure 17–17).

Ammonium Nitrate Explosives   In recent years, nitroglycerin-based dynamite has all but disappeared from the industrial explosives market. Commercially, these explosives have been replaced mainly by ammonium nitrate–based explosives, that is, water gels, emulsions, and ANFO explosives. These explosives mix oxygen-rich ammonium nitrate with a fuel to form a low-cost, stable explosive.

Typically, water gels have a consistency resembling that of set gelatin or gel-type toothpaste. They are characterized by their water-resistant nature and are employed for all types of blasting under wet conditions. These explosives are based on formulations of ammonium nitrate and sodium nitrate gelled with a natural polysaccharide such as guar gum. Commonly, a combustible material such as aluminum is mixed into the gel to serve as the explosive's fuel.

Emulsion explosives differ from gels in that they consist of two distinct phases, an oil phase and a water phase. In these emulsions, a droplet of a supersaturated solution of ammonium nitrate is surrounded by a hydrocarbon serving as a fuel. A typical emulsion consists of water, one

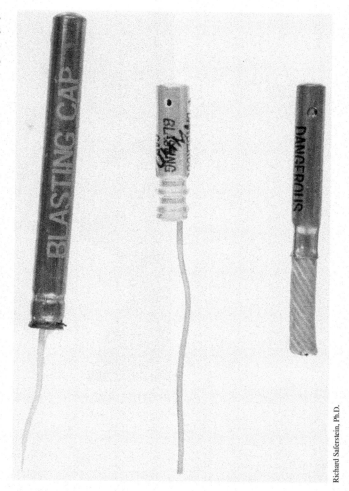

Richard Saferstein, Ph.D.

FIGURE 17–16

Blasting caps. The left and center caps are initiated by an electrical current; the right cap is initiated by a safety fuse.

high explosive
An explosive with a velocity of detonation greater than 1,000 meters per second.

primary explosive
A high explosive that is easily detonated by heat, shock, or friction.

secondary explosive
A high explosive that is relatively insensitive to heat, shock, or friction.

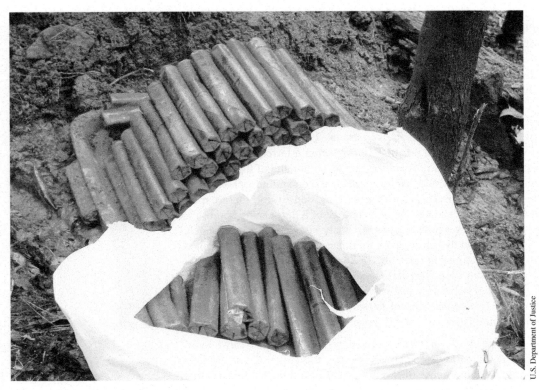

U.S. Department of Justice

FIGURE 17–17
Sticks of dynamite.

or more inorganic nitrate oxidizers, oil, and emulsifying agents. Commonly, emulsions contain micron-sized glass, resin, or ceramic spheres known as *microspheres* or *microballoons*. The size of these spheres controls the explosive's sensitivity and detonation velocity.

Ammonium nitrate soaked in fuel oil is an explosive known as *ANFO*. Such commercial explosives are inexpensive and safe to handle and have found wide applications in blasting operations in the mining industry. Ammonium nitrate in the form of fertilizer makes a readily obtainable ingredient for homemade explosives. Indeed, in an incident related to the 1993 bombing of New York City's World Trade Center, the FBI arrested five men during a raid on their hideout in New York City, where they were mixing a "witches' brew" of fuel oil and an ammonium nitrate–based fertilizer.

TATP   *Triacetone triperoxide* (TATP) is a homemade explosive that has been used as an improvised explosive by terrorist organizations in Israel and other Middle Eastern countries. It is prepared by reacting the common ingredients of acetone and hydrogen peroxide in the presence of an acid catalyst, such as hydrochloric acid.

TATP is a friction- and impact-sensitive explosive that is extremely potent when confined in a container such as a pipe. The 2005 London transit bombings were caused by TATP-based explosives and provide ample evidence that terrorist cells have moved TATP outside the Middle East. A London bus destroyed by one of the TATP bombs is shown in Figure 17–18. The ease of preparation has made TATP a choice explosive for Middle-East operatives. TATP was responsible for inflicting casualties at the Brussels airport bombings in 2016. Also, in Brussels, investigators recovered TATP packed into suitcases also containing ammonium nitrate, metal bolts, and nails.

A plot to blow up 10 international plane flights leaving Britain for the United States with a "liquid explosive" apparently involved plans to smuggle the peroxide-based TATP explosive onto the planes. This plot has prompted authorities to prohibit airline passengers from carrying liquids and gels onto planes.

Military High Explosives   No discussion of high explosives would be complete without a mention of military high explosives. In many countries outside the United States, the accessibility of high explosives to terrorist organizations makes them common constituents of homemade

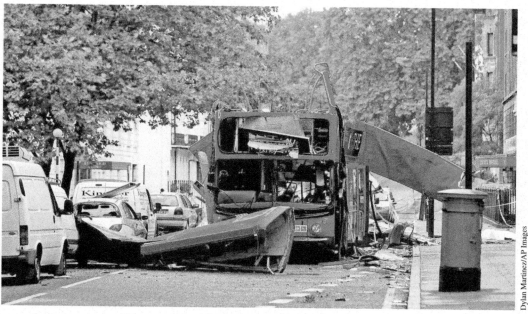

Dylan Martinez/AP Images

FIGURE 17–18

A London bus destroyed by a TATP-based bomb.

bombs. RDX, the most popular and powerful military explosive, is often encountered in the form of a pliable plastic of doughlike consistency known as *composition C–4* (a U.S. military designation).

TNT was produced and used on an enormous scale during World War II and may be considered the most important military bursting charge explosive. Alone or in combination with other explosives, it has found wide application in shells, bombs, grenades, demolition explosives, and propellant compositions. Interestingly, military "dynamite" contains no nitroglycerin but is actually composed of a mixture of RDX and TNT. Like other military explosives, TNT is rarely encountered in bombings in the United States.

PETN is used by the military in TNT mixtures for small-caliber projectiles and grenades. Commercially, the chemical is used as the explosive core in a **detonating cord** or *primacord*. Instead of the slower-burning safety fuse, a detonating cord is often used to connect a series of explosive charges so that they will detonate simultaneously.

detonating cord
A cordlike explosive containing a core of high-explosive material, usually PETN; also called primacord.

Detonators   Unlike low explosives, bombs made of high explosives must be detonated by an initiating explosion. In most cases, detonators are blasting caps composed of copper or aluminum cases filled with lead azide as an initiating charge and PETN or RDX as a detonating charge. Blasting caps can be initiated by means of a burning safety fuse or by an electrical current.

Homemade bombs camouflaged in packages, suitcases, and the like are usually initiated with an electrical blasting cap wired to a battery. An unlimited number of switching-mechanism designs have been devised for setting off these devices; clocks and mercury switches are favored. Bombers sometimes prefer to employ outside electrical sources. For instance, most automobile bombs are detonated when the ignition switch of a car is turned on.

Collection and Analysis of Evidence of Explosives

The most important step in the detection and analysis of explosive residues is the collection of appropriate samples from the explosion scene. Invariably, undetonated residues of the explosive remain at the site of the explosion. The detection and identification of these explosives in the laboratory depends on the bomb-scene investigator's skill and ability to recognize and sample the areas most likely to contain such materials.

> > > > > > > > >

Liquid Explosives

In 2006, security agencies in the United States and Great Britain uncovered a terrorist plot to use liquid explosives to destroy commercial airlines operating between the two countries. Of the hundreds of types of explosives, most are solid. Only about a dozen are liquid. But some of those liquid explosives can be readily purchased and others can be made from hundreds of different kinds of chemicals that are not difficult to obtain. After the September 11 attacks, worries about solid explosives became the primary concern. In 2001, Richard Reid was arrested for attempting to destroy an American Airlines flight out of Paris. Authorities later found a high explosive with a TATP detonator hidden in the lining of his shoe. It is therefore not surprising that terrorists turned to liquids in this latest plot. A memo issued by federal security officials about the plot to blow up 10 international planes highlighted a type of liquid explosive based on peroxide.

The most common peroxide-based explosive is TATP (triacetone triperoxide), which is made up of acetone and hydrogen peroxide, two widely available substances. TATP can be used as a detonator or a primary explosive and has been used in al Qaeda–related bomb plots and by Palestinian suicide bombers. TATP itself is a white powder made up of crystals that form when acetone and hydrogen peroxide are mixed together, usually with a catalyst added to speed the chemical reactions. Acetone is the main ingredient in nail polish remover, while hydrogen peroxide is a popular antiseptic. When the two main ingredients are mixed, they form a white powder that can be easily detonated using an electrical spark.

Commercially available hydrogen peroxide, however, is not concentrated enough to create TATP. The solution sold in stores contains about 3 percent hydrogen peroxide, compared to the approximately 70 percent concentration need for TATP. However, hydrogen peroxide solutions of up to 30 percent can be obtained from chemical supply houses. According to explosives experts, a mixture of 30 percent hydrogen peroxide and acetone can create a fire hot enough to burn though the fuselage of an aircraft.

In theory, scientists know how to detect peroxide-based explosives. The challenge is to design machines that can perform scans quickly and efficiently on thousands of passengers passing through airport security checks. Current scanning machines at airports are designed to detect nitrogen-containing chemicals and are not designed to detect peroxide-containing explosive ingredients. Since 9/11, security experts have worried about the possibility of liquid explosives in the form of liquids and gels getting onto airliners.

Without the luxury of waiting for newly designed scanning devices capable of ferreting out dangerous liquids to be in place at airports, experts decided to use a commonsense approach—that is, to restrict the types and quantities of liquids that a passenger can carry onto a plane.

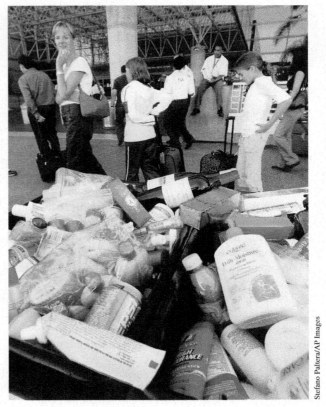

Stefano Paltera/AP Images

Gels and liquids discarded by airline passengers before boarding.

Detecting and Recovering Evidence of Explosives

The most obvious characteristic of a high or contained low explosive is the presence of a crater at the origin of the blast. Once the crater has been located, all loose soil and other debris must immediately be removed from the interior of the hole and preserved for laboratory analysis. Other good sources of explosive residues are objects located near the origin of detonation. Wood, insulation, rubber, and other soft materials that are readily penetrated often collect traces of the explosive. However, nonporous objects near the blast must not be overlooked. For instance, residues can be found on the surfaces of metal objects near the site of an explosion. Material blown away from the blast's origin should also be recovered because it, too, may retain explosive residues.

The entire area must be systematically searched, with great care given to recovering any trace of a detonating mechanism or any other item foreign to the explosion site. Wire-mesh screens are best used for sifting through debris. All personnel involved in searching the bomb scene must take appropriate measures to avoid contaminating the scene, including dressing in disposable gloves, shoe covers, and overalls.

COLLECTION AND PACKAGING   All materials collected for examination by the laboratory must be placed in airtight sealed containers and labeled with all pertinent information. In pipe-bomb explosions, particles of the explosive are frequently found adhering to the pipe cap or to the pipe threads, as a result of either being impacted into the metal by the force of the explosion or being deposited in the threads during the construction of the bomb. Soil and other soft loose materials are best stored in metal airtight containers such as clean paint cans. Debris and articles collected from different areas are to be packaged in separate airtight containers. Plastic bags should not be used to store evidence suspected of containing explosive residues. Some explosives can actually escape through the plastic. Sharp-edged objects should not be allowed to pierce the sides of a plastic bag. It is best to place these types of items in metal containers.

Inside the Science

Analysis of Evidence of Explosives

When the bomb-scene debris and other materials arrive at the laboratory, everything is first examined microscopically to detect particles of unconsumed explosive. Portions of the recovered debris and detonating mechanism, if found, are carefully viewed under a low-power stereoscopic microscope in a painstaking effort to locate particles of the explosive. Black powder and smokeless powder are relatively easy to locate in debris because of their characteristic shapes and colors (see Figure 17–15). However, dynamite and other high explosives present the microscopist with a much more difficult task and often must be detected by other means.

One approach for screening objects for the presence of explosive residues in the field or the laboratory is the ion mobility spectrometer (IMS).[5] A portable IMS is shown in the figure.

This handheld detector uses a vacuum to collect explosive residues from suspect surfaces. Alternatively, the surface suspected of containing explosive residues is wiped down with a Teflon-coated fiberglass disc and the collected residues are then drawn into the spectrometer off the disc. Once in the IMS, the explosive residues are vaporized by the application of heat. These vaporized substances are exposed to a beam of electrons or beta rays emitted by radioactive nickel and converted into electrically charged molecules or ions. The ions are then allowed to move through a tube (drift region) under the influence of an electric field. A schematic diagram of an IMS is shown in the figure.

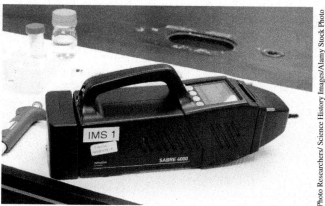

Hardened MobileTrace®, a portable ion mobility spectrometer used to rapidly detect and tentatively identify trace quantities of explosives.

[5] Keller et al., "Application of Ion Mobility Spectrometry in Cases of Forensic Interest," *Forensic Science International* 161 (2006): 130.

(continued)

Sample is bombarded
by radioactive particles
emitted by an isotope
of nickel to form ions

Sample is
drawn into
ionization
chamber

Drift rings

^{63}Ni

Collection
electrode

Shutter

Ionization chamber

Drift region

(a)

Sample is converted into ions
of different sizes and structures

Drift rings

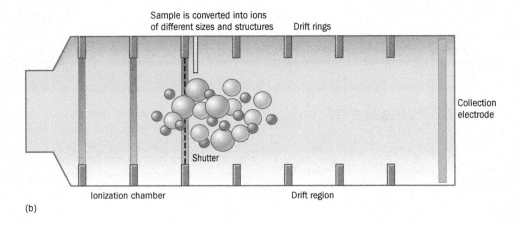

Collection
electrode

Shutter

Ionization chamber

Drift region

(b)

Explosive substances can
be characterized by the
speed at which they move
through the electric field

Drift rings

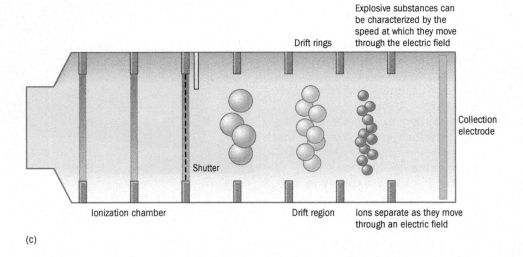

Collection
electrode

Shutter

Ionization chamber

Drift region

Ions separate as they move
through an electric field

(c)

Schematic diagram of an ion mobility spectrometer. A sample is introduced into an ionization chamber, where bombardment with radioactive particles emitted by an isotope of nickel converts the sample to ions. The ions move into a drift region where ion separation occurs based on the speed of the ions as they move through an electric field.

The preliminary identification of an explosive residue can be made by noting the time it takes the explosive to move through the tube. Because ions move at different speeds depending on their size and structure, they can be characterized by the speed at which they pass through the tube. Used as a screening tool, this method rapidly detects a full range of explosives, even at low detection levels. However, all results need to be verified through confirmatory tests.

Following microscopic examination, the recovered debris is thoroughly rinsed with acetone. The high solubility of most explosives in acetone ensures their quick removal from the debris. When a water-gel explosive containing ammonium nitrate or a low explosive is suspected, the debris should be rinsed with water so that water-soluble substances (such as nitrates and chlorates) will be extracted. Table 17–3 lists a number of simple color tests the examiner can perform on the acetone and water extracts to screen for the presence of organic and inorganic explosives, respectively.

Once collected, the acetone extract is concentrated and analyzed using color spot tests, thin-layer chromatography (TLC), high-performance liquid chromatography (HPLC), and gas chromatography/mass spectrometry. The presence of an explosive is indicated by a well-defined spot on a TLC plate corresponding to a known explosive—for example, nitroglycerin, RDX, or PETN.

The high sensitivity of HPLC also makes it useful for analyzing trace evidence of explosives. HPLC operates at room temperature and hence does not cause explosives, many of which are temperature sensitive, to decompose during their analysis. When a water-gel explosive containing ammonium nitrate or a low explosive is suspected, the debris should be rinsed with water so that water-soluble substances (such as nitrates and chlorates) will be extracted.

When sufficient quantities of explosives are recoverable, confirmatory tests may be performed by infrared spectrophotometry. The former produces a unique "fingerprint" pattern for an organic explosive, as shown by the IR spectrum of RDX in the figure.

TABLE 17–3
Color Spot Tests for Common Explosives

Substance	Reagent		
	Griess[a]	Diphenylamine[b]	Alcoholic KOH[c]
Chlorate	No color	Blue	No color
Nitrate	Pink to red	Blue	No color
Nitrocellulose	Pink	Blue-black	No color
Nitroglycerin	Pink to red	Blue	No color
PETN	Pink to red	Blue	No color
RDX	Pink to red	Blue	No color
TNT	No color	No color	Red
Tetryl	Pink to red	Blue	Red-violet

[a] Griess reagent: Solution 1—Dissolve 1 g sulfanilic acid in 100 mL 30 percent acetic acid. Solution 2—Dissolve 0.5 g N-(1-napthyl) ethylenediamine in 100 mL methyl alcohol. Add solutions 1 and 2 and a few milligrams of zinc dust to the suspect extract.
[b] Diphenylamine reagent: Dissolve 1 g diphenylamine in 100 mL concentrated sulfuric acid.
[c] Alcoholic KOH reagent: Dissolve 10 g of potassium hydroxide in 100 mL absolute alcohol.

(continued)

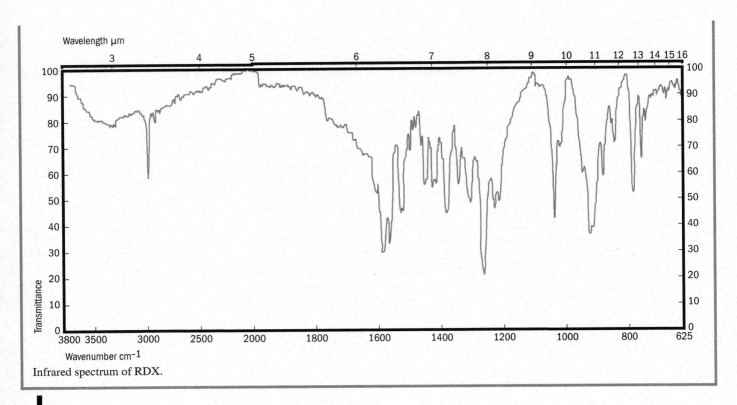

Infrared spectrum of RDX.

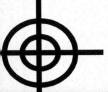

Chapter Summary >>>>>>>>>>>

When a fire occurs, oxygen combines with a fuel to produce noticeable quantities of heat and light (flames). Three requirements must be satisfied to initiate and sustain combustion: (1) a fuel must be present, (2) oxygen must be available in sufficient quantity to combine with the fuel, and (3) sufficient heat must be applied to initiate the combustion and generated to sustain the reaction. A fuel achieves a reaction rate with oxygen sufficient to sustain a fire only when it is in the gaseous state.

As a fire progresses, the heat created by the combustion process tends to move from a high-temperature region to one at a lower temperature. Understanding heat transfer from one location to another is important for reconstructing the origin of a fire, as well as for understanding why and how fire spreads through a structure. The three mechanisms of heat transfer are conduction, radiation, and convection.

The arson investigator must begin examining a fire scene for signs of arson as soon as the fire has been extinguished. Some telltale signs of arson include evidence of separate and unconnected fires, the use of "streamers" to spread the fire from one area to another, and evidence of severe burning found on the floor as opposed to the ceiling of a structure.

The search of the fire scene must focus on finding the fire's origin. There are no fast and simple rules for identifying a fire's origin. Normally, a fire tends to move upward, and thus the probable origin is most likely closest to the lowest point that shows the most intense characteristics of burning. Sometimes as the fire burns upward, a V-shaped pattern forms against a vertical wall. At the suspect point of origin of a fire, porous materials should be collected and stored in airtight containers.

In the laboratory, the gas chromatograph is the most sensitive and reliable instrument for detecting and characterizing flammable residues. Most arsons are initiated by petroleum distillates such as gasoline and kerosene. The gas chromatograph separates the hydrocarbon components and produces a chromatographic pattern characteristic of a particular petroleum product. By comparing select gas chromatographic peaks recovered from fire-scene debris to known flammable liquids, a forensic analyst may be able to identify the accelerant used to initiate the fire.

Explosives are substances that undergo a rapid oxidation reaction with the production of large quantities of gases. This sudden buildup of gas pressure constitutes an explosion. The speed at which explosives decompose permits their classification as high or low explosives.

The most widely used low explosives are black powder and smokeless powder. Among the high explosives, primary explosives are ultrasensitive to heat, shock, or friction and provide the major ingredients found in blasting caps. Secondary explosives normally constitute the main charge of a high explosive.

Among the high explosives, nitroglycerin-based dynamite has all but disappeared from the industrial explosives market and has been replaced by ammonium nitrate–based explosives (such as water gels, emulsions, and ANFO explosives). In many countries outside the United States, the accessibility of military high explosives to terrorist organizations makes them common constituents of homemade bombs. RDX is the most popular and powerful of the military explosives.

The entire bomb site must be systematically searched, with great care given to recovering any trace of a detonating mechanism or any other item foreign to the explosion site. Objects located at or near the origin of the explosion must be collected for laboratory examination. Volatile items should be packaged in airtight containers, such as clean paint cans, for transport to the laboratory.

Typically, in the laboratory, debris collected at explosion scenes is examined microscopically for unconsumed explosive particles. Recovered debris may also be thoroughly rinsed with organic solvents and analyzed by testing procedures that include color spot tests, thin-layer chromatography, high-performance liquid chromatography, and gas chromatography/mass spectrometry.

Review Questions

1. True or False: The absence of chemical residues always rules out the possibility of arson. _____

2. The combination of oxygen with other substances to produce new chemical products is called _____.

3. True or False: All oxidation reactions produce noticeable quantities of heat and light. _____

4. _____ is the capacity for doing work.

5. Burning methane for the purpose of heating water to produce steam in order to drive a turbine is an example of converting _____ energy to _____ energy.

6. The quantity of heat evolved from a chemical reaction arises out of the _____ and _____ of chemical bonds.

7. Molecules must (absorb, liberate) energy to break their bonds and (absorb, liberate) energy when their bonds are reformed.

8. All oxidation reactions (absorb, liberate) heat.

9. Reactions that liberate heat are said to be _____.

10. Excess heat energy liberated by an oxidation reaction is called the _____.

11. A chemical reaction in which heat is absorbed from the surroundings is said to be _____.

12. True or False: All reactions require an energy input to start them. _____

13. The minimum temperature at which a fuel burns is known as the _____ temperature.

14. A fuel achieves a sufficient reaction rate with oxygen to produce a flame only in the (gaseous, liquid) state.

15. The lowest temperature at which a liquid fuel produces enough vapor to burn is the _____.

16. _____ is the chemical breakdown of a solid material to gaseous products.

17. _____ is a phenomenon in which a fuel burns without the presence of a flame.

18. The rate of a chemical reaction (increases, decreases) as the temperature rises.

19. _____ describes a fire caused by a natural heat-producing process.

20. True or False: An immediate search of a fire scene can commence without obtaining a search warrant. _____

21. A search of the fire scene must focus on finding the fire's _____.

22. True or False: The probable origin of a fire is most likely closest to the lowest point that shows the most intense characteristics of burning. _____

23. The collection of debris at the origin of a fire should include all (porous, nonporous) materials.

24. _____ containers must be used to package all materials suspected of containing hydrocarbon residues.

25. The most sensitive and reliable instrument for detecting and characterizing flammable residues is the (gas chromatograph, infrared spectrophotometer).

26. The identity of a volatile petroleum residue is determined by the (size, pattern) of its gas chromatogram.

27. True or False: The major advantage of using the vapor concentration technique in combination with gas chromatography is its extreme sensitivity for detecting volatile residues from fire-scene evidence. _____

28. True or False: A forensic analyst typically compares the gas chromatographic pattern generated from a fire-scene sample to a library of patterns in order to identify the accelerant. _____

29. The criminalist (can, cannot) identify gasoline residues by brand name.

30. Rapid combustion accompanied by the creation of large volumes of gases describes a(n) _____.

31. True or False: Chemicals that supply oxygen are known as oxidizing agents. _____

32. Explosives that decompose at relatively slow rates are classified as _____ explosives.

33. The speed at which low explosives decompose is called the speed of _____.

34. Three ingredients of black powder are_____, _____, and _____.

35. _____ explosives detonate almost instantaneously to produce a smashing or shattering effect.

36. The most widely used low explosives are _____ and _____.

37. A low explosive becomes explosive and lethal only when it is _____.

38. True or False: Air and a gaseous fuel burn when mixed in any proportions. _____

39. High explosives can be classified as either _____ or _____ explosives.

40. The most widely used explosive in the military is _____.

41. The explosive core in detonating cord is _____.

42. A high explosive is normally detonated by a(n) _____ explosive contained within a blasting cap.

43. An obvious characteristic of a high explosive is the presence of a(n) _____ at the origin of the blast.

44. The three mechanisms of heat transfer are _____, _____, and _____.

45. True or False: Debris and articles at an explosion scene that are collected from different areas are to be packaged in separate airtight containers _____.

Review Questions for Inside the Science

1. A fire moves away from the original point of ignition because the _____ created by the combustion process tends to move from a high-temperature region to one at a lower temperature.

2. Electrons and atoms within a solid object exposed to heat collide with one another, causing movement of heat through the object in a process called _____.

3. In a process known as _____, a heated surface emits electromagnetic radiation of various wavelengths that moves in a straight line from one surface to another, helping the fire to spread throughout a structure.

4. Complex chromatographic patterns can be simplified by passing the components emerging from the gas chromatographic column through a(n) _____.

5. To screen objects for the presence of explosive residues in the field or the laboratory, the investigator may use a handheld _____.

6. Unconsumed explosive residues may be detected in the laboratory through a careful _____ examination of the debris.

7. Debris recovered from the site of an explosion is routinely rinsed with _____ in an attempt to recover high-explosive residues.

8. Once collected, the acetone extract is initially analyzed by _____, _____, and _____.

9. The technique of _____ produces a unique absorption spectrum for an organic explosive.

Application and Critical Thinking

1. Indicate which method of heat transfer is most likely to be responsible for each of the following:
   a. Ignition of papers in the room where a fire starts
   b. Ignition of electrical wiring in a room adjoining the fire's point or origin
   c. Ignition of roof timbers
   d. Ignition of a neighboring house

2. It is late August in Houston, Texas, and you are investigating a fire that occurred at a facility that stores motor oils and other lubricating oils. A witness

points out a man who allegedly ran from the structure about the same time that the fire started. You question the man, who turns out to be the owner of the facility. He tells you that he was checking his inventory when barrels of waste motor oil stored in an unventilated back room spontaneously burst into flames. The owner claims that the fire spread so rapidly that he had to flee the building before he could call 911. After speaking with several employees, you learn that the building has no air conditioning and that the oil had been stored for almost a year in the cramped back room. You also learn from a detective assisting on the case that the owner increased his insurance coverage on the facility within the past three months. Should you believe the owner's story, or should you suspect arson? On what do you base your conclusion?

3. Criminalist Mick Mickelson is collecting evidence from a fire scene. He gathers about a quart of ash and soot debris from several rooms surrounding the point of origin. He stores the debris in a new, clean paint can, filled about three-quarters full. Seeing several pieces of timber that he believes may contain accelerant residues, he cuts them and places them in airtight plastic bags. A short time later, a suspect is arrested and Mick searches him for any signs of an igniter or accelerants. He finds a cigarette lighter on the suspect and seizes it for evidence before turning the suspect over to the police. What mistakes, if any, did Mick make in collecting evidence?

4. Classify the following chromatograms of ignitable liquids as low, medium, or high petroleum distillates. Refer to Figure 17–10.

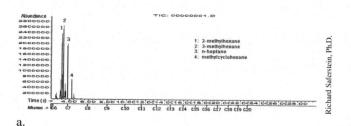

a. _____

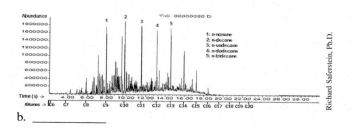

b. _____

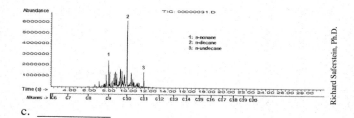

c. _____

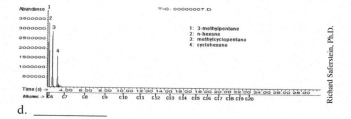

d. _____

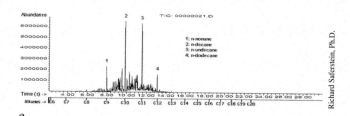

e. _____

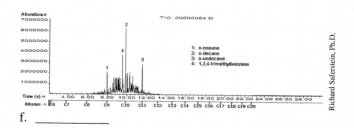

f. _____

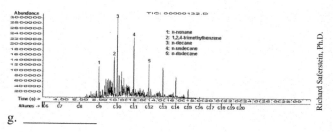

g. _____

5. The following pieces of evidence were found at separate explosion sites. For each item, indicate whether the explosion was more likely caused by low or high explosives, and explain your answer:

a. Lead azide residues

b. Nitrocellulose residues

c. Ammonium nitrate residues

d. Scraps of primacord

e. Potassium chlorate residues

6. Which color test or tests would you run first on a suspect sample to test for evidence of each of the following explosives? Explain your answers.

a. Tetryl

b. TNT

c. Chlorate

d. Nitrocellulose

7. Criminalist Matt Weir is collecting evidence from the site of an explosion. Arriving on the scene, he immediately proceeds to look for the crater caused by the blast. After finding the crater, he picks through the debris at the site by hand, looking for evidence of detonators or foreign materials. Matt collects loose soil and debris from the immediate area, placing the smaller bits in paper folded into a druggist fold. Larger items he stores in plastic bags for transportation to the laboratory. What mistakes, if any, did Matt make in collecting and storing this evidence?

Further References

DeHaan, John D., and D. J. Icove, *Kirk's Fire Investigation*, 7th ed. Upper Saddle River, NJ: Pearson Educational, 2012.

Hendrikse, J., M. Grutters, and F. Schafer, Identifying *Ignitable Liquids in Fire Debris*. London Wall, UK: Elsevier Academic Press, 2016.

Icove, David J., J. D. DeHaan, and G. A. Haynes, *Forensic Fire Scene Reconstruction*, 3rd ed. Upper Saddle River, NJ: Prentice Hall, 2013.

Lentini, J. J., *Scientific Protocols for Fire Investigation*, 2nd ed. Boca Raton, FL: CRC Press, 2013.

Midkiff, C. R., "Arson and Explosive Investigation," in R. Saferstein, ed., *Forensic Science Handbook*, vol. 1, 2nd ed. Upper Saddle River, NJ: Prentice Hall, 2002.

NFPA 921 Guide for Fire and Explosion Investigations. Quincy, MA: National Fire Protection Association, 2014.

Stauffer, Eric, Julia A. Dolan, and Reta Newman, *Fire Debris Analysis*. Burlington, MA: Academic Press, 2008.

Thurman, J. T., *Practical Bomb Scene Investigation*, 2nd ed. Boca Raton, FL: CRC Press, 2011.

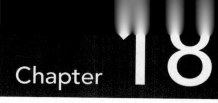

Document Examination

KEY TERMS

Learning Objectives

After studying this chapter, you should be able to:

18.1 Define the term *questioned document*

18.2 Explain the factors considered when comparing variations in handwriting and the challenges associated with it

18.3 List some important guidelines for the collection of known writings for comparison to a questioned document

18.4 Recognize some of the class and individual characteristics of printers and photocopiers

18.5 List some of the techniques document examiners use to uncover alterations, erasures, and obliterations

18.6 Summarize some of the other problems faced by document examiners

The Life and Deaths of Robert Durst

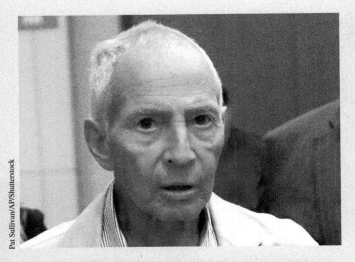

Trail heats up in missing wife mystery

Robert Durst married Kathleen McCormack in April of 1973. The two lived busy lives in Manhattan, where Kathie was a medical student and Robert worked for his family's real estate business. By all accounts, their relationship started as a loving one, but after nearly 10 years of marriage, the union was in decline. Kathie was treated at a Bronx hospital for facial bruises and told a friend that Robert had beat her. One night after dinner with friends in January 1982, Kathie went missing. She was never seen or heard from again.

After the disappearance of his wife, many people—including the police—focused on Durst as a suspect. He often sought solace and counsel from his close friend, Susan Berman. Berman acted as a representative for Durst, making statements on his behalf to the news media following Kathie's disappearance and even providing police with an alibi for his whereabouts on the night she went missing. Some 20 years later, Berman had fallen on hard times. Police believed that she knew too much about the disappearance of Kathie, and began extorting Durst, who began providing her with checks for large sums of money. On December 24, 2000, Susan Berman was found murdered execution-style in her home in California. Durst is known to have been in Northern California days before Berman was killed, and to have flown from San Francisco to New York the night before Berman's body was discovered.

Police discovered the crime after they received an anonymous letter written to the Beverly Hills Police Department alerting them to a "cadaver" at Berman's address. The handwriting in the letter was compared to other documents authored by Durst, including letters mailed to Berman. A curious misspelling of the word "Beverley" appeared in both the "cadaver" letter to police and letters known to be authored by Durst. Handwriting experts, as well as Durst himself, have acknowledged the similarity between his handwriting and the handwriting on the letter to the Beverly Hills Police. Robert Durst was arrested and indicted on charges of first degree murder related to the death of Susan Berman in March of 2015 based in part on the handwriting analysis performed on the "cadaver" letter. His trial is set to begin in late 2019.

Document Examiner

Ordinarily, the work of the document examiner involves examining handwriting and typescript to ascertain the source or authenticity of a questioned document. However, document examination is not restricted to a mere visual comparison of words and letters. The document examiner must know how to use the techniques of microscopy, photography, and even such analytical methods as chromatography to uncover successfully all efforts, both brazen and subtle, designed to change the content or meaning of a document.

Alterations of documents through overwriting, erasures, or the more obvious crossing out of words must be recognized and characterized as efforts to alter or obscure the original meaning of a document. The document examiner uses their special skills to reconstruct the written contents of charred or burned paper or to uncover the meaning of indented writings found on a paper pad after the top sheet has been removed.

Any object that contains handwritten or typewritten markings whose source or authenticity is in doubt may be referred to as a **questioned document**. Such a broad definition covers all of the written and printed materials we normally encounter in our daily social and business activities. Letters, checks, driver's licenses, contracts, wills, voter registrations, passports, petitions, and even lottery tickets are the more common specimens received in crime laboratories to be examined. However, we need not restrict our examples to paper documents. Questioned documents may include writings or other markings found on walls, windows, doors, or any other objects.

Document examiners possess no mystical powers or scientific formulas for identifying the authors of writings. They apply knowledge gathered through years of training and experience to recognize and compare the individual characteristics of questioned and known authentic writings. For this purpose, the gathering of documents of known authorship or origin is critical to the outcome of the examination. Collecting known writings may entail considerable time and effort, and their collection may be further hampered by uncooperative or missing witnesses. However, the uniqueness of handwriting makes this type of physical evidence, like fingerprints, one of few definitive individual characteristics available to the investigator, a fact that certainly justifies an extensive investigative effort.

questioned document
Any document about which some issue has been raised or that is the subject of an investigation.

Handwriting Comparisons

Document experts continually testify that no two individuals write exactly alike. This is not to say that there cannot be marked resemblances between two individuals' handwritings because many factors make up the total character of a person's writing.

General Style

Perhaps the most obvious feature of handwriting to the layperson is its general style. As children, we all learn to write by attempting to copy letters that match a standard form or style shown to us by our teachers. The style of writing acquired by the learner is that which is fashionable for the particular time and locale. In the United States, for example, the two most widely used systems are the Palmer method, first introduced in 1880, and the Zaner-Bloser method, introduced in about 1895 (see Figure 18–1). To some extent, both of these systems are taught in nearly all 50 states.

The early stages that accompany the learning and practicing of handwriting are characterized by a conscious effort on the part of the student to copy standard letter forms. It is not surprising that many pupils in a handwriting class tend at first to have writing styles that are similar to one another, with minor differences attributable to skill in copying. However, as initial writing skills improve, a child normally reaches the stage where the nerve and motor responses associated with the act of writing become subconscious. The individual's writing now begins to take on innumerable habitual shapes and patterns that distinguish it from all others. The document examiner looks for these unique writing traits.

Variations in Handwriting

The unconscious handwriting of two different individuals can never be identical. Individual variations associated with mechanical, physical, and mental functions make it extremely unlikely that all of these factors can be exactly reproduced by any two people. Thus, variations are expected in angularity, slope, speed, pressure, letter and word spacings, relative dimensions of letters, connections, pen movement, writing skill, and finger dexterity.

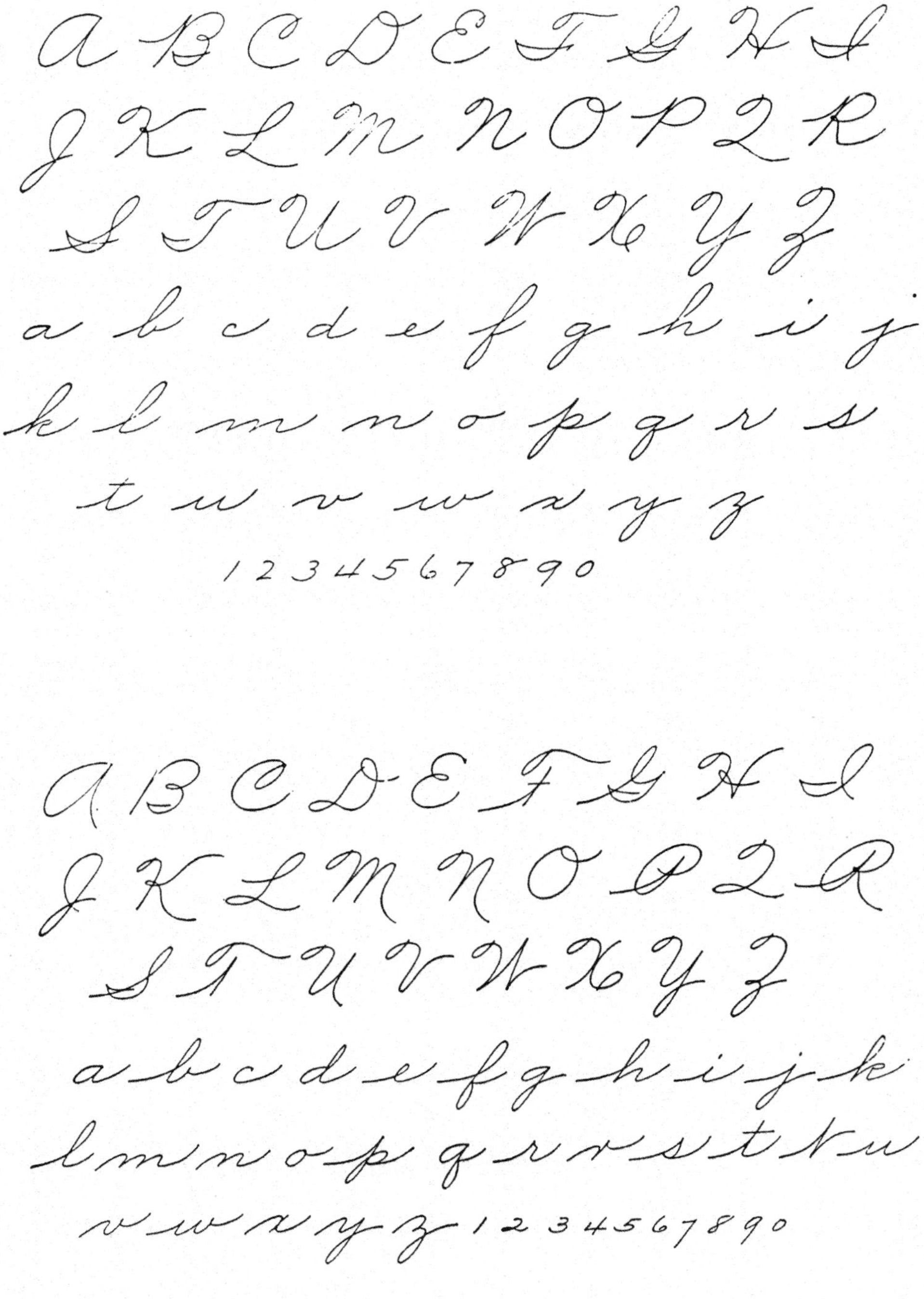

FIGURE 18–1
(Top) An example of Zaner-Bloser handwriting; (bottom) an example of Palmer handwriting.

Courtesy Robert J. Phillips, Document Examiner, Audubon, NJ

Furthermore, many other factors besides pure handwriting characteristics should be considered. The arrangement of the writing on the paper may be as distinctive as the writing itself. Margins, spacings, crowding, insertions, and alignment are all results of personal habits. Spelling, punctuation, phraseology, and grammar can be personal and, if so, combine to individualize the writer.

In a problem involving the authorship of handwriting, all characteristics of both the known and questioned documents must be considered and compared. Dissimilarities between the two writings are a strong indication of two writers, unless these differences can logically be accounted for by the facts surrounding the preparation of the documents. Because any single characteristic, even the most distinctive one, may be found in the handwriting of other individuals, no single handwriting characteristic can by itself be taken as the basis for a positive comparison. The final conclusion must be based on a sufficient number of common characteristics between the known and questioned writings to effectively preclude the chance of their having originated from two different sources.

What constitutes a sufficient number of personal characteristics? Here again, there are no hard and fast rules for making such a determination. The expert examiner can make this judgment only in the context of each particular case.

Challenges to Handwriting Comparison

When the examiner receives a reasonable amount of known handwriting for comparison, there is usually little difficulty in finding sufficient evidence to determine the source of a questioned document. Frequently, however, circumstances may prevent a positive conclusion or may permit only the expression of a qualified opinion. Such situations usually develop when an insufficient number of known writings are made available for comparison. Although nothing may be found that definitely points to the questioned and known handwriting being of a different origin, not enough personal characteristics may be present in the known writings that are consistent with the questioned materials.

Difficulties may also arise when the examiner receives questioned writings containing only a few words, all deliberately written in a crude, unnatural form or all very carefully written and thought out so as to disguise the writer's natural style—a situation usually encountered with threatening or obscene letters. It is extremely difficult to compare handwriting that has been very carefully prepared to a document written with such little thought for structural details that it contains only the subconscious writing habits of the writer. However, although it may be relatively easy to change one's writing habits for a few words or sentences, the task of maintaining such an effort grows more difficult with each additional word.

When an adequate amount of writing is available to the examiner, the attempt at total disguise may fail. This was illustrated in the attempt by Clifford Irving to forge letters in the name of the late industrialist Howard Hughes in order to obtain lucrative publishing contracts for Hughes's life story. Figure 18–2 shows the forged signatures of Howard Hughes along with Clifford Irving's known writings. By comparing these signatures, document examiner R. A. Cabbane of the U.S. Postal Inspection Service detected many examples of Irving's personal characteristics in the forged signatures.

For example, note the formation of the letter *r* in the word *Howard* on lines 1 and 3, as compared with the composite on line 6. Observe the manner in which the terminal stroke of the letter *r* tends to terminate with a little curve at the baseline of Irving's writing and the forgery. Notice the way the bridge of the *w* drops in line 1 and also in line 6. Also, observe the similarity in the formation of the letter *g* as it appears on line 1 as compared with the second signature on line 5.

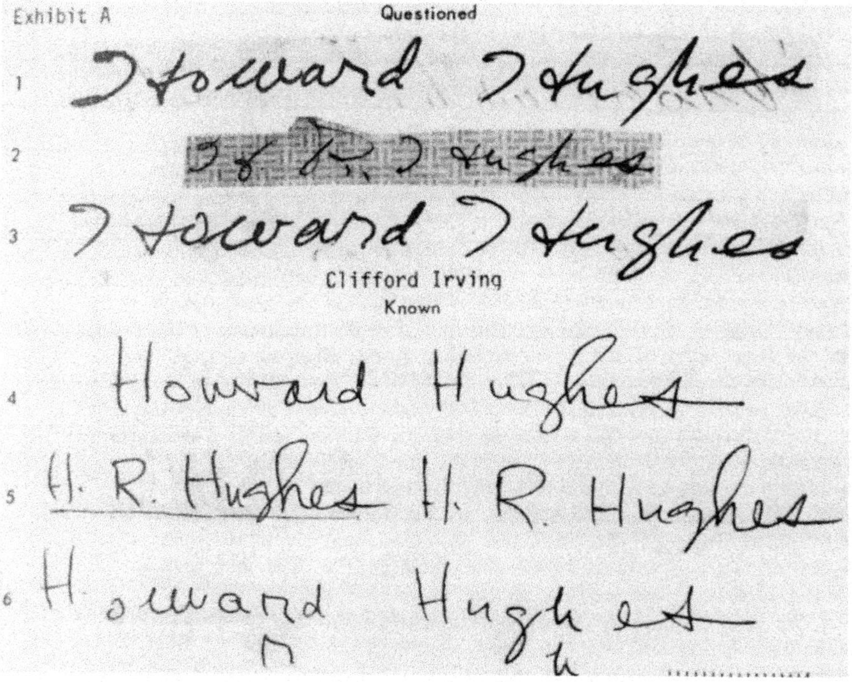

FIGURE 18–2

Forged signatures of Howard Hughes and examples of Clifford Irving's writing.

The document examiner must also be aware that writing habits may be altered beyond recognition by the influence of drugs or alcohol. Under these circumstances, it may be impossible to obtain known writings of a suspect written under conditions comparable to those at the time the questioned document was prepared.

Collection of Handwriting Exemplars

exemplar
An authentic sample used for comparison purposes, such as handwriting.

It should be fairly obvious by now that collection of an adequate number of known writings (**exemplars**) is most critical for determining the outcome of a comparison. Generally, known writings of the suspect furnished to the examiner should be as similar as possible to the questioned document. This is especially true with respect to the writing implement and paper. Styles and habits may be somewhat altered if a person switches from a pencil to a ballpoint pen or to a fountain pen. The way the paper is ruled, or the fact that it is unruled, may also affect the handwriting of a person who has become particularly accustomed to one type or the other. Known writings should also contain some of the words and combinations of letters present in the questioned document.

natural variations
Normal deviations found between repeated specimens of an individual's handwriting or any printing device.

DETERMINING AUTHENTICITY The known writings must be adequate in number to show the examiner the range of **natural variations** in a suspect's writing characteristics. No two specimens of writing prepared by one person are ever identical in every detail. Variation is an inherent part of natural writing. In fact, a signature forged by tracing an authentic signature can often be detected even if the original and tracing coincide exactly because no one ever signs two signatures exactly alike (see Figures 18–3 and 18–4).

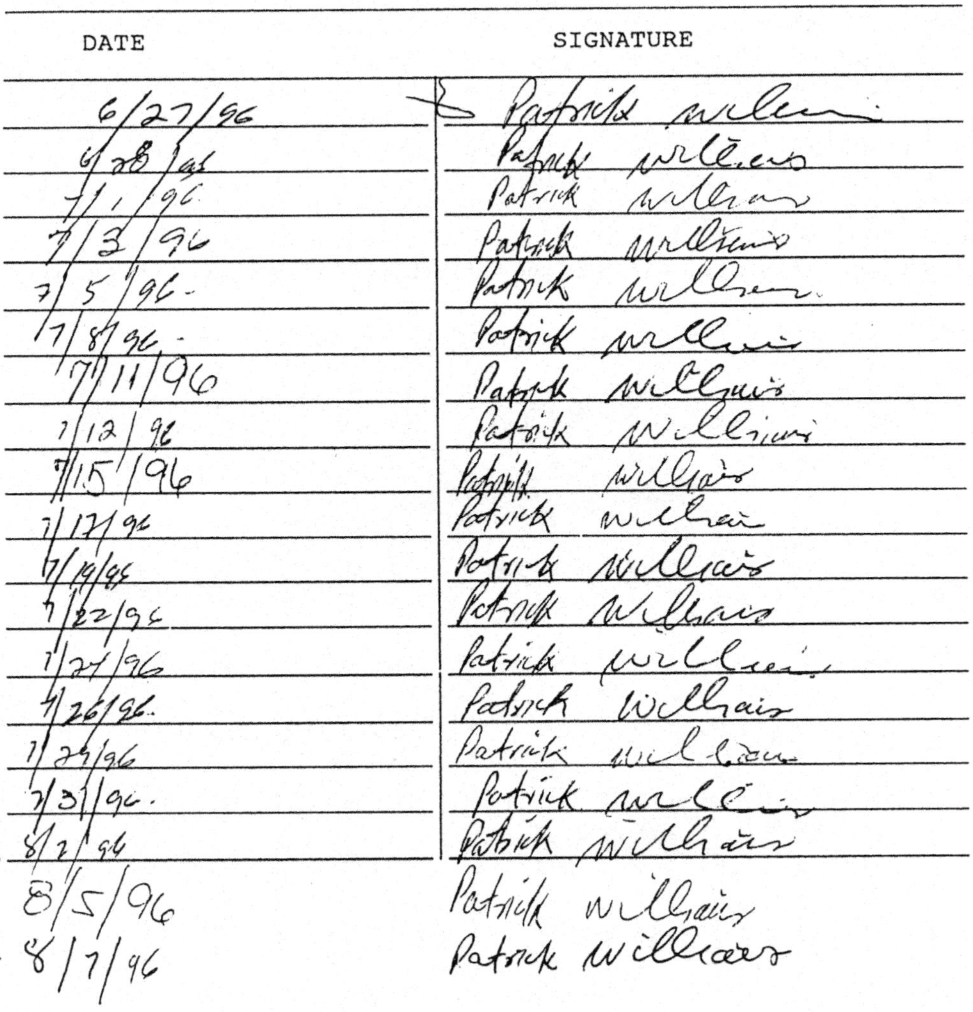

FIGURE 18–3
Examples of handwriting from the same individual over an extended period of time.

DATE	SIGNATURE

Courtesy Rober J. Phillips, Document Examiner, Audubon, NJ

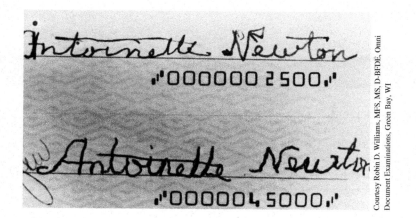

Courtesy Robin D. Williams, MFS, MS, D-BFDE, Omni Document Examinations, Green Bay, WI

FIGURE 18–4
Forged signature. The top signature is genuine. The bottom signature is a simulated forgery. The adaption to the space is incorrect; there are numerous pen lifts and overwrites. The forged signature is awkward and drawn.

Many sources are available to the investigator for establishing the authenticity of the writings of a suspect. An important consideration in selecting sample writings is the age of the genuine document relative to the questioned one. It is important to try to find standards that date closely in time to the questioned document. For most typical adults, basic writing changes are comparatively slow. Therefore, material written within two or three years of the disputed writing is usually satisfactory for comparison; as the age difference between the genuine and unknown specimens becomes greater, the standard tends to become less representative.

OBTAINING WRITING SAMPLES Despite the many potential sources of handwriting exemplars, it may be difficult or impossible to obtain an adequate set of collected standards. In these situations, handwriting may have to be obtained voluntarily or under court order from the suspect. There is ample case law to support the constitutionality of taking handwriting specimens. In the case of *Gilbert* v. *California*,[1] the Supreme Court upheld the taking of handwriting exemplars before the appointment of counsel. The Court also reasoned that handwriting samples are identifying physical characteristics that lie outside the protection privileges of the Fifth Amendment. Furthermore, in the case of *United States* v. *Mara*,[2] the Supreme Court ruled that taking a handwriting sample did not constitute an unreasonable search and seizure of a person and hence did not violate Fourth Amendment rights.

As opposed to nonrequested specimens (written without the thought that they may someday be used in a police investigation), requested writing samples may be consciously altered by the writer. However, the investigator can take certain steps to minimize attempts at deception. The requirement of several pages of writing normally provides enough material that is free of attempts at deliberate disguise or nervousness for a valid comparison. In addition, the writing of dictation yields exemplars that best represent the suspect's subconscious style and characteristics.

Other steps that can be taken to minimize a conscious writing effort, as well as to ensure conditions approximating those of the questioned writing, can be summarized as follows:

1. The writer should be allowed to write sitting comfortably at a desk or table and without distraction.
2. The suspect should not under any conditions be shown the questioned document or be told how to spell certain words or what punctuation to use.
3. The suspect should be furnished a pen and paper similar to those used in the questioned document.
4. The dictated text should be the same as the contents of the questioned document, or at least should contain many of the same words, phrases, and letter combinations found in the document. In handprinting cases, the suspect must not be told whether to use uppercase (capital) or lowercase (small) lettering. If after writing several pages the writer fails to use the desired type of lettering, they can then be instructed to include it. Altogether, the text must be no shorter than a page.

[1] 388 U.S. 263 (1967).
[2] 410 U.S. 19 (1973).

Inside the Science

Hitler's Diaries

In 1981, a spectacular manuscript attributed to Adolf Hitler was disclosed by the brother of an East German general. These documents included Hitler's 27-volume diary and an unknown third volume of his autobiography, *Mein Kampf*. The existence of these works was both culturally and politically significant to the millions who were affected by World War II.

Authentication of the diaries was undertaken by two world-renowned experts, one Swiss and one American. Both declared that the handwritten manuscripts were identical to the known samples of Adolf Hitler's handwriting that they were given. Bidding wars began for publishing rights, and a major national newspaper in the United States won with a price near $4 million.

The publishing company that originally released the documents to the world market undertook its own investigation, which ultimately revealed a clever but devious plot. The paper on which the diaries were written contained a whitener that didn't exist until 1954, long after Hitler committed suicide. The manuscript binding threads contained viscose and polyester, neither of which was available until after World War II. Further, the inks used in the manuscript were all inconsistent with those in use during the year these pages were allegedly written.

Moreover, the exemplars sent to the Swiss and American experts as purportedly known examples of Hitler's handwriting were actually from the same source as the diaries. Thus, the experts were justified in proclaiming that the documents were authentic because they were written by the same hand—it just wasn't Hitler's. Chemical analysis of the inks later determined that the "Hitler diaries" were in fact less than one year old—spectacular, but fake!

5. Dictation of the text should take place at least three times. If the writer is trying to disguise the writing, noticeable variations should appear among the three repetitions. Discovering this, the investigator must insist on continued repetitive dictation of the text.
6. Signature exemplars can best be obtained when the suspect is required to combine other writings with a signature. For example, instead of compiling a set of signatures alone, the writer might be asked to fill out completely 20 to 30 separate checks or receipts, each of which includes a signature.
7. Before requested exemplars are taken from the suspect, a document examiner should be consulted and shown the questioned specimens.

Typescript Comparisons

With the emergence of digital technology, document examiners are confronted with a new array of machines capable of creating documents subject to alteration or fraudulent use. Personal computers use daisy wheel, dot-matrix, ink-jet, and laser printers. More and more, the document examiner encounters problems involving these machines, which often produce typed copies that have only inconspicuous defects.

Photocopier, Fax, and Printer Examination

In the cases of photocopiers, fax machines, and computer printers, an examiner may need to identify the make and model of a machine that may have been used in printing a document. Alternatively, the examiner may need to compare a questioned document with test samples printed from a suspect machine. Typically, the examiner generates approximately 10 samples through each machine to obtain a sufficient representation of a photocopier's characters. A side-by-side comparison is then made between the questioned document and the printed exemplars to compare markings produced by the machine.

PHOTOCOPIERS Transitory defect marks originating from random debris on the glass platen, inner cover, or mechanical portions of a copier produce images. These images are often

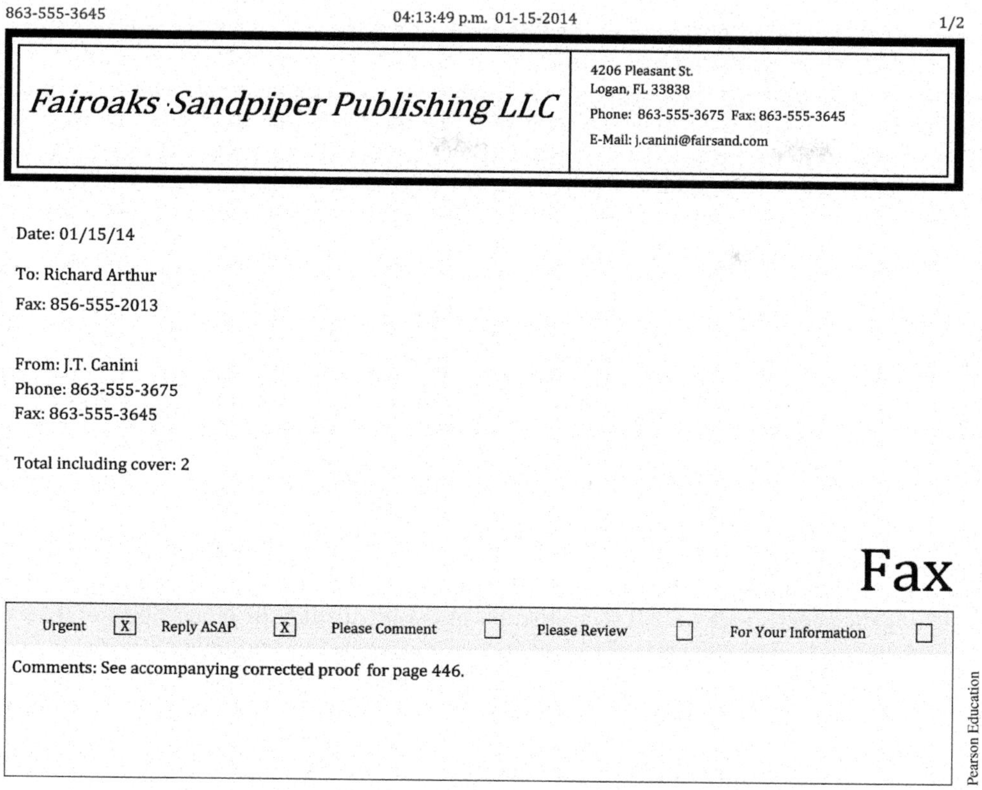

Fairoaks Sandpiper Publishing LLC

4206 Pleasant St.
Logan, FL 33838
Phone: 863-555-3675　Fax: 863-555-3645
E-Mail: j.canini@fairsand.com

Date: 01/15/14

To: Richard Arthur
Fax: 856-555-2013

From: J.T. Canini
Phone: 863-555-3675
Fax: 863-555-3645

Total including cover: 2

Fax

| Urgent | [X] | Reply ASAP | [X] | Please Comment | [ ] | Please Review | [ ] | For Your Information | [ ] |

Comments: See accompanying corrected proof for page 446.

Pearson Education

FIGURE 18–5

A fax page showing a transmitting terminal identifier (TTI).

irregularly shaped and sometimes form distinctive patterns. Thus, they become points of comparison as the document examiner attempts to link the document to suspect copiers. The gradual change, shift, or duplication of these marks may aid the examiner in dating the document.

FAX MACHINES In analyzing computer printouts and faxes, examiners use the same approach for comparing the markings on a questioned document to exemplar documents generated by a suspect machine. These markings include all possible transitory patterns arising from debris and other extraneous materials. Interestingly, fax machines print a header known as the *transmitting terminal identifier* (TTI) at the top of each fax page. For the document examiner, the TTI is an important point of comparison (see Figure 18–5). The header and the document's text should have different type styles. TTIs can be fraudulently prepared and placed in the appropriate position on a fax copy. However, a microscopic examination of the TTI's print quickly reveals significant characteristics that distinguish it from a genuine TTI.

In determining the fax machine's model type, the examiner most often begins by analyzing the TTI type style. The fonts of that line are determined by the sending machine. The number of characters, their style, and their position in the header are best evaluated through a collection of TTI fonts organized into a useful database. One such database is maintained by the American Society of Questioned Document Examiners.

COMPUTER PRINTERS Computer printer model determination requires an extensive analysis of the specific printer technology and type of ink used. Visual and microscopic techniques provide useful information in determining the technology and toner used. Generally, printers are categorized as impact and nonimpact printers by the mechanism of their toner application. Nonimpact printers, such as ink-jet and laser printers, and impact printers, such as thermal and dot-matrix printers, all have characteristic ways of printing documents. Character shapes, toner differentiation, and toner application methods are easily determined with a low-power microscope and help the examiner narrow the possibilities of model type.

When the suspect machine is not available, the examiner may need to analyze the document's class characteristics to identify the make and model of the machine. It is important to identify the printing technology, the type of paper, the type of toner or ink used, the chemical composition of the toner, and the type of toner-to-paper fusing method used in producing the document. Examination of the toner usually involves microscopic analysis to characterize its surface morphology, followed by identification of the inorganic and organic components of the toner. These results separate model types into categories based on their mechanical and printing characteristics. Typically, document examiners access databases to help identify the model type of machine used to prepare a questioned document. The resulting list of possibilities produced by the database hopefully reduces the number of potential machines to a manageable number. Obviously, once a suspect machine is identified, the examiner must perform a side-by-side comparison of questioned and exemplar printouts as described previously.

Alterations, Erasures, and Obliterations

Documents are often altered or changed after preparation so that their original intent may be hidden or so that a forgery may be perpetrated. Documents can be changed in several ways, and for each way, the application of a special discovery technique is necessary.

Erasures and Alterations

erasure
The removal of writing, typewriting, or printing from a document; it is normally accomplished by either chemical means or an abrasive instrument.

One of the most common ways to alter a document is to try to erase parts of it, using an India rubber eraser, sandpaper, a razor blade, or a knife to remove writing or type by abrading or scratching the paper's surface. All such attempts at erasure disturb the upper fibers of the paper. These changes are apparent when the suspect area is examined under a microscope using direct light or by allowing the light to strike the paper obliquely from one side (side lighting) (see Figure 18–6). Although microscopy may reveal whether an **erasure** has been made, it does not necessarily indicate the original letters or words present. Sometimes so much of the paper has been removed that identifying the original contents is impossible.

In addition to abrading the paper, the perpetrator may also choose to obliterate words with a chemical erasure. In this case, strong oxidizing agents are placed over the ink, producing a colorless reaction product. Although such an attempt may not be noticeable to the naked eye, examination under the microscope reveals a discoloration on the treated area of the paper. Sometimes examination of the document under ultraviolet or infrared lighting reveals the chemically treated portion of the paper. Interestingly, examination of documents under ultraviolet light may also reveal the presence of fluorescent ink markings that go unnoticed in room light, as seen in Figure 18–7.

FIGURE 18–6
Erasure in a check book deposit stub revealed by photography with the use of oblique lighting. The amount of cash deposited was changed and the difference was pocketed by the bookkeeper.

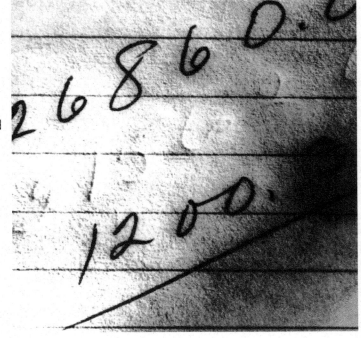

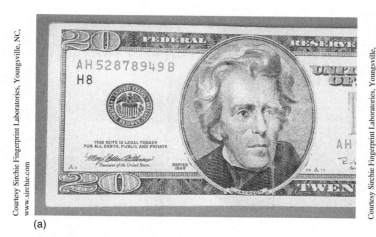

(a)

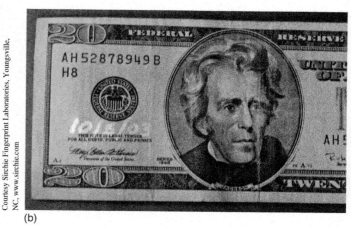

(b)

FIGURE 18–7

(a) A 20-dollar bill as it appears under room light. (b) The bill illuminated with ultraviolet light reveals ink writing.

Some inks, when exposed to blue-green light, absorb the radiation and reradiate infrared light. This phenomenon is known as **infrared luminescence**. Thus, if an alteration is made to a document with ink differing from the original, it can sometimes be detected by illuminating the document with blue-green light and using infrared-sensitive film to record the light emanating from the document's surface. In this fashion, any differences in the luminescent properties of the inks are observed. Infrared luminescence has also revealed writing that has been erased. Such writings may be recorded by invisible residues of the original ink that remain embedded in the paper even after an erasure.

Another important application of infrared photography arises from the observation that inks may differ in their ability to absorb infrared light. Thus, illuminating a document with infrared light and recording the light reflected off the document's surface with infrared-sensitive film may enable the examiner to differentiate inks of a dissimilar chemical composition (see Figure 18–8).

infrared luminescence
A property exhibited by some dyes that emit infrared light when exposed to blue-green light.

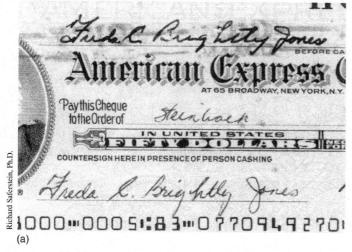

(a)

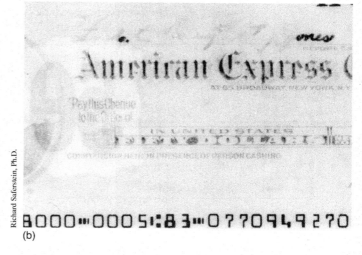

(b)

FIGURE 18–8

(a) This photograph, taken under normal illumination, shows the owner of an American Express check to be "Freda C. Brightly Jones." Actually, this signature was altered. The check initially bore the signature "Fred C. Brightly Jr."
(b) This photograph taken under infrared illumination, using infrared-sensitive film, clearly shows that the check was altered by adding a to Fred and ones to Jr. The ink used to commit these changes is distinguishable because it absorbs infrared light, whereas the original ink does not.

FIGURE 18–9

An order number was obliterated with magic marker to cover up a theft. Infrared photography was used to penetrate the covering ink to reveal the original writing.

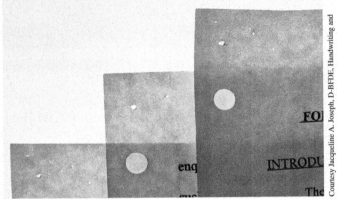

Courtesy Robin D. Williams, MFS, MS, D-BFDE, Omni Document Examinations, Green Bay, WI

FIGURE 18–10

Staple hole exam. The middle sheet was substituted based on the evidence of staple hole pattern differences.

Courtesy Jacqueline A. Joseph, D-BFDE, Handwriting and Document Forensics, Portland, OR, www.jjhandwriting.com

Obliterations

obliteration
The blotting out or smearing over of writing or printing to make the original unreadable.

Intentional **obliteration** of writing by overwriting or crossing out is seldom used for fraudulent purposes because of its obviousness. Nevertheless, such cases may be encountered in all types of documents. Success at permanently hiding the original writing depends on the material used to cover the writing. If it is done with the same ink as was used to write the original material, recovery will be difficult if not impossible. However, if the two inks are of a different chemical composition, photography with infrared-sensitive film may reveal the original writing. Infrared radiation may pass through the upper layer of writing while being absorbed by the underlying area (see Figure 18–9).

Close examination of a questioned document sometimes reveals staple holes, crossing strokes, or strokes across folds or perforations in the paper that are not in a sequence that is consistent with the natural preparation of the document. Again, these differences can be shown by microscopic or photographic scrutiny (see Figure 18–10).

charred document
Any document that has become darkened and brittle through exposure to fire or excessive heat.

Infrared photography sometimes reveals the contents of a document that has been accidentally or purposely charred in a fire. Another way to decipher **charred documents** involves reflecting light off the paper's surface at different angles in order to contrast the writing against the charred background (see Figure 18–11).

Digital image processing is the method by which the visual quality of digital pictures is improved or enhanced. *Digitizing* is the process by which the image is stored in memory. This is commonly done by scanning an image with a flatbed scanner or a digital camera and converting the image by computer into an array of digital intensity values called *pixels*, or picture elements (see page 147). Once the image has been digitized, an image editing program, such as Adobe Photoshop, is used to adjust the image. An image may be enhanced through lightening, darkening, and color and contrast controls. An example of how the technology is applied to forensic document examination is shown in Figures 18–12 and 18–13.

Other Document Problems

Indented Writings

indented writings
Impressions left on papers positioned under a piece of paper that has been written on.

Indented writings are the partially visible depressions on a sheet of paper underneath the one on which the visible writing was done. Such depressions are caused by the application of pressure on the writing instrument and would appear as a carbon copy of a sheet if carbon paper had been inserted between the pages.

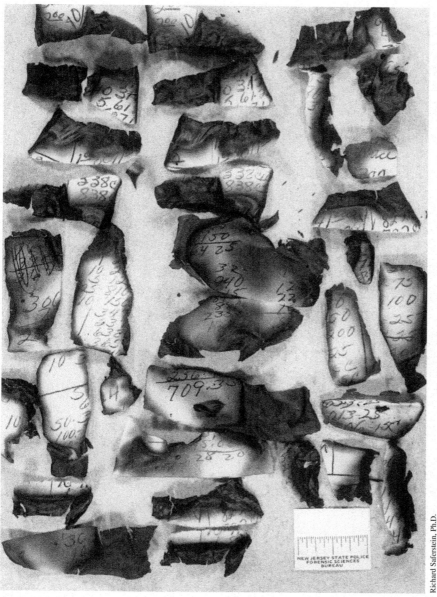

Richard Saferstein, Ph.D.

FIGURE 18–11

Decipherment of charred papers seized in the raid of a suspected bookmaking establishment. The charred documents were photographed with reflected light.

Indented writings have proved to be valuable evidence. For example, the top sheet of a bookmaker's records may have been removed and destroyed, but it still may be possible to determine the writing by the impressions left on the pad. These impressions may contain incriminating evidence supporting the charge of illegal gambling activities. When paper is studied under oblique or side lighting, its indented impressions are often readable.

An innovative approach to visualizing indented writings has been developed at the London College of Printing in close consultation with the Metropolitan Police Forensic Science Laboratory.[3] The method involves applying an electrostatic charge to the surface of a polymer film that has been placed in contact with a questioned document, as shown in Figure 18–14. Indented impressions on the document are revealed by applying a toner powder to the charged film. For many documents examined by this process, clearly readable images have been produced from impressions that could not be seen or were barely visible under normal illumination. An instrument that develops indented writings by electrostatic detection is commercially available and is routinely used by document examiners.

[3] D. M. Ellen, D. J. Foster, and D. J. Morantz, "The Use of Electrostatic Imaging in the Detection of Indented Impressions," *Forensic Science International* 15 (1980): 53.

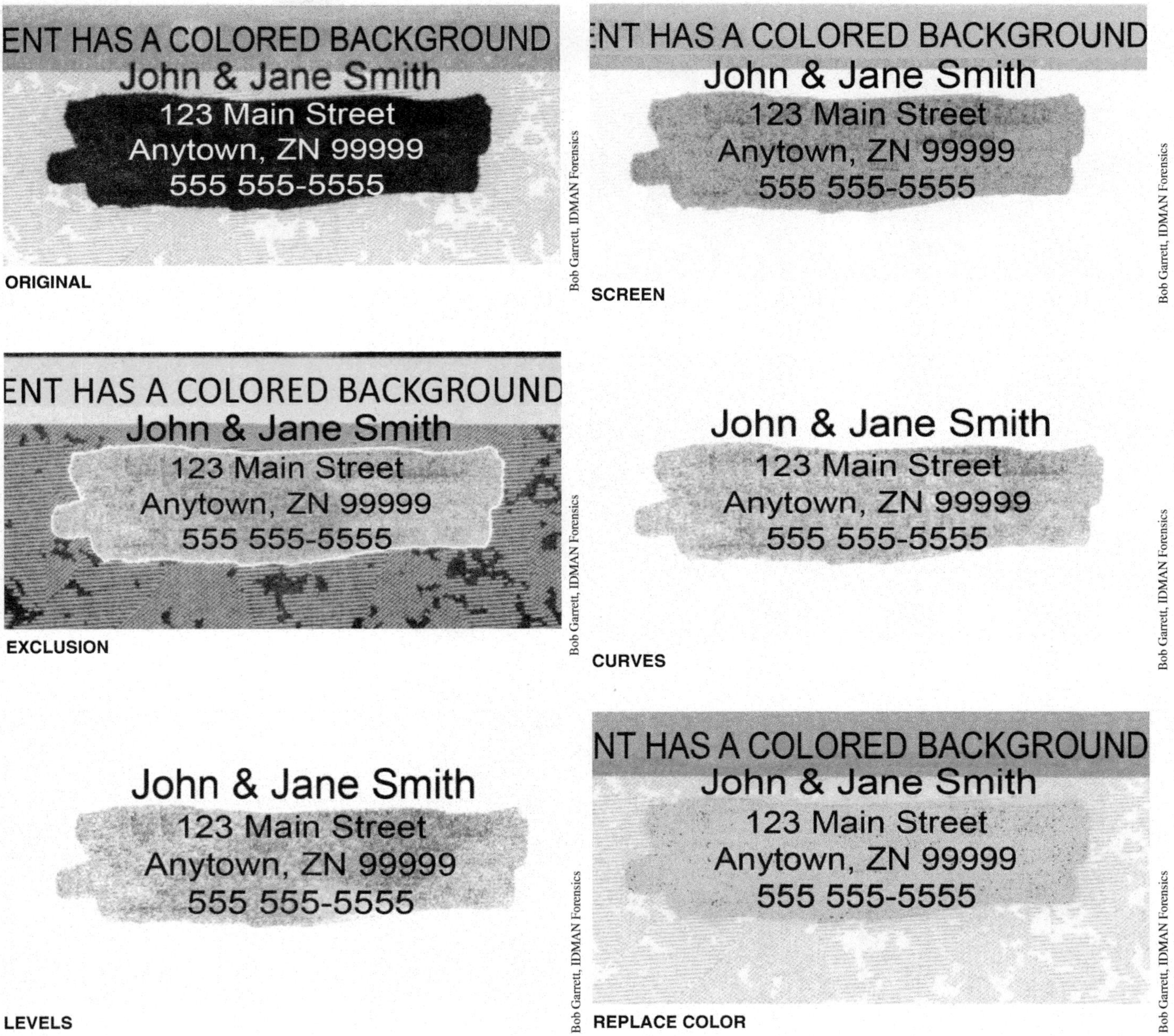

ENT HAS A COLORED BACKGROUND
John & Jane Smith
123 Main Street
Anytown, ZN 99999
555 555-5555

ORIGINAL

Bob Garrett, IDMAN Forensics

ENT HAS A COLORED BACKGROUND
John & Jane Smith
123 Main Street
Anytown, ZN 99999
555 555-5555

SCREEN

Bob Garrett, IDMAN Forensics

ENT HAS A COLORED BACKGROUND
John & Jane Smith
123 Main Street
Anytown, ZN 99999
555 555-5555

EXCLUSION

Bob Garrett, IDMAN Forensics

John & Jane Smith
123 Main Street
Anytown, ZN 99999
555 555-5555

CURVES

Bob Garrett, IDMAN Forensics

John & Jane Smith
123 Main Street
Anytown, ZN 99999
555 555-5555

LEVELS

Bob Garrett, IDMAN Forensics

NT HAS A COLORED BACKGROUND
John & Jane Smith
123 Main Street
Anytown, ZN 99999
555 555-5555

REPLACE COLOR

Bob Garrett, IDMAN Forensics

FIGURE 18–12

This composite demonstrates the various changes that can be applied to a digitized image in order to reveal information that has been obscured. Using a photo editor (Adobe Photoshop), the original was duplicated and pasted as a second layer. Colors were changed in selected areas of the image using the "screen" and "exclusion" options. "Replace color" allows the user to choose a specific color or range of colors and lighten, darken, or change the hue of the colors selected. "Level" and "curves" tools can adjust the lightest and darkest color ranges and optimize contrast, highlights, and shadow detail of the image for additional clarity.

Ink and Paper Comparison

A study of the chemical composition of writing ink present on documents may verify whether known and questioned documents were prepared by the same pen. A nondestructive approach to comparing ink lines is accomplished with a visible microspectrophotometer (see pages 177–178).[4] A case example illustrating the application of this approach to ink analysis appears in Figure 18–11.

[4] P. W. Pfefferli, "Application of Microspectrophotometry in Document Examination," *Forensic Science International* 23 (1983): 129.

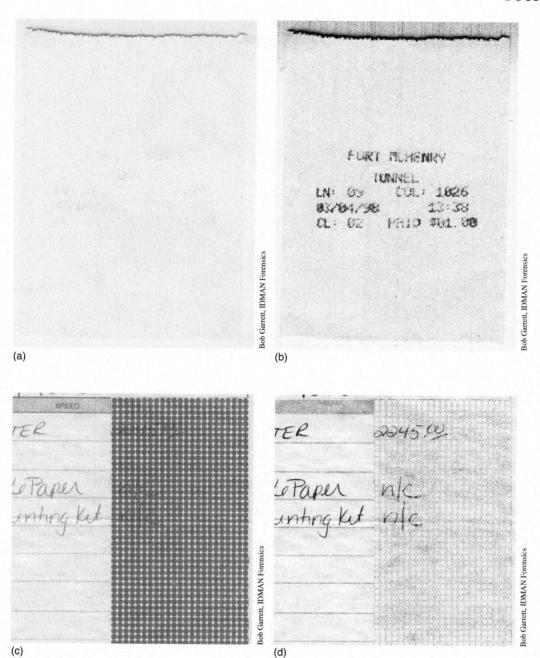

(a)

(b)

FURT MCHENRY

TUNNEL

LN: 69   CUL: 1026

03/04/98   13:38

CL: 02   PAID $01.00

(c)

SPEED

TER

'Paper

nting Kit

(d)

TER   2245.00

'Paper   n/c

nting Kit   n/c

Bob Garrett, IDMAN Forensics

FIGURE 18–13

(a) Receipts have been used in investigations to establish a victim's whereabouts, provide suspects with alibis, and substantiate a host of personal conduct. Unfortunately, many times because of wear, age, or poor printing at the register, the receipt may be unreadable. This can be corrected using photo-editing software. In this example, the original toll receipt was scanned at the highest color resolution, which allows more than 16 million colors to be reproduced. The image was then manipulated, revealing the printed details, by adjusting the lightest and darkest levels and the color content of the image. (b) Invoices may contain details about a transaction that are important to an investigation. The copy that ships with the merchandise may have that information blocked out. This information may be recovered using digital imaging. The left figure shows the original shipping ticket. The right figure shows the information revealed after replacing the color of the blocking pattern.

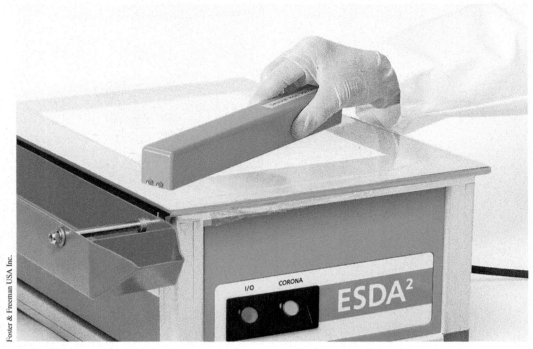

Foster & Freeman USA Inc.

FIGURE 18–14

An electrostatic detection apparatus (ESDA) works by applying an electrostatic charge to a document suspected of containing indented writings. The indentations are then visualized by the application of charge-sensitive toner.

Thin-layer chromatography is also suitable for ink comparisons. Most commercial inks, especially ballpoint inks, are actually mixtures of several organic dyes. These dyes can be separated on a properly developed thin-layer chromatographic plate. The separation pattern of the component dyes is distinctly different for inks with different dye compositions and thus provides many points of comparison between a known and a questioned ink.

Ink can be removed from paper with a hypodermic needle with a blunted point to punch out a small sample from a written line. About 10 plugs or microdots of ink are sufficient for chromatographic analysis. The U.S. Secret Service and the Internal Revenue Service jointly maintain the United States International Ink Library. This collection includes more than 9,200 inks, which date back to the 1920s. Each year new pen and ink formulations from writing pens, ink-jets, and toners are added to the reference collection. These inks have been systematically cataloged according to dye patterns developed by thin-layer chromatography (TLC; see Figure 18–15). On several occasions, this approach has been used to prove that a document has been fraudulently backdated. For example, in one instance, it was possible to establish that a document dated 1958 was backdated because a dye identified in the questioned ink had not been synthesized until 1959.

To further aid forensic chemists in ink-dating matters, several ink manufacturers, at the request of the U.S. Treasury Department, voluntarily tag their inks during the manufacturing process. The tagging program allows inks to be dated to the exact year of manufacture by changing the tags annually.

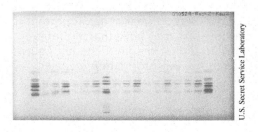

U.S. Secret Service Laboratory

FIGURE 18–15

Chart demonstrating different TLC patterns of blue ballpoint inks.

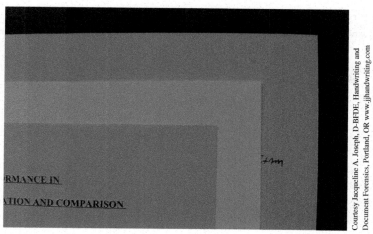

Courtesy Jacqueline A. Joseph, D-BFDE, Handwriting and Document Forensics, Portland, OR www.jjhandwriting.com

FIGURE 18–16

The results of an ultraviolet light exam revealing a substituted document. The middle sheet was differentiated from the upper and lower sheets by exposure to UV light.

Another area of inquiry for the document examiner is the paper on which a document is written or printed. Paper is often made from cellulose fibers found in wood and fibers recovered from recycled paper products. The most common features associated with a paper examination are general appearance, color, weight, and watermarks (see Figure 18–16). Other areas of examination include fiber identification and the characterization of additives, fillers, and pigments present in the paper product.

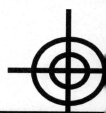

Chapter Summary > > > > > > > > > > >

Any object with handwriting or print whose source or authenticity is in doubt may be referred to as a questioned document. Document examiners apply knowledge gathered through years of training and experience to recognize and compare the individual characteristics of questioned and known authentic writings. For this purpose, gathering documents of known authorship or origin is critical to the outcome of the examination. Many factors compose the total character of a person's writing. The unconscious handwriting of two different individuals can never be identical. Furthermore, the writing style of one individual may be altered beyond recognition by the influence of drugs or alcohol. The collection of an adequate number of known writings is critical for determining the outcome of a handwriting comparison. Known writing should contain some of the words and combinations of letters present in the questioned document.

The two requests most often made of the examiner in connection with the examination of typewriters and printing devices are to determine whether the make and model of the typewriter and printing devices used to prepare the questioned document can be identified and whether a particular

suspect typewriter or printing device can be identified as having prepared the questioned document. The individual type character's style, shape, and size are compared to a complete reference collection of past and present typefaces. As is true for any mechanical device, use of a printing device results in wear and damage to the machine's moving parts. These changes occur both randomly and irregularly, thereby imparting individual characteristics to the printing device. The document examiner has to deal with problems involving business and personal computers, which often produce printed copies that have only subtle defects.

Document examiners must deal with evidence that has been changed in several ways, such as through alterations, erasures, and obliterations. Indented writings have proved to be valuable evidence. It may be possible to determine what was written by the impressions left on a paper pad. Applying an electrostatic charge to the surface of a polymer film that has been placed in contact with a questioned document visualizes indented writings. A study of the chemical composition of writing ink on documents may verify whether known and questioned documents were prepared by the same pen.

Review Questions

1. Any object that contains handwriting or typescript and whose source or authenticity is in doubt is referred to as a(n) _____.

2. Variations in mechanical, physical, and mental functions make it (likely, unlikely) that the writing of two different individuals can be distinguished.

3. In a problem involving the authorship of handwriting, all characteristics of both the _____ and _____ documents must be considered and compared.

4. True or False: A single handwriting characteristic by itself can be taken as a basis for a positive comparison. _____

5. True or False: Normally, known writings need not contain words and combinations of letters present in the questioned document. _____

6. As the age difference between genuine and unknown specimens becomes greater, the standard tends to become (more, less) representative of the unknown.

7. In the case of _____, the Supreme Court held handwriting to be nontestimonial evidence not protected by Fifth Amendment privileges.

8. When requested writing is being given by a suspect, care must be taken to minimize a(n) _____ writing effort.

9. Examination of a document under _____ or _____ lighting may reveal chemical erasures of words or numbers.

10. Some inks, when exposed to blue-green light, absorb _____ radiation and emit light.

11. Handwriting containing inks of different chemical compositions may be distinguished by photography with _____ film.

12. _____ writings are partially visible impressions appearing on a sheet of paper underneath the one on which the visible writing was done.

13. Many ink dyes can be separated by the technique of _____ chromatography.

14. Transitory defect marks originating from random debris on the _____, _____, or _____ of a copier produce images.

Application and Critical Thinking

1. Criminalist Julie Sandel is investigating a series of threatening notes written in pencil and sent to a local politician. A suspect is arrested and Julie directs the suspect to prepare writing samples to compare to the writing on the notes. She has the suspect sit at a desk in an empty office and gives him a pen and a piece of paper. She begins to read one of the notes and asks the suspect to write the words she dictates. After reading about half a page, she stops, then dictates the same part of the note a second time for the suspect. At one point, the suspect indicates that he does not know how to spell one of the words, so Julie spells it for him. After completing the task, Julie takes the original notes and the dictated writing from the suspect to a document examiner. What mistakes, if any, did Julie make?

2. In each of the following situations, indicate how you would go about recovering original writing that is not visible to the naked eye.

   a. The original words have been obliterated with a different ink than was used to compose the original.

   b. The original words have been obliterated by chemical erasure.

   c. The original writing was made with fluorescent ink.

   d. The original documents have been charred or burned.

3. You have been asked to determine whether a handwritten will, supposedly prepared 30 years ago, is authentic or a modern forgery. What aspects of the document would you examine to make this determination? Explain how you would use thin-layer chromatography to help you come to your conclusion.

Further References

Brunelle, Richard L., "Questioned Document Examination," in R. Saferstein, ed., *Forensic Science Handbook*, vol. 1, 2nd ed. Upper Saddle River, NJ: Prentice Hall, 2002.

Ellen, David, *The Scientific Examination of Documents—Methods and Techniques*, 3rd ed. Boca Raton, FL: CRC Press, 2005.

Held, D. A. E., "Handwriting, Typewriting, Shoeprints, and Tire Treads: FBI Laboratory's Questioned Documents Unit," *Forensic Science Communications*, 3, no. 2 (2001), https://www2.fbi.gov/hq/lab/fsc/backissu/april2001/index.htm

Kelly, J. S., and B. S. Lindblom, *Scientific Examination of Questioned Documents*, 2nd ed. Boca Raton, FL: CRC Press, 2006.

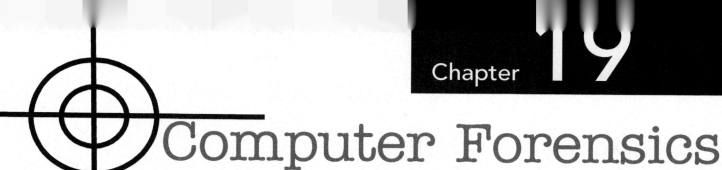

Chapter 19

Computer Forensics

by Andrew W. Donofrio

Andrew W. Donofrio is a retired detective lieutenant from the prosecutor's office in Bergen County, New Jersey, and is a leading computer forensic examiner for Bergen County, with more than 23 years' experience in the field of law enforcement. He has conducted hundreds of forensic examinations of computer evidence and frequently lectures on the subject throughout the state, as well as teaching multiday courses on computer forensics and investigative topics at police academies, colleges, and corporations throughout the United States. Mr. Donofrio now owns Cyberology Consultants, which provides IT investigation, computer and network forensic, and business continuity and disaster recovery planning services.

Go to www.pearsonhighered.com/careersresources to access Webextras for this chapter.

KEY TERMS

bit
bookmark
byte
central processing unit (CPU)
cluster
cookies
file slack
firewall
hacking
hard disk drive (HDD)
hardware
Internet cache
Internet history
latent data
Message Digest 5 (MD5)/Secure Hash Algorithm (SHA)
motherboard
operating system (OS)
partition
random-access memory (RAM)
sector
software
swap file
temporary files
unallocated space
visible data

The BTK Killer

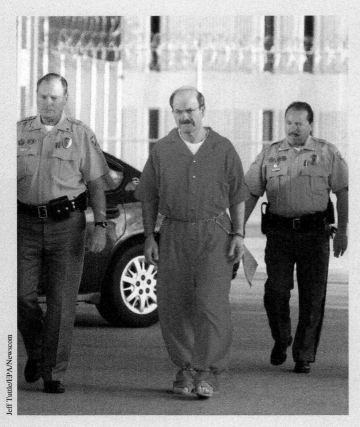

Jeff Tuttle/EPA/Newscom

Dennis Rader was arrested in February 2005 and charged with committing 10 murders since 1974 in the area around Wichita, Kansas. The BTK killer, whose nickname stands for "bind, torture, kill," hadn't murdered since 1991 but resurfaced in early 2004 when he sent a letter to a local newspaper taking credit for a 1986 slaying. Included with the letter were a photocopy of the victim's driver's license and three photos of her body. The BTK killer was back to his old habit of taunting the police. Three months later, another letter surfaced. This time the letter detailed some of the events surrounding BTK's first murder victims. In 1974, he had strangled Joseph and Julie Otero along with two of their children. Shortly after committing those murders, BTK had also sent a letter to a local newspaper in which he gave himself the name BTK. In December 2004, a package found in a park contained the driver's license of another BTK victim along with a doll whose hands were bound with pantyhose and that was covered with a plastic bag.

The major break in the case came when BTK sent a message on a floppy disk to a local TV station. "Erased" information on the disk was recovered and restored by forensic computer specialists, and the disk was traced to the Christ Lutheran Church in Wichita. The disk was then quickly linked to Dennis Rader, the church council president. The long odyssey of searching for the BTK killer was finally over.

Since the 1990s, few fields have progressed as rapidly as computer technology. Computers are no longer a luxury, nor are they in the hands of just a select few. Technology and electronic data are a part of everyday life and permeate all aspects of society. Consequently, computers have become increasingly important as sources of evidence in an ever-widening spectrum of criminal activities. Moreover, on the corporate side, issues of regulatory compliance, such as HIPAA and the Sarbanes–Oxley Act, and problems of employee misconduct have made IT investigations and data forensics a necessary component of a company's security program.

Police investigators frequently encounter computers and other digital devices in all types of cases. As homicide investigators sift for clues, they may inquire, for example, whether the method for a murder was researched on the Internet, whether signs of an extramarital affair can be found in e-mails or remnants of instant messages (which may provide a motive for a spouse killing or murder for hire), or whether threats were communicated to the victim before a murder by an obsessed stalker. Arson investigators may want to know whether financial records on a computer show a motive for an arson-for-profit fire. A burglary investigation would certainly be aided if law enforcement could show that the proceeds from a theft were being sold online— perhaps through eBay or a similar online auction site.

In addition, the use of computers poses some threats of its own. The accessibility of computers to children and the perception of anonymity in online interactions has given sexual predators a way to seek out child victims online. The vulnerability of computers to hacker attacks is a constant reminder of security issues surrounding digitally stored data. Finally, the fact that computers control most of our critical infrastructure makes technology an appetizing target for would-be terrorists.

Computer forensics involves the preservation, acquisition, extraction, analysis, and interpretation of computer data. Although this is a simple definition, it gets a bit more complicated. Part of this complication arises from technology itself. More and more devices are capable of storing electronic data: cell phones, personal digital assistants (PDAs), iPods, digital cameras, flash memory cards, smart cards, jump drives, and many others. Further complicating matters is the cross-pollination of devices. Cell phones now have the same capabilities of personal computers, and personal computers are often used to facilitate communications. Methods for extracting data from these devices each present unique challenges. However, sound forensic practices apply to all of these devices. The most logical place to start to examine these practices is with the most common source of electronic data: the personal computer.

From Input to Output: How Does the Computer Work?

Hardware Versus Software

Before we get into the nuts and bolts of computers, we must establish the important distinction between hardware and software. **Hardware** comprises the physical components of the computer: the computer chassis, monitor, keyboard, mouse, hard disk drive, random-access memory (RAM), central processing unit (CPU), and so on (see Figure 19–1). The list is extensive, but generally speaking, if it is a computer component or peripheral that you can see, feel, and touch, then it is hardware.

Software, on the other hand, is a set of instructions compiled into a program that performs a particular task. Software consists of programs and applications that carry out a set of instructions on the hardware. Operating systems (e.g., Windows, Mac OS, Linux, and Unix), word-processing programs (e.g., Microsoft Word and WordPerfect), web-browsing applications (e.g., Internet Explorer, Safari, and Firefox), and accounting applications (e.g., Quicken, QuickBooks, and Microsoft Money) are all examples of software.

It is important not to confuse software with the physical media that it comes on. When you buy an application such as Microsoft Office, it comes on a compact disc (CD). The CD containing this suite of applications is typically referred to as software, but this is technically wrong. The CD is external computer media that contains the software; it is a container for a set of instructions and a medium from which to load the instructions onto the hard disk drive (i.e., the hardware).

Hardware Components

COMPUTER CASE/CHASSIS   The case is the physical box holding the fixed internal computer components in place. Cases come in many shapes and sizes: a full upright tower chassis, a slim model sitting on a desktop, or an all-in-one monitor/computer case like the iMac. For our purposes, the term *system unit* is probably most appropriate when describing a chassis seized as evidence. The term *system unit* accurately references the chassis, including the motherboard and other internal components.

hardware
The physical components of a computer: case, keyboard, monitor, motherboard, RAM, HDD, mouse, and so on; generally speaking, if it is a computer component you can touch, it is hardware.

software
A set of instructions compiled into a program that performs a particular task; software consists of programs and applications that carry out a set of instructions on the hardware.

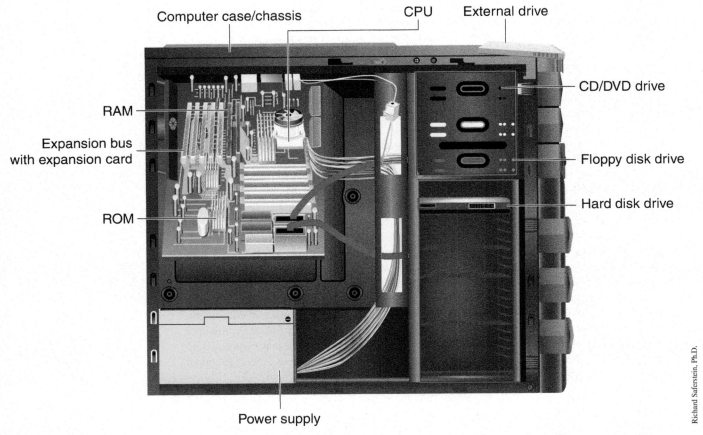

FIGURE 19–1

Cutaway diagram of a personal computer showing the tangible hardware components of a computer system.

POWER SUPPLY The term *power supply* is actually a misnomer because it doesn't actually supply power—the power company does that. Rather, a computer's power supply converts power from the wall outlet to a usable format for the computer and its components. Different power supplies have different wattage ratings. The use or, more specifically, the components of the computer dictate the appropriate power supply.

MOTHERBOARD The main circuit board in a computer (or other electronic device) is referred to as the **motherboard**. Motherboards contain sockets for chips and slots for add-on cards. Examples of add-on cards are the video card to connect the computer to the monitor, a network card or modem to connect to an internal network or the Internet, and a sound card to connect to speakers. Sockets on the motherboard typically accept things like RAM or the CPU. The keyboard, mouse, CD-ROM drives, floppy disk drives, monitor, and other peripherals or components connect to the motherboard in some fashion through a wired or wireless connection.

SYSTEM BUS Contained on the motherboard, the system bus is a vast, complex network of wires that carry data from one hardware device to another. This network is analogous to a complex highway. Data is sent along the bus in the form of ones and zeros (or, to be accurate, as electrical impulses representing an "on" or "off" state); this two-state form of data is known as *binary computing*.

READ-ONLY MEMORY (ROM) This rather generic term describes special chips on the motherboard. ROM chips store programs called *firmware*, used to start the boot process and

motherboard
The main system board of a computer (and many other electronic devices), which delivers power, data, and instructions to the computer's components; every component in the computer connects to the motherboard, either directly or indirectly.

configure a computer's components. Today's ROM chips, termed *flash ROM*, are a combination of two types of chips used in past motherboard technologies. The first was known as the *system ROM*, which was responsible for booting the system and handling the "assumed" system hardware present in the computer. As the system ROM, generally speaking, could not be altered, and because as technology matured changes to the "assumed" hardware were more common, a different type of chip was introduced. The *complementary metal-oxide semiconductor* (CMOS) was a separate chip that allowed the user to exercise setup control over several system components. Regardless of how this technology is present on the motherboard, it can be referred to as the BIOS, for *basic input–output system*. The operation of the BIOS is relevant to several computer forensic procedures, particularly the boot sequence. It is the set of routines associated with the BIOS in ROM that initiates the booting process and enables the computer to communicate with various devices in the system such as disk drives, keyboard, monitor, and printer. As this chapter will make clear, it is important not to boot the actual computer under investigation to the original hard disk drive. This would cause changes to the data, thus compromising the integrity of evidence. The BIOS allows investigators to control the boot process to some degree.

CENTRAL PROCESSING UNIT (CPU)

The **central processing unit (CPU)**, also referred to as a processor, is essentially the brain of the computer. It is the main (and typically the largest) chip that plugs into a socket on the motherboard. The CPU is the part of the computer that actually computes. Basically, all operations performed by the computer are run through the CPU. The CPU carries out the program steps to perform a requested task. That task can range from opening and working in a Microsoft Word document to performing advanced mathematical algorithms. CPUs come in various shapes, sizes, and types. Intel Pentium chips and Advanced Micro Devices (AMD) chips are among the most common.

central processing unit (CPU)
The main chip within the computer, also referred to as the brain of the computer, which handles most of the operations (i.e., code and instructions) of the computer.

RANDOM-ACCESS MEMORY (RAM)

This is one of the most widely mentioned types of computer memory. **Random-access memory (RAM)** takes the burden off the computer's processor and hard disk drive (HDD). If the computer had to access the HDD each time it wanted data, it would run slowly and inefficiently. Instead the computer, aware that it may need certain data at a moment's notice, stores the data in RAM. It is helpful to envision RAM as chips that create a large spreadsheet, with each cell representing a memory address that the CPU can use as a reference to retrieve data. RAM is referred to as *volatile memory* because it is not permanent; its contents undergo constant change and are lost once power is taken away from the computer. RAM takes the physical form of chips that plug into the motherboard; SIMMs (single inline memory modules), DIMMs (dual inline memory modules), and SDRAM (synchronous dynamic random-access memory) are just a few of the types of chips. Today's computers come with varying amounts of RAM: 4 to 8 GB (gigabytes) is the most common capacity.[1]

random-access memory (RAM)
The volatile memory of a computer, where programs and instructions that are in use are stored; when power is turned off, its contents are lost.

INPUT DEVICES

Input devices are used to get data into the computer or to give the computer instructions. Input devices constitute part of the "user" side of the computer. Examples include the keyboard, mouse, joystick, and scanner.

OUTPUT DEVICES

Output devices are equipment through which data is obtained from the computer. Output devices are also part of the "user" side of the computer and provide the results of the user's tasks. They include the monitor, printer, and speakers.

HARD DISK DRIVE (HDD)

Generally speaking, the **hard disk drive (HDD)** is the primary component of storage in the personal computer (see Figure 19–2). It typically stores the operating system (e.g., Windows, Mac OS, Linux, or Unix), the programs (e.g., Microsoft Word, Internet Explorer, Open Office for Linux), and data files created by the user (i.e., documents, spreadsheets, accounting information, the company database). Unlike RAM, the HDD is permanent storage and retains its information even after the power is turned off.

hard disk drive (HDD)
Typically the main storage location within the computer, which consists of magnetic platters contained in a case (usually 3.5" long in a desktop computer and 2.5" in a laptop) and is usually where the operating system, applications, and user data are stored.

---

[1] A megabyte (MB) is approximately one million bytes; a gigabyte (GB) is approximately one billion bytes, or 1,000 megabytes.

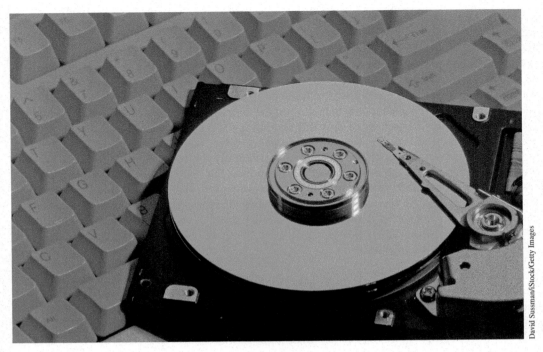

FIGURE 19–2

An inside view of the platter and read/write head of a hard disk drive.

HDDs work off a controller that is typically part of the motherboard, but they sometimes take the form of an add-on (expansion) card plugged into the motherboard. The most common types of HDD controllers are integrated drive electronics (IDE), small computer system interface (SCSI), and serial ATA (SATA). Each HDD type has a different interface that connects it to the controller. Regardless of the type of controller, the data is stored in basically the same fashion. HDDs are mapped, or formatted, and have a defined layout. They are logically divided into sectors, clusters, tracks, and cylinders (see the section titled "Storing and Retrieving Data").

Putting It All Together

A person approaches the computer, sits down, and presses the power button. The power supply wakes up and delivers power to the motherboard and all of the hardware connected to the computer. At this point, the flash ROM chip on the motherboard (the one that contains the BIOS) conducts a power-on self test (POST) to make sure everything is working properly.

The flash ROM also polls the motherboard to check the hardware that is attached and follows its programmed boot order, thus determining from what device it should boot. Typically, the boot device is the HDD, but it can also be a CD or USB drive. If it is the HDD, the HDD is then given control. It locates the first sector of its disk (known as the master boot record), determines its layout (i.e., (partition[s]), and boots an operating system (e.g., Windows, Mac OS, Linux, or Unix). The person is then presented with a computer work environment, commonly referred to as a *desktop*.

Now ready to work, the user double-clicks an icon on the desktop, such as a Microsoft Word shortcut, to open the program and begins to type a document. The CPU processes this request, locates the Microsoft Word program on the HDD (using a predefined map of the drive called a *file system table*), carries out the programming instructions associated with the application, loads Microsoft Word into RAM via the system bus, and sends the output to the monitor by way of the video controller, which is either located on or attached to the motherboard.

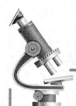

Inside the Science

Other Common Storage Devices

Although the HDD is the most common storage device for the personal computer, many others exist. Methods for storing data and the layout of that data can vary from device to device. A CD-ROM, for example, uses a different technology and format for writing data than a smart media card or USB thumb drive. Fortunately, regardless of the differences among devices, the same basic forensic principles apply for acquiring the data. Common storage devices include the following:

CD-R/RW (Compact Disc—Record/Rewrite) and DVD-R/RW (DVD—Record/Rewrite) Compact discs (CDs) and digital video discs (DVDs) are two of the most common forms of external data storage. They are used to store a wide variety of information, such as music, video, and data files. They are discs made largely of plastic, with an aluminum layer that is read by laser light in a CD/DVD reader. Blu-Ray discs have also emerged in the market offering larger storage capacity than their predecessor optical media. In addition to larger storage capacities, Blu-Ray discs are read by a blue laser light instead of the red laser that reads CDs and DVDs. Different optical media are encoded in different ways, making the job of the forensic examiner difficult at times.

USB Thumb Drives and Smart Media Cards These devices can store a large amount of data—some as much as 64 GB. They are known as solid-state storage devices because they have no moving parts. Smart media cards are typically found in digital cameras, mobile devices, and PDAs, but USB thumb drives come in many shapes, sizes, and storage capacities.

Tapes Tapes come in many different formats and storage capacities. Each typically comes with its own hardware reader and, sometimes, a proprietary application to read and write its contents. Tapes and thumb drives are typically used for backup purposes and consequently have great forensic potential.

Network Interface Card (NIC) Very rarely does one encounter a computer today that doesn't have a NIC. Whether they are on a local network or the Internet, when computers need to communicate with each other, they typically do so through a NIC. NICs come in many different forms: add-on cards that plug into the motherboard, hard-wired devices on the motherboard, add-on cards (PCMCIA) for laptops, and universal serial bus (USB) plug-in cards, to name a few. Some are wired cards, meaning they need a physical wired connection to participate on the network, and others are wireless, meaning they receive their data via radio waves.

The user then begins to type, transferring data from the keyboard into RAM. When finished, the user may print the document or simply save it to the HDD for later retrieval. If printed, the data is taken from RAM, processed by the CPU, placed in a format suitable for printing, and sent through the system bus to the external port where the printer is connected. If the document is saved, the data is taken from RAM, processed by the CPU, passed to the HDD controller (i.e., IDE, SCSI, or SATA) by way of the system bus, and written to a portion of the HDD. The HDD's file system table is updated so it knows where to retrieve that data later. In actuality, the boot process is more complex than this, and the forensic examiner must possess an in-depth knowledge of the process.

The preceding example illustrates how three components perform most of the work: the CPU, RAM, and system bus. The example can get even more complicated as the user opens more applications and performs multiple tasks simultaneously (i.e., *multitasks*). Several tasks can be loaded into RAM at once, and the CPU is capable of juggling them all. This allows for a multitasking environment and the ability to switch back and forth between applications. All of this is orchestrated by the operating system and is written in the language of the computer—ones and zeros. The only detail missing, one that is important from a forensic standpoint, is a better understanding of how data is stored on the HDD. This is discussed next.

Storing and Retrieving Data

Before beginning to understand how data is stored on a HDD, it is first important to understand the role of the **operating system (OS)**. An OS, such as Windows, Mac OS, Linux, or Unix, is the bridge between the human user and the computer's electronic components. It provides the user with a working environment and facilitates interaction with the system's components. Each OS supports certain types of file systems that store data in different ways.

Formatting and Partitioning the HDD

Generally speaking, before an OS can write to an HDD, it must first be formatted. But even before it can be formatted, a partition must be defined. A **partition** is nothing more than a contiguous set of blocks that are defined and treated as an independent disk. This means that a HDD can hold several partitions, making a single HDD appear as several disks.

Partitioning a drive can be thought of as dividing a container that begins as nothing more than six sides. We then cut a hole in the front of the container and insert two drawers and the hardware required to open and close them. We have just created a two-drawer filing cabinet and defined each drawer as contiguous blocks of storage. A partitioning utility such as Disk Manager or fdisk defines the drawer or drawers (i.e., partitions) that will later hold the data on the HDD. Just as the style, size, and shape of filing cabinet drawers can vary, so too can partitions.

After a hard drive is partitioned, typically it is formatted. (At this point, this would be high-level formatting, not to be confused with low-level formatting, which is generally done by the manufacturer of the HDD.) The formatting process initializes portions of the HDD and creates the structure of the file system. The file system can be thought of as the system for storing and locating data on a storage device. Some of the file system types are FAT12 (typically on floppy disks), FAT16 (older DOS and older Windows partitions), FAT32 (Windows file systems), NTFS (most current Windows systems—Windows 7 and 8), EXT2 and EXT3 (Linux systems), and HPFS (some Macintosh systems).

Each of these file systems has a different way of storing, retrieving, and allocating data. In summary, a drive is prepared in three processes: low-level formatting (typically done by the manufacturer, dividing the platters into tracks and sectors), partitioning (accomplished through a utility such as fdisk or Disk Manager, defining a contiguous set of blocks), and formatting (i.e., initializing portions of the disk and creating the file system structure). The process is a bit more technical and detailed than this, but at the conclusion of these basic steps, the drive is logically defined. (We say "logically" because no real divisions are made. That is, if you were to crack open the HDD before or after partitioning and formatting, to your naked eye the platters would look the same.)

Mapping the HDD

As shown in Figure 19–3, HDDs contain several platters stacked vertically that are logically divided into sectors, clusters, tracks, and cylinders. **Sectors** are typically 512 bytes in size (a **byte** is eight bits; a **bit** is a single one or zero). (Currently, work is being done on HDDs with increased minimum sector sizes, in an effort to increase drive performance. However, at this time, 512 bytes is still the standard for most HDDs.) **Clusters** are groups of sectors; their size is defined by the file system, but they are always in sector multiples of two. (Although an NTFS partition does permit a one-sector-per-cluster scenario, such a scenario is not usually chosen.) A cluster, therefore, consists of two, four, six, or eight sectors, and so on. (With modern file systems, the user can exercise some control over the number of sectors per cluster.) *Tracks* are concentric circles that are defined around the platter. *Cylinders* are groups of tracks that reside directly above and below each other.

Additionally, the HDD has a file system table, or map, of the layout of the defined space in that partition. FAT file systems use a *file allocation table* (which is where the acronym *FAT* comes from) to track the location of files and folders (i.e., data) on the HDD, whereas NTFS file systems (used by most current Windows systems—Windows 7 and 8) use, among other things, a *master file table (MFT)*. Each file system table tracks data in different ways, and computer forensic examiners should be versed in the technical nuances of the HDDs they examine. It is sufficient for our purposes here, however, to merely visualize the file system table as a map where the data is located. This map uses the numbering of sectors, clusters, tracks, and cylinders to keep track of the data.

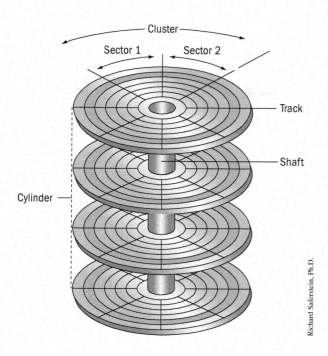

Richard Saferstein, Ph.D.

FIGURE 19–3

Partitions of a hard disk drive.

One way to envision a partition and file system is as a room full of safe-deposit boxes. The room itself symbolizes the entire partition, and the boxes symbolize clusters of data. In order to determine who rented which box, and where each renter's property is, a central database is needed. This would be especially necessary if a person rented two boxes located in opposite ends of the room (this would be noncontiguous data on the HDD). The database tracking the locations of the safe-deposit boxes is much like a file system table tracking the location of data within the clusters.

This example is also useful for understanding the concept of reformatting an HDD. If the database managing the locations of the safe-deposit boxes were wiped out, the property in them would still remain; we just wouldn't know what was where. It is the same with the HDD. If a user were to wipe the file system table clean—for example, by reformatting it—the data itself would not be gone. Both the database tracking the locations of the safe-deposit boxes and the file system table tracking the location of the data in the cluster are maps—they are not actual contents. (Exceptions exist with some file systems, such as an NTFS file system, which stores data for very small files right in its file system table, known as the master file table).

Processing the Electronic Crime Scene

Processing the electronic crime scene has a lot in common with processing a traditional crime scene. The investigator must first ensure that the proper legal requirements (e.g., search warrant and consent) have been met so that the scene can be searched and the evidence seized. The investigator should then devise a plan of approach based on the facts of the case and the physical location. The scene should be documented in as much detail as possible before disturbing any evidence and before the investigator lays a finger on any computer components. Of course, there are circumstances in which an investigator may have to act quickly and pull a plug before documenting the scene, such as when data is in the process of being deleted.

Documenting the Crime Scene

Typical crime-scene documentation is accomplished through two actions: sketching and photographing. The electronic crime scene is no different. First, the scene should be sketched in the style of a floor plan (see Figure 19–4), and then overall photographs of the location should be taken. In the case of a network, a technical network sketch should also be included if possible.

After photographs have been taken of the overall layout, close-up photographs should be shot. A close-up photograph of any running computer monitor should be taken. All the

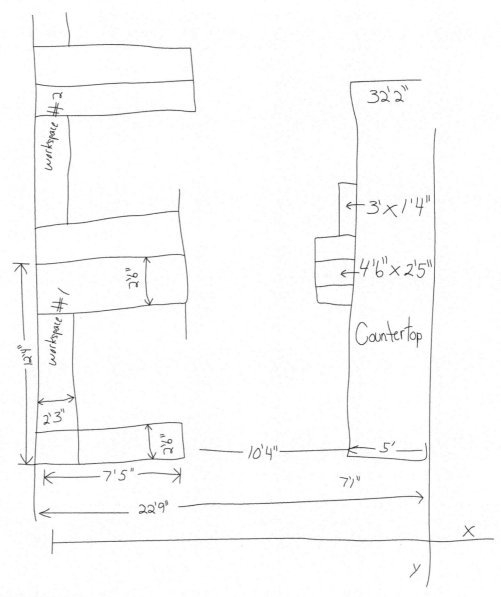

FIGURE 19–4

Rough sketch made at a crime scene with necessary measurements included.

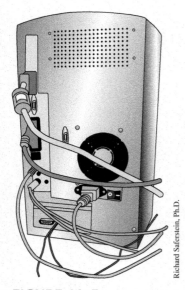

Richard Saferstein, Ph.D.

FIGURE 19–5

Back of a computer showing all connections.

connections to the main system unit, such as peripheral devices (e.g., keyboard, monitor, speakers, and mouse), should be photographed. If necessary, system units should be moved delicately and carefully to facilitate the connections photograph (see Figure 19–5). Close-up photographs of equipment serial numbers should be taken if practical.

Live Computer Acquisition

At this point, investigators must decide whether to perform a live acquisition of the data, perform a system shutdown (as in the case of server equipment), pull the plug from the back of the computer, or do a combination of these things. Pulling the plug should always be done by removing the plug from the back of the computer. If the plug is removed from the wall and a battery backup (UPS) is in place, the UPS will cause an alert to the system and keep the unit "powered on." Several factors influence this decision. For example, if encryption is being used and by pulling the plug, the data will encrypt, rendering it unreadable without a password or key, pulling the plug would not be prudent. Similarly, if crucial evidentiary data exists in RAM and has not been saved to the HDD, the data will be lost. Hence, if power to the system is discontinued, another option must be considered. Regardless, the equipment will most likely be seized. Exceptions exist in the corporate environment, where servers are fundamental to business operations.

A computer can be found in several states. Among these is live (i.e., running or powered on) and dead (i.e., not running or powered off). The traditional approach for dealing with a live, running computer in computer forensics was to pull the plug from the back. By doing this, the examiner froze the data in time, thus preventing any additions or modifications to the HDD contained within. Although this methodology still has its limited place, several traits of today's computer technology and some evidentiary considerations necessitate consideration of performing a live examination prior to disconnecting power. By examining one of many instances in which a live examination might be considered, we can get a good view of how this process works.

Let's say an investigator responds to the scene of a missing 14-year-old girl. The investigator notices a laptop computer on a desk in the girl's bedroom. Closer scrutiny reveals that the laptop is live and what appears to be an instant message conversation is on the screen. Additionally, what can be seen of the conversation discusses a meeting with what appears to be an older man. The investigator needs to start the process of identifying the individual in the conversation. Almost simultaneously, the investigator needs to preserve the evidence that probably exists only in RAM. Here, a consideration of "order of volatility" must be made. The fact that the investigator needs to work with the computer system means that changes to the data (i.e., the electronic crime scene) will be made. Considering order of volatility allows the investigator to develop a sequence of steps that will limit the effects of each change on the subsequent steps and collection methods, thus affording the collection of the greatest amount of unaltered evidentiary data. In this example, steps might be completed in the following order:

1. Photograph all sections of the conversation screen to document the conversation in the same form the user sees. Merely scrolling through the conversation to afford photographing the entire conversation is minimally intrusive, and limited (and arguably inconsequential) changes will occur.
2. Depending on their skill level, the investigator may want to acquire the contents of RAM at this point. This would be accomplished by running a controlled application that the investigator already possesses and that is designed for such a purpose. Of course, the resulting content needs to be written somewhere, and it should not be written to the computer's hard drive. Rather, the examiner should use a clean piece of media that can handle the size of the output. There are several options for this.
3. Next, the investigator may want to consider copying the text and pasting it to a new document or using a save command in the chat application to save the conversation in text format. Again, this conversation should not be saved to the hard drive of the system being examined.
4. If the investigator feels that encryption is being used, he or she may consider imaging the entire hard drive in this live environment. Because shutting down the computer with encryption in place renders the hard drive's contents unreadable without a password, it may be a good idea to get an image of the hard drive while it is still decrypted. This requires special response tools and external media that can handle the large image size.

This is just one way to approach this and other live examinations. The order of steps can also be debated among forensic examiners. The following questions are important for the forensic examiner to consider:

1. What is the type of case I am investigating?
2. What is the evidence I seek?
3. How best can I completely acquire that evidence without contaminating other aspects of the electronic crime scene?
4. In what order should I take those steps? (order of volatility)
5. Do I have the training, education, experience, equipment, and tools to accomplish this, or do I need assistance?

Finally, the only perfect crime scene is one that has not been entered. The minute investigators enter a crime scene, there will be changes to the environment, but obviously, entering the physical crime scene is a necessary function of evidence collection. Processing it should be done in a certain order so that, for example, the collection of fingerprints won't prevent the proper collection of blood, hair, fiber, and so on. The same applies to the electronic crime scene.

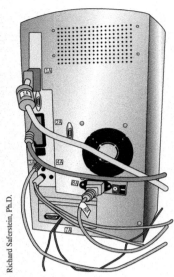

Richard Saferstein, Ph.D.

FIGURE 19–6

Back of a computer with each component correlated with its port through the use of a labeling scheme.

Message Digest 5 (MD5)/ Secure Hash Algorithm (SHA)

A software algorithm used to "fingerprint" a file or contents of a disk; used to verify the integrity of data. In forensic analysis, it is typically used to verify that an acquired image of suspect data was not altered during the process of imaging.

After the photographs and sketches are complete and, if appropriate, the live examination has been performed, but before disconnecting the peripherals from the computer, a label should be placed on the cord of each peripheral, with a corresponding label placed on the port to which it is connected. A numbering scheme should be devised to further identify each system unit if several computers are at the scene (Figure 19–6). The combination of sketching, photographing, and labeling should adequately document the scene, prevent future confusion about which component went with which system unit, and facilitate reconstruction if necessary for lab or courtroom purposes.

Forensic Image Acquisition

Now that the items have been seized, the data must be obtained for analysis. The number of electronic items that potentially store evidentiary data is too vast to cover in this section. The HDD will be used as an example, but the same "best practices" principles apply for other electronic devices as well.

Throughout the entire process, the computer forensic examiner must use the least intrusive method. The goal in obtaining data from an HDD is to do so without altering even one bit of data. Because booting an HDD to its operating system changes many files and could potentially destroy evidentiary data, obtaining data is generally accomplished by removing the HDD from the system and placing it in a laboratory forensic computer so that a forensic image can be created. However, the BIOS of the seized computer sometimes interprets the geometry of the HDD differently than the forensic computer does. In these instances, the image of the HDD must be obtained using the seized computer. Regardless, the examiner must ensure that the drive to be analyzed is in a "write-blocked," or read-only, state when creating the forensic image. Furthermore, the examiner needs to be able to prove that the forensic image he or she obtained includes every bit of data and caused no changes, or writes, to the HDD.

To this end, a sort of fingerprint of the drive is taken before and after imaging. This fingerprint is taken through the use of a **Message Digest 5 (MD5)/Secure Hash Algorithm (SHA)**, or similar validated algorithm. Before imaging the drive, the algorithm is run and a 32-character alphanumeric string is produced based on the drive's contents. The algorithm is then run against the resulting forensic image; if nothing changed, the same alphanumeric string is produced, thus demonstrating that the image is all-inclusive of the original contents and that nothing was altered in the process.

A forensic image of the data on an HDD (as well as on floppy disks, CDs, DVDs, tapes, flash memory devices, and any other storage medium) is merely an exact duplicate of the entire contents of the drive. In other words, all portions of the drive are copied, from the first bit (i.e., one or zero) to the last. Why would investigators want to copy what appears to be blank or unused portions of the HDD? The answer is simple: to preserve latent data, which is discussed later in the chapter. It suffices to say here that data exists in areas of the drive that are, generally speaking, unknown and inaccessible to most end users. This data can be valuable as evidence. Therefore, a forensic image—one that copies every single bit of information on the drive—is necessary. A forensic image differs from a backup or standard copy in that it takes the entire contents, not only data the operating system is aware of.

Many forensic software packages come equipped with a method for obtaining the forensic image. The most popular software forensic tools—EnCase, Forensic Toolkit (FTK), Forensic Autopsy (Linux-based freeware), and SMART (Linux-based software by ASR Data)—all include a method for obtaining a forensic image. All produce self-contained image files that can then be interpreted and analyzed. They also allow image compression to conserve storage. The fact that forensic imaging results in self-contained, compressed files allows many images from different cases to be stored on the same forensic storage drive. This makes case management and storage much easier (see Figure 19–7).

Analysis of Electronic Data

Analysis of electronic data is virtually limitless and bound only to the level of skill of the examiner. The more familiar an examiner is with computers, operating systems, application software, data storage, and a host of other disciplines, the more prepared he or she will be to look for evidentiary data.

Because computers are vast and complex, discussing each area, file, directory, log, or computer process that could potentially contain evidentiary data is beyond the scope of one chapter—and may be beyond the scope of an entire book. What follows are some of the more common

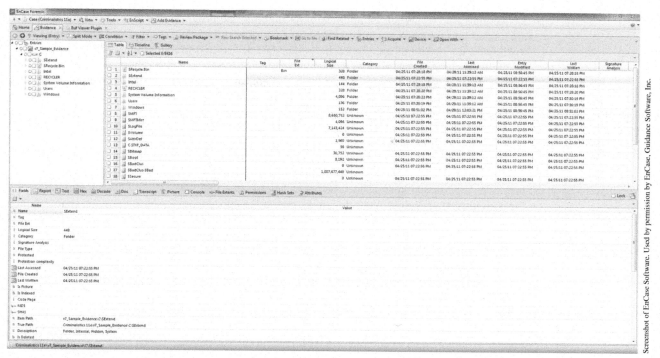

FIGURE 19–7

Screenshot of EnCase Software. EnCase is a common forensic software application capable of imaging and assisting in the analysis of data.

areas of analysis. While reading this section, reflect on your own knowledge of computers and consider what other data might be of evidentiary value and where it might be found.

Visible Data

The category of **visible data** includes all information that the operating system is presently aware of and thus is readily accessible to the user. Here, we present several common types of visible data considered in many investigations. This list is by no means exhaustive and can include any information that has value as evidence.

visible data
All data that the operating system is presently aware of and thus is readily accessible to the user.

DATA/WORK PRODUCT FILES   One place to find evidence is in documents or files produced by the suspect. This category is extremely broad and can include data from just about any software program. Microsoft Word and WordPerfect word-processing programs typically produce text-based files such as typed documents and correspondence. These programs, and a host of other word-processing programs, have replaced the typewriter. They are common sources of evidence in criminal cases, particularly those involving white-collar crime.

Also relevant in white-collar crime and similar financial investigations is any data related to personal and business finance. Programs such as QuickBooks and Peachtree accounting packages can manage the entire financial portion of a small to midsize business. Similarly, it is not uncommon to find personal bank account records in the computer that are managed with personal finance software such as Microsoft Money and Quicken. Moreover, people who commit crimes sometimes use these programs as well as spreadsheet applications to track bank accounts stolen from unsuspecting victims. Computer forensic examiners should familiarize themselves with these programs, the ways in which they store data, and methods for extracting and reading the data.

Advances in printer technology have made high-quality color printing both affordable and common in many homes. Although this is a huge benefit for home office workers and those interested in graphic arts, the technology has been used for criminal gain. Counterfeiting and check and document fraud are easily perpetrated on most home computers. All that is required is a decent ink-jet printer and a scanner. Including the computer, an individual could set up a counterfeiting operation for less than $1500. Examiners must learn the graphics and photo-editing applications used for nefarious purposes. Being able to recognize the data produced by these applications and knowing how to display the images is key to identifying this type of evidence.

SWAP FILE DATA   When an application is running, the program and the data being accessed are loaded into RAM. A computer's RAM is much faster than the "read" speed of the HDD, and that's why the programs are loaded here—for fast access and functioning. RAM, however, has its limits. Some computers have a gigabyte or two of RAM, and still others as much as four to eight gigabytes. Regardless of the amount, though, most operating systems (Windows, Linux, and so on) are programmed to conserve RAM when possible. This is where the **swap file** comes in. The operating system attempts to keep only data and applications that are presently being used in RAM. Other applications that were started, but are currently waiting for user attention, may be swapped out of RAM and written to the swap space on the HDD.[2]

For example, a manager of a retail store may want to type a quarterly report based on sales. The manager starts up Microsoft Word and begins his report. Needing to incorporate sales figures from a particular spreadsheet, he opens Microsoft Excel. Depending on what is running on the computer, the original Word document may be swapped from RAM to the swap space on the HDD to free up space for Excel. As the manager goes back and forth between the programs (and maybe checks his e-mail in between) this swapping continues. Data that is swapped back and forth is sometimes left behind in the swap space. Even as this area is constantly changed, some of the data is orphaned in unallocated space, an area of the HDD discussed later in this chapter.

A *swap file* or *space* can be defined as a particular file or even a separate HDD partition, depending on the operating system and file system type (e.g., FAT, NTFS, EXT2). For Windows systems, either the swap file *Win386.sys* or *pagefile.sys* is used, depending on the specific Windows version and file system type. Linux and current Mac OS systems can create partitions just for swapping data in and out of RAM. Data in the swap space can be read by examining the HDD through forensic software or a utility that provides a binary view, such as Norton Disk Editor or WinHex (see Figure 19–8).

TEMPORARY FILES   Any user who has suffered a sudden loss of power in the middle of typing a document can attest to the value of a **temporary file**. Most programs automatically save a copy of the file being worked on in a temporary file. After typing a document, working on a spreadsheet, or working on a slide presentation, the user can save the changes, thus promoting the temporary copy to actual file status. Temporary files are created as a sort of backup on the fly. If the computer experiences a sudden loss of power or other catastrophic failure, the temporary file can be recovered, limiting the amount of data lost. The loss is limited, but not altogether prevented,

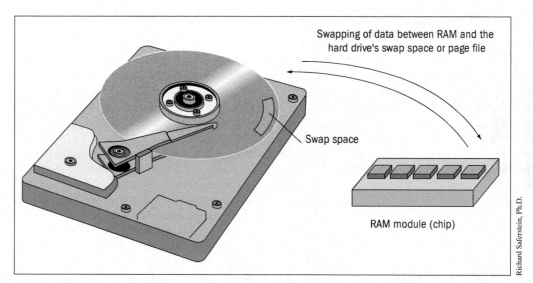

FIGURE 19–8

As a user switches between applications and performs multiple tasks, data is swapped back and forth between RAM and the computer's hard drive. This area on the hard drive is referred to as either swap space or a paging file.

---

[2] Actually, the more appropriate term is probably paging as opposed to *swapping*. This is because entire programs are typically not swapped in and out of memory to the swap space; rather, *pages* of memory are placed there.

because the temporary file is not updated in real time. Rather, it is updated periodically, depending on the application's settings. The default interval in most programs is every 10 minutes.

Temporary files can sometimes be recovered during a forensic examination. Additionally, some of the data that may have been orphaned from a previous version may be recoverable, if not the complete file. This is true even when a document has been typed and printed but never saved. The creation of the temporary file makes it possible for some of this "unsaved" data to be recovered during analysis.

Another type of temporary file valuable to the computer investigator is the print spool file. When a print job is sent to the printer, a spooling process delays the sending of the data to the printer. This happens so the application can continue to work while the printing takes place in the background. To facilitate this, a temporary print spool file is created; this file typically includes the data to be printed and information specific to the printer. There are different methods for accomplishing this, and thus the files created as a result of this process vary. It is sometimes possible to view the data in a readable format from the files created during the spooling process.

Latent Data

The term **latent data** includes data that is obfuscated (not necessarily intentionally) from a user's view. It includes areas of files and disks that are typically not apparent to the computer user but that contain data nonetheless. Latent data is one of the reasons a forensic image of the media is created. If a standard copy were all that is produced, only the logical data (i.e., that which the operating system is aware of) would be captured. Getting every bit of data ensures that potentially valuable evidence in latent data is not missed.

Once the all-inclusive forensic image is produced, how is the latent data viewed? Utilities that allow a user to examine a HDD on a binary (ones and zeros) level are the answer. Applications such as Norton Disk Editor and WinHex provide this type of access to a HDD or other computer media. Thus these applications, sometimes also referred to as *hex editors* (for the hexadecimal shorthand of computer language), allow all data to be read on the binary level independent of the operating system's file system table. Utilities such as these can write to the media under examination, thus changing data. Consequently, a software or hardware write-blocker should be used.

A more common option in data forensics is to use specialized forensic examination software. EnCase and Forensic Toolkit for Windows and SMART and Forensic Autopsy for Linux are examples of forensic software. Each allows a search for evidence on the binary level and provides automated tools for performing common forensic processing techniques. Examiners should be cautious, however, about relying too heavily on automated tools. To merely use an automated tool without understanding what is happening in the background and why evidentiary data may exist in particular locations would severely impede the investigator's ability to testify to the findings.

SLACK SPACE   Slack space is empty space on a HDD created because of the way the HDD stores files. Recall that although the smallest unit of data is one bit (either a one or a zero), an HDD cannot address or deal with such a small unit. In fact, not even a byte (eight bits) can be addressed. Rather, the smallest unit of addressable space by an HDD is the sector. HDDs typically assign sectors in 512-byte increments, whereas CD-ROMs allocate 2,048 bytes per sector.

If the minimum addressable unit of the HDD is 512 bytes, what happens if the file is only 100 bytes? In this instance there are 412 bytes of slack space. It does not end here, however, because there is also a minimum cluster requirement. As you may recall, clusters are groups of sectors used to store files and folders. The cluster is the minimum storage unit defined and used by the logical partition. It is because of the minimum addressable sector of the HDD and the minimum-unit-of-storage requirement of the volume that we have slack space.

Minimum cluster allocation must be defined in sectors in multiples of two. Thus, a cluster includes two, four, six, or eight sectors or more. Returning to our initial example of the 100-byte file, suppose an HDD has a two-sectors-per-cluster volume requirement. This means that the HDD will allocate a minimum of two 512-byte sectors (a total of 1,024 bytes) of storage space for that 100-byte file. The remaining 924 bytes would be slack space (see Figure 19–9).

To illustrate this point, let us expand on the previous example of safe-deposit boxes. The bank offers safe-deposit boxes of a particular size. This is the equivalent of the HDD's clusters. A person wanting to place only a deed to a house in the box gets the same size box as a person who wants to stuff it full of cash. The former would have empty space should he or she desire to place additional items in the box. This empty space is the equivalent of slack space. But what

latent data
Areas of files and disks that are typically not apparent to the computer user (and often not to the operating system) but contain data nonetheless.

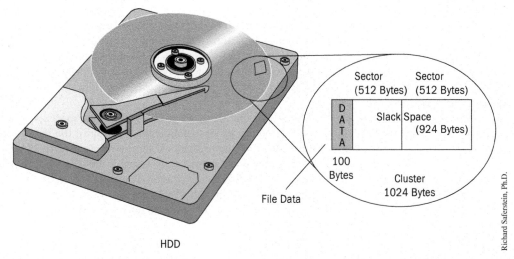

FIGURE 19–9

Slack space illustrated in a two-sector cluster. Cluster sizes are typically greater than two sectors, but two sectors are displayed here for simplicity.

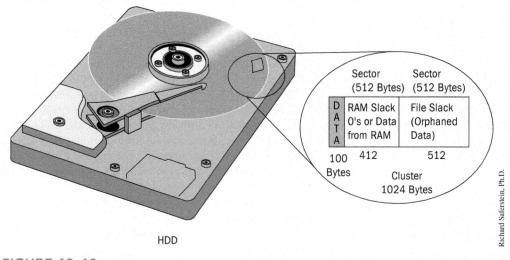

FIGURE 19–10

File slack.

if the box becomes full and the person needs more space? That person must then get a second box. Similarly, if a file grows to fill one cluster and beyond, a second cluster is allocated. The remaining space in the second cluster is slack space. This continues as more and more clusters are allocated to accommodate the size of the growing file.

There are actually two types of slack space: *RAM slack* and file slack. *RAM slack* occupies the space from where the actual (i.e., logical) data portion of the file ends to where the first allocated sector in the cluster terminates. **File slack**, therefore, occupies the remaining space of the cluster. RAM slack is a concept that was more relevant in older operating systems. Remember that the minimum amount of space the HDD can address is the 512-byte sector. Therefore, if the file size is only 100 bytes, the remaining space must be padded. Some older operating systems pad this area with data contained in RAM. This could include web pages, passwords, data files, or other data that existed in RAM when the file was written. Modern Windows operating systems pad this space with zeros, but some examinations may still yield valuable data in this area.

Let us go back to the 100-byte file with the two-sectors-per-cluster minimum requirement. Following the end of the logical data (i.e., beyond the 100 bytes), the remaining 412 bytes of that sector is RAM slack; the additional 512 bytes completing the cluster is then file slack. See Figure 19–10 for a visual depiction. The question now becomes, What can I expect to find in slack space, and why is this important? The answer: junk—valuable junk.

file slack

The area that begins at the end of the last sector that contains logical data and terminates at the end of the cluster.

File slack, on the other hand, can contain a lot of orphaned data. To illustrate this point, let's take the 100-byte file example a bit further. Let's say that before the 100-byte file was written to the HDD, occupying one cluster (two sectors totaling 1,024 bytes), a 1,000-byte file occupied this space but was deleted by the user. When a file is "deleted," the data still remains behind, so it is probably a safe bet that data from the original 1,000-byte file remains in the slack space of the new 100-byte file now occupying this cluster. This is just one example of why data exists in file slack and why file slack may be valuable as evidence.

In one final attempt to illustrate this point, let us again build on our safe-deposit box analogy. Suppose a person rents two safe-deposit boxes, each box representing a sector and the two combined representing a cluster. If that person places the deed to her house in the first box, the remaining space in that box would be analogous to RAM slack. The space in the second box would be the equivalent of file slack. The only difference is that, unlike the empty spaces of the safe-deposit box, the slack space of the file probably contains data that may be valuable as evidence.

The data contained in RAM and file slack is not really the concern of the operating system. As far as the OS is concerned, this space is empty and therefore ready to be used. Until that happens, however, an examination with one of the aforementioned tools will allow a look into these areas, thus revealing the orphaned data. The same is true for unallocated space.

UNALLOCATED SPACE   Latent evidentiary data also resides in **unallocated space**. What is unallocated space, how does data get in there, and what is done to access this space? If we have an 80 GB hard drive and only half of the hard drive is filled with data, then the other half, or 40 GB, is unallocated space (see Figure 19–11). Returning to our safe-deposit box analogy, if the entire bank of safe-deposit boxes contains 100 boxes, but only 50 are currently in use, then the other 50 would be the equivalent of unallocated space. The HDD's unallocated space typically contains a lot of useful data. The constant shuffling of files on the HDD causes data to become orphaned in unallocated space as the logical portion of the file is rewritten to other places. Some examples of ways in which data can become orphaned are through fragmentation, during the creation of swap files or swap space, or in the process of deleting files.

DEFRAGMENTING   Defragmenting an HDD involves moving noncontiguous data back together. Remember that the HDD has minimum space reservation requirements. Again, if the file requires only 100 bytes of space, the operating system may allocate much more than that. If the file grows past what has been allocated for it, another cluster is required. If, however, a different

unallocated space
The unused area of the HDD that the operating system file system table sees as empty (i.e., containing no logical files) but that may contain old data.

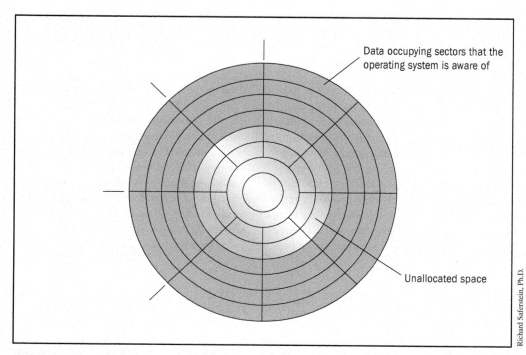

Data occupying sectors that the operating system is aware of

Unallocated space

Richard Saferstein, Ph.D.

FIGURE 19–11

A simplistic view of a hard drive platter demonstrating the concept of unallocated space.

file occupies the next cluster in line, then the operating system will have to find another place for that additional data on the drive. In this scenario, the file is said to be *fragmented* because data for the same file is contained in noncontiguous clusters. In the case of the HDD, the shuffling of files causes data to be orphaned in unallocated space.

Ultimately fragmentation of numerous files can degrade the performance of an HDD, causing the read/write heads to have to traverse the platters to locate the data. Defragmenting the HDD rearranges noncontiguous data into contiguous clusters. Building yet again on our safe-deposit box analogy, if our renter eventually needs to store more property than her original box can hold, the bank will rent her a second box. If, however, all the boxes around hers are occupied and the only free one is in another section of the room, then her property is "fragmented." The bank would have to "defrag" the safe-deposit boxes to get the property of users with more than one box into adjacent boxes.

SWAP FILE/SWAP SPACE   Recall that a computer uses the HDD to maximize its amount of RAM by constantly swapping data in and out of RAM to a predetermined location on the HDD, thus freeing valuable RAM. The constant read and write operations of RAM cause a constant change in the swap file—*WIN386.swp* or *pagefile.sys*—in Windows or in the swap space on a Linux system. Data can become orphaned in unallocated space from this constant swapping to and from the HDD.

DELETED FILES   The deletion of files is another way that data becomes orphaned in unallocated space. Data from deleted files can manifest itself in different ways during a forensic examination. The actions that occur when a file is deleted vary among file systems. What is fairly consistent, though, is that generally the data is not truly removed. For example, consider what happens when a user or program deletes a file in a Windows operating system with a FAT file system. When a file is deleted, the first character in the file's directory entry (i.e., in its name) is replaced with the Greek letter sigma. When the sigma replaces the first character, the file is no longer viewable through conventional methods and the operating system views the space previously occupied by the file as available. The data, however, is still there.

This example doesn't account for the actions of the Windows Recycle Bin. When the Windows operating system is set up to merely place the deleted file in the Recycle Bin, the original directory entry is deleted and one is created in the Recycle folder for that particular user. The new Recycle folder entry is linked to another file, the *info* or *info2* file, which includes some additional data, such as the location of the file before its deletion should the user wish to restore it to that location. Detailed discussions of the function of the Recycle Bin are beyond the scope of this chapter, but suffice it to say that even when the Recycle Bin has been "emptied," the data usually remains behind until overwritten. Although Windows NTFS partitions and Linux EXT partitions handle deleted files differently, in both cases the data typically remains.

What if a new file writes data to the location of the original file? Generally speaking, the data is overwritten. This is, of course, unless the new file only partially overwrites the original: If a file that occupied two clusters is deleted, and a new file overwrites one of the clusters, then the data in the second cluster is orphaned in unallocated space. Of course, yet a third file can overwrite the second cluster entirely, but until then the data remains in unallocated space.

Let us once again look to our safe-deposit box analogy. If, for example, the owner of two safe-deposit boxes stopped renting them, the bank would list them as available. If the owner didn't clean them out, the contents would remain unchanged. If a new owner rented one of the boxes, the contents from the former owner would be replaced with the new owner's possessions. The second box would therefore still contain orphaned contents from its previous owner. The contents would remain in this "unallocated box" until another renter occupies it.

Forensic Analysis of Internet Data

It's important from the investigative standpoint to be familiar with the evidence left behind regarding a user's Internet activity. A forensic examination of a computer system reveals quite a bit of data about a user's Internet activity. The data described next would be accessed and examined using the forensic techniques outlined in the previous sections of this chapter.

Internet Cache

Evidence of web browsing typically exists in abundance on the user's computer. Most web browsers (e.g., Internet Explorer and Firefox) use a caching system to expedite web browsing and make it more efficient. This was particularly true in the days of dial-up Internet access. When a user accesses a website, such as the *New York Times* home page, the data is fed from that server (in this example, that of the *New York Times*), via the Internet service provider and over whatever type of connection the user has, to the user's computer. If that computer is accessing the Internet via a dial-up connection, the transfer of the *New York Times* home page may take a while because the data transfer rate and capabilities (bandwidth) of the telephone system are limited. Even with the high-speed access of a fiber or cable connection, conservation of bandwidth is always a consideration. Taking that into account, web browsers store, or cache, portions of the pages visited on the local HDD. This way, if the page is revisited, portions of it can be reconstructed more quickly from this saved data, rather than having to use precious bandwidth to pull it yet again from the Internet.

This **Internet cache** is a potential source of evidence for the computer investigator. Portions of, or in some cases entire, visited web pages can be reconstructed. For security purposes, modern Internet browsers take steps to clear out, or erase, the web cache. But in some cases, even after being deleted, these cached files can be recovered (see the section titled "Deleted Files"). Investigators must know how to search for this data within the particular web browser used by a suspect.

Internet cache
Portions of visited web pages placed on the local hard disk drive to facilitate quicker retrieval when a web page is revisited.

Internet Cookies

Cookies provide another area where potential evidence can be found. To appreciate the value of cookies, you must first understand how they get onto the computer and their intended purpose. **Cookies** are placed on the local HDD by websites the user has visited, if the user's web browser (such as Internet Explorer) is set to allow this to happen. Microsoft Internet Explorer places cookies in a dedicated directory. Websites use cookies to track certain information about their visitors. This information can be anything, such as history of visits, purchasing habits, passwords, and personal information used to recognize the user for later visits.

Consider a user who registers for an account at the Barnes and Noble bookstore website, then returns to the same site from the same computer a few days later. The site will then display "Welcome, [*User Name*]." This data was retrieved from the cookie file placed on the user's HDD by the website during the initial visit and registration with the site.

It is helpful to think of cookies almost like a Caller ID for websites. The site recognizes and retrieves information about the visitor, as when a salesperson recognizes a caller from a Caller ID display and quickly pulls the client's file. Cookie files can be a valuable source of evidence. In Internet Explorer, they take the form of plain text files, which can typically be opened with a standard text viewer or word-processing program. The existence of the files themselves, regardless of the information contained within, can be of evidentiary value to show a history of Web visits. A typical cookie may resemble the following: rsaferstein@forensicscience.txt. From this we can surmise that someone using the local computer login *rsaferstein* accessed the forensic science website. It is possible that the cookie was placed there by an annoying pop-up ad, not a website the user visited, but considered against other evidence in the computer data, the presence of a particular cookie may have corroborative value.

cookies
Files placed on a computer from a visited website that are used to track visits to and usage of that site.

Internet History

Most web browsers track the history of web page visits for the computer user. This is probably done merely for convenience. Like the "recent calls" list on a cell phone, the **Internet history** provides an accounting of sites most recently visited, with some storing weeks' worth of visits. Users can go back and access sites they recently visited just by going through the browser's history. Most web browsers store this information in one particular file; Internet Explorer uses the *index.dat* file. On a Windows system, an *index.dat* file is created for each login user name on the computer.

The history file can be located and read with most popular computer forensic software packages. It displays the uniform resource locator (URL) of each website, along with the date and time the site was accessed. An investigation involving Internet use almost always includes an examination of Internet history data.

Internet history
An accounting of websites visited; different browsers store this information in different ways.

FIGURE 19–12

The Internet history displays more than just web browsing activity. Here we see Microsoft Word documents and a picture accessed on the current day.

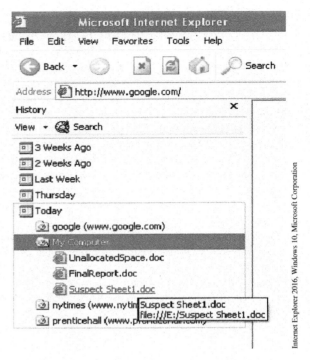

In some respects, the term *Internet history* is wrong because it doesn't encompass all of these files' functions. Several browsers—Internet Explorer, for one—store other valuable evidence independent of Internet access. It is not uncommon to see files accessed over a network listed in the history. Similarly, files accessed on external media, such as CDs or thumb drives, may also appear in the history. Regardless, the Internet history data is a valuable source of evidence worthy of examination (see Figure 19–12).

Bookmarks and Favorite Places

bookmark

A feature that enables the user to designate favorite sites for fast and easy access.

Another way users can access websites quickly is to store them in their **bookmarks** or Favorite Places. Like presetting radio stations, web browsers allow users to bookmark websites for future visits (see Figure 19–13). A lot can be learned from a user's bookmarked sites. You may learn what online news a person is interested in or what type of hobbies he or she has. You may also see that person's favorite child pornography or computer hacking sites bookmarked.

In Internet Explorer, the favorite places are kept in a folder with link files, or shortcuts, to particular URLs. They can be organized in subfolders or grouped by type. The same is true for the Firefox web browser, except that Firefox bookmarks are stored in a document written in hypertext markup language (HTML), the same language interpreted by the web browsers themselves.

Forensic Investigation of Internet Communications

Computer investigations often begin with or are centered on Internet communication. Whether it is a chat conversation among many people, an instant message conversation between two individuals, or the back-and-forth of an e-mail exchange, human communication has long been a source of evidentiary material. Regardless of the type, investigators are typically interested in communication.

Role of the IP

With all of the computer manufacturers and software developers out there, some common rules are necessary for computers to be able to communicate on a global network. Just as any human language needs rules for communication to be successful, so does the language of computers.

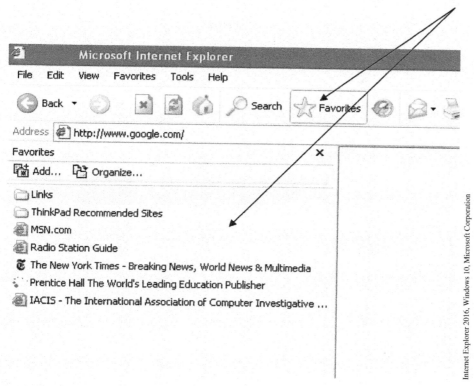

Internet Explorer 2016, Windows 10, Microsoft Corporation

FIGURE 19–13

Bookmarks or favorite places can be saved for quick access in most web browsers.

Computers that participate on the Internet, therefore, must be provided with an address known as an Internet protocol (IP) address from the Internet service provider to which they connect.

IP addresses take the form *###.###.###.###*, in which, generally speaking, *###* can be any number from 0 to 255. A typical IP address might look like this: 66.94.234.13. Not only do IP addresses provide the means by which data can be routed to the appropriate location, but they also provide the means by which most Internet investigations are conducted (see Figure 19–14). Thus the IP address may lead to the identity of a real person. If an IP address is the link to the identity of a real person, then it is quite obviously valuable for identifying someone on the Internet.

To illustrate, let's assume that a user of the Internet, fictitiously named John Smith, connects to the Internet from his home by way of a Verizon FIOS connection. Verizon in this case would be responsible for providing Smith with his IP address. Verizon was issued a bank of IP addresses with which to service its customers from a regulatory body designed to track the usage of IP addresses (obviously so no one address is used by two different users at the same time).

Suppose that Smith, while connected to the Internet, decides to threaten an ex-girlfriend by sending her an e-mail telling her he is going to kill her. That e-mail must first pass through Smith's Internet service provider's routers (in this case, Verizon's) on its way to its destination—Smith's girlfriend. The e-mail would be stamped by the servers that it passes through, and this stamp would include the IP address given to Smith by Verizon for his session on the Internet.

An investigator responsible for tracking that e-mail would locate the originating IP address stamped in the e-mail header. That IP address could be researched using one of many Internet sites (e.g., *www.centralops.net*) to determine which Internet service provider was given this IP as part of the block it was assigned for serving its customers. The investigator then files a subpoena with the Internet service provider (i.e., Verizon) asking which of its customers was using that IP address on that date and time.

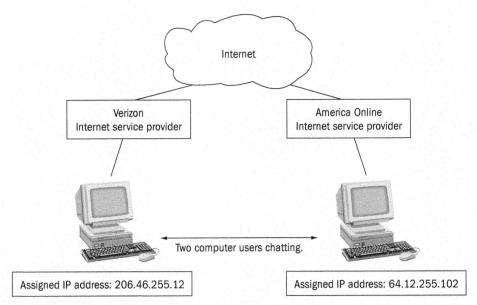

FIGURE 19–14
Two computers communicating by sending data to each other's IP address via the Internet. An IP address is assigned to each computer by their respective Internet service providers.

IP addresses are located in different places for different methods of Internet communications. E-mail has the IP address in the header portion of the mail. This may not be readily apparent and may require a bit of configuration to reveal. Each e-mail client is different and needs to be evaluated on a case-by-case basis. For an instant message or chat session, the provider of the chat mechanism—AOL, Yahoo!, and so on—would be contacted to provide the user's IP address.

E-Mail, Chat, and Instant Messaging

E-mail files can be read by a number of *clients*, or software programs. Two of the most popular ways to access, read, and store e-mail in today's Internet environment, however, are Microsoft Outlook and through an Internet browser. Some people even use a combination of the two.

If an e-mail account is linked through Microsoft Outlook, then the e-mail is stored in a compound file (i.e., a file with several layers). Typically, compound files exist for received e-mail (i.e., the inbox), sent e-mail, and deleted e-mail. Users can also create new categories (shown as folders in Outlook) and categorize saved e-mail there. Most computer forensic software applications can view, or mount, these compound files so that the e-mail can be seen, including any file attachments. These files can also be imported into a clean copy of Microsoft Outlook (i.e., one not attached to an account), and the e-mail can be viewed there. Investigators must also be aware that in a computer network environment, the user's Outlook files may not reside on the user's workstation computer but rather on a central mail or file server.

Most accounts offer the ability to access e-mail through a web-based interface as well. This way, users can access their e-mail remotely from other computers. For e-mail accessed through a web browser, the information presented earlier on Internet-based evidence applies. The web interface converts the e-mail into a document suitable for reading in a web browser. Consequently, web-based e-mail is sometimes found in the Internet cache. This is particularly true of free Internet e-mail providers such as Hotmail and Yahoo!.

Much of the evidence from Internet communication is also derived from chat and instant message technology. This is particularly true in the world of child sexual exploitation over the Internet. Various technologies provide chat and instant messaging services. Most chat and instant message conversations are not saved by the parties involved. Although most of the software does allow for conversation archiving, it is typically turned off by default. Therefore, conversations of this nature typically exist in the volatile memory space of RAM.

Recall that RAM is termed *volatile* because it holds data only while the computer has power. Unplugging the computer will cause the data located in RAM to be lost. If, however, chat or instant message conversations occurred that are relevant as evidence, even if the computer was turned off, thus erasing the data in RAM, all may not be lost. Remember that there is an interaction between the computer system's RAM and the HDD. RAM is a commodity, and therefore the computer's operating system makes an effort to conserve it as much as possible. This is done by swapping/paging that information back and forth into the swap space or paging file. Therefore, remnants of chat conversations are often found in the swap space or paging file during a forensic examination of the HDD. These remnants, however, are typically fragmented, disconnected, and incomplete. Therefore, if the chat or instant message is still present on the screen (and thus probably still in RAM), the investigator needs a method by which to preserve and collect it.

A detailed discussion of capturing volatile data from RAM is beyond the scope of this chapter, but considerations for dealing with a live (running) computer have been discussed in the section titled "Live Computer Acquisition." Note that several commercial forensic software packages can capture this data. Similarly, Linux-based tools can accomplish this as well. The examiner may even be able to export the data remotely to another device. Regardless of the method, the data must be acquired.

Furthermore, many programs such as AOL Instant Messenger, Yahoo! Messenger, and mIRC (Internet Relay Chat) create files regarding the rooms or channels a user chatted in or the screen names with which a user sent instant messages. Each application should be researched, and the computer forensic examination should be guided by an understanding of how each functions.

WEBEXTRA 19.1
Follow the Trail of an E-Mail as It Travels Through the Internet

Hacking

Unauthorized computer intrusion, more commonly referred to as **hacking**, is the concern of every computer administrator. Hackers penetrate computer systems for a number of reasons. Sometimes the motive is corporate espionage; other times it is merely for bragging rights within the hacker community. Most commonly, though, a rogue or disgruntled employee with some knowledge of the computer network is looking to cause damage. Whatever the motivation, U.S. corporations frequently turns to law enforcement to investigate and prosecute these cases.

Generally speaking, when investigating an unauthorized computer intrusion, investigators concentrate their efforts in three locations: *log files, volatile memory*, and *network traffic*. Logs typically document the IP address of the computer that made the connection. Logs can be located in several locations on a computer network. Most servers on the Internet track connections made to them through the use of logs. Additionally, the router (i.e., the device responsible for directing data) may contain log files detailing connections.

Similarly, devices known as **firewalls** may contain log files listing computers that were allowed (or that merely attempted) access to the network or an individual system. Firewalls are devices (taking the form of either hardware or software) that permit only requested traffic to enter a computer system or, more appropriately, a network. In other words, if a user didn't send out a request for Internet traffic from a specific system, the firewall should block its entry unless previously configured to allow that traffic through. If the log files have captured the IP address of the intruder, then revealing the user behind the IP is the same process as for e-mail. Investigating a computer intrusion, however, does get a bit more complicated.

Frequently, in cases of unlawful access to a computer network, the perpetrator attempts to cover the tracks of their IP address. In these instances, advanced investigative techniques may be necessary to discover the hacker's true identity. When an intrusion is in progress, the investigator may have to capture volatile data, or data in RAM. The data in RAM at the time of an intrusion may provide valuable clues to the identity of the intruder or, at least, about the intruder's method or tools of attack. As in the case of an instant message or chat conversation, the data in RAM has to be acquired.

Another standard tactic for investigating intrusion cases is to document all programs installed and running on a system in order to discover any additional malicious software installed

hacking
A slang term frequently used to refer to performing an unauthorized computer or network intrusion.

firewall
Hardware or software designed to protect intrusions into an Internet network.

by the perpetrator to facilitate entry. The investigator uses specialized software to document running processes, registry entries, open ports, and any installed files.

Additionally, the investigator may want to capture live network traffic as part of the evidence-collection and investigation process. Traffic that travels the network does so in the form of data packets. In addition to data, these packets also contain source and destination IP addresses. If the attack requires two-way communication, as in the case of a hacker stealing data, then data has to be transmitted back to the hacker's computer using the destination IP address. Once this is learned, the investigation can focus on that system. However, care must be taken to ensure that the destination IP address does not belong to an unwitting and previously compromised computer under the control of the hacker. Moreover, the type of data that is being transmitted on the network may be a clue to what type of attack is being launched; whether any important data is being stolen; or what types of malicious software, if any, are involved in the attack.

Mobile Forensics

This section could just as well be titled "Cell Phone Forensics," but because of the technological advances in mobile technology, handheld devices are much more than just phones. There truly has been cross-pollination between traditional computers and cell phones. In addition to

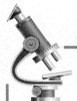

Inside the Science

Mobile Services

The following is a list of the more common services available on today's mobile devices, along with several examples of the potential evidentiary value they hold:

1. *Short Message Service (SMS)—Text Messaging* Text messages are another form of communication. They can be used to establish a link between two people simply by showing they have "messaged" each other. There have been cases where a person has entered a business to commit robbery while a lookout remains in a vehicle parked outside, and text messages were used to communicate between the two.
2. *Multimedia Message Service (MMS)* Can be thought of as text messaging with attachments such as video clips, sound files, or pictures. In one particular case, an individual took a video of himself sexually assaulting an incapacitated girl and then sent the video clip to friends via MMS.
3. *Contact Lists and Call History* The names, phone numbers, addresses, and/or e-mail addresses of people who are associated with the owner of the mobile device and the log of recent contacts he

or she has had are generally available and are of use in an investigation.
4. *Calendars, Appointments, and Tasks* This information may provide evidence of a suspect's actions on a particular date.
5. *Internet Access/Internet History/Internet Communication* Much as on a traditional computer, Internet activity on a mobile device can be of great evidentiary value. For example, it may link a suspect to a specific social networking site or screen name in a child sexual exploitation case. Often, mobile devices contain the same Internet artifacts as computers, such as cookies, browser history, and bookmarks.
6. *Digital Camera/Video* There have been numerous cases where individuals have exploited this technology to take surreptitious, candid photographs of unsuspecting women in malls and stores.
7. *E-Mail* Full e-mail access and clients (i.e., e-mail software) are available on most mobile devices, offering another source of potential evidence.
8. *Global Positioning System (GPS) and Map Data* Many devices, such as the Droid and iPhone, offer full GPS capabilities. The information in these applications can be extremely valuable in documenting the travel history of a suspect.

traditional cell phone services, mobile devices offer many services that are offered by computers and other devices. These devices can provide a vast amount of useful and evidentiary data in an investigation.

The list of services available for mobile devices, although comprehensive, is certainly not exhaustive. It should be apparent, however, that aside from size and structure, little distinction can be made between the services offered by a computer system and those of a mobile device. As such, forensic examinations of mobile devices have much in common with computer forensics, at least in principle. Although there is a great deal of standardization in the computer market, the same is not true in the world of mobile devices. The operating systems that run mobile devices vary from manufacturer to manufacturer and device to device. Moreover, their inherent remote capabilities and constant connection and communication with service providers make collection and preservation difficult.

Recall from our early discussion that one of the principal goals in electronic evidence collection and analysis is to avoid alteration of data. With mobile devices, which are constantly registering their location with the service provider and potentially receiving GPS location updates, protecting against alteration is challenging. Compounded by the fact that many mobile devices offer remote kill and clear capabilities, investigators have their hands full. It may seem logical to merely shut the mobile device off to preserve data, but this is typically not recommended because it can clear out unsaved data existing in volatile memory (much like a computer's RAM contents).

Leaving the mobile device running but placing it in something that will block its communication is the preferred method. A Faraday shield is frequently used for mobile device evidence collection. Such a shield, often designed by mobile forensics manufacturers, will prevent the device from communicating (in or out) with the service provider. It has also been observed that other devices, such as the type of unlined paint can typically used for collecting arson-related evidence, can work as well. However, the effectiveness of alternatives should be tested in advance.

Another consideration in the collection of these devices is maintaining power so that the device can be transported, stored, and ultimately analyzed. Mobile forensics manufacturers provide battery devices that can be used to keep a unit running while it is being transported to the lab. The investigator, if possible, should always seize the mobile device's charger and any associated cables. Because of the lack of standardization mentioned earlier, chargers and cables vary greatly between devices, and it is nearly impossible for examiners to stock every one.

Ultimately, data from the mobile device must be extracted and analyzed. Unlike computer forensics, however, the approach to mobile devices is more complicated. This complication arises because of the divergent ways that different devices store and manage data. Moreover, manufacturers vary in the type of memory used to store data, involving a combination of expansion cards and internal memory structures (RAM/ROM). Similarly, operating systems vary between devices. The Motorola Droid, for example, uses Google's Android operating system, while today's iPhone uses Apple's iPhone operating system, typically referred to as iOS. The two vary in their partition, file, and directory structure. These are just two of the overwhelming number of devices on the market and thus encountered by investigators. Consequently, mobile device examiners need a multitude of equipment and a significant amount of knowledge.

There are numerous approaches to mobile forensics data extraction and analysis. Extraction of data can be done on the physical level, generally affording the greatest amount of total data collection but also, at times, presenting challenges in analysis. Extraction can also be done on a logical level, which limits the data acquired, but the data is often easier to analyze. The examiner generally makes these determinations based on the type of case, the evidence sought, their own training, and the technological limitations of the mobile device or the tools available for analysis. It is the experience of most mobile forensic examiners that a lab must be equipped with several varied tools for acquisition and analysis.

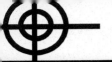

Chapter Summary >>>>>>>>>>>

Computers have permeated society and are used in countless ways with innumerable applications. Similarly, the role of electronic data in investigative work has realized exponential growth in the last decade. Users of computers and other electronic data storage devices leave footprints and data trails behind. Computer forensics involves the preservation, acquisition, extraction, analysis, and interpretation of computer data. In today's world of technology, many devices are capable of storing data and could thus be grouped into the field of computer forensics.

The central processing unit (CPU) is the brain of the computer—the main chip responsible for doing the actual computing. Random-access memory (RAM) is volatile memory containing data that is forever lost when the power is turned off. Programs are loaded into RAM because of its faster read speed. The hard disk drive (HDD) is typically the primary location of data storage within the computer. Different operating systems map out HDDs differently, and examiners must be familiar with the file system they are examining. Evidence exists in many different locations and in numerous forms on an HDD. This evidence can be grouped into two major categories: visible and latent data.

Visible data is data that the operating system is aware of and consequently is easily accessible to the user. From an evidentiary standpoint, it can encompass any type of user-created data, such as word-processing documents, spreadsheets, accounting records, databases, and pictures. Temporary files, created by programs as a sort of backup on the fly, can also prove valuable as evidence. Finally, data in the swap space (used to conserve the valuable RAM within the computer system) can yield evidentiary visible data.

Latent data, on the other hand, is data that the operating system typically is not aware of. Evidentiary latent data can exist in both RAM slack and file slack. RAM slack is the area from the end of the logical file to the end of the sector. File slack is the remaining area from the end of the final sector containing logical data to the end of the cluster. Another area where latent data may be found is in unallocated space. Unallocated space is space on an HDD that the operating system sees as empty and ready for data. The constant shuffling of data through deletion, defragmentation, and swapping is one of the ways data is orphaned in latent areas. Finally, when a user deletes files, the data typically remains behind. Deleted files are therefore another source of latent data to be examined during forensic analysis.

Investigators seeking a history of an Internet user's destinations can take advantage of the fact that computers store or cache portions of web pages visited, and websites often create cookies to track certain information about website visitors. An investigator tracking the origin of an e-mail seeks out the sender's IP address in the e-mail's header. Chat and instant messages are typically located in a computer's RAM. Finding the origin of unauthorized computer intrusions (hacking) requires investigation of a computer's log file, RAM, and network traffic, among other things.

Mobile devices offer many of the services that are offered by computers and other devices. These devices can provide a vast amount of useful and evidentiary data in an investigation. Leaving a mobile device running but placing it in something that will block its communication is the preferred method for preserving data on a mobile device. Complications arise in extracting and evaluating data from mobile devices because of the variety of ways that different devices store and manage data.

Review Questions

1. Computer forensics involves the _____, _____, _____, _____, and _____ of computer data.

2. True or False: Hardware comprises the physical components of the computer. _____

3. _____ is a set of instructions compiled into a program that performs a particular task.

4. (ROM, RAM) chips store programs used to start the boot process.

5. The term used to describe the chassis, including the motherboard and any other internal components of a personal computer, is _____.

6. True or False: The motherboard is a complex network of wires that carry data from one hardware device to another. _____

7. True or False: The first thing you should do when you encounter a computer system in a forensic investigation is to connect the power supply and boot the system. _____

8. RAM is referred to as volatile memory because it is not _____.

9. The brain of the computer is referred to as the _____.

10. The _____ is the primary component of storage in a personal computer.

11. Personal computers typically communicate with each other through a(n) _____.

12. The computer's _____ permits the user to manage files and applications.

13. A hard drive's partitions are typically divided into _____, _____, _____, and _____.

14. A(n) _____ is a single one or zero in the binary system and the smallest term in the language of computers.

15. A(n) _____ is a group of eight bits.

16. A group of sectors, always units in multiples of two, is called a(n) _____.

17. An exact duplicate of the entire contents of a hard disk drive is known as a(n) _____.

18. All data readily available to a computer user is known as _____ data.

19. A(n) _____ file is created when data is moved from RAM to the hard disk drive to conserve space.

20. Most programs automatically save a copy of a file being worked on into a(n) _____ file.

21. The existence of _____ data is why a forensic image of the media is created.

22. The smallest unit of addressable space on a hard disk drive is the _____.

23. The two types of slack space are _____ slack and _____ slack.

24. _____ slack is the area from the end of the data portion of the file to the end of the sector.

25. The portion of a disk that does not contain stored data is called _____.

26. True or False: Defragmenting a hard disk drive involves moving noncontiguous data back together. _____

27. True or False: A portion of a "deleted" file may be found in a computer's unallocated space. _____

28. A(n) _____ takes the form of a series of numbers to route data to an appropriate location on the Internet.

29. A user's hard disk drive will _____ portions of web pages that have been visited.

30. A(n) _____ is placed on a hard disk drive by a website to track certain information about its visitors.

31. E-mails have the _____ address of the sender in the header portion of the mail.

32. True or False: Chat and instant messages conducted over the Internet are typically stored in RAM storage. _____

33. When investigating a hacking incident, investigators concentrate their efforts on three locations: _____, _____, and _____.

34. Devices that permit only requested traffic to enter a computer system are known as _____.

35. A(n) _____ is a device that can prevent a mobile phone from communicating with a service provider.

36. True or False: Extracting and analyzing data from mobile devices is complicated because manufacturers of these devices store and manage data in a variety of ways. _____

Application and Critical Thinking

1. If a file system defines a cluster as six sectors, how many bits of information can be stored on each cluster? Explain your answer.

2. Criminalist Tom Parauda is investigating the scene of a crime involving a computer. After he arrives, he photographs the overall scene and takes close-up shots of all the connections to the single computer involved, as well as photos of the serial numbers of the computer and all peripheral devices. Tom then labels the cord to each peripheral device, then disconnects them from the computer. After making sure that all data in RAM has been saved to the hard disk drive, he unplugs the computer from the wall. What mistakes, if any, did Tom make?

3. You are investigating a case in which an accountant is accused of keeping fraudulent books for a firm. Upon examining his computer, you notice that the suspect uses two different accounting programs that are capable of reading the same types of files. Given this information, where would you probably begin to search for latent data on the computer and why?

4. You are examining two computers to determine the IP address from which several threatening e-mails were sent. The first computer uses Microsoft Outlook as an e-mail client and the second uses a web-based e-mail client. Where would you probably look first for the IP addresses in each of these computers?

Further References

Digital Evidence in the Courtroom: A Guide for Law Enforcement and Prosecutors. Washington, D.C.: National Institute of Justice, 2007, http://www.nij.gov/pubs-sum/211314.htm

Electronic Crime Scene Investigation: A Guide for First Responders, 2nd ed. Washington, D.C.: National Institute of Justice, 2008, https://www.ncjrs.gov/pdffiles1/nij/219941.pdf

Forensic Examination of Digital Evidence: A Guide for Law Enforcement. Washington, D.C.: National Institute of Justice, 2004, https://www.ncjrs.gov/pdffiles1/nij/199408.pdf

Chapter 20

Mobile Device Forensics

Peter Stephenson, Ph.D.

KEY TERMS

analog
architecture
broadband
CDMA (Code Division Multiple Access)
file system
geolocation
GSM (Global System for Mobile Communication)
GPS (Global Positioning System)
logical extraction
operating system (OS)
physical extraction
SIM (Subscriber Identification Module) card
SD (Secure Digital) card
SMS (Short Message Service)
Wi-Fi

Learning Objectives

After studying this chapter, you should be able to:

20.1   Identify the types of computing devices categorized as "mobile devices"

20.2   Explain the forensic challenges in examining mobile devices in comparison with personal computers

20.3   Explain the two procedures used to extract useful data from mobile devices

20.4   Explain the architecture of mobile devices that provides forensically valuable artifacts

20.5   Describe the types of evidence that can be found on mobile devices and how it is recovered

20.6   Explain how mobile devices fit into a digital investigation

Dr. Peter Stephenson, a cybercriminologist and educator with 50 years of technology experience, has written, edited, or contributed to 18 books and several hundred articles in major national and international trade, technical, and scientific publications. Dr. Stephen-son joined On Point Cyber after retiring from Norwich University where he served as an associate professor teaching network attack and defense, digital forensics, and cyber investigation at both the graduate and undergraduate levels. He also served as the Chief Information Security Officer for the University and Director of the Norwich University Center for Advanced Computing and Digital Forensics. Dr. Stephenson has received the Distinguished Faculty Award in the College of Graduate and Continuing Studies. He holds one of the first PhDs in the world in digital investigation and was one of the first recipients of the prestigious Certified Cyber Forensics Professional designation from (ISC). In addition, he holds the CISSP and CISM designations and is a member of the American Academy of Forensic Sciences and the Vidocq Society. He holds a master's degree in diplomacy with a concentration in terrorism.

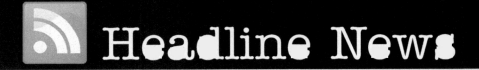

Michelle Carter: The Texting Suicide Case

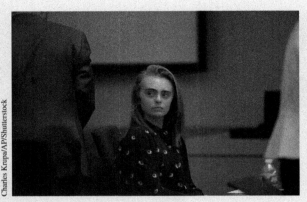

On Sunday, July 13, 2014, 18-year-old Conrad Roy was found dead of carbon monoxide poisoning. When police began investigating the circumstances surrounding his death, they uncovered a series of text messages between Roy and his long distance girlfriend, Michelle Carter. From at least July 6 to July 12, 2014, Carter counseled him to overcome his doubts, devised a plan to run a combustion engine within his truck in order to poison him with carbon monoxide, and by directed him to go back in his truck after he exited it when he became frightened that the plan was working.

She told him that he was "strong" enough to execute the suicide plan and that he would be happy once he was dead. In a text to Conrad, she wrote that he would go "straight to heaven guided by God." Conrad replied: "And I will be happy again." Carter wrote: "Yes, you will, (smiley face)...there is no way you can fail ... You're strong ... I love you to the moon and back and deeper than the ocean and higher than the pines, too, babe, forever and always. It's painless and quick." Below are excerpts of text messages exchanged between Michelle Carter and Conrad Roy on the day that he died:

CONRAD: Like, why am I so hesitant lately. Like two weeks ago I was willing to try everything and now I'm worse, really bad, and I'm LOL not following through. It's eating me inside.

CARTER: You're so hesitant because you keeping over thinking it and keep pushing it off. You just need to do it, Conrad. The more you push it off, the more it will eat at you. You're ready and prepared. All you have to do is turn the generator on and you will be free and happy. No more pushing it off. No more waiting.

CONRAD: You're right.

CONRAD: I don't know. I'm freaking out again. I'm over thinking.

CARTER: I thought you wanted to do this. This time is right and you're ready. You just need to do it. You can't keep living this way. You just need to do it like you did the last time and not think about it and just do it, babe. You can't keep doing this every day.

CONRAD: I do want to but I'm like freaking for my family I guess. I don't know.

CARTER: Conrad, I told you I'll take care of them. Everyone will take care of them to make sure they won't be alone and people will help them get through it. We talked about this and they will be okay and accept it. People who commit suicide don't think this much. They just could do it.

CONRAD: I'm ready.

CARTER: Good because it's time, babe. You know that. When you get back from them (sic) beach you've gotta go do it. You're ready. You're determined. It's the best time to do it.

CONRAD: Okay, I will.

CARTER: Are you back?

CONRAD: No more thinking.

CARTER: Yes. No more thinking. You need to just do it. No more waiting.

CONRAD: I don't know. I'm stressing.

CARTER: You're fine. It's gonna be okay. You just gotta do it, babe. You can't think about it.

CONRAD: Okay. Okay. I got this.

CARTER: Yes, you do. I believe in you. Did you delete the messages?

CONRAD: Yes. But you're going to keep messaging me.

CARTER: I will until you turn on the generator.

Michelle Carter was charged and convicted of involuntary manslaughter in the death of Conrad Roy and sentenced to 15 months in prison.

Of all of the areas of digital forensics, mobile device forensics may be the most complicated. It is complicated for several reasons. First, there is a huge number—growing daily—of mobile devices. Second, these devices often have little in common, even those from the same manufacturer. Additionally, the proliferation of mobile devices as substitutes for full-size or laptop computers is significant and increasing rapidly. Finally, these devices are an amalgam of radio and computing technologies and may in some cases be treated differently under the law. The forensics involved certainly is complicated by this paradigm.

Mobile devices began as an outgrowth of ship-to-shore radios in the Second World War. Additionally, handheld radio transceivers, or walkie-talkies, were available then, and they evolved into mobile phones for cars in the 1940s. The real explosion in mobile devices came much later. Before that, we saw the Motorola handheld phone debuting in 1973. From that point on, advances in cellular technology enabled the mobile phone boom that followed. Early mobile phone systems were **analog** (1G). They were followed by digital networks (2G).

When mobile **broadband** networks (3G) arrived on the scene in Japan in 2001, the mobile device landscape changed forever. Now, it was possible to do much more than talk on a cell phone. Now, the cell phone had the possibility of behaving like a small computer and could transfer data—at Internet speeds. The smartphone was born. When native IP networks arrived (4G), the smartphone became a node on the Internet just like any other computing device. With the proliferation of **Wi-Fi** networking, smartphones evolved into tablets, and products such as the iPad became viable substitutions for small computers.

The Mobile Device Neighborhood: What Makes a Mobile Device "Mobile"?

We start with the notion of cellular systems. A *cellular system* is a network of relatively short-distance transceivers that are spaced strategically so that low-power transmitters can reach the phones in their coverage areas and the very-low-power transmitters in the cell phones can reach the cell tower. Since the 1960s, the concepts of *handoff* and *frequency reuse* allowed users to move between cells without dropping a call. Usually, as we will see, 1G networks suffered from this problem, much to the consternation of their users. Figure 20–1 shows the layout of cell towers and their coverage areas. Although there is overlap as indicated by the red circles, the transmitting patterns are hexagonal because of the transmission patterns of the tower's antenna array.

Returning to the early (1G) analog phones, we have several issues that laid the groundwork for modern mobile devices. Some of these are still with us and can bedevil the forensic examiner. 1G networks are analog. That means that they behave in exactly the same way as older radio stations behave. A mobile device is made up of a computer and one or more radios. The computer may be quite primitive and the radios may communicate with a network of some type. Because cellular networks are much different from Wi-Fi networks, devices that communicate with both need two radios. 1G devices usually could communicate only with the cellular system.

Digital (2G) cellular networks appeared in the 1990s using two standards: **GSM (Global System for Mobile Communications)** and **CDMA (Code Division Multiple Access)**. This new generation moved phones into the small, handheld form, and, because they were digital, the new networks opened the door for practical data communications and the beginning of what was referred to as "feature phones." These phones had more features than simply being

analog
The traditional method of modulating radio signals so that they can carry information.

broadband
A communication channel that can provide higher-speed data communication than a standard telephone circuit.

Wi-Fi
A term describing a wireless local area network.

GSM (Global System for Mobile Communication)
A set of standards for second-generation cellular networks.

CDMA (Code Division Multiple Access)
A spread-spectrum technology for cellular networks.

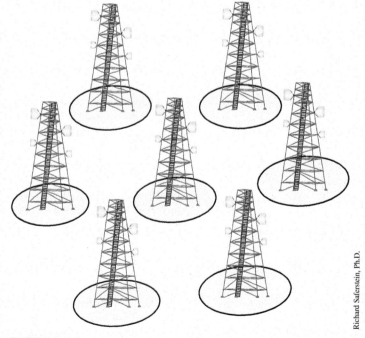

FIGURE 20–1

Cell tower geographic configuration.

Richard Saferstein, Ph.D.

able to make and receive phone calls, hence the name. Feature phones could send and receive SMS (text) messages, synchronize with e-mail, and provide other features that were heading the mobile device genre in the direction of smartphones and tablets.

Communications were slow, however, and such things as surfing the web and transferring photos were not particularly practical. Smaller radios were, however, practical because of the increased density of cell tower installations, and that saved battery life, further reducing the physical size of the phones.

Mobile broadband (3G) data opened the floodgates for mobile communications and, thus, the explosion of mobile devices on the market. The architectural functionality that distinguishes 2G from 3G is that 2G systems were circuit switched and 3G systems are packet switched. Without delving too deeply into the technical differences between the two, we may say that, fundamentally, circuit switching is similar to landline telephone systems and packet switching is like the Internet. Indeed, one of the benefits of packet switching is the ability to connect more readily to the Internet.

The advent of packet-switched mobile phone networks allowed virtually any kind of data to be accessed by the mobile device, and the smartphone was born. Moving photos over the network, streaming video and television, video chat, and other advanced services now could be supported. 3G was launched in Japan in 2001.

Native IP (4G) networks differ technologically from 3G networks in that they access the Internet directly, increasing speed and bandwidth dramatically. With 4G, virtually any form of communication possible with a PC was now possible from a smartphone or tablet. The age of the mobile device was now in full swing.

Forensic Challenges: Mobile Devices as Small Computers—Sort Of

Modern mobile devices are, in many respects, little more than small PCs. However, they do have some unique aspects that complicate the digital forensic process a bit. Let's begin by going back to those 1G devices. They still exist in some parts of the world and even with die-hard users in the United States in regions where 1G networks still exist. While those are extremely rare, the more common occurrence is getting a 1G phone tied to a 15-year-old crime. The problem with these old devices is that they do not have the capabilities that we are used to with a computer. Virtually none have what we would classify as an **operating system (OS)**, and about the most you can hope to get off them is the phone directory. Some may keep a call log, but the number of calls retained is fairly small. Anything that has been deleted is no longer available. Unlike many OSs, we are unable to recover deleted material.

When we get to 2G, the ballgame changes considerably. These phones still exist, mostly with people who are satisfied with their limited capabilities and who live in a 2G network area. The capabilities of these phones, while considerably fewer than smartphones, are well ahead of 1G phones, and most of the 2G devices have real OSs. Mostly these OSs are custom designed for the phones—such as Palm and BlackBerry—but in some cases they are the forerunners of smartphone OSs.

Some 2G phones, such as feature phones, come closer to smartphones than others. However, the ability to recover deleted messages, for example, varies significantly from phone model to model. However, just because a phone has an OS does not mean that the OS is the same as a PC's. While the OS performs many of the same functions as that of a PC, it does not necessarily follow that it performs them in the same way or, in many cases, even as well. The most popular OSs for mobile devices—including phones and tablets—are Apple iOS, Google Android, and Microsoft Windows Phone OS. Primitive versions of these were widely available for 2G devices.

Some had other features, but the higher the bandwidth requirement, the poorer these devices performed. From a forensic perspective, it is a toss-up as to how much data you will be able to extract from a 2G device. More important, during this time, the manufacturers of mobile devices started to go wild with new product releases. The problem with that was—and still is—that even

operating system (OS)
A custom-designed program that controls the components of mobile devices and facilitates how they function.

if two phones looked a lot alike, had the same functionality, and used the same OS, there was no guarantee that they were the same, and if your mobile device forensic tool did not have a driver specifically designed for that particular phone, you were out of luck forensically. This continues to be the single most difficult issue plaguing mobile device forensics: it is nearly impossible to stay current with the available mobile device models.

3G and 4G phones are the closest in **architecture** and design to a PC. They behave the same way—especially 4G devices—and they have the ability to download and install applications ("apps") the same as any PC or Mac. They are the same in architectural issues such as processors and file systems, but the nature of those architectures are different between mobile devices and computers. This is because mobile devices have special requirements such as multiple radios (Wi-Fi and 4G, for example), size restrictions, and storage space. Apps are both a boon and a devilment to the forensic examiner. Apps each have their own specific operating parameters, and how they communicate with the outside—*if* they communicate—is inconsistent from app to app. Apple has taken major steps to standardize the development of apps for its iPad and iPhone, but Android apps are far less constrained. Furthermore, just because an app is written for the iOS OS does not mean that it runs equally well or behaves the same on iPad and iPhone. In that regard Android apps are a bit less forgiving.

For the forensic analyst, understanding what is running on the mobile device under examination is a key issue, and one that is nontrivial to figure out. Once the examiner understands what is running, it is equally difficult to figure out what the app is doing and how it is interacting with the user and the outside. One interesting aspect of mobile device forensics is **geolocation**. Some devices and many apps report out the geographical location of the device (see Figure 20–2). That can make it much easier to track the owner's movements.

Additionally, mobile devices that offer geolocation include not just smartphones and tablets, but we also can analyze **GPS (Global Positioning System)** devices such as Garmin or TomTom. However, special tools and drivers are required, as with other mobile devices, and GPS units are becoming as prolific and ever-changing as smartphones and tablets.

Another forensic challenge with phones, particularly, is the chipset used to build the phone. This adds another variable to the mix along with OS, model, manufacturer, and apps.

architecture
The basic components of a mobile device.

geolocation
Assessment of the actual geographical location of a mobile device.

GPS (Global Positioning System)
A system for determining position by comparing radio signals from several satellites.

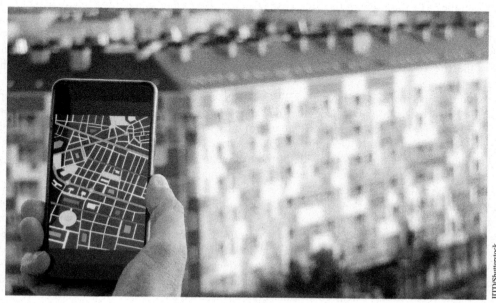

FIGURE 20–2
Representation of geolocation using a mobile device.

The chipset is the hardware that makes the device work. Today, there is quite a large number of chipsets, and the most difficult to deal with are knock-offs of American chips manufactured in China. Not all of these behave the same as American chips, and special driver sets for mobile device forensic tools are required.

The big problem, of course, is that even though some of these devices are really small computers with computer-like OSs, they usually cannot be examined using typical computer forensic tools. Each device has its own quirks, and each device needs special connectors and special device drivers on the tool that is examining it to decipher what is on the device's storage. Device storage also takes several forms, such as onboard nonvolatile memory and mini-SD cards that add storage in a modern smartphone or tablet. This does not include devices that predate the computer-like architectures. They need special drivers and connectors as well, but the amount of information that can be gleaned from them is much less because the amount of information they store is much less.

Extracting Useful Data: The Differences in Various Types of Mobile Devices

When working on a mobile device, the investigator has several sources of information available. Probably the most useful is web searching. Doing a search on the phone model often reveals a wealth of information such as other investigators' experiences, battery charging techniques (discussed momentarily), and what can and cannot be recovered if it was deleted. Some phones and tablets are fairly modern and rather straightforward. With those, connection to the forensic tool and extraction are fairly simple to do. But some devices—both very old and very new—are not so obvious. Some research before connecting is important. All mobile devices should be kept in a Faraday bag or box. This prevents changes from being made to the device remotely. These changes might be initiated by the owner of the device, such as a remote wipe to preserve a picture of innocence by destroying evidence, or unintentional, such as changes made by the device's carrier that could overwrite evidence. The efficacy of Faraday enclosures has been debated by experts, but the consensus still is to use them.

physical extraction
A duplicate of data located on a mobile device.

logical extraction
A snapshot of the file system of a mobile device.

So, the examiner's first step is to determine what they are working with. Is it a very old feature phone, a typical iPad or iPhone, or a state-of-the-art, just-announced-last-week smartphone? The examiner must do a little research, select a tool, and then make the next decision: physical or logical extraction (or both)? Just as with computers, **physical extraction** is the best bet. Physical forensic images are bit-by-bit copies of the file system (discussed later), including deleted data. **Logical extraction** is a snapshot of the file system showing what the file system wants the user to see. Here, the examiner gets the same view that the user gets.

Some tools, such as Cellebrite's UFED Touch, are quite clear about which devices support physical extraction. For a device that supports physical extraction, that is the way to image the device. Logical extractions are useful only when the physical option is not available because of the device itself. On some cell phones, an exchange of text messages may hold evidence in a murder. However, one side of the exchange may be missing—obviously someone deleted it—and because of the architecture of the phone, retrieving the deleted messages is not possible. The only solution is to acquire the other phone in the conversation and extract it from that phone. If that phone is not available, the examiner is left with a tantalizing snippet that may include evidence—or not.

Tools such as UFED and MPE+ greatly simplify analysis. And these are not the only available tools for mobile device analysis. Others include Parabin's product, Device Seizure, a forensic tool that started mobile device analysis and an excellent tool by Oxygen. When selecting a tool for mobile device forensics, one should look at the field and pick more than one, in the same way that most digital forensic labs use more than one computer forensic tool.

Mobile device forensic analysis can provide an overlay to physical evidence and timelines as well as computer forensic timelines to give a clearer picture of the events preceding and following a crime event. However, the efficacy with which the examiner can gather this information depends a lot on the generation of mobile device being tested. Technological capabilities vary widely from first- through fourth-generation devices, though third- and fourth-generation devices tend to have a lot of power.

When you analyze the device, be sure to follow the recommendations of the tool you are using for analysis. Do an Internet search to learn as much about the device make and model as you can before attempting acquisition and analysis if you are unfamiliar with the specific device.

YouTube has a remarkable number of videos that show detailed step-by-step procedures for device disassembly. Special tools may be required. Working on a carpeted surface often raises the danger of static electricity. That can damage the chips in a device. It may be wise to wear a grounded antistatic wristband when working on a mobile device, especially if disassembly will be required.

When the examiner has identified the device and the procedures to extract its data, the next step is to run the tools and take a forensic image. Examiners make it a practice to run the imager twice, taking one of the images and treating it as evidence. The other is the working image. This ensures that if necessary, the examiner can make another copy of the evidence original as a new work copy if the working copy is inadvertently damaged.

Logical images are fairly fast for most devices, depending on how much memory the device has and how much of the memory is full. Physical images can take a very long time to make because on a large storage device, even if the storage is not full, the imager must look at the entire memory footprint, not just the part that has something save to it. The examiner should decide, based on what can be done for the particular device, whether to obtain a physical or logical extraction or both. The logical extraction is fairly fast, and one may want to examine it for obvious evidence while the tool is making a physical image of the target.

It's important that the examiner select the proper connector—or "pigtail"—for the device from his or her tool kit.

Inside the Science

Analysis of Submerged Devices

Many people go to great lengths to conceal their mobile activity. Some even go as far as to physically destroying their phone altogether by submerging it in oil, drain cleaner, fuel, or some other flammable liquid. However, digital evidence can be very resilient, and digital forensics practitioners equipped with the right tools and knowledge can still find valuable information from a damaged smartphone.

A team of scientists from VTO Labs, which included interns from Marshall University's Forensic Science Graduate Program, studied the effects of submerging smartphones in different liquids. In their study, they submerged 49 phones, of the same model and operating system, in a variety of oil-based, flammable and clandestine chemical liquids for seven days. Their results showed that a full forensic image could still be extracted from all of them—even when circuit board components were severely corroded.

Even in the most severe case of physical damage—the drain cleaner trial—the team was able to image all 3,909,091,328 bytes of data on the phones, which is the same exact amount imaged before the phones were submerged. Trials of all other liquids yielded the same results. The other liquids were vegetable oil, new motor oil, used motor oil, regular gasoline, diesel fuel, kerosene heating oil, ammonia, and hydrogen peroxide.

Due to the damage to each phone's exterior and circuit board, researchers had to remove and repair the memory chips from the drain-cleaner-drenched devices, and take the data directly from the chips, a technique known as "chip-off." But before this, the devices were cleaned using specific methods—the methods that they determined to be most effective.

The lab had previously tested to see how digital evidence fared after devices were submerged in various types of water—including fresh water, salt water, tap water and chlorinated pool water—for varying amounts of time. In the previous study, the team had managed to extract data from phones submerged for as long as three years. They found that salt water was actually more damaging to phones than oil-based liquids, gasoline, or drain cleaner.

Mobile Device Architecture: What Is Inside the Device and What Is It Used For?

All mobile devices have an architecture. Just like computers, the architecture defines the basic components of the device. How and where is data stored? What kind of processor is used? What does the file system look like? Is there a formal file system? These and other questions form the basis of the analysis. Extraction is affected only if there is additional storage—such as an extra plug-in SD card—that must be analyzed. Most analysis tools acquire these add-in storage modules, but it is helpful to know which so data won't be missed.

SIMs and SDs

SD (Secure Digital) card
A storage expansion card for a mobile device.

SIM (Subscriber Identification Module) card
The card that is inserted into a mobile device that identifies the user account to the network, handles authentication, and provides storage for basic user data and network information.

SD (Secure Digital) cards are storage expansion cards that many mobile devices can accept. The SD card adds memory for storing such things as photos and music. SD cards are *nonvolatile*, meaning that even if the power is turned off on the device, you won't lose your favorite tunes or your pictures of Great Aunt Susie just as she was going down the water slide at the local swimming pool (see Figure 20–3).

SIM (Subscriber Identification Module) cards are different. Each SIM has an international mobile subscriber identity (IMSI) number that associates the phone with the subscriber's mobile network. In many cases, you can keep all of your subscriber information when you change mobile phones simply by switching the SIM to the new phone. SIMs may also store text messages and other user data as well as the user's phone book and the phone number of the device. Not all mobile devices use SIMs. The information on the SIM may be stored in the device itself. However, for forensic purposes, the examiner must be able to access that information because it is a way to identify the target device unambiguously during a forensic analysis.

Also on each SIM is the integrated circuit card identifier (ICCID). That number also is printed on the SIM. The ICCID contains the issuer identification number (IIN), the individual account identification, and a check digit. The forensic image of the mobile device is acquired and the tool will extract and record the ICCID. That is usually the way that the examiner identifies the phone, but if it is a SIM and not embedded in the mobile device, the examiner must bear in mind that he or she is seeing only the SIM and not necessarily the device itself. Figure 20–4 shows the SIM ready for placement in the cell phone. Note that this information is embedded in the tablet, not in an external card.

It often is desirable to clone the SIM in much the same way as one would take a physical image of the mobile device or a computer. By cloning the SIM, the investigator retains a perfect copy for evidentiary purposes. Some mobile device forensics vendors, such as AccessData, developer of the MPE+, provide forensic SIMs for use as targets to which the investigator may clone the evidence SIM for preservation.

In addition to memory, the typical mobile device contains a digital signal processor, a microprocessor, a radio frequency transmitter/receiver, audio components, and a power supply that

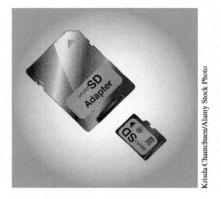

FIGURE 20–3
32 GB Micro SD Card (right) and adapter.

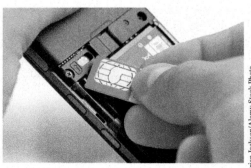

FIGURE 20–4
A SIM inserted in a cell phone.

Krisda Chamchuen/Alamy Stock Photo

Brian Jackson/Alamy Stock Photo

takes battery power to run the device as well as providing the ability to charge the battery. Thus, the mobile device is a simple radio transceiver with a few digital twists and turns that make it more like a computer in some regards.

This hybrid construction—a radio and a computer—means that forensic investigators must focus on the laws that cover both. In some regards, thinking from the computer side, they must be concerned about such things as privacy. From the radio side, there also are protections of which to be aware that vary greatly from jurisdiction to jurisdiction.

File Systems—or Not

To say that every mobile device has a **file system** is both correct and incorrect. Certainly, there needs to be a way to keep track of such things as phone books, but in some cases, the examiner is simply looking at a flat file database. A *flat file database* is a single file, usually human-readable, that contains some collection of data, in this case names and phone numbers. The earliest, most primitive mobile devices had such a file structure.

file system
A software mechanism that defines the way files are named, stored, organized, and accessed.

When we think of a file system, though, we usually think of some organized method of collecting files of various types and keeping track of them. In computers, we have file tables that track both the files in the file system and their physical location on the computer's hard drive. A real file system must be able to do those two things: track the logical location of the files on the device and tie them to the files' physical locations. More modern mobile devices do both of those things, sometimes with a proprietary file system and occasionally with a more open one.

Tracking the location of files, both physically and logically, is done with some sort of database. Sometimes the database is proprietary and tied to the file structure itself, and sometimes it is a standard database such as SQL Lite (SQLite). In either case, the analysis tool must know what file system structure the device uses, and it must know how to address files on the device both physically and logically. Extracting file information from such a data structure is critical to the analysis of mobile devices just as it is on computers. And the extraction and analysis are quite similar.

One important aspect of file system analysis is accessibility. Can the examiner access deleted files, for example? Is there some indication, as is the case with the Windows OS on a computer (in the link or .lnk files), that a file existed even if it has been deleted? The answer, unfortunately, is "maybe." As shown in Table 20–1, different types of OSs have different types of file systems, some more recoverable than others.

It may not be possible to recover deleted file items such as e-mails, texts, and photos from a mobile device. For example, BlackBerrys cannot be recovered directly. To recover deleted files, the examiner must go to the backup—usually on a PC somewhere—and recover from that. One can also recover from the BlackBerry server if available. Recovery of deleted items from iOS devices is somewhat easier, and tools such as Cellebrite's UFED can do that with a physical extraction. Androids are usually recoverable as well since they are, at heart, a form of the Linux OS.

Analyzing Mobile Devices: Finding Forensically Valuable Artifacts

The detailed analysis of mobile devices is a book in itself. There are so many different devices (between 50,000 and 100,000 by some counts) and multiple generations of devices that a full analysis addressing all of these possibilities is not attainable in a single chapter. As well, a detailed understanding of computer and mobile device architecture is necessary to grasp many of the finer points of analysis. It suffices here to discuss the process and give some examples that are at opposite ends of the mobile device spectrum. We have introduced the Apple iPad and the Samsung SCH R350.

TABLE 20–1

Example Mobile Device File Systems (Not Exhaustive)

BlackBerry	SQLite or MS exFAT
Android	Ext4, YAFFS, or vendor proprietary
iOS	HFSX

Let's start with our Samsung phone. The R350 is a feature phone popular around 2009. It had a lot of features but some, such as its music player, required an optional memory card. Overall, the R350 was a very good stepping-stone to today's smartphones if you deployed all of its features. The file system is EFS (encrypting file system). By looking at the Project Tree on the UFED extraction report, it's possible to find out if the user browsed the web and the history of web browsing. Further, by browsing down the Project Tree on the UFED extraction report, one may find folders associated with a phone book and calendar.

The iPhone is replete with data for one's perusal. The calendar is referred to as *Calendar* rather than *task list*. That is because *Calendar* is the phone's terminology and the UFED simply uses it for consistency.

In addition to the calendar, we can follow the project tree in the UFED report and see several other resources that our iPhone gives up to our analysis. There is a call log with details, chats including deleted messages, contacts including those who were recently contacted, cookies, **SMS (Short Message Service)** messages (texts), voice mails, and more. This is a veritable treasure trove of data on the phone's user and the user's behavior. But there is much more if we look a bit deeper. For example, it would be nice to take all of the phone's activities and place them on a timeline. Digital forensic investigations depend on timelines for their success. Indeed, when overlaid on the timelines of a physical crime, the timelines from mobile devices and computers provide an excellent yardstick by which to measure the play of events surrounding the crime itself. Because of the vast amount of data the iPhone 4S smartphone offers, we can create just such a timeline.

The UFED also provides us with the ability to analyze phone activity by caller, giving us incoming, outgoing, missed, and SMS (text) calls.

Another useful type of mobile device is the GPS. GPS can locate the user's activities and, when used with a timeline, can place the user in the vicinity of a crime. Timelines are the meat and potatoes of digital forensic investigations. Because computers and mobile devices have a fairly accurate clock, examiners can match the activities on these devices to physical crime activities to do a precrime, pericrime (during the crime event), and postcrime analysis of a suspect's behavior.

For example, with the Garmin nuvi 40 GPS, the UFED provides a timeline, but since this is a GPS the timeline is associated with a specific location. In addition to the timeline graph, there are specific entries noting where the GPS was located at a particular latitude and longitude at a particular time.

Following the track of locations using Google Maps and these coordinates is a straightforward way to track the progress of the GPS during some particular period of time. To make the tracking easier, the GPS provides a list of journeys, each with the coordinates of waypoints over the course of the trip. That can be correlated back to the timeline view for devices that have been used heavily, simplifying the tracking of the GPS on specific dates of interest.

SMS (Short Message Service) A cellular network facility that allows users to send and receive text messages.

Case File

The FBI v. Apple: The Encryption Dispute

In December, 2015, Syed Rizwan Farook and his wife Tashfeen Malik killed 14 people and injured 22 others in a mass shooting and attempted bombing attack at the Inland Regional Center in San Bernardino, California. The couple were killed in a shootout with the police shortly after their attack. Farook's work phone, an Apple iPhone 5C, was recovered intact. The phone had been locked with a four digit password. Two-month effort by the FBI to unlock the phone failed due to the phone's advanced encryption system. As a result, the FBI asked Apple, Inc. to create a version of the iPhone operating system to allow the FBI to disable certain security features. Apple declined citing its policy of never undermining the security systems of it products. The FBI then proceeded to have a court order issued requiring that Apple comply with the government's request. However, two months later, the FBI withdrew the request stating that it had unlocked the phone with the help of a third party.

The use of mobile devices are playing an increasing role in criminal investigations. In addition to the San Bernardino case, Apple has received at least 10 different requests from federal courts to extract data like contacts, photos and calls from locked iPhones. Apple has consistently objected to these requests taking the position that to make access easier for law enforcement will also make it easier for criminal hackers to access personal data placed on their customer's phone.

The standoff between Apple and the FBI is at the center of an escalating battle between technology companies that are encrypting data in order to safeguard their customers' privacy and government's desires to access encrypted data to secure criminal investigative information.

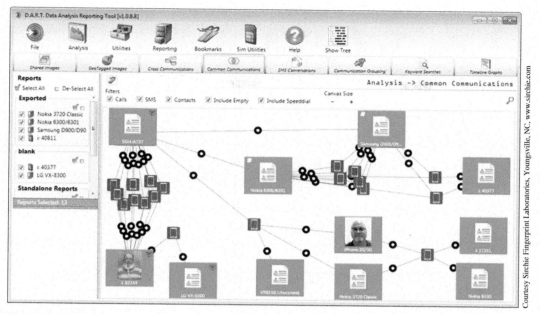

FIGURE 20–5

Graphic representation of communications between subjects and devices.

Additionally, the GPS provides a list of favorite destinations with their coordinates.

Software tools exist to aid in extracting and compiling information from various devices. These analytic aids sort the data and generate graphic interpretations that illustrate location, relationships, call records, geographical locations, timeline analysis, and other critical information (see Figures 20–5 to 20–8).

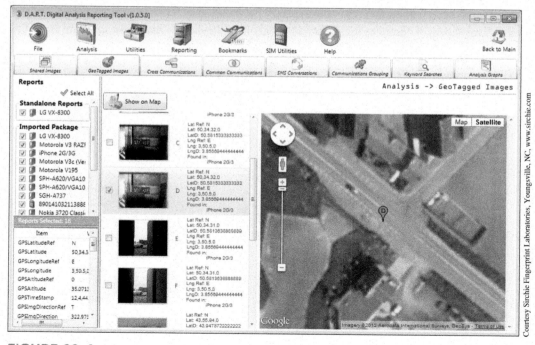

FIGURE 20–6

Locations of images GeoTagged in devices.

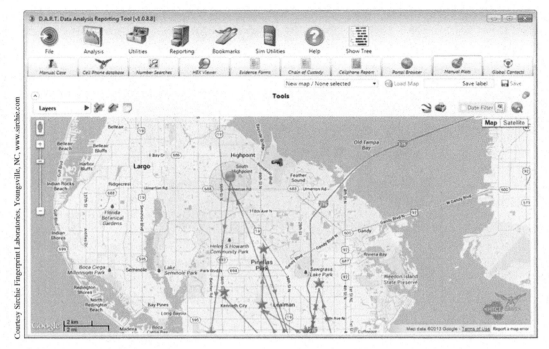

FIGURE 20–7

Mapping analysis from cell tower information showing locations for usage of a mobile device.

Hybrid Crime Assessment: Fitting the Mobile Device into the Digital Forensic Investigation

Now that we've gotten a look at how digital forensics is performed on mobile devices, it would be useful to fit that process into the investigative process as a whole. In any investigation, chain of evidence is very important. *Chain of evidence* (as opposed to *chain of custody*, which describes access to evidence) describes the events and concomitant evidence that make up the events of the

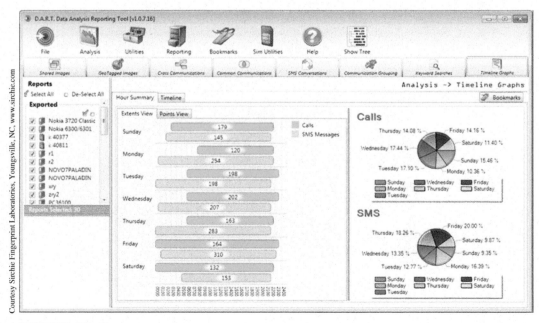

FIGURE 20–8

Timeline analysis calls and text messages between several mobile devices.

crime. There are two types of chains of evidence. *Temporal chains* show events in the order in time in which they occurred. This commonly is called a timeline and is the easiest way for lay-people, such as triers of fact, to visualize a crime, especially a complicated one.

Causal chains of evidence describe the events of a crime in terms of cause and effect. The links in the chain are the pieces of evidence, and they are tied together based upon how one link affects one or more other links. We could say that our first link causes the next link to occur, which in turn causes two other links—events—to happen, and so on, until the events of the crime fully describe the crime itself. For our purposes—and to keep this manageable—we will stick with the temporal chain. This is where a technique called *hybrid crime assessment* enters the picture.

Hybrid crime assessment is a technique that investigators can use when faced with a physical crime—such as murder, rape, or robbery—that has a digital element to it: a computer, a cell phone, or some other mobile device. The idea is to tie all of these elements together into a single crime scene and use the timelines to build a picture and describe the events, and supporting evidence, of the crime. This works very well. So well, in fact, that it has been used in at least one case to describe the last few minutes of a shooting victim's life when the closest physical event that could be corroborated occurred more than a half hour before the shooting and had nothing to do with the crime itself.

In that regard, it is important to recognize that there are events in the timeline that have little or nothing to do with the actual crime but can act as markers—rather like quarter-hour chimes on a clock that simply happen but do not play any role beyond marking time. In the case of the shooting, the activities of the victim on his computer ended moments before he was murdered. Given the physical crime scene and the position of the body, the activities surrounding his use of the computer were very important. They placed, with little question, the time of the event within an eight-minute period, which corroborated a witness account. They also allowed some level of description of the events immediately following the event, since the computer was turned back on after it had been shut down briefly.

This is a simplistic example of correlating the events of a physical crime with a timeline of events on a computer. In this case, the period of inactivity on the computer could be measured, and that timeline—very accurate since it was based upon the computer's clock—could be laid against the physical timeline to fill in gaps and corroborate witness accounts. When we add the dimension of a mobile device, which works in essentially the same manner as the computer for our purposes, we have a layered view of the timeline of an event and the pre-event and post-event elements/evidence that make up the layers. The mobile device is one of the layers and, in most cases, the most accurate one.

Mobile devices may be synchronized to the network clock. That means that the network provider—such as AT&T, Verizon, or T-Mobile—is sending the clock signal to the mobile device. Since the network provider is likely to use a time standard such as the U.S. Naval Observatory to obtain time signals, it is likely that the mobile device is extremely accurate as a yardstick for measuring when events happen. How the user behaves with the mobile device can be measured precisely against that yardstick.

Mobile devices, like most computers, perform various types of housekeeping. That means that the device is constantly doing things on its own to maintain its own operation. For example, it must continue to stay in contact with the mobile network (or the Wi-Fi network if it is set up to connect to one). It must make sure that all of its internal functions are working properly, so it is constantly testing parts of itself. When the device is in use, it does more. When it is in standby, it does less. When it is off, obviously, it does none. There are variations on that as well. For example, if you put the device in "airplane mode," the radio is off but the rest of the computer (in the phone) still is working. By checking logs, when they are present, we can see when the radio was turned off or on.

As we have seen, the amount of information that we can get from a mobile device varies greatly with the device. Unfortunately, most books that deal with mobile device forensics assume that the digital investigator will invariably encounter a fairly recent device. That means that the oldest devices are likely to be feature phones. That, as it turns out, is not a practical position to take. Feature phones of widely varying capabilities are generally available, and there are mobile phones that are little more than that: mobile phones. These and older phones often have very little to offer in the way of establishing timelines but should be examined in any event.

However, when a mobile device has information to give up, it can be extremely useful. For example, when a mobile device is set to use Wi-Fi, it will recognize any Wi-Fi network in its range. It may not be able to join the network because of the security settings on the Wi-Fi access point, but the mobile device will see it and note that it exists. When that happens, the device takes note of the network and logs it. This is a function of today's mobile devices such as smartphones, of course. The iPhone 4S can look at its timeline, expand it to get maximum resolution, and see, for example, that at 15:42:30 on 6/12/2012 the phone was in a Best Buy store. We see that because the timeline shows that it joined the Best Buy network at that time.

Taken with other evidence, such as GPS information, witness interviews, or the individual's own timeline as reported during an interview/interrogation, this becomes a good corroborator and may, in some cases, provide an alibi as well as it might otherwise place the individual near the crime scene. If one opts to take a bit more complicated look, the mobile device can be examined for everything happening on it at a particular time. Then the investigator can put all of the pieces together from both the mobile device logs—which are quite precise—and the physical evidence, which may not be as precise.

Inside the Science

What Is a StingRay?

A StingRay is an international mobile subscriber identity catcher (IMSI) device designed in 2013 by the Harris Corporation. This technology is used by military, intelligence, and law enforcement agencies across the world for cellphone surveillance. It allows these agencies to intercept mobile phone traffic, send fake text messages, inject malware, and track the movements of mobile phone users. StingRays act as cell site simulators that collect data from users by mirroring cell towers. The StingRay equipment has two operating modes: active and passive. In the active mode the device simply mimics the behavior of a cell tower in order to force all nearby mobile phones and other cellular data devices to connect to it. In the passive mode, however, the StingRay actively interacts with cellular devices and performs functions like data extraction and location tracking. The StingRay family of devices can be mounted in vehicles, on airplanes, helicopters, and drones. Hand-carried versions are referred to under the trade name KingFish. Currently over 70 state and local law enforcement agencies in 24 states along with 13 federal agencies across the United States use StingRay technology to monitor mobile phone users.

Case File

Carpenter v. United States

Carpenter v. United States was a landmark United States Supreme Court case that involved the process of obtaining call logs and cell site location information (CSLI) from cellphone companies as part of a police investigation. Prior to *Carpenter*, government entities could obtain cellphone location records by court order by claiming the information was required as part of an investigation. Law enforcement agencies could compel a third party entity (cell phone provider) to provide those records because they kept them in the normal course of their business in the cell phone industry.

In *Carpenter*, the Supreme Court determined what type of legal authorization is required by a government entity in order to compel third-party wireless service providers to turn over historical records containing the physical locations of cellphones. Attorneys for Carpenter argued that the authorization should be a search warrant. Attorneys for the United States argued that the authorization should be a court order for disclosure. Requirements to obtain an "order for disclosure" are less stringent than the requirements to obtain a warrant.

An order for disclosure is a type of court order typically instructing a third party to turn over information in its possession related to an investigation. To obtain an order for disclosure from a court, a governmental entity must provide specific and articulable facts showing that there are reasonable grounds to believe that the information sought is relevant and material to an ongoing criminal investigation. Government entities are not required to show probable cause to obtain an order for disclosure.

Under the Fourth Amendment to the United States Constitution, people have the right to be free from unreasonable searches of their "persons, houses, papers, and effects" unless the government entity obtains a search warrant supported by probable cause. Probable cause to search exists when facts and circumstances known to the government entity provide the basis for a reasonable person to believe that a crime was committed and the items to be searched are relevant to the crime.

The Court held, in a 5–4 decision authored by Chief Justice Roberts, that obtaining the records without a warrant supported by probable cause and signed by a judge or magistrate violated the Fourth Amendment to the United States Constitution. After *Carpenter*, government entities must obtain a warrant in order to access these records for domestic criminal investigations.

Chapter Summary 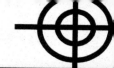 > > > > > > > > > >

Mobile devices began as an outgrowth of ship-to-shore radios in the Second World War. Additionally, hand-held radio transceivers, or walkie-talkies, were available then and they evolved into mobile phones for cars in the 1940s. Early mobile phone systems were analog (1G), which means that they behaved in exactly the same way as older radio stations behave. They were followed by 2G, or digital cellular networks which appeared in the 1990s using two standards: GSM (Global System for Mobile Communications) and CDMA (Code Division with Multiple Access). This ultimately set the generation of "Feature Phones." The smartphone was born with the advent of 3G and 4G phones. With the popularity of Wi-Fi networking, smartphones evolved into tablets, and products such as the iPad became practical substitutions for small computers because they have the ability to download and install applications ("apps") the same as any PC or Mac. Geolocation is a major aspect of mobile forensics.

The basic and detailed architecture of the mobile device consists of hardware and software. The main hardware components of the mobile phone is the application processor that controls all other components of the device such as display, keypad, power, audio, and video. Mobile architecture allows maintaining this connection whilst during transit.

SD or Secure Digital cards are storage expansion cards that many mobile devices can accept. The SD adds memory for storing. SIM cards are different. SIM means "subscriber identity (or 'identification') module." Each SIM has an international mobile subscriber identity (IMSI) number that associates the phone with the subscriber's mobile network. In many cases you can keep all of your subscriber information when you change mobile phones simply by switching the SIM to the new phone. Also on each SIM is the integrated circuit card identifier (ICCID). That number also is printed on the SIM. The ICCID contains the issuer identification number (IIN), the individual account identification, and a check digit.

Another very useful tool for mobile devices is the GPS because it locates the user's activities and when used with a timeline, can place the user in the vicinity of a crime. Chain of evidence describes the events and concomitant evidence that make up the events of the crime. There are two types of chains of evidence. Temporal chains show events in the order in time in which they occurred—commonly called a timeline. Causal chains of evidence describe the events of a crime in terms of cause and effect.

When the examiner has identified the device and procedures to extract its data, the next step is to run the tools and take a forensic image. Examiners make it a practice to run the imager twice, taking one of the images and treating it as evidence. The other is the working image. The examiner should decide, based on what can be done for the particular device, whether to obtain a physical or logical extraction, or both. The logical extraction is fairly fast, and one may want to examine it for obvious evidence while the tool is making a physical image of the target.

Mobile device forensic analysis can provide an overlay to physical evidence and timelines as well as computer forensic timelines to give a clearer picture of the events preceding and following a crime event. However, the efficacy with which you can gather this information depends a lot on the generation of mobile device under test. Technological capabilities vary widely from first- through fourth-generation devices.

Review Questions

1. Early mobile phone systems were followed by digital _____ networks.

2. True or False: The architectural functionality that distinguishes 2G from 3G is that 2G systems were circuit switched and 3G systems are packet switched _____.

3. True or False: One of the benefits of packet switching is the ability to connect more readily to the Internet _____.

4. It's (easy, difficult) to stay current with the available mobile device models.

5. Apple has taken major steps to standardize the development of apps for its _____ and _____.

6. Some devices and many apps report the _____ of the device. That can make it much easier to track the owner's movements.

7. When working on a mobile device, the investigator has several sources of information available. Probably the most useful source of information available to an investigator is _____.

8. An examiner should decide whether to obtain a(n) _____ extraction or _____ extraction or both of a mobile device.

9. True or False: If the examiner has a device that supports physical extraction, that is the way to image the device. Logical extractions are useful only when the physical option is not available because of the device itself _____.

10. True or False: Logical extractions are bit-by-bit copies of the file system, including deleted data _____.

11. Examiners make it a practice to run an extracted image (once, twice).

12. The _____ extraction is fairly fast, and one may want to examine it for obvious evidence while a tool is making a physical image of the target.

13. Just like computers, the _____ defines the basic components of the mobile device.

14. _____ are storage expansion cards that many mobile devices can accept.

15. True or False: SD cards are *nonvolatile*, meaning that even if the power is turned off on the device, you won't lose your music or photos _____.

16. In many cases, users can keep their subscriber information when changing mobile phones by simply switching the _____ card to the new phone.

17. It often is desirable to _____ the SIM in much the same way as one would take a physical image of the mobile device or a computer in order to retain a copy for evidentiary purposes.

18. True or False: It's always possible to recover deleted file items such as e-mails, texts, and photos from a mobile device _____.

19. _____ describes the events and concomitant evidence that make up the events of the crime.

20. _____ chains of evidence show events in the order in time in which they occurred.

21. _____ chains of evidence describe the events of a crime in terms of cause and effect.

22. _____ crime assessment attempts to tie elements of a crime together into a single crime scene and use the timelines to build a picture and describe the events and supporting evidence of the crime.

23. It is likely that the mobile device is extremely accurate as a yardstick for measuring when events happen, as the device may be synchronized to a(n) _____ clock.

24. When a mobile device is set to use _____, it will recognize any _____ network in its range.

25. True or False: Mobile device forensic analysis can provide an overlay to physical evidence and timelines, as well as computer forensic timelines, to give a clearer picture of the events preceding and following a crime event _____.

26. EFS stands for _____.

Application and Critical Thinking

1. What precautions should the examiner take when seizing/analyzing a live, turned-on mobile device?

2. Differentiate chain of evidence and chain of custody and give examples of both in the context of an investigation where mobile devices play an important part.

3. How can law enforcement make use of the locations of cell phone towers?

4. How are today's generations of mobile devices different from and the same as personal computers?

5. What are SIMs and SD cards and why does a mobile device need them? Do all mobile devices have one or both of these? If not, what substitutes?

6. What is the IMSI, where might it reside, and what is it used for? How would the digital forensic investigator use it?

7. If there is a GPS capability on a smartphone, how might the investigator make use of it? Is it useful for correlation? What kind and how would such correlation be accomplished?

Further References

Ayers, R., S. Brothers, and W. Jansen, Guidelines on Mobile Device Forensics, http://nvlpubs.nist.gov/nist-pubs/SpecialPublications/NIST.SP.800-101r1.pdf

Ayers, R. et al., Cell phones Forensic Tools: An Overview and Analysis Update, http://csrc.nist.gov/publications/nistir/nistir-7387.pdf

Digital Evidence and Forensics, 2010, http://www.nij.gov/topics/forensics/evidence/digital/welcome.htm

Electronic Crime Scene Investigation: A Guide for First Responders, 2nd ed., 2008, https://www.ncjrs.gov/pdf-files1/nij/219941.pdf

Appendixes

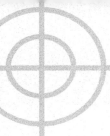

Appendix I
Department of Justice

Code of Professional Responsibility for the Practice of Forensic Science

The following Code of Professional Responsibility for the Practice of Forensic Science defines a framework for promoting integrity and respect for the scientific process. Forensic science providers—both practitioners and agencies, including its managers—must meet requirements 1 to 15 enumerated below. Requirement 16 specifically refers to the responsibility of forensic science management rather than individual practitioners.

1. Accurately represent relevant education, training, experience, and areas of expertise.
2. Be honest and truthful in all professional affairs including not representing the work of others as one's own.
3. Foster and pursue professional competency through such activities as training, proficiency testing, certification, presentation, and publication of research findings.
4. Commit to continuous learning in relevant forensic disciplines and stay abreast of new findings, equipment, and techniques.
5. Conduct research and forensic casework using the scientific method or agency best practices. Where validation tools are not known to exist or cannot be obtained, conduct internal or interlaboratory validation tests in accordance with the quality management system in place.
6. Handle evidentiary materials to prevent tampering, adulteration, loss, or nonessential consumption of evidentiary materials.
7. Avoid participation in any case in which there is a conflict of interest.
8. Conduct examinations that are fair, unbiased, and fit-for-purpose.
9. Make and retain contemporaneous, clear, complete, and accurate records of all examinations, tests, measurements, and conclusions, in sufficient detail to allow meaningful review and assessment by an independent professional proficient in the discipline.
10. Ensure interpretations, opinions, and conclusions that are supported by sufficient data and minimize influences and biases for or against any party.
11. Render interpretations, opinions, or conclusions only when within the practitioner's proficiency or expertise.
12. Prepare reports and testify using clear and straightforward terminology, clearly distinguishing data from interpretations, opinions, and conclusions. Reports should disclose known limitations that are necessary to understand the significance of the findings.
13. Do not alter reports and other records or withhold information for strategic or tactical advantage.
14. Document and, if appropriate, inform management or quality assurance personnel of nonconformities and breaches of law or professional standards.
15. Honestly communicate with all parties (the investigator, prosecutor, defense, and other expert witnesses) about all information relating to their analyses, when communications are permitted by law and agency practice.
16. Inform the prosecutors involved through proper laboratory management channels of material nonconformities or breaches of law or professional standards that adversely affect a previously issued report or testimony.[4]

Appendix II
Handbook of Forensic Services—FBI

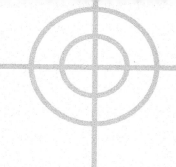

The Handbook of Forensic Services provides guidance and procedures for the safe and efficient methods of collecting, preserving, packaging, and shipping evidence and describes the forensic examinations performed by the FBI's Laboratory Division and Operational Technology Division. The contents of the Handbook are to be found by the reader on either the iPhone app entitled "FBI Handbook" or the Android app entitled "Handbook of Forensic Services."

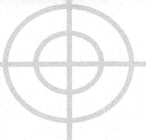

Appendix III
Instructions for
Collecting Gunshot
Residue (GSR)

INSTRUCTIONS FOR COLLECTING GUNSHOT RESIDUE (GSR)
for Scanning Electron Microscopy and Atomic Absorption Analysis

---

NOTE

In control test firings, it has been shown that the concentration of gunshot residue significantly declines on living subjects after approximately 4 hours. In view of these findings, if more than 4 hours have passed since the shooting, it is recommended that you check with your crime laboratory before submitting samples for analysis.

S.E.M. COLLECTION PROCEDURE

(A) When the covering is removed from the metal stubs, the adhesive collecting surface is exposed and care must be used to not drop the stub or contaminate the collecting surface by allowing this exposed surface to come in contact with an object other than the area that is to be sampled. (See Figure 1.)

(B) *Do not* return paper stub cover to stubs after collection. (*Discard stub covers.*)

(C) Heavily soiled or bloody areas should be avoided if possible.

(D) When pressing the stubs on the questioned areas, use enough pressure to cause a mild indentation on the surface of the subject's hand.

STEP 1   Fill out all information requested on the enclosed Gunshot Residue Analysis Information Form.

STEP 2   Put on the disposable plastic gloves provided in this kit. *Do not substitute with other gloves!*

> NOTE: If there is blood on the subject's hands or clothing, the investigating officer should put on latex or other approved barrier gloves to protect him/her from bloodborne pathogens, then put on the plastic gloves provided in this kit.

STEP 3   <u>RIGHT BACK:</u>

     (A) Carefully remove the cap from the vial labeled RIGHT BACK, then remove the paper covering from the metal sample stub.

     (B) While holding the vial cap, press the collecting surface of the stub onto the back of the subject's right hand until the area shown below in Figure 2 has been covered.

     (C) After sampling the back of the subject's right hand, return the cap, with metal stub, to the RIGHT BACK vial. *Do not return paper covering to metal stub!*

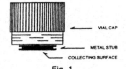

Fig. 1

STEP 4   <u>RIGHT PALM:</u>

     Repeat the procedure described in Step 3, using the metal stub in the vial marked RIGHT PALM. Make sure to sample the area shown below in Figure 3.

STEP 5   <u>LEFT BACK and LEFT PALM:</u>

     For collection from the left hand, repeat Steps 3 and 4 using the vials labeled LEFT BACK and LEFT PALM.

STEP 6   After sampling all four areas, return capped vials to kit envelope.

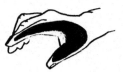

Fig. 2 (BACK)

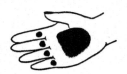

Fig. 3 (PALM)

A.A. COLLECTION PROCEDURE

NOTE: (A) This second part of the GSR collection is *ONLY* to be performed *AFTER* sampling with the SEM stubs.

(B) If you feel that during the SEM collection procedure you have contaminated the gloves, discard contaminated gloves, then thoroughly wash your hands with soap and water and dry with a clean towel. At no time during the collection process should your hands (with or without gloves) come into contact with the cotton tip of the swab.

(C) When dispensing nitric acid, use 2 - 3 drops of 5% nitric acid solution to moisten each swab (do not over-moisten). In order to dispense an appropriate amount of the nitric acid solution, hold the acid dispenser in a horizontal position above and *almost* touching the top of the swab, and squeeze gently.

(D) To swab the subject's hands, the investigator should grasp the subject's arm above the wrist with one hand and swab with the other. The subject's hand should be in a "spread" position. Thorough swabbing of the hands is carried out by using moderate pressure while swabbing. The swab should be rotated during this procedure to insure that all of the surface of the cotton tip is utilized. At least 30 seconds per swab is required.

(E) When placing swabs in tubes, always place cotton tips *FACE DOWN*.

STEP 7   **CONTROL SWABS:** Remove *two* of the swabs from the unmarked ziplock bag. Moisten both swabs with 2 - 3 drops of the 5% nitric acid solution supplied in kit (do not substitute). Place both swabs in the tube labeled CONTROL. Then recap tube and set it aside.

STEP 8   **RIGHT BACK:**

(A) Moisten the tip of *ONE* swab with 2 - 3 drops of nitric acid solution, then thoroughly swab the back of the subject's right hand including the back of the fingers and all of the web area which would be exposed while holding a weapon. Fig. 4 illustrates the area of hand for swabbing. Place swab used in the tube labeled RIGHT BACK.

(B) Repeat the above procedure using a *SECOND* swab. Place the second swab used in the RIGHT BACK tube, then recap tube and set it aside.

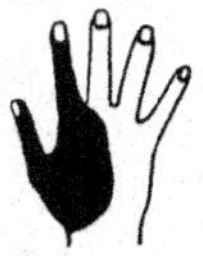

Fig. 4 (BACK)

STEP 9   **RIGHT PALM:**

(A) Moisten the tip of *ONE* swab with 2 - 3 drops of nitric acid solution, then thoroughly swab the palm of the subject's right hand as shown in Fig. 5. Place swab used in the tube labeled RIGHT PALM.

(B) Repeat the above procedure using a *SECOND* swab. Place the second swab used in the RIGHT PALM tube, then recap tube and set it aside.

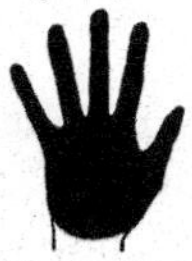

Fig. 5 (PALM)

STEP 10   **LEFT BACK/LEFT PALM:** Follow the same procedures described in Steps 8 and 9, but swabbing the subject's left hand.

STEP 11   **CARTRIDGE CASE:**

NOTE: For .22 cal and foreign manufactured ammunition, it is necessary that either Steps A and B described below be completed <u>OR</u> the casings be submitted to the laboratory. If latent prints are required on the expended casing(s), Steps A and B should be omitted and the casings should be submitted for latent print processing. If for any reason the CARTRIDGE CASE swabs are not used, mark the tube "*NOT USED*".

(A) Moisten the tip of *ONE* swab with 2 - 3 drops of nitric acid solution, then thoroughly swab the inside of the cartridge case. Place swab used in the tube labeled CARTRIDGE CASE.

(B) Repeat the above procedure using a *SECOND* swab. Place second swab used in the CARTRIDGE CASE tube, and then recap tube and set it aside.

FINAL INSTRUCTIONS

(A) Fill out all information requested on the front of the kit envelope.

(B) With the exception of the 5% nitric acid dispenser and the disposable gloves, return all other kit components, used or unused, to kit envelope.

(C) Moisten kit envelope flap, then seal envelope. Affix Police Evidence Seal where indicated, then initial seal.

(D) Mail or hand deliver sealed kit to the crime laboratory for analysis. (If mailed, package kit in a cardboard box to prevent damage in transit.)

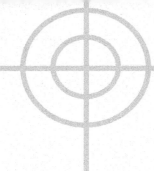

Appendix IV
Chemical Formulas for Latent Fingerprint Development

Iodine Spray Reagent

1. Prepare the following stock solutions:

   Solution A

   Dissolve 1 g of iodine in 1 L of cyclohexane

   Solution B

   Dissolve 5 g of α-Naphthoflavone in 40 mL of methylene chloride (dichloromethane)

2. Add 2 mL of Solution B to 100 mL of Solution A. Using a magnetic stirrer, mix thoroughly for 5 minutes.
3. Filter the solution through a facial tissue, paper towel, and then filter paper, into a beaker. The solution should be lightly sprayed on the specimen using an aerosol spray unit or a mini spray gun powered with compressed air.
4. Lightly spray the suspect area with several applications until latent prints sufficiently develop.

Remarks

- Solution A may be stored at room temperature. Shelf life is in excess of 30 days.
- Solution B must be refrigerated. Shelf life is in excess of 30 days.
- The combined working solution (A and B) should be used within 24 hours after mixing.
- The iodine spray solution is effective on most surfaces (porous and nonporous).
- A fine spray mist is the most effective form of application.
- The cyanoacrylate (Super Glue) process cannot be used prior to the iodine spray reagent process. Cyanoacrylate may be used, however, after the iodine spray reagent.
- On porous surfaces, DFO and/or ninhydrin may be used after the iodine spray.
- Propanol may be used to remove the staining of the iodine spray reagent.
- 1,1,2 Trichlorotrifluoroethane may be substituted for cyclohexane.

1,8-Diazafluoren-9-one (DFO)

Step 1: Stock solution: Dissolve 1 g DFO in 200 mL methanol, 200 mL ethyl acetate, and 40 mL acetic acid.

Step 2: Working solution (make as needed): Start with stock solution and dilute to 2 L with petroleum ether (40° to 60° boiling point fraction). Pentane can also be used. Solution should be clear.

Dip the paper document into the working solution and allow it to dry. Dip again and allow it to dry. When completely dry, apply heat (200° for 10 to 20 minutes). An oven, hair dryer, or dry iron can be used.

Visualize with an alternate light source at 450, 485, 525, and 530 nm and observe through orange goggles. If the surface paper is yellow, such as legal paper, it may be necessary to visualize the paper at 570 nm and view it through red goggles.

Source: In part from *Processing Guide for Developing Latent Prints*, Revised 2000. Washington, D.C.: FBI; http://www.fbi.gov/about-us/lab/forensic-science-communications/fsc/jan2001/lpu.pdf

1,2-Indanedione
2.0 g 1,2-Indanedione
70 mL Ethyl Acetate
930 mL HFE 7100 (3M Company)

Ninhydrin

20 g Ninhydrin
3,300 mL Acetone
Shelf life is approximately one month

or

5 g Ninhydrin
30 mL Methanol
40 mL 2-Propanol
930 mL Petroleum Ether
Shelf life is approximately one year

Dip the paper document in the working solution and allow it to dry. Dip again and allow it to dry. When completely dry, heat may be applied. A steam iron should be used on the steam setting. Do not touch the iron directly to the paper. Rather, hold the iron above the paper and allow the steam to heat it.

Zinc Chloride Solution (Post-Ninhydrin Treatment)

5 g of Zinc Chloride crystals
2 mL of Glacial Acetic Acid
100 mL of Methyl Alcohol
Add 400 mL of 1,1,2 trichlorotrifluoroethane to the mixture and stir.
Add 2 mL of 5 percent sodium hypochlorite solution (commercially available liquid bleach such as Clorox, Purex, and others).

Lightly spray the paper with the zinc solution. Repeat the spraying as needed. Do not overdo the spraying.

The ninhydrin-developed prints treated with this solution may fluoresce at room temperature with an alternate light source. For maximum fluorescence, place the paper in a bath of liquid nitrogen and examine again with an alternate light source.

Physical Developer

When mixing and using these solutions, make sure the glassware, processing trays, stirring rods, and stirring magnets are absolutely clean. Do not use metal trays or tweezer.

Stock Detergent Solution: 3 g of N-dodecylamine acetate is combined with 4 g of Synperonic-N mixed in 1 L of distilled water.
Silver Nitrate Solution: 20 g of silver nitrate crystals is mixed in 100 mL of distilled water.
Redox Solution: 60 g of ferric nitrate is mixed in 1,800 mL of distilled water. After this solution is thoroughly mixed, add 160 g of ferrous ammonium sulfate, mix thoroughly and add 40 g of citric acid and mix thoroughly.
Maleic Acid Solution: Put 50 g of maleic acid into 2 L of distilled water.
Physical Developer Working Solution: Begin with 2,125 mL of the redox solution and add 80 mL of the stock detergent solution, mix well, then add 100 mL of the silver nitrate solution and mix well. Appropriate divisions can be used if smaller amounts of the working solution are desired.

Immerse specimen in maleic acid solution for 10 minutes. Incubate item in physical developer (PD) working solution for 15 to 20 minutes. Thoroughly rinse specimen in tap water for 20 minutes. Air-dry and photograph.

Cyanoacrylate Fluorescent Enhancement Reagents

Rhodamine 6G

Stock Solution

100 mg Rhodamine 6G

100 mL Methanol (Stir until thoroughly dissolved.)

Working Solution

3 mL Rhodamine 6G Stock Solution

15 mL Acetone

10 mL Acetonitrile

15 mL Methanol

32 mL 2-Propanol

925 mL Petroleum Ether (Combine in order listed.)

Ardrox

2 mL Ardrox P-133D

10 mL Acetone

25 mL Methanol

10 mL 2-Propanol

8 mL Acetonitrile

945 mL Petroleum Ether

MBD

7-(p-methoxybenzylaminol)-4-nitrobenz-2-oxa-1,3-diazole

Stock Solution

100 mg MBD

100 mL Acetone

Working Solution

10 mL MBD Stock Solution

30 mL Methanol

10 mL 2-Propanol

950 mL Petroleum Ether (Combine in order listed.)

Basic Yellow 40

2 g Basic Yellow 40

1 L Methanol

RAM Combination Enhancer*

3 mL Rhodamine 6G Stock Solution

2 mL Ardrox P-133D

7 mL MBD Stock Solution

20 mL Methanol

10 mL 2-Propanol

8 mL Acetonitrile

950 mL Petroleum Ether (Combine in order listed.)

RAY Combination Enhancer*

To 940 mL of either isopropyl alcohol or denatured ethyl alcohol add:

1.0 g of Basic Yellow 40

1.1 g of Rhodamine 6G

8 mL of Ardrox P-133D

50 mL of Acetonitrile (optional, but dye stain of prints will appear more brilliant)

Source: John H. Olenik, Freemont, OH.

MRM 10 Combination Enhancer

3 mL Rhodamine 6G Stock Solution
3 mL Basic Yellow 40 Stock Solution
7 mL MBD Stock Solution
20 mL Methanol
10 mL 2-Propanol
8 mL Acetonitrile
950 mL Petroleum Ether
(Combine in order listed.)

The above solutions are used on evidence that has been treated with cyanoacrylate (Super Glue) fumes. These solutions dye the cyanoacrylate residue adhering to the latent print residue. Wash the dye over the evidence. It may be necessary to rinse the surface with a solvent, such as petroleum ether, to remove the excess stain.

CAUTION: These solutions contain solvents that may be respiratory irritants, so they should be mixed and used in a fume hood or while wearing a full-face breathing apparatus. Also, these solvents may damage some plastics, cloth, wood, and painted surfaces.

Because of the respiratory irritation possible and the general inefficiency of spraying, it is *not* recommended to spray these solutions. To obtain the maximum benefit and coverage, it is recommended that evidence be soaked, submerged, or washed with these types of solutions.

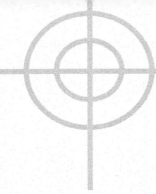

Appendix V
Chemical Formulas for Development of Footwear Impressions in Blood

Amido Black

Staining Solution:
1.2 g Naphthalene 12B or Naphthol Blue
Black 10 mL Glacial Acetic Acid
90 mL Methanol

Rinsing Solution:
90 mL Methanol
10 mL Glacial Acetic Acid

Stain the impression by spraying or immersing the item in the staining solution for approximately 1 minute. Next, treat with the rinsing solution to remove stain from nonimpression area. Then rinse well with distilled water.

Coomassie Blue

Staining Solution (add in this order):
0.44 g Coomassie Brilliant Blue
200 mL Methanol
40 mL Glacial Acetic Acid
200 mL Distilled Water

Rinsing Solution:
40 mL Glacial Acetic Acid
200 mL Methanol
200 mL Distilled Water

Spray object with the staining solution, completely covering the area of interest. Then spray the object with rinsing solution, clearing the background. Then rinse with distilled water.

Crowle's Double Stain

Developer:
2.5 g Crocein Scarlet 7B
150 mg Coomassie Brilliant Blue R
50 mL Glacial Acetic Acid
30 mL Trichloroacetic Acid

Combine the above ingredients, then dilute to 1 L with distilled water. Place the solution on a stirring device until all the Crocein Scarlet 7B and Coomassie Brilliant Blue R are dissolved.

Rinse:
30 mL Glacial Acetic Acid
970 mL Distilled Water

Apply the developer to the item(s) by dipping. Completely cover the target area, leaving the developer on for approximately 30 to 90 seconds, then rinse. Finally, rinse well with distilled water.

Diaminobenzidine (DAB)

Solution A (Fixer Solution):
20 g 5-Sulphosalicylic Acid
Dissolved in 1 L Distilled Water

Solution B:
100 mL 1M Phosphate Buffer (pH 7.4)
800 mL Distilled Water

Solution C:
1 g Diaminobenzidine
Dissolved in 100 mL Distilled Water

Working Solution (Mix Just Prior to Use):
900 mL Solution B
100 mL Solution C
5 mL 30% Hydrogen Peroxide

Immerse impression area in fixer solution A for approximately 4 minutes. Remove and rinse in distilled water. Immerse impression area for approximately 4 minutes in the working solution or until print is fully developed. Remove and rinse in distilled water.

Fuchsin Acid

20 g Sulfosalicylic Acid
2 g Fuchsin Acid
Dissolved in 1 L Distilled Water

Stain the impression by spraying or immersing the item in the dye solution for approximately 1 minute. Rinse well with distilled water.

Leucocrystal Violet

10 g 5-Sulfosalicylic Acid
500 mL 3% Hydrogen Peroxide
3.7 g Sodium Acetate
1 g Leucocrystal Violet

If Leucocrystal Violet crystals are yellow instead of white, do not use. This indicates crystals are old and solution will not work.

Spray the object until completely covered. Then allow object to air-dry. Development of impressions will occur within 30 seconds. Store the solution in amber glassware and refrigerate.

Leucocrystal Violet Field Kit*

When the reagents are separated in the listed manner below, a "field kit" can be prepared. The field kit separation will allow for an extended shelf life.

Bottle A:
10 g 5-Sulfosalicylic Acid
500 mL Hydrogen Peroxide 3%

Bottle B:
1.1 g Leucocrystal Violet
Weigh out reagent and place in an amber 60 mL (2 ounce) bottle.

Bottle C:
4.4 g Sodium Acetate
Weigh out reagent and place in an amber 60 mL (2 ounce) bottle.

Add approximately 30 mL of Bottle A reagent to Bottle B. Secure cap and shake Bottle B for 2 to 3 minutes. Pour contents of Bottle B back into Bottle A.

Add approximately 30 mL of Bottle A reagent to Bottle C. Secure cap and shake Bottle C for approximately 2 to 3 minutes. Pour contents of Bottle C into Bottle A. Secure Bottle A's cap and shake thoroughly.

Spray the target area; development will occur within 30 seconds. After spraying, blot the area with a tissue or paper towel. Then allow object to air-dry.

Patent Blue

20 g Sulfosalicylic Acid
2 g Patent Blue V (VF)
Dissolved in 1 L Distilled Water

Stain object by spraying or immersing the item in the dye solution for approximately 1 minute. Rinse well with distilled water.

Tartrazine

20 g Sulfosalicylic Acid
2 g Tartrazine
Dissolved in 1 L Distilled Water

Stain object by spraying or immersing the item in the dye solution for approximately 1 minute. Rinse well with distilled water.

Index